THE CLINICIAN'S HANDBOOK OF

NATURAL MEDICINE

THE CLINICIAN'S HANDBOOK OF NATURAL MEDICINE

THIRD EDITION

Joseph E. Pizzorno, ND
Michael T. Murray, ND
Herb Joiner-Bey, ND

ELSEVIER

ELSEVIER

3251 Riverport Lane
St. Louis, Missouri 63043

THE CLINICIAN'S HANDBOOK OF NATURAL MEDICINE,
THIRD EDITION

ISBN: 978-0-7020-5514-0

Library of Congress Cataloging-in-Publication Data

Pizzorno, Joseph E., Jr., author.
The clinician's handbook of natural medicine / Joseph E. Pizzorno, Jr., Michael T. Murray, Herb Joiner-Bey. — Third edition.
p. ; cm.
Includes index.
ISBN 978-0-7020-5514-0 (pbk.)
I. Murray, Michael T., author. II. Joiner-Bey, Herb, author. III. Title.
[DNLM: 1. Naturopathy—Handbooks. WB 39]
RZ440
615.5′35—dc23

2015025026

Content Strategist: Shelly Stringer
Content Development Manager: Jolynn Gower
Content Coordinator: Rachel Allen
Publishing Services Manager: Jeff Patterson
Project Manager: Lisa A. P. Bushey
Designer: Ashley Miner

Printed in India
Last digit is the print number: 13 12 11

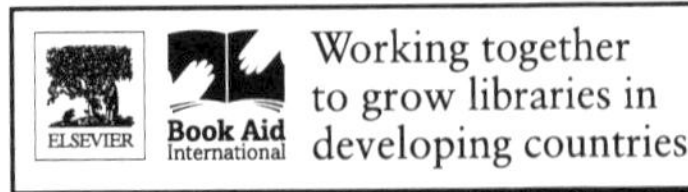

In loving memory of the late

Dr. Bill Mitchell,

whose faith, passion, dedication, vision, and compassion made him the living embodiment of the spirit and essence of naturopathic holistic healing

Preface

We are excited to see the continuing blossoming of natural medicine by many names. No matter the term used (e.g., *integrative, holistic,* or *functional*), the philosophic precepts kept alive in the culture by natural medicine physicians are informing and transforming medicine. Treating the person, rather than the disease, seems an obvious concept, yet it has struggled to be heard. As Dr. Bastyr taught us as students, "Despite the obstacles, the truth of our medicine will win out."

The Clinician's Handbook of Natural Medicine, third edition, was created as a companion to the *Textbook of Natural Medicine,* fourth edition. It was written for several audiences: students, clinicians, and researchers. For the busy clinician it provides concise guidance for the care of patients who may have one or more of over 75 of the most common diseases effectively treated with natural medicine. Although Sections 4 and 6 of the *Textbook* provide an in-depth discussion of the pathophysiology, causes, documented natural medicine interventions, and full references for these diseases, the *Handbook* provides only the most pertinent information needed for intervention for the typical patient. Together, these books provide the clinician with the best of both worlds: easily accessible advice for quick guidance for the less-complicated patient, and in-depth understanding when needed. (Of course, the *Textbook* also contains considerable additional information in its other four sections.)

For students, this resource helps them understand more deeply the patient who has the disease. One of the challenges for those learning natural medicine is the pitfall of "green drug" medicine—that is, simply substituting an herb or a natural therapy for the synthetic drug to treat the symptoms. Our best practice of medicine is to understand the true causes of disease and then to help the patient restore normal function. By carefully studying the comprehensive flowcharts offered in the *Handbook,* the student can more profoundly understand the uniqueness of each patient. The guidance on when to refer to (or use, depending on the student's training and licensure) more conventional approaches will also help the student recognize the limitations of natural therapies.

For the researcher wanting to truly evaluate the efficacy of natural medicine, we hope the special flowcharts in the *Handbook* will help him or her progress beyond the false homogeneity of disease. Although the standardization of disease works for symptom relief–oriented health care, it is an oversimplification and is inconsistent with the curative medicine we believe is possible. With recognition that multiple interventions are needed for each disease, depending on the patient, algorithms can be developed that lead to more accurate research on how we actually care for patients.

Each chapter of the *Handbook* is composed of several parts: Diagnostic Summary, General Considerations, Flowchart, Therapeutic Considerations, and Therapeutic Approach. We believe that this format is unique, and we are unaware of any other textbook in which the flowchart approach is used to provide guidance for integrative and natural medicine care.

The flowcharts separate the diagnostic and therapeutic deliberation into three phases: (1) determine the need for conventional intervention, (2) minimize obstacles to healing, and (3) tailor natural interventions to patient needs. The first phase is provided to assist the clinician in understanding which patients may immediately require a more-conventional intervention or those whose condition has progressed beyond the capabilities of natural therapies. The other phases present the most relevant diagnostic and therapeutic differentiations needed to determine which cause(s) must be controlled and which interventions are needed to provide each patient highly personalized natural medicine care. Carefully following this thoughtfully constructed logic chain will efficiently provide key therapeutic insights.

The astute reader may notice a few inconsistencies between the recommendations found in the *Handbook* and those in the *Textbook*. Because the *Handbook* was written approximately 3 years after the *Textbook*, we have worked to ensure that the latest research has been incorporated.

This third edition closely follows the format of the second edition. The main differences are the inclusion of several additional diseases.

We are excited to provide clinicians with this special resource, which we believe will substantially aid their efforts to provide their patients with the best care possible.

Joseph E. Pizzorno, ND
Michael T. Murray, ND
Herb Joiner-Bey, ND

Acknowledgments

I would like to acknowledge all my students over the years for the health and healing they have brought to millions of people. You made the hard work of creating Bastyr University worth every sacrifice.

Dr. Michael Murray, with your many books and tireless teaching to the public, you have played a major role in transforming medicine. I am made speechless by your accomplishments.

I would like to acknowledge Dr. Herb Joiner-Bey for his tireless work making natural medicine understandable to both clinicians and consumers. His conversion of the much more complex *Textbook of Natural Medicine* into this concise, insightful, and extremely accessible resource is very impressive, and his expansion of this work with several new chapters for the third edition is a true gift to all.

As ever, this work would not have been possible without the love and care of my family: Lara, my dear wife, and Galen and Raven, my beloved children. Thank you for bringing such joy and fullness to my life.

Joseph E. Pizzorno, ND

Most of all I would like to acknowledge that inner voice that has guided me in my life, providing me with inspiration, strength, and humility at the most appropriate times. My motivation has been largely the good that I know can come from using natural medicine appropriately. It can literally change people's lives. I know it changed mine.

There are many things that I am thankful for. I am especially thankful for my wife and best friend, Gina. I have also been blessed by having wonderful parents whose support and faith have never waned. I now have the opportunity to carry on their legacy of love with my own children, Alexa, Zachary, and Addison.

In addition to my family, those people who have truly inspired me include Dr. Ralph Weiss, Dr. Ed Madison, Dr. Bill Mitchell,

Dr. Gaetano Morello, my classmates and the entire Bastyr University community, and all the special people I am lucky enough to call friends who have helped me on my life's journey.

And finally, I am deeply honored to have Dr. Joe Pizzorno and Dr. Herb Joiner-Bey, not only as my coauthors, but also as truly valued friends.

Michael T. Murray, ND

I wish to extend to Dr. Joseph Pizzorno and Dr. Michael Murray my deep appreciation for the high honor and privilege of preparing the third edition of this handbook, based on the fourth edition of their *Textbook of Natural Medicine.* Because of my declining visual acuity, the challenges of preparing this new edition have been far greater than encountered for the first and second. It is with deep gratitude that I wish to thank Rachel Allen, Content Coordinator, and Elsevier for their patience, understanding, and generosity in providing whatever support they could to make my task easier. It is also with great appreciation that I wish to thank Dr. Pizzorno for his gracious willingness to lighten my load by preparing a number of the chapters himself. Thank you so very much, Kim and Joe. Without your help, this project could not have been finished in a timely fashion.

Herb Joiner-Bey, ND

Finally, we would like to acknowledge the outstanding professional staff at Elsevier, whose creative talents and expertise have been indispensable to the publishing of this book. Thank you to Shelly Stringer, Jolynn Gower, and Rachel Allen who worked on this new edition. Thanks also to the individuals who worked to make the previous editions of this text successful, including Kellie White, Claire Kramer, Kim Fons, and Kelly Milford. (We still miss you too, Inta Ozols.)

Contents

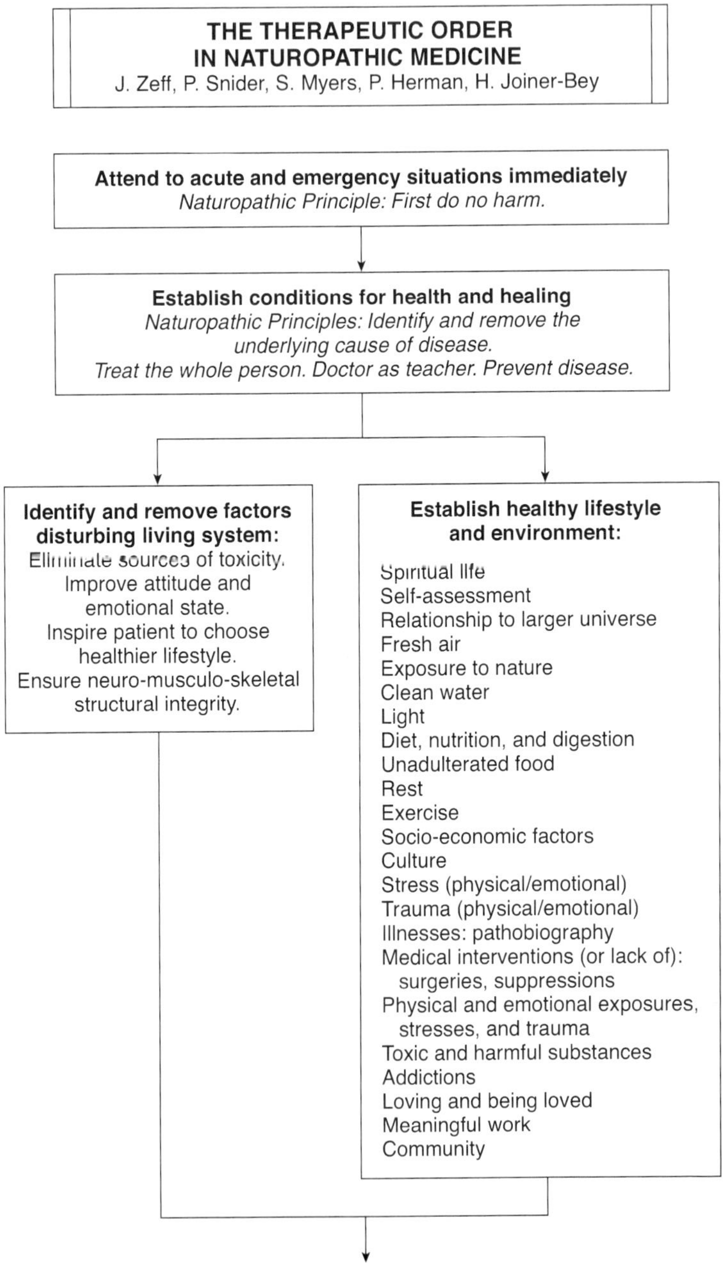

THE THERAPEUTIC ORDER IN NATUROPATHIC MEDICINE
J. Zeff, P. Snider, S. Myers, P. Herman, H. Joiner-Bey

Attend to acute and emergency situations immediately
Naturopathic Principle: First do no harm.

↓

Establish conditions for health and healing
Naturopathic Principles: Identify and remove the underlying cause of disease.
Treat the whole person. Doctor as teacher. Prevent disease.

↓

Identify and remove factors disturbing living system:
Eliminate sources of toxicity.
Improve attitude and emotional state.
Inspire patient to choose healthier lifestyle.
Ensure neuro-musculo-skeletal structural integrity.

Establish healthy lifestyle and environment:

- Spiritual life
- Self-assessment
- Relationship to larger universe
- Fresh air
- Exposure to nature
- Clean water
- Light
- Diet, nutrition, and digestion
- Unadulterated food
- Rest
- Exercise
- Socio-economic factors
- Culture
- Stress (physical/emotional)
- Trauma (physical/emotional)
- Illnesses: pathobiography
- Medical interventions (or lack of): surgeries, suppressions
- Physical and emotional exposures, stresses, and trauma
- Toxic and harmful substances
- Addictions
- Loving and being loved
- Meaningful work
- Community

↓

THE THERAPEUTIC ORDER
IN NATUROPATHIC MEDICINE
J. Zeff, P. Snider, S. Myers, P. Herman, H. Joiner-Bey

Mobilize self-healing processes:
Naturopathic Principles: The healing power of nature.
Treat the whole person. Identify and treat the cause of disease.
Constitutional hydrotherapy
Classical homeopathy
Traditional Chinese medicine
Spiritual healing

↓

Repair weakened tissues:
Naturopathic Principles: The healing power of nature.
Treat the whole person. Identify and treat the cause of disease.
Improve digestion
Optimize elimination
Optimize metabolism
Modulate immune function as indicated
Normalize inflammatory responses
Correct endocrine imbalances
Support natural regeneration function
Guide patient in harmonizing with life-force

↓

Treat specific tissue pathological states:
Naturopathic Principles: First, do no harm.
Treat the whole person. Prevent future disease.
Preferred order of interventions:
Natural modalities
Pharmaceuticals
Surgery, chemotherapy, radiotherapy

Acne Vulgaris and Acne Conglobata

DIAGNOSTIC SUMMARY

- Open comedones: dilated follicles with central dark, horny plugs (blackheads)
- Closed comedones: small follicular papules with (red papules) or without (whiteheads) inflammatory changes
- Superficial pustules: collections of pus at follicular opening
- Nodules: tender collections of pus deep in dermis
- Cysts: nodules that fail to discharge contents to the surface
- Large, deep pustules: nodules that break down adjacent tissue, leading to scars

GENERAL CONSIDERATIONS

Most common skin problem. A key factor is genetics; acne is inherited autosomal dominant pattern with incomplete penetrance. If both parents had acne, three of four children will have acne. If one parent had acne, then one of four children will have acne. Lesions are mainly on the face, but also back, chest, and shoulders. More common in males; onset during puberty but later for conglobata. Acne vulgaris onset from increased size of pilosebaceous glands and sebum secretion by androgenic stimulation. Severity and progression arise from interactions of hormones, keratinization, sebum, and bacteria.

- **Progression:** hyperkeratinization of upper portion of follicle, blockage of canal, dilation and thinning, formation of comedones (open or closed based on degree of keratinization and blockage of duct), purulent exudate in pustules and cysts.
- **Bacteria:** normal skin species (*Propionibacterium acnes* [*Corynebacterium acnes*] and *Staphylococcus albus*). *P. acnes* releases lipases, hydrolyzing sebum triglycerides into free fatty acid lipoperoxides, promoting inflammation.

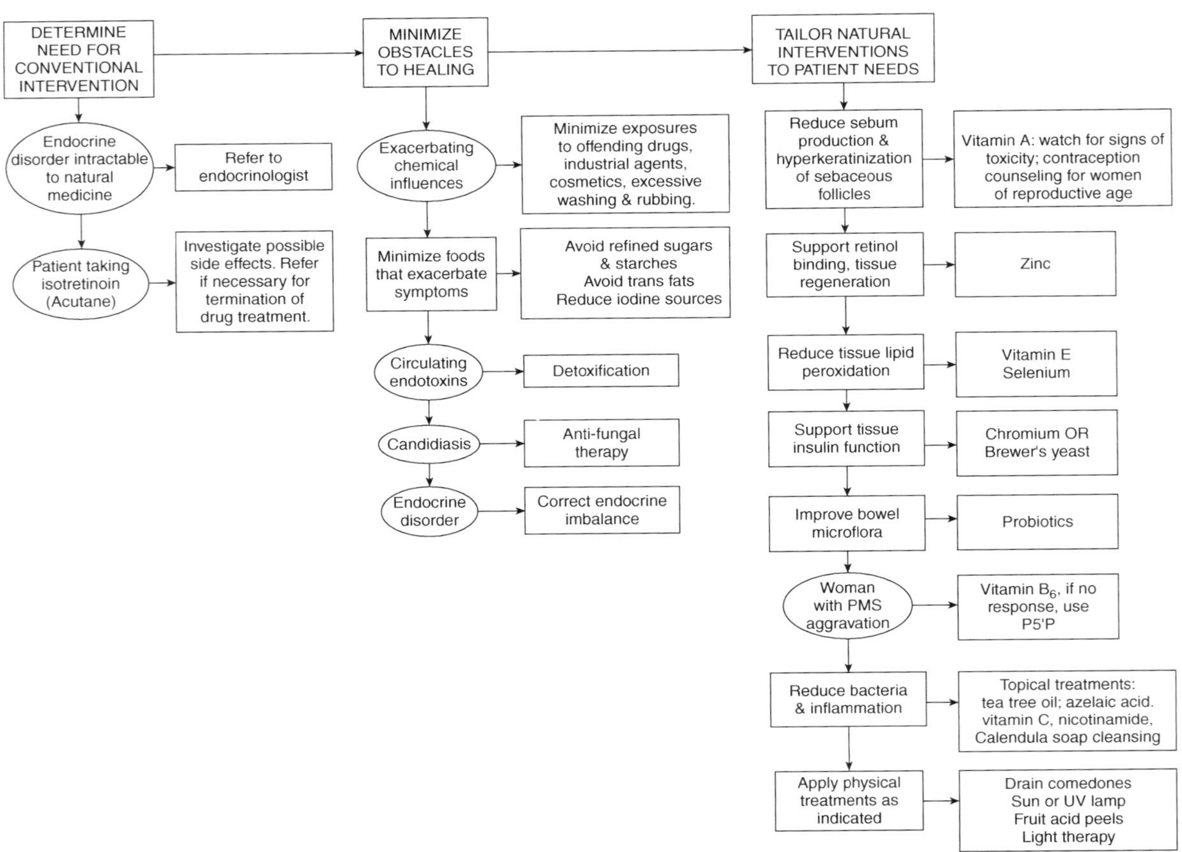
ACNE VULGARIS AND CONGLOBATA
DETERMINE NEED FOR CONVENTIONAL INTERVENTION
Endocrine disorder intractable to natural medicine
Refer to endocrinologist
Patient taking isotretinoin (Acutane)
Investigate possible side effects. Refer if necessary for termination of drug treatment.
MINIMIZE OBSTACLES TO HEALING
Exacerbating chemical influences
Minimize exposures to offending drugs, industrial agents, cosmetics, excessive washing & rubbing.
Minimize foods that exacerbate symptoms
Avoid refined sugars & starches
Avoid trans fats
Reduce iodine sources
Circulating endotoxins
Detoxification
Candidiasis
Anti-fungal therapy
Endocrine disorder
Correct endocrine imbalance
TAILOR NATURAL INTERVENTIONS TO PATIENT NEEDS
Reduce sebum production & hyperkeratinization of sebaceous follicles
Vitamin A: watch for signs of toxicity; contraception counseling for women of reproductive age
Support retinol binding, tissue regeneration
Zinc
Reduce tissue lipid peroxidation
Vitamin E
Selenium
Support tissue insulin function
Chromium OR Brewer's yeast
Improve bowel microflora
Probiotics
Woman with PMS aggravation
Vitamin B_6, if no response, use P5'P
Reduce bacteria & inflammation
Topical treatments: tea tree oil; azelaic acid. vitamin C, nicotinamide, Calendula soap cleansing
Apply physical treatments as indicated
Drain comedones
Sun or UV lamp
Fruit acid peels
Light therapy

- **Inducing compounds and habits:** corticosteroids, halogens, isonicotinic acid, diphenylhydantoin, lithium carbonate, machine oils, coal tar derivatives, chlorinated hydrocarbons, cosmetics, pomades, overwashing, and repetitive rubbing.
- **Endocrinologic aspects:** androgen-dependent condition. Androgens control sebaceous secretion and exacerbate follicular hyperkeratinization. Endocrine disorders producing excess androgens induce acne development: idiopathic adrenal androgen excess, 21-hydroxylase, polycystic ovaries, free testosterone (T), dehydroepiandrosterone (DHEA), DHEA sulfate, deficient sex-hormone binding globulin. Skin of patient with acne has greater activity of 5-alpha-reductase, elevating more-active male hormone dihydrotestosterone (DHT) locally in skin tissue. Receptors for growth hormone and insulin-like growth factor 1 (IGF-1) reside on sebaceous gland; these hormones stimulate sebum production. Conditions of growth hormone excess (e.g., acromegaly) are associated with increased sebum production and acne. Insulin at high levels can interact with IGF-1 receptors. IGF-1 promotes expression of enzymes responsible for androgen biosynthesis and conversion. Elevated cortisol from chronic stress thickens sebum. The stress of acne compounds this problem.

THERAPEUTIC CONSIDERATIONS

Nutrition

- **Diet/incidence ratio:** linked to Western diet. Recommend high-protein diet (45% protein, 35% carbohydrate [CHO], 20% fat) to decrease 5-alpha-reductase activity and increase cytochrome p450 degradation of estradiol. High CHO diet (10% protein, 70% CHO, 20% fat) has opposite effect. Limit foods high in iodine and milk. Milk contains estrogens, progesterone, and androgens as well as glucocorticoids and IGF-1. Eliminate *trans* fats and high-fat foods.
- **Sugar, insulin, and chromium:** insulin efficacy in treating acne suggests cutaneous glucose intolerance and/or insulin insensitivity. Impaired skin glucose tolerance suggests that acne may be called "skin diabetes." Eliminate concentrated CHOs to minimize immunosuppression. High-chromium yeast improves glucose tolerance and may help acne. A diet that encourages high insulin response chronically could promote acne by elevating IGF-1.

- **Vitamin A:** retinol reduces sebum production and hyperkeratinization of sebaceous follicles. Effective at toxic dosage of 300,000-400,000 international units (IU) q.d. × 5 to 6 months. Toxicity: cheilitis (chapped lips) and xerosis (dry skin), especially in dry weather; headache then fatigue, emotional lability, and muscle and joint pain. Laboratory tests are unreliable to monitor toxicity—serum vitamin A correlates poorly with toxicity, whereas serum glutamicoxaloacetic transaminase (SGOT) and serum glutamicpyruvic transaminase (SGPT) are elevated only in symptomatic patients. Massive doses are teratogenic—women of child-bearing age must use birth control during and for at least 1 month after treatment. Reserve massive doses for intractable cases, in which it should not be used alone. Contraception counseling is mandatory, and two negative pregnancy test results are required before initiation of vitamin A therapy in women of child-bearing potential. Baseline laboratory examination should include cholesterol and triglycerides, hepatic transaminase, and complete blood count. Conduct pregnancy tests and laboratory examinations monthly during treatment. Vitamin A at 150,000 IU daily in emulsified form for short duration is reliable and safe in bringing acne under control.
- **Zinc (Zn):** vital to acne treatment. Involved in production of local hormones and retinol-binding protein, wound healing, tissue regeneration, and immune function. Absorption characteristics of Zn salts used may affect results; requires 12 weeks to show good results. Prefer Zn picolinate, acetate, or monomethionine. Zn is essential to normal skin function (e.g., Zn-deficient syndrome acrodermatitis enteropathica). Zn is essential for retinol-binding protein and serum retinol levels. Low Zn levels increase 5-alpha reduction of T, and high Zn inhibits this reaction. Serum Zn is lower in 13- and 14-year-old boys than in any other age group.
- **Vitamin E and selenium:** vitamin E regulates retinol levels. Male patients with acne have decreased red blood cell (RBC) glutathione peroxidase, which normalizes with vitamin E and selenium. Acne of men and women improves with this treatment—inhibiting lipid peroxide formation—suggesting use of other free-radical quenchers.
- **Pyridoxine:** helpful for women with premenstrual acne because of effect on steroid hormone metabolism. B_6 deficiency causes increased uptake and sensitivity to T. In some patients, thyroid therapy markedly improves acne.

Topical Treatments

Goal is to reduce bacteria and inflammation.

- **Tea tree oil *(Melaleuca alternifolia)*:** from leaves of small trees in New South Wales, Australia; antiseptic properties; ideal skin disinfectant. Effective against wide range of organisms (including 27 of 32 strains of *P. acnes*); good penetration without skin irritation. Therapeutic uses are based on antiseptic and antifungal properties; prefer strong solutions (up to 15% tea tree oil) for best results; occasionally produces contact dermatitis.
- **Azelaic acid:** natural 9-carbon dicarboxylic antibiotic against *P. acnes*. Twenty percent azelaic acid cream has an effect in all forms of acne. Must be applied b.i.d. to affected areas for 4 weeks and must be continued for 6 months. Twenty percent azelaic acid cream is as effective as 5% benzoyl peroxide, 4% hydroquinone cream, 0.05% tretinoin, 2% erythromycin, and 0.5 to 1 g/day oral tetracycline at ameliorating comedonal, papulopustular, and nodulocystic acne but less effective than oral isotretinoin 0.5 to 1 mg/kg q.d. at reducing conglobate acne; few side effects; no overt systemic toxicity; plus lower incidence of allergic sensitization, exogenous ochronosis, and residual hypopigmentation—better clinical choice.
- **Vitamin C:** sodium L-ascorbyl-2-phosphate 5% lotion is stable vitamin C derivative and highly effective in improving symptoms.
- **Nicotinamide:** topical nicotinamide inhibits release of lysosomal enzymes, vasoactive amines, and activity of *P. acnes* lipase. It is well tolerated, does not induce bacterial resistance, and is superior to 1% clindamycin gel for moderate inflammatory acne.

Procedural Treatments

- **Nonmedical treatment of acne:** Older acne procedures: comedone extraction, intralesional injections, epidermal exfoliation (cryotherapy, peels, microdermabrasion). Newer procedures: use of various types of lights and lasers. Blue light may be anti-inflammatory, reducing cytokine-induced production of IL-1α in keratinocytes.

Other Considerations

- Psychological support may be necessary: depression is twofold to threefold more common compared with general population.

Acne is cause of emotional distress and maladjustment between parents and children, and general insecurity and feelings of inferiority.

- Emotional stress also plays a role in disease progression. Some researchers have proposed a gastrointestinal mechanism for the overlap among depression, anxiety, and acne. Emotional states might alter the normal intestinal microflora, increase intestinal permeability, and contribute to systemic inflammation. As many as 40% of those with acne have hypochlorhydria; inadequate stomach acid can allow migration of bacteria from colon toward distal small intestine, and permits alteration of normal intestinal microflora. Consider *Lactobacillus acidophilus* cultures. This "gut-brain-skin unifying theory" has recently been validated. The ability of gut microflora and oral probiotics to influence systemic inflammation, oxidative stress, glycemic control, tissue lipid content, and even mood itself may have implications in acne. Probiotic supplementation is often indicated, given common use of antibiotics to treat acne.

THERAPEUTIC APPROACH

- Acne is multifactorial disease requiring integrated therapeutic approach to avoid supplement toxicity. Check patients for treatable causes and underlying hormonal abnormalities before specific therapies are initiated.
- Most effective acne pharmaceutical is isotretinoin (Accutane), a derivative of vitamin A, approved only for severe and recalcitrant nodular acne. Concern over its safety and widespread use is growing. Side effects: intracranial hypertension, depression, and suicidal ideation.
- A U.S. Food and Drug Administration–mandated registry exists for all individuals prescribing, dispensing, or taking isotretinoin, to decrease risk of pregnancy and potentially dangerous adverse effects during a course of isotretinoin therapy.
- **Diet:** eliminate refined and/or concentrated CHOs and foods containing *trans* fats and iodine.
- **Supplements:**
  - Vitamin A: 150,000 IU q.d. for 3 months (monitor closely for side effects)
  - Vitamin E: 400 IU q.d. (mixed tocopherols)
  - Vitamin C: 1000 mg q.d.

— Zn: 30 to 45 mg q.d. (picolinate, acetate, or monomethionine)
— Selenium: 200 mcg q.d.
— Chromium: 200 to 400 mcg q.d. or brewer's yeast 1 tablespoon b.i.d.
— Probiotic: 5 to 10 billion live bacteria q.d. (multistrain)

- **Physical medicine:**
  — Sun or ultraviolet lamp
  — Fruit acid peels
  — Light therapy (blue and red light), intense pulsed light, laser, photodynamic therapy, fractionated light (for acne scars)
- **Topical medicine:**
  — Tea tree oil (5% to 15%) preparations
  — Azelaic acid (20%) preparations
  — Nicotinamide gel (4%)
  — Daily cleansing with *Calendula* soap
  — Expression of comedones with comedone extractor

Affective Disorders

DIAGNOSTIC SUMMARY

Depression (major or unipolar depression):

- Poor appetite with weight loss or increased appetite with weight gain
- Insomnia or hypersomnia
- Physical hyperactivity or inactivity
- Loss of interest or pleasure in usual activities, decrease in sexual drive
- Loss of energy and feelings of fatigue
- Feelings of worthlessness, self-reproach, or inappropriate guilt
- Diminished ability to think or concentrate
- Recurrent thoughts of death or suicide

Presence of five of these for at least 1 month indicates clinical depression; presence of four means depression probable.

Dysthymia: patient depressed most of the time at least 2 years (1 year for children or adolescents) plus at least three of following:

- Low self-esteem, lack of self-confidence
- Pessimism, hopelessness, despair
- Lack of interest in ordinary pleasures and activities
- Withdrawal from social activities
- Fatigue, lethargy
- Guilt, ruminating about past
- Irritability, excessive anger
- Lessened productivity
- Difficulty in concentrating or making decisions

Manic phase:

- Mood typically elation, but irritability and hostility not uncommon
- Signs and symptoms: inflated self-esteem, grandiose delusions, boasting, racing thoughts, decreased need for sleep, psychomotor acceleration, weight loss from increased activity and lack of attention to dietary habits

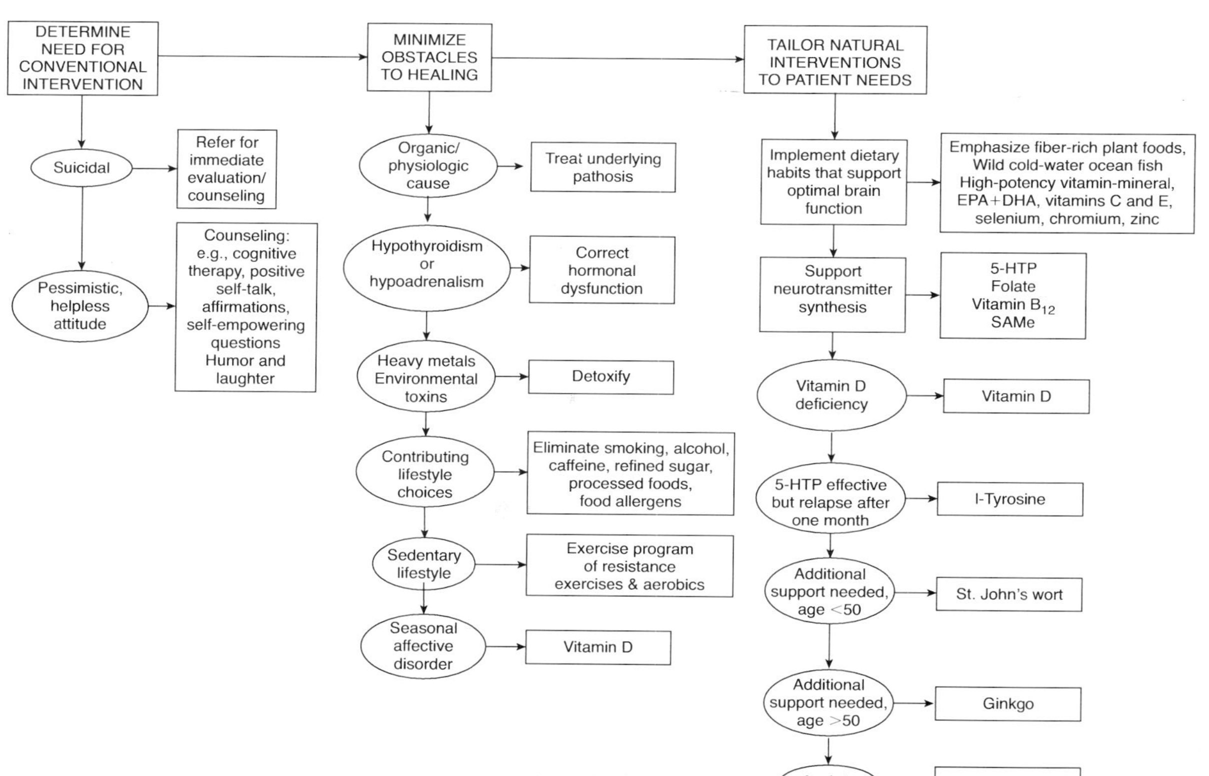
AFFECTIVE DISORDERS: DEPRESSION
DETERMINE NEED FOR CONVENTIONAL INTERVENTION
MINIMIZE OBSTACLES TO HEALING
TAILOR NATURAL INTERVENTIONS TO PATIENT NEEDS
Suicidal
Refer for immediate evaluation/ counseling
Pessimistic, helpless attitude
Counseling: e.g., cognitive therapy, positive self-talk, affirmations, self-empowering questions Humor and laughter
Organic/ physiologic cause
Treat underlying pathosis
Hypothyroidism or hypoadrenalism
Correct hormonal dysfunction
Heavy metals Environmental toxins
Detoxify
Contributing lifestyle choices
Eliminate smoking, alcohol, caffeine, refined sugar, processed foods, food allergens
Sedentary lifestyle
Exercise program of resistance exercises & aerobics
Seasonal affective disorder
Vitamin D
Implement dietary habits that support optimal brain function
Emphasize fiber-rich plant foods, Wild cold-water ocean fish High-potency vitamin-mineral, EPA+DHA, vitamins C and E, selenium, chromium, zinc
Support neurotransmitter synthesis
5-HTP Folate Vitamin B_{12} SAMe
Vitamin D deficiency
Vitamin D
5-HTP effective but relapse after one month
l-Tyrosine
Additional support needed, age <50
St. John's wort
Additional support needed, age >50
Ginkgo
Anxiety
Kava kava

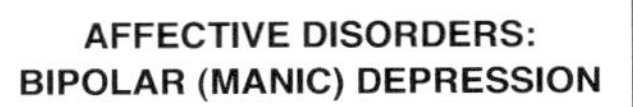

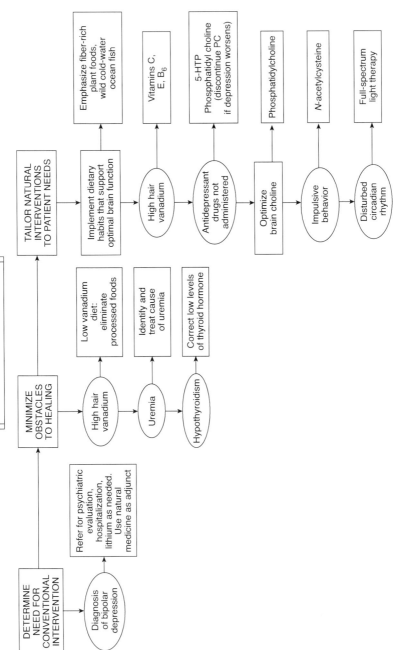

DETERMINE NEED FOR CONVENTIONAL INTERVENTION

- Diagnosis of bipolar depression → Refer for psychiatric evaluation, hospitalization, lithium as needed. Use natural medicine as adjunct

MINIMIZE OBSTACLES TO HEALING

- High hair vanadium → Low vanadium diet: eliminate processed foods
- Uremia → Identify and treat cause of uremia
- Hypothyroidism → Correct low levels of thyroid hormone

TAILOR NATURAL INTERVENTIONS TO PATIENT NEEDS

- Implement dietary habits that support optimal brain function → Emphasize fiber-rich plant foods, wild cold-water ocean fish
- High hair vanadium → Vitamins C, E, B_6
- Antidepressant drugs not administered → 5-HTP Phospphatidyl choline (discontinue PC if depression worsens)
- Optimize brain choline → Phosphatidylcholine
- Impulsive behavior → *N*-acetylcysteine
- Disturbed circadian rhythm → Full-spectrum light therapy

Seasonal affective disorder (SAD): regularly occurring winter depression frequently associated with summer hypomania

Affective disorders are mood disturbances; mood with prolonged emotional tone dominating outlook; transient moods (e.g., sadness, grief, elation) are part of daily life—demarcation of "pathologic" difficult to determine; depression and mania, alone or in alternation, are the most common disorders, and depression alone is much more common; unipolar is depression alone; bipolar is either mania alone or mania alternating with depression.

Eight factors modify functional state of brain and affect mood and behavior:

- Genetic inheritance
- Age of neuronal development (age-specific variability)
- Functional plasticity of brain during development
- Motivational state affected by biologic drives, channeling behavior toward goals by priorities or prejudicing context of incoming information
- Memory-stored information and processing strategies
- Environment that adjusts incoming input according to momentary significance
- Brain disease or lesion causing aberrant function
- Metabolic or hormonal system or biochemical environment of central nervous system (CNS)

Chapter focus: nutritional, environmental, and lifestyle factors affecting mood and therapies to alter brain neurotransmitter levels

DEPRESSION

General Considerations

- **Six theoretical models:**
  - — "Aggression turned inward" (apparent in many cases but no substantial proof).
  - — "Loss model" (depression is a reaction to loss of person, thing, status, self-esteem, or habit pattern).
  - — "Interpersonal relationship" (depressed person uses depression to control other people, including doctors, by pouting, silence, or ignoring something or someone).
  - — "Learned helplessness" (habitual feelings of pessimism and hopelessness).

— "Biogenic amine" hypothesis (biochemical derangement of biogenic amines).
— Analytical (or adaptive) rumination hypothesis: ruminative cognitive processes of a person with depression facilitate solution of complex social problems.

Learned helplessness model (Martin Seligman, PhD) is most useful.

- **Biogenic amine model:** dominant medical conception of depression. Counseling is valuable, especially with clear psychological cause.
- **Learned helplessness (Seligman):** Animals and human beings can be experimentally conditioned to feel and act helpless. Animals conditioned to be helpless have alteration of brain monoamine content; teaching them how to gain environmental control normalizes brain chemistry. Altered brain monoamines in animals with learned helplessness mirror altered brain monoamine biochemistry in human beings during depression. This model revolutionized psychopharmacology; animals conditioned to be helpless and then given antidepressant drugs unlearn helplessness and exercise control over environment. Antidepressants restore monoamine balance and thereby alter behavior. Helping patients gain control over their lives produces greater brain biochemical changes than drugs. Powerful technique—teach optimism. Determining factor for person's reaction to uncontrollable events is "explanatory style" (how patient explains events to self). Optimistic people are immune to helplessness and depression; they have positive, optimistic explanatory style. Pessimists are susceptible to depression when "bad" things happen; they have negative, fatalistic explanatory style. Direct correlation between level of optimism and risk for depression and other illnesses.

Therapeutic Considerations

Although the use of antidepressants may be important in treating severe depressive illness and threatened suicide, antidepressants have not been shown to work any better than placebo in cases of mild to moderate depression, the most common reason for prescription medication. In fact, 25% of patients taking antidepressants do not even have a diagnosable psychiatric problem. The bottom line is that millions of people are using antidepressants for a problem they do not have, and for the people who do have a diagnosable condition, these medications generally do not work. This is a clear mandate to consider natural medicine therapeutics to address the underlying causes of these mood disorders.

Ascertain what nutritional, environmental, social, and psychological factors are involved. Rule out simple organic factors known to contribute to depression: nutrient deficiency or excess, drugs (e.g., prescription, illicit, alcohol, caffeine, nicotine), hypoglycemia, stress and feelings of being overwhelmed, hormonal derangement, allergy, environmental factors, microbial factors.

Organic and Physiologic Factors that May Underlie Depression

Preexisting Physical Conditions	Prescription Drugs
Diabetes	Antihypertensives
Heart disease	Anti-inflammatory agents
Lung disease	Birth control pills
Rheumatoid arthritis	Antihistamines
Chronic inflammation	Corticosteroids
Chronic pain	Tranquilizers and sedatives
Cancer	
Liver disease	
Multiple sclerosis	
Premenstrual syndrome	
Stress or low adrenal function	
Heavy metal toxicity	
Food allergies	
Hypothyroidism	
Hypoglycemia	
Nutritional deficiencies	
Sleep disturbances	

Psychiatry focuses on manipulating neurotransmitters rather than identifying and eliminating psychological factors. Regardless of whether there is underlying organic cause, always recommend counseling for patients with depression.

- **Counseling:**
  - **Cognitive behavioral therapy (CBT):** most merit and support in medical literature. CBT is as effective as antidepressants for moderate depression with lower rate of relapse. Patient is taught new skills to change the way he or she consciously thinks about failure, defeat, loss, and helplessness. Five basic tactics: (1) recognize negative automatic thoughts when patient feels worst, (2) dispute negative thoughts by focusing on contrary evidence, (3) generate different explanation to dispute negative thoughts, (4) avoid

rumination (constant churning of negative thoughts in mind) by consciously controlling thoughts, (5) question negative thoughts and beliefs and replace with empowering positive thoughts and beliefs. Does not involve long psychoanalysis; solution oriented.
- — **Interpersonal therapy (IPT):** focuses on improving communication skills and increasing self-confidence and self-esteem. IPT is often used with depression caused by loss of loved one, during life transitions (becoming a parent or changing careers), feelings of isolation, and relationship conflicts. Once-monthly frequency appears to be as effective as once weekly in preventing recurrence of depressive symptoms. Attrition rate for twice-monthly therapy is the lowest, raising the idea that patient preferences for treatment frequency may be a factor in determining effectiveness of treatment.
- **Organic or physiologic causes:** preexisting physical condition, diabetes, heart disease, lung disease, rheumatoid arthritis, chronic inflammation, chronic pain, cancer, liver disease, multiple sclerosis, prescription drugs, antihypertensives, anti-inflammatories, birth control pills, antihistamines, corticosteroids, tranquilizers and sedatives, premenstrual syndrome, stress or low adrenal function, heavy metals, food allergies, hypothyroidism, hypoglycemia, nutritional deficiencies, sleep disturbances.
- **Conduct comprehensive clinical evaluation:** ascertain nutritional, environmental, social, and psychological factors; rule out organic factors: nutrient deficiency or excess, drugs (prescription, illicit, alcohol, caffeine, nicotine), hypoglycemia, hormonal derangement, allergy, environmental factors, microbes; counseling recommended regardless of underlying organic cause.

Hormonal Factors

The focus of this text is on thyroid and adrenal hormones.

- **Thyroid:** depression is an early manifestation of thyroid disease: subtle decreases in thyroid hormone can be symptomatic. Whether hypothyroidism results from depression-induced hypothalamic-pituitary-thyroid dysfunction or from thyroid hypofunction is uncertain, but it may be a combination. Screen for hypothyroidism, particularly with suggestive symptoms (e.g., fatigue).
- **Stress and adrenal function:** adrenal dysfunction associated with depression can result from stress. Adrenal stress index measures cortisol and DHEA in saliva. Depression signs: elevated

morning cortisol and decreased DHEA. Cortisol elevation reflects disturbed hypothalamic-pituitary-adrenal (HPA) axis and is the basis of the dexamethasone suppression test (DST). HPA dysregulation affecting mood results in excessive cortisol independent of stress responses, abnormal nocturnal cortisol release, and inadequate suppression by dexamethasone. CNS effects of increased endogenous cortisol include depression, mania, nervousness, insomnia, and schizophrenia (high levels). Glucocorticoid effects on mood are related to induction of tryptophan oxygenase, shunting tryptophan to kynurenine pathway at the expense of serotonin and melatonin synthesis.

- **Tests of hypothalamic-pituitary function:** DST and thyroid stimulation test—determine whether mood is caused by hypothalamic dysfunction and categorize psychiatric illness (e.g., severe major affective disorders versus severe psychotic disorders). DST—little clinical value for screening and no better than urinary free cortisol. Thyroid hormone assays do not detect all cases of hypothyroidism—not an effective screening procedure. Thyrotropin releasing hormone (TRH) stimulation test is more sensitive, diagnosing subclinical hypothyroidism. TRH test has wide clinical usefulness because thyroid dysfunction is implicated in many disorders.

  TRH grading system for hypothyroidism is as follows:
  - Grade 3 (subclinical hypothyroidism, 4%): patients without classic hypothyroid signs; normal T3RU, T_4, and thyroid-stimulating hormone (TSH); abnormal TSH response to TRH test
  - Grade 2 (mild hypothyroidism, 3.6%): mild isolated clinical signs or symptoms; normal T3RU and T_4; baseline TSH elevated; abnormal TRH test
  - Grade 1 (overt hypothyroidism, 1%): classic hypothyroid signs and symptoms; abnormal laboratory values (reduced T3RU and T_4, increased TSH, abnormal TRH response)

Environmental Toxins

- **Heavy metals** (lead [Pb], mercury [Hg], cadmium [Cd], arsenic [As], nickel [Ni], aluminum [Al]), solvents (e.g., cleaning materials, formaldehyde, toluene, benzene), pesticides, herbicides—affinity for nervous tissue; associated symptoms include depression, headache, mental confusion, mental illness, tingling in extremities, abnormal nerve reflexes, other signs of impaired nervous function (*Textbook,* "Environmental Medicine" and "Metal Toxicity: Assessment of Exposure and Retention").

- **Detailed medical history and hair mineral analysis** screen for environmental toxins. If hair mineral analysis is inconclusive, a more-sensitive test is the 8-hour Pb mobilization test—chelating agent ethylenediaminetetraacetic acid (EDTA)—measure Pb excreted in urine for 8 hours after injection of EDTA.

Lifestyle Factors

Eliminate smoking, excess alcohol consumption, sugar abuse, caffeine. Add regular exercise and healthful diet—better clinical results than antidepressants with no side effects or monetary cost.

- **Smoking:** major factor contributing to premature death. Nicotine stimulates adrenal secretion (cortisol), a feature of depression. Cortisol and stress activate tryptophan oxygenase, reducing tryptophan delivery to the brain. Brain serotonin depends on amount of tryptophan delivered—cortisol reduces levels of serotonin and melatonin. Cortisol downregulates brain serotonin receptors, reducing sensitivity to available serotonin. Smoking induces relative vitamin C deficiency; vitamin C helps detoxify smoke. Low levels of brain vitamin C can cause depression and hysteria.
- **Alcohol:** brain depressant; increases adrenal hormone output; interferes with brain cell processes; disrupts sleep cycles; depletes nutrients and mood-enhancing prostaglandin E_1, all of which will disrupt mood; leads to hypoglycemia and craving for sugar, which aggravates hypoglycemia and mental and emotional problems.
- **Caffeine:** stimulant. Intensity of response varies greatly—people prone to depression or anxiety are sensitive to caffeine. "Caffeinism" is a clinical syndrome of nervousness, palpitations, irritability, and recurrent headache. Students with moderate to high coffee intake score higher on depression scale and have lower academic performance than low users. Patients with depression have high caffeine intake (more than 700 mg/day). Caffeine intake is positively correlated with degree of mental illness in patients with psychiatric disorders. Caffeine plus refined sugar is worse than either alone—combination has clinical link to depression. Average American intake: 150 to 225 mg caffeine q.d., or 1 to 2 cups coffee. Some people are more sensitive to effects than others, even small amount in decaffeinated coffee. Patients with psychological disorders should avoid caffeine completely.
- **Exercise:** most powerful natural antidepressant. Benefit in heart health may be related as much to improved mood as to cardiovascular fitness. Profound antidepressive effects—decreased anxiety, depression, and malaise plus higher self-esteem and more happiness;

increases endorphins, which are directly correlated with mood. Sedentary men are more depressed, perceive greater life stress, have higher cortisol and lower beta-endorphins than joggers. Depression is responsive to exercise, firming up biochemical link between physical activity and depression. Exercise improves self-esteem and work behavior; can be as effective as antidepressant drugs and psychotherapy. Best exercises: strength training (weight lifting) or aerobics (walking briskly, jogging, bicycling, playing basketball, cross-country skiing, swimming, aerobic dance, and racquet sports).

Nutrition

Any single nutrient deficiency can alter brain function, inducing depression or anxiety. Nutrition powerfully influences cognition, emotion, and behavior. Even in the absence of laboratory validation of deficiency, nutritional supplementation can be of benefit. Full-range high-potency multiple vitamins are the foundation. Nutrient deficiencies are common in depressed individuals; most common are folate, B_{12}, and B_6.

Behavioral Effects of Some Vitamin Deficiencies

Deficient Vitamins	Behavioral Effects
Thiamine	Korsakoff's psychosis, mental depression, apathy, anxiety, irritability
Riboflavin	Depression, irritability
Niacin	Apathy, anxiety, depression, hyperirritability, mania, memory deficits, delirium, organic dementia, emotional lability
Biotin	Depression, extreme lassitude, somnolence
Pantothenic acid	Restlessness, irritability, depression, fatigue
Vitamin B_6	Depression, irritability, sensitivity to sound
Folic acid	Forgetfulness, insomnia, apathy, irritability, depression, psychosis, delirium, dementia
Vitamin B_{12}	Psychotic states, depression, irritability, confusion, memory loss, hallucinations, delusions, paranoia
Vitamin C	Lassitude, hypochondriasis, depression, hysteria

- **Diet:** brain requires constant sugar supply; hypoglycemia must be avoided. Hypoglycemia symptoms: psychological disturbances (e.g., depression, anxiety, irritability), fatigue, headache, blurred vision, excessive sweating, mental confusion, incoherent speech, bizarre behavior, convulsions. Hypoglycemia is common in depressed individuals; eliminate refined carbohydrates; health promotion diet rich in whole, natural, unprocessed foods, especially high in plant foods (fruits, vegetables, whole grains, beans, seeds, nuts). People who eat healthful Mediterranean diet are half as likely to develop depression as those who do not.

- **Folate and B_{12}:** function together in many pathways. Folate deficiency is the most common nutrient deficiency worldwide; 31% to 35% of patients with depression are folate deficient, 35% to 92.6% among the elderly. Depression is the most common symptom of folate deficiency. B_{12} deficiency is less common but can also cause depression, especially in the elderly. Folate, B_{12}, and SAM (*S*-adenosyl-methionine) are "methyl donors"; SAM is the major methyl donor in the body. Antidepressant effects of folate increase brain SAM. The key brain compound dependent on methylation is tetrahydrobiopterin (BH4), a coenzyme in the manufacture of monoamine neurotransmitters (e.g., serotonin and dopamine) from respective amino acids. Patients with recurrent depression have reduced BH4 synthesis, probably from low SAM levels. BH4 synthesis is stimulated by folate, B_{12}, and C; supplementation can increase BH4 and serotonin content. Folate doses as antidepressant are very high: 15 to 50 mg is safe (except in epilepsy) and is as effective as antidepressant drugs. Doses of 800 mcg folate and 800 mcg B_{12} are sufficient to prevent deficiencies. Folate supplements should always be accompanied by B_{12} to prevent masking B_{12} deficiency.
- **Vitamin B_6:** low in patients with depression, especially women on birth control pills or Premarin; essential to manufacture of all monoamines; dose is 50 to 100 mg q.d.
- **Zinc (Zn):** cofactor in 70 metalloenzymes. Severe deficiency symptoms: bullous-pustular dermatitis, diarrhea, alopecia, recurrent infections. Derangement of Zn homeostasis is linked to mood disorders. Antidepressant drugs increase Zn in hippocampus of patients with depression with low baseline Zn. Zn may act as antagonist of *N*-methyl-D-aspartate NMDA glutamate receptor. Small study: Zn reduced scores on Hamilton and Beck depression scales in patients taking antidepressant drugs. Balance with copper during long-term use.
- **Selenium (Se):** levels are low in alcoholics. Low Se status encourages depressed mood; high dietary Se or supplementation improves mood. Low Se is linked to depression, anxiety,

confusion, hostility. Alcoholism combined with depression in the same person increases risk for suicide.

- **Chromium (Cr):** increased sugar intake is correlated with depression. Cr may balance insulin levels. Atypical depression (one fifth of all depressive illness) is characterized by mood reactivity, increased appetite and weight gain, hypersomnia, leaden paralysis, interpersonal rejection sensitivity, earlier onset, and greater chronicity, disability, and suicidality than other forms of depression. Cr picolinate may help some atypical patients with depression at 400 to 600 mcg daily. Mechanism of action: alteration of brain serotonin levels and increase in insulin insensitivity.
- **Vitamin D:** helps treat a critical underlying deficiency. Low levels may be involved in pathogenesis of depression. Distribution of vitamin D receptors is in high concentration in the hypothalamus, suggesting a neuroendocrine role. Distribution of target neurons of vitamin D suggests an influence on nerve growth factor, acetylcholine, serotonin, testosterone, thyroid hormone, and tyrosine hydroxylase messenger RNA. All these have been implicated in the pathogenesis of depression. Prevention of depression in the adult may even occur by treating pregnant women; gestational deficiency may cause depression-like behavior in offspring. The laboratory test indicative of functional vitamin D status measures 25-hydroxy (OH) vitamin D, an intermediate metabolite. Doses of 4000 international units (IU) daily in depressed patients tend to improve well-being. This may be a good place to start for depressed patients; higher levels may be needed for some. Dosage level that induces hypervitaminosis over time is unknown; be cautious at 20,000 IU daily or blood levels of 100 ng/mL. Main sources: wild ocean fish, exposure to sunlight. Vitamin D deficiency is likely the primary cause of SAD.
- **Omega-3 fatty acids:** insufficiency linked to depression; affect phospholipid composition of neuronal cell membranes. The brain is the richest source of phospholipids in the body; lack of essential fatty acids (EFAs) (omega-3 oils) and excess saturated fats induce formation of cell membranes with less fluid than optimal and impair membrane regulation of passage of molecules into and out of cell, disrupting homeostasis and proper nerve cell function, affecting behavior, mood, and mental function. Biophysical properties, including fluidity of brain cell membranes, influence neurotransmitter synthesis, signal transmission, neurotransmitter binding and uptake, and activity of monoamine oxidase (MAO)—factors implicated in depression. Omega-3 EFAs may inhibit development of depression as they do cardiovascular

disease. Lowering plasma cholesterol by diet and medications increases suicide, homicide, and depression. The quantity and type of dietary fats consumed alter biophysical and biochemical properties of cell membranes. Dietary efforts to lower cholesterol tend to increase the n-6/n-3 ratio and decrease eicosapentaenoic acid (EPA) and docosahexaenoic acid (DHA). Decreased consumption of omega-3 EFAs correlates with increasing rates of depression. Consistent association between depression and coronary artery disease, also linked to omega-3 deficits.
- **Food allergies:** depression and fatigue are linked to food allergies. "Allergic toxemia" is a syndrome with symptoms of depression, fatigue, muscle and joint aches, drowsiness, difficulty concentrating, and nervousness.

Monoamine Metabolism and Precursor Therapy

Monoamine precursors (tryptophan, 5-hydroxytryptophan [5-HTP], and tyrosine) offer natural alternative to monoamine oxidase (MAO) inhibitors and tricyclics for influencing monoamine metabolism.
- **Tryptophan catastrophe:** for more than 30 years, L-tryptophan has been used by millions in the United States and around the world safely and effectively for insomnia and depression. In October 1989, one Japanese manufacturer, Showa Denko, the largest supplier to the United States (50% to 60%), produced batches contaminated with substances now linked to eosinophilia-myalgia syndrome (EMS) caused by changes in the bacteria used to produce L-tryptophan and the filtration process. Patients with EMS have the following signs and symptoms: more than 1000 eosinophils per cubic millimeter (twice normal); allergic and inflammatory symptoms from release of histamine by eosinophils—severe muscle and joint pain, high fever, weakness, swelling of arms and legs, skin rashes, and shortness of breath. EMS affected 144 of every 50,000 men and 268 of every 50,000 women, or 1 in 250 people taking contaminated L-tryptophan. Only those with an abnormal activation of kynurenine pathway reacted to the contaminant; kynurenine and its metabolites (quinolinic acid) are linked to other EMS-related illnesses (e.g., Spain's 1991 toxic oil syndrome, one of the largest food-related epidemics ever); people who took multiple vitamin preparation were somewhat protected against EMS; vitamins (B_6 and niacin) shunted tryptophan away from the kynurenine pathway or contaminants were somehow metabolized by vitamin-dependent enzymes.

- **L-Tryptophan:** increases brain serotonin and melatonin. Many depressed individuals have low tryptophan and serotonin. Supplementation provides mixed clinical results; only two of eight studies indicated superiority compared with placebo, but nine of 11 studies indicated equivalence to antidepressant drugs. Factors to consider: study size, severity of depression, duration, and dose. Hormones (estrogen and cortisol) and tryptophan itself stimulate tryptophan oxygenase, which converts tryptophan to kynurenine with less tryptophan delivered to brain. Summary: L-tryptophan only modestly effective when used alone; must be used with B_6 and niacinamide to block kynurenine pathway; better results with 5-HTP. Because dehydration may limit amount of tryptophan available to the brain, optimal water intake is also important.
- **5-HTP:** cannot be converted to kynurenine and easily crosses the blood-brain barrier. Only 3% of oral L-tryptophan is converted to serotonin, whereas more than 70% of oral 5-HTP is converted. 5-HTP causes increased endorphins and catecholamine; equipotency with serotonin reuptake inhibitors and tricyclics; advantages—less expensive, better tolerated, fewer and milder side effects.
- **Phenylalanine and tyrosine:** phenylalanine is hydroxylated to tyrosine and degraded to phenylketonic acids, but also decarboxylated to phenylethylamine (PEA). PEA is an amphetamine-like endogenous stimulatory and antidepressive substance in human beings. (PEA is a biogenic amine in high concentrations in chocolate.) Low urinary PEA is found in patients with depression, high levels in schizophrenics. D-Phenylalanine and L-phenylalanine increase urinary and CNS PEA. Phenylalanine is a tyrosine hydroxylase inhibitor; shunting phenylalanine to PEA synthesis occurs with supplementation. Tyrosine increases trace amines (octopamine, tyramine, and PEA), enhances catecholamine synthesis, stimulates thyroid hormone synthesis. L-Dopa alone is ineffective in affective disorders. Central norepinephrine turnover is decreased in patients with depression—may result from low serum tyrosine seen in some depressed individuals. Brain tyrosine is best determined by ratio of serum tyrosine to sum of its brain-uptake competitors (leucine, isoleucine, valine, tryptophan, and phenylalanine). Tyrosine ratios increase with high-protein meals. Tyrosine supplements increase urine 3-methoxy-4-hydroxyphenethylene glycol (MHPG), the principal breakdown product of norepinephrine in CNS and a biochemical marker for

determining which amino acid to supplement. Phenylalanine and tyrosine are encouraging alternatives to tricyclics and MAO inhibitors. Van Praag study: 20% of patients who responded well to 5-HTP relapsed after 1 month despite the fact that blood 5-HTP and presumably brain serotonin remained the same as when experiencing benefit; other monoamine neurotransmitters (dopamine and norepinephrine) declined; patients responded to supplemental tyrosine.

- **SAM:** involved in methylation of monoamines, neurotransmitters, and phospholipids. The brain manufactures SAM from methionine; SAM synthesis is impaired in patients with depression. SAM supplementation in patients with depression increases serotonin, dopamine, and phosphatides and improves binding of neurotransmitters to receptors, increasing serotonin and dopamine activity and improving neuron membrane fluidity and clinical symptoms. SAM is an effective natural antidepressant but expensive; oral dose 400 mg q.i.d. (1600 mg total). Better tolerated with quicker action than tricyclics; study comparing SAM with tricyclic desipramine: 62% of SAM patients and 50% of desipramine patients significantly improved. Regardless of type of treatment, patients with 50% decrease in Hamilton depression scale had significant increase in plasma SAM. No significant side effects with oral SAM; nausea and vomiting in some people. Start dosage at 200 mg b.i.d. first day, 400 mg b.i.d. day 3, 400 mg t.i.d. day 10, and 400 mg q.i.d. after 20 days. Bipolar (manic) patients should not take SAM—susceptible to hypomania or mania.

Botanical Medicines

- ***Hypericum perforatum*** (St. John's wort): extracts standardized for hypericin and hyperforin are the most thoroughly researched natural antidepressants. Mechanisms of action may include serotonin reuptake modulation, increases in interleukin-6 activity, and agonist action of sigma receptors. Improves many symptoms: depression, anxiety, apathy, sleep disturbances, insomnia, anorexia, feelings of worthlessness. Advantages over antidepressant drugs are fewer side effects, lower cost, and greater patient tolerance. Beware of hyperforin's enhancement of drug degradation, including contraceptives, by liver cytochrome p450 enzymes (*Textbook*, "*Hypericum perforatum* [St. John's Wort]").
- ***Piper methysticum* (kava kava):** approved in Germany, United Kingdom, Switzerland, and Austria for treatment of nervous

anxiety, insomnia, depression, and restlessness based on detailed pharmacologic data and favorable clinical studies; efficacy compares favorably with benzodiazepines without drug side effects (impaired mental acuity, addictiveness). Prefer extracts standardized for kava lactones (30% to 70%). High incidence of improper dosage of kava extract; know how to use this botanical properly for best efficacy; most useful for depression with severe anxiety. Rare but serious side effects may have occurred owing to poor-quality kava and other risk factors—overdose, prolonged therapy, and co-medication. A review of clinical trial participants taking kava (some at high doses) showed no liver toxicity. Hepatotoxicity is rare side effect (*Textbook, "Piper methysticum* [Kava]").
- ***Ginkgo biloba:*** leaf extract standardized to 24% ginkgo flavon glycosides and 6% terpenoids; exerts good antidepressant effects, especially for those older than 50; improves mood in patients with cerebrovascular insufficiency; can be used with antidepressant drugs and may enhance their efficacy in patients older than 50. Counteracts one of the major brain chemistry changes associated with aging—reduction in number of serotonin receptors. Mechanism of effect: correcting or preventing impaired receptor synthesis or changes in cerebral neuronal membranes or receptors as a result of free radical damage; increases protein synthesis and acts as a potent antioxidant (*Textbook, "Ginkgo biloba* [Ginkgo Tree]").

Therapeutic Approach

Accurately determine which factors contribute to patient's depression; balance errant neurotransmitter levels and optimize patient's nutrition, lifestyle, and psychological health.
- **Diet:** increase fiber-rich plant foods (fruits, vegetables, grains, legumes, raw nuts and seeds); avoid caffeine, nicotine, other stimulants, sugar, and alcohol; identify and control food allergies; increase consumption of small wild cold-water fish to at least twice per week.
- **Lifestyle:** refer to counselor or counsel patient to develop positive, optimistic mental attitude—help patient set goals, use positive self-talk and affirmations, identify self-empowering questions, and find ways to inject humor and laughter into life. Exercise at least 30 minutes at least three times a week; apply relaxation and stress reduction techniques 10 to 15 minutes daily.

- **Supplements:**
  - — High-potency multiple vitamins and minerals
  - — Vitamin C: 500 to 1000 mg t.i.d.
  - — Vitamin D: 2000 to 4000 IU q.d. or more, depending on laboratory values until normal levels reached. (If patient's serum $25(OH)D_3$ does not increase proportionately to dose, measure $1,25(OH)2D_3$ for overconversion.)
  - — Vitamin E (mixed tocopherols): 200 to 400 IU q.d.
  - — Se: 200 mcg q.d.
  - — Cr: 400 to 600 mcg q.d.
  - — Zn: 25 mg q.d.
  - — Omega-3 fatty acids: 2000 mg combined EPA + DHA q.d.
  - — 5-HTP: 100 to 200 mg t.i.d.
  - — Folic acid and vitamin B_{12}: 800 mcg of each q.d.
  - — SAM: 200 mg b.i.d. up to 400 mg t.i.d. (especially indicated for those with a catechol-O-methyltransferase [COMT] polymorphism with decreased activity)
- **Botanical medicines:**
  - — Younger than 50: St. John's wort extract (0.3% hypericin, 4% hyperforin), 300 mg t.i.d.; severe cases, St. John's wort in combination with 5-HTP
  - — Older than 50: *G. biloba* extract (24% ginkgo flavon glycosides, 6% terpenoids), 80 mg t.i.d.; severe cases, use in combination with St. John's wort and/or 5-HTP
  - — Significant anxiety: kava extract (standardized to kava lactones), 45 to 70 mg kava lactones t.i.d.

BIPOLAR (MANIC) DEPRESSION AND HYPOMANIA

Diagnostic Summary

Diagnostic criteria for bipolar depression—at least three of following symptoms:

- Excessive self-esteem or grandiosity
- Reduced need for sleep
- Extreme talkativeness, excessive telephoning
- Extremely rapid flight of thoughts along with the feeling that the mind is racing
- Inability to concentrate, easily distracted
- Increase in social or work-oriented activities, often with a 60- to 80-hour work week
- Poor judgment, as indicated by sprees of uncontrolled spending, increased sexual indiscretions, and misguided financial decisions

General Considerations

Bipolar depression is characterized by periods of major depression alternating with periods of elevated mood. If elevated mood is relatively mild and lasts 4 days or less, it is called hypomania. Mania is longer and more intense. Full-blown manic attack requires hospitalization: loss of self-control, may hurt themselves or others. Standard treatment is lithium—stabilizes mood, prevents manic phase—used either alone or with antidepressant. Antidepressant drugs can occasionally induce mania and hypomania; difficult to control lows in bipolar depressives with drugs.

Therapeutic Considerations

Initially hospitalize 2 weeks under sedation with antipsychotic drugs until blood lithium levels are acceptable. Refer for conventional therapy until mood stabilizes. Principles outlined for depression also apply to mania; seriousness of condition—use nutritional therapy as adjunct rather than primary therapy. Selective serotonin reuptake inhibitors are helpful in combination with lithium; 5-HTP and St. John's wort may be useful as adjuncts to lithium but without side effects.

- **Tryptophan**: effective doses are generally quite large: 12 g q.d. L-tryptophan. Better choice is 5-HTP, in combination with lithium, at 100 mg t.i.d.
- ***N*-acetylcysteine (NAC):** precursor to amino acid cysteine, which contributes to cell glutathione production and to general antioxidant activities. As a modulator of glutamatergic system, cysteine influences reward-reinforcement pathway. NAC may exert therapeutic effect on psychiatric disorders allegedly related to oxidative stress—schizophrenia and bipolar disorder. It is used in psychiatric syndromes characterized by impulsive and compulsive symptoms—trichotillomania, pathologic nail biting, gambling, and substance misuse. NAC appears to be a promising intervention posing very little risk. In bipolar patients, NAC at 2000 mg/day for 6 months showed large decreases in depressive symptoms—global improvement, severity, and function scales. NAC treatment needs to be ongoing. For those rare patients who are sulfur intolerant, add molybdenum.
- **Phosphatidylcholine (PC):** large amounts of PC (15 to 30 g q.d. in both pure form and lecithin)—better results for mania than monoamine precursors. Lithium promotes increased CNS cholinergic activity by inhibition of choline flux across the

blood-brain barrier; mania is associated with reduced CNS cholinergic activity. Using PC to increase CNS choline may improve symptoms in some patients.

- **Omega-3 fatty acids:** one 4-month, double-blind, placebo-controlled study found marked therapeutic efficacy and no side effects. Dose: 9.6 g of omega-3 fatty acids per day. Benefits: longer period of remission and may inhibit neuronal signal transduction pathways in a manner similar to that of lithium carbonate and valproate.
- **Vanadium (Va):** increased Va found in hair of manic patients; levels normalize with recovery. Patients with depression have normal hair Va, with whole blood and serum Va elevated and returning to normal on recovery. Vanadate ion is a strong inhibitor of Na^+,K^+-ATPase; lithium reduces this inhibition. Therapies to reduce vanadate to less-inhibitory vanadyl form include ascorbic acid, methylene blue, and EDTA separately and in combination. Ascorbic acid (3 g q.d.) provides significant clinical improvement. Low-Va diet—low-Va foods (1 to 5 ng/g) include fats, oils, fresh fruits, vegetables; range of 5 to 30 ng/g includes whole grains, seafood, meat, dairy; range of 11 to 93 ng/g includes prepared foods (peanut butter, white bread, breakfast cereals). Other correctable factors known to inhibit Na^+,K^+-ATPase are uremia, hypothyroidism, and catecholamine insensitivity. Vitamins E and B_6 increase Na^+,K^+-ATPase activity in vitro; vitamin E also stabilizes membranes.
- **Circadian rhythms:** patients with manic depression have disturbed circadian rhythms, seasonal patterns of exacerbations, and supersensitivity to light. Alteration of circadian light-dark cycles with light therapy may help (see later section on SAD).

Therapeutic Approach

Same dietary and lifestyle guidelines as for depression.

- **Diet**: low-Va diet—eliminate all refined and processed foods; promote fresh fruits and vegetables.
- **Supplements**:
  - PC: 10 to 25 g q.d. (PC may induce depression in some patients; if this occurs, discontinue immediately.)
  - NAC: 1 g b.i.d.
  - Vitamin C: 3 to 5 g q.d. in divided doses
  - Vitamin E: 400 to 800 IU q.d.
  - Pyridoxine: 100 mg q.d.

SEASONAL AFFECTIVE DISORDER

General Considerations

Associated with winter depression and summer hypomania. Typically patients feel depressed, slow down, oversleep, overeat, and crave carbohydrates in winter. In summer, they feel elated, active, energetic.

Therapeutic Considerations

- **Melatonin:** light exposure is the main contributing factor. Key hormonal changes are reduced melatonin from pineal and increased cortisol from adrenals. Melatonin supplementation may improve SAD; it increases brain melatonin and suppresses cortisol secretion.
- Synthesis and secretion and reestablishing circadian rhythm. Place full-spectrum fluorescent tubes in regular fluorescent fixtures (eight tubes total). Patients sit 3 feet away from light from 5:00 to 8:00 AM and 5:30 to 8:30 PM. Patients are free to engage in activities as long as they glance at the light at least once per minute. Protocol restricts social life; replacing standard bulbs with full-spectrum light may help. Commercially made lights at a concentration of 10,000 lux yield exposure to full-spectrum white light (10,000 lux) for at least 30 minutes every day in the morning.
- ***H. perforatum:*** St. John's wort extract (standardized to 0.3% hypericin, 4% hyperforin) (*Textbook, "Hypericum perforatum* [St. John's Wort]") at dose of 300 mg t.i.d. improves SAD but is more effective in combination with light therapy. Beware of enhanced drug degradation by liver cytochrome p450 enzymes.

Therapeutic Approach

Extend light exposure on winter days; use full-spectrum lighting throughout indoor environment; nighttime melatonin (3 mg 45 minutes before retiring); daytime St. John's wort or 5-HTP.

Alcohol Dependence

DIAGNOSTIC SUMMARY

- Alcohol dependence manifests when alcohol is withdrawn: tremulousness, convulsions, hallucinations, delirium
- Alcoholic binges, benders (48 hours or more of drinking associated with failure to meet usual obligations), or blackouts
- Evidence of alcohol-induced illnesses: cirrhosis, gastritis, pancreatitis, myopathy, polyneuropathy, cerebellar degeneration
- Physical signs of excess alcohol consumption: alcohol odor on breath, flushed face, tremor, ecchymoses
- Psychological or social signs of excess alcohol consumption: depression, loss of friends, arrest for driving while intoxicated, surreptitious drinking, drinking before breakfast, frequent accidents, unexplained work absences

GENERAL CONSIDERATIONS

Alcohol dependence, alcohol-use disorder, or, as it was formerly known, alcoholism, is a disabling addictive disorder characterized by alcohol consumption that exceeds acceptable cultural limits or injures health or social relationships. Alcohol dependence is more prevalent among men, whites, Native Americans, younger and unmarried adults, and those with lower incomes.

- **Consequences:** increased mortality: 10- to 12-year-lower life expectancy; twice death rate in men, three times in women; six times the suicide rate; major factor in four leading causes of death in men aged 25 to 44 (accidents, homicides, suicides, cirrhosis); economic toll; health effects: metabolic damage to every cell; intoxication; abstinence and withdrawal syndromes; nutritional deficiency diseases; cerebellar degeneration; cerebral atrophy; psychiatric disorders; esophagitis, gastritis, ulcer; increased risk of cancer of mouth, pharynx, larynx, esophagus; pancreatitis; liver fatty degeneration and cirrhosis; arrhythmias; myocardial degeneration; hypertension; angina; hypoglycemia;

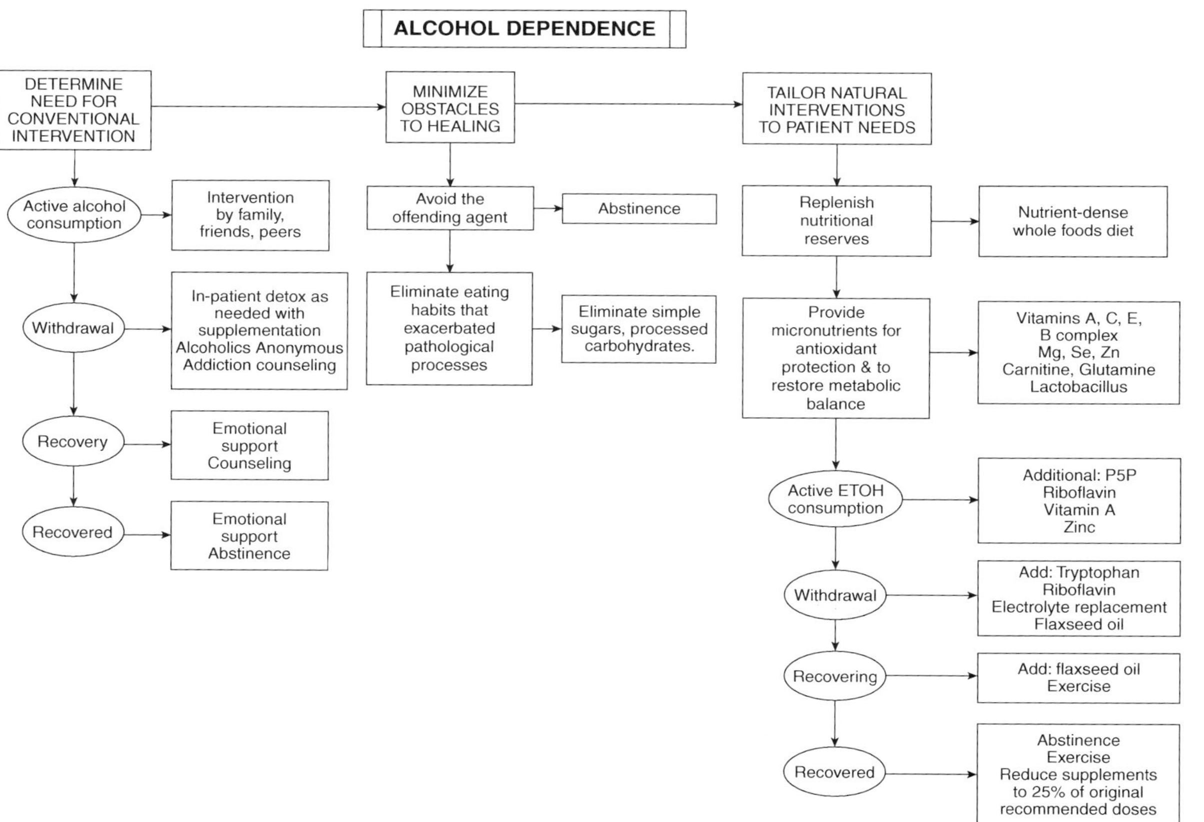
ALCOHOL DEPENDENCE
DETERMINE NEED FOR CONVENTIONAL INTERVENTION
Active alcohol consumption
Intervention by family, friends, peers
Withdrawal
In-patient detox as needed with supplementation Alcoholics Anonymous Addiction counseling
Recovery
Emotional support Counseling
Recovered
Emotional support Abstinence
MINIMIZE OBSTACLES TO HEALING
Avoid the offending agent
Abstinence
Eliminate eating habits that exacerbated pathological processes
Eliminate simple sugars, processed carbohydrates.
TAILOR NATURAL INTERVENTIONS TO PATIENT NEEDS
Replenish nutritional reserves
Nutrient-dense whole foods diet
Provide micronutrients for antioxidant protection & to restore metabolic balance
Vitamins A, C, E, B complex Mg, Se, Zn Carnitine, Glutamine Lactobacillus
Active ETOH consumption
Additional: P5P Riboflavin Vitamin A Zinc
Withdrawal
Add: Tryptophan Riboflavin Electrolyte replacement Flaxseed oil
Recovering
Add: flaxseed oil Exercise
Recovered
Abstinence Exercise Reduce supplements to 25% of original recommended doses

decreased protein synthesis; increased serum and liver triglycerides; decreased serum testosterone; myopathy; osteoporosis; rosacea, spider veins; coagulation disorders.
- **Effects on fetus:** growth retardation; mental retardation; fetal alcohol syndrome; teratogenicity.
- 18 million alcoholics in United States; often a "hidden" disease disguised by sympathetic family and friends.

The Brief Michigan Alcohol Dependence Screening Test

1. Do you feel you are a normal drinker?	Yes (0)	No (2)
2. Do friends or relatives think you are a normal drinker?	Yes (0)	No (2)
3. Have you ever attended a meeting of Alcoholics Anonymous (AA)?	Yes (5)	No (0)
4. Have you ever lost friends or girlfriends or boyfriends because of drinking?	Yes (2)	No (0)
5. Have you ever gotten into trouble at work because of drinking?	Yes (2)	No (0)
6. Have you ever neglected your obligations, your family or your work for 2 or more days in a row because you were drinking?	Yes (2)	No (0)
7. Have you ever had delirium tremens (DTs), severe shaking, heard voices, or seen things that were not there after heavy drinking	Yes (2)	No (0)
8. Have you ever gone to anyone for help about your drinking?	Yes (5)	No (0)
9. Have you ever been in a hospital because of drinking?	Yes (5)	No (0)
10. Have you ever been arrested for drunk driving or driving after drinking?	Yes (2)	No (0)

Modified from Hyman SE, Cassem NH. Alcoholism. In Dale DC, Federman DD, eds. Scientific American medicine. New York: Scientific American, 1997: III, 1–12, 13

- **Etiology:** obscure; multifactorial: genetic, physiologic, psychological, and social factors equally important; 35% of alcoholics start at ages 15 to 19 years, 80% before age 30; most common in men; female/male ratio is rising to 1:2. Women become addicted at lower intake than men. Genetic features:
  — Family condition.

— Adopted children of alcoholic parents raised by foster parents have higher risk.
— Differences between identical and nonidentical twins.
— Association with genetic markers: color vision, nonsecretor ABH, HLA-B13, and low platelet monoamine oxidase (MAO).
— Importance of alcohol dehydrogenase (ADH) polymorphism in racial susceptibility.

Intoxication and Withdrawal

- **Intoxication signs:** central nervous system depression: drowsiness, errors of commission, disinhibition, dysarthria, ataxia, and nystagmus; 15 mL pure alcohol (1 oz whiskey, 4 oz wine, or 10 oz beer) raises blood alcohol level by 25 mg/dL in 70-kg person; effects of varying levels of blood alcohol are shown in table.

Effects of Varying Levels of Blood Alcohol

BLOOD LEVEL (MG/DL)	EFFECT
<50	No significant motor dysfunction
100	Mild intoxication—decreased inhibitions, slight visual impairment, slight muscular incoordination, slowing of reaction time Legally intoxicated in most jurisdictions
150	Ataxia, dysarthria, slurring of speech, nausea and vomiting
350	Marked muscular incoordination, blurred vision, approaching stupor
500	Coma and death

- **Withdrawal symptoms:** 1 to 3 days after last drink; anxiety, tremulousness, mental confusion, tremor, sensory hyperactivity, visual hallucinations, autonomic hyperactivity, diaphoresis, dehydration, electrolyte disturbances, seizures, and cardiovascular abnormalities.

Metabolic Effects of Alcohol and Alcohol Dependence

- **Ethanol metabolism:** factors influencing alcohol catabolism are rate of alcohol absorption, concentration and activity of liver ADH and aldehyde dehydrogenase (ALDH), and ratio of reduced to oxidized nicotinamide adenine dinucleotide ($NADH/NAD^+$)

in liver mitochondria. Availability and regeneration of NAD^+ are rate-limiting factors for alcohol oxidation. Alcohol is converted to acetaldehyde by ADH, with cofactor NAD^+. Aldehyde is responsible for harmful effects and addictive process; high blood aldehyde found in alcoholics and relatives after alcohol consumption—either increased ADH activity or depressed ALDH activity in people susceptible to alcohol dependence. Acetaldehyde is converted by ALDH to acetate, with little entering Krebs cycle; most is converted to long-chain fatty acids, leading to fatty liver.

- **Fatty liver:** in all alcoholics, even with minimal consumption; severity proportional to duration and degree of alcohol excess. Pathogenesis arises from increased endogenous fatty acid synthesis, diminished triglyceride utilization, impaired lipoprotein excretion, direct damage to endoplasmic reticula by free radicals produced by ethanol metabolism, and high-fat diet typical of alcoholics. Leptin is peptide hormone helping regulate appetite and energy metabolism. Circulating leptin levels are increased in a dose-dependent manner in chronic alcohol dependence regardless of nutritional status. Elevated leptin contributes to liver pathology: increased fibrosis, a known factor in liver steatosis.
- **Hypoglycemia:** alcohol induces reactive hypoglycemia and produces craving for foods that quickly elevate blood sugar (sugar and alcohol). Sugar aggravates reactive hypoglycemia, particularly with alcohol-induced impairment of gluconeogenesis. Hypoglycemia aggravates mental and emotional problems of alcoholics and withdrawal with sweating, tremor, tachycardia, anxiety, hunger, dizziness, headache, visual disturbance, decreased mental acuity, confusion, depression.

THERAPEUTIC CONSIDERATIONS

Nutrition

Nutritional problems are related to alcohol and the fact that alcoholics tend not to eat. Alcohol is substitute for food.

- **Zinc (Zn):** ADH and ALDH are Zn-dependent enzymes, with ALDH more sensitive to deficiency. Short- and long-term alcohol abuse induces Zn deficiency from decreased dietary intake, decreased ileal absorption (interference with Zn-binding ligand, picolinic acid, and nonspecific mucosal damage), hyperzincuria. Higher hair Zn and copper (Cu) are found in male alcoholics. Hair Cu is related to amount of alcohol consumed; hair Zn is higher with distilled beverages; observations may indicate abnormal metabolism and loss of these minerals. Low serum Zn is associated with impaired alcohol metabolism, risk of cirrhosis, and impaired testicular function. Zn supplementation, particularly with ascorbate, greatly increases alcohol detoxification and survival in rats.

- **Vitamin A:** deficiency is common in alcoholics and works with Zn deficiency to produce major complications of alcohol dependence. Mechanism is reduced intestinal absorption of vitamin A and Zn, with impaired liver function (reduced extraction of Zn, mobilization of retinol-binding protein [RBP], and storage of vitamin A); results in reduced blood Zn, vitamin A, RBP, and transport proteins and a shift to nonprotein ligands. Effects: reduced tissue vitamin A and Zn, abnormal enzyme activities and glycoprotein synthesis, and impaired DNA and RNA metabolism with increased kidney Zn loss. Results: symptoms of alcohol dependence—night blindness, skin disorders, liver cirrhosis, reduced skin healing, decreased testicular function, impaired immunity. Endocrine influences: supplementation with vitamin A inhibits alcohol consumption in female but not male rats, and the effect is inhibited by exogenous testosterone; ovariectomized and adrenalectomized rats show decreased preference for alcohol; corticosterone injections increase preference. Supplementation in alcoholic corrects vitamin A deficiency: improved night blindness and sexual function. *Caution:* excessive amounts of vitamin A are contraindicated because alcohol-damaged liver loses ability to store vitamin A; risk of vitamin A toxicity at dose greater than dietary allowance of 5000 international units (IU) daily.
- **Antioxidants:** alcohol increases lipid peroxidation, causing increased lipoperoxide in liver and serum. Alcoholics are deficient in antioxidants and nutrients: vitamin E, Se, and vitamin C. Significant correlation between serum lipid peroxide, serum glutamic-oxaloacetic transaminase (SGOT) activity, and liver cell necrosis. Antioxidants, before or simultaneously with alcohol intake, inhibit lipoperoxide formation and prevent fatty liver infiltration. Effective antioxidants: vitamin C, vitamin E, Zn, Se, and cysteine.
- **Carnitine (Crn):** common lipotropic agents (choline, niacin, cysteine) are indicated but of little value. Crn significantly inhibits alcohol-induced fatty liver disease. Long-term alcohol abuse causes functional Crn deficiency. Crn facilitates fatty acid transport and oxidation in mitochondria; high liver Crn is needed for increased fatty acid produced from alcohol. Crn supplements

reduce serum triglycerides and SGOT levels while elevating high-density lipoprotein (HDL).

- **Amino acids (AAs):** chromatography patterns are aberrant in alcoholics; normalization greatly assists alcoholics (liver is the primary site for AA metabolism). AAs are particularly indicated in hepatic cirrhosis and depression. Branched-chain amino acids (BCAAs) (valine, isoleucine, leucine) inhibit hepatic encephalopathy and protein catabolism (sequelae of cirrhosis). Deranged neurotransmitter profiles (from very low plasma tryptophan) cause depression, encephalopathy, and coma—aggravated by low-protein diet in standard therapy for cirrhosis and avoided by free-form AAs without risk of hepatic encephalopathy (see chapter on affective disorders—depression). Individualized approach indicated because of differences in nutritional status, biochemistry, and amount of liver damage. AA chromatography is helpful for best results.
- **Vitamin C:** deficiency of ascorbate found in 91% of patients with alcohol-related diseases. Vitamin C helps ameliorate effects of alcohol toxicity in human beings and guinea pigs (species unable to synthesize own ascorbate). Direct correlation between white blood cell (WBC) ascorbate (good index of body ascorbate status), rate of alcohol blood clearance, and activity of hepatic ADH. Vitamin C is strong reducing agent: acts as electron donor similar to NAD in alcohol metabolism, increasing alcohol conversion to acetaldehyde and catabolism of acetaldehyde.
- **Selenium (Se):** plasma, serum, WBC, and red blood cell (RBC) Se is lower in alcoholics. Low Se encourages depression, anxiety, confusion, and hostility; supplementation improves mood. Alcohol dependence and depression in same patient increase risk for suicide. Se supplementation is warranted to ameliorate untoward comorbid psychological and physical profiles.
- **B vitamins:** alcoholics are deficient in most B vitamins. Mechanisms: low dietary intake, deactivation of active form, impaired conversion to active form by alcohol or acetaldehyde, impaired absorption, decreased storage capacity. Alcohol decreases absorption and use of B vitamins by liver and/or increases urinary excretion of B vitamins (especially folate). Vitamin B_1 deficiency is the most common (55%) and most serious, leading to beriberi and Wernicke-Korsakoff syndrome and greater intake of alcohol. (Vitamin B_1 deficiency may predispose to alcohol dependence.) Functional B_6 deficiency is also common, leading to impaired conversion to active form, pyridoxal-5-phosphate, and enhanced degradation.

- **Magnesium (Mg):** deficiency common in alcoholics (60%), strongly linked to delirium tremens, and major reason for increased cardiovascular disease in alcoholics. Deficiency is caused by reduced intake plus alcohol-induced renal hyperexcretion, which continues during withdrawal despite hypomagnesemia. Alcoholic cardiomyopathy has been linked to vitamin B_1 deficiency but may instead be from Mg deficiency.
- **Essential fatty acids (EFAs):** alcohol interferes with EFA metabolism; alcohol abuse may produce symptoms of EFA deficiency. Alcohol abuse in rhesus monkeys leads to alcoholic amblyopia, a rare neuropathy characterized by blurred vision, diminished retinal function, and reduced visual acuity. Docosahexaenoic acid (DHA) deficits found in brain and retinal tissues.
- **Glutamine:** supplementation (1 g q.d.) reduces voluntary alcohol consumption in uncontrolled human studies and experimental animal studies. This preliminary research is over 40 years old, but there has been no follow-up despite efficacy, safety, and low cost.

Psychosocial Aspects

Physicians must be nonjudgmental, but not passive, in their attitude toward their patients. Alcohol dependence is a chronic, progressive, addictive, and potentially fatal disease. Social support for patient and family is essential. Success is often proportional to involvement with Alcoholics Anonymous, counselors, and social agencies. Maintain close working relationships with experienced counselors, Alcoholics Anonymous, Al-Anon, and Ala-Teen. Requirements for successful initiation of treatment: patient realization that he or she has alcohol problem; education of patient and/or family about physical and psychosocial aspects of alcohol dependence; and immediate patient involvement in treatment program. Elements of successful programs: strict control of alcohol plus replacement with another addiction that is nonchemical, time-consuming, and heavily supported by family, friends, and peers; strict abstinence safest and most effective choice.

Depression: common in alcoholics; leads to high suicide rate. Many are depressed first then become alcoholic (primary depressives); others are alcoholic first then develop depression in context of alcohol dependence (secondary depressives). Alterations in serotonin metabolism and availability of precursor (tryptophan) are implicated in some forms of depression; other forms are linked to catecholamine metabolism and tyrosine availability. Alcoholics have severely depleted tryptophan, leading to depression and sleep disturbances. Alcohol impairs tryptophan transport into brain. Enzyme tryptophan pyrolase is rate limiting in tryptophan catabolism and more active in rats during alcohol withdrawal. Plasma tryptophan is depleted in withdrawing alcoholics but normalizes after 6 days of treatment and abstinence. Brain tryptophan uptake is also influenced by competition from AAs sharing the same transport (tyrosine, phenylalanine, valine, leucine, isoleucine, methionine), which are elevated in malnourished alcoholics. Depressed alcoholics have lowest ratios of tryptophan to these AAs; AAs that lower ratio are catecholamine precursors (tyrosine and phenylalanine). Elevated plasma catecholamines are common in alcoholics and may contribute to depression. Taurine is also low in depressed alcoholics, with lowest levels in psychotic alcoholics.

Miscellaneous Factors

- **Intestinal flora:** severely deranged in alcoholics. Endotoxin-producing bacteria may colonize small intestine, inducing malabsorption of fats, carbohydrates, protein, folate, and vitamin B_{12}. Alcohol increases intestinal permeability to endotoxins and macromolecules, increasing toxic and antigenic effects, contributing to complications of alcohol dependence. Addictive tendency of food allergies may contribute to alcohol cravings.
- **Exercise:** graded, individualized fitness program improves likelihood of maintaining abstinence. Regular exercise alleviates anxiety and depression and enables better response to stress and emotional upset.
- **Kudzu *(Pueraria lobata)***: one of earliest medicinal plants used in traditional Chinese medicine. Pharmacologic actions: antidipsotropic (anti–alcohol abuse) activity, owing to isoflavones daidzin and daidzein. It acts by inhibiting ALDH-2. Deficiency of this enzyme reduces risk of alcohol dependence. Decreased drinking because of ALDH-2 inhibition is attributed to aversive properties of acetaldehyde accumulated during alcohol consumption. However, daidzin can reduce drinking in some rodents without necessarily increasing acetaldehyde. In humans, results have been mixed. It may be that kudzu reduces alcohol intake without significantly affecting cravings. Dose: kudzu root extract 1.2 g b.i.d.
- Silybum marianum **(milk thistle):** flavonoid complex (silymarin) effective in treatment of full spectrum of alcohol-related liver disease; extends life span of alcoholics. Silymarin can improve immune function in patients with cirrhosis.

THERAPEUTIC APPROACH

Alcohol dependence is difficult to treat; little documented long-term success, except for Alcoholics Anonymous (overall success of Alcoholics Anonymous is highly controversial); requires integrated, whole-person, stage-oriented program designed for four stages of alcohol dependence: (1) active consumption, (2) withdrawal, (3) recovery, (4) recovered. Recovery stage is period between withdrawal and full reestablishment of normal metabolism. Complete diagnostic workup required because of high risk for wide variety of clinical and subclinical diseases. Therapeutic support is needed in all stages.

- **Diet:** stabilize blood sugar; eliminate simple sugars (sucrose, fructose, glucose; fruit juice; dried fruit; low-fiber fruits: grapes and citrus); limit processed carbohydrates (e.g., white flour, instant potatoes, white rice); increase unprocessed complex carbohydrates (e.g., whole grains, vegetables, beans).
- **Supplements:**
  - — Vitamin A: 5000 IU q.d.
  - — B complex: 20 times the recommended daily allowances
  - — Vitamin C: 1 g b.i.d.
  - — Vitamin E: 400 IU q.d. (mixed tocopherols)
  - — Mg: 250 mg b.i.d.
  - — Se: 200 mcg q.d.
  - — Zn: 30 mg elemental Zn q.d. (picolinate)
  - — L-Carnitine: 500 mg b.i.d.
  - — L-Glutamine: 1 tsp q.d.
  - — *Lactobacillus acidophilus:* 1 tsp q.d.
- **Exercise:** graded program using heart rate response to determine intensity; five to seven times weekly for 20 to 30 minutes at intensity raising heart rate to 60% to 80% of age group maximum.
- **Counseling:** Alcoholics Anonymous and experienced counselor with alcohol addiction expertise.
- **Additional recommendations for four stages:**
  1. Active alcohol *consumption:* family, peers, social group support to elicit patient's recognition of alcohol problem and willingness to enter treatment program; additional supplements:
     a. Pyridoxal-5-phosphate: 20 mg q.d.
     b. Riboflavin: 100 mg q.d.
     c. Vitamin A: 5000 IU q.d.
     d. Zn: 30 mg q.d.

2. *Withdrawal:* symptom severity variable, proportional to degree of dependence and duration of disease. Milder cases—within a few hours after cessation of drinking and resolve within 48 hours; more-severe cases—in patients older than 30 and develop after 48 hours of abstinence—need in-patient facility, additional supplements (obtain institutional permission before admission):
   a. L-Tryptophan: 3 g q.d.
   b. Riboflavin: 100 mg q.d.
   c. Electrolyte replacement as needed
   d. Flaxseed oil: 1 tbsp t.i.d.
3. *Recovering:* strong emotional support network; involve patient in intense, people-oriented activities; help patient reject alcohol as destructive response to stress and develop more-effective ways of handling adversity; additional supplement:
   a. flaxseed oil: 1 tbsp t.i.d.
4. *Recovered:* maintain emotional support network; continue total abstinence; slowly reduce supplement doses, after 6 months of abstinence, to 25% of aforementioned recommendations.

Alzheimer's Disease

DIAGNOSTIC SUMMARY

- Progressive mental deterioration, loss of memory and cognitive functions, inability to carry out activities of daily life
- Characteristic symmetric, usually diffuse, pattern on electroencephalography (EEG)
- Diagnosis usually made by exclusion
- Definitive diagnosis can be made only by postmortem biopsy of brain, demonstrating atrophy, senile plaques, and neurofibrillary tangles

GENERAL CONSIDERATIONS

Alzheimer's disease (AD) is a neurodegenerative disorder of progressive deterioration of memory and cognition or dementia. Five percent of U.S. population older than 65 have severe dementia; another 10% have mild to moderate dementia. Frequency rises with increasing age: 50% to 60% of all cases of dementia (senile and presenile) are caused by AD. "The disease of the twentieth century": tenfold increase in AD in U.S. population older than 65.

Neuropathology

Distinctive neuropathologic features: plaque formation, amyloid deposition, neurofibrillary tangles, granulovascular degeneration, massive loss of telencephalic neurons; particularly evident in cerebral cortex and hippocampal formation. Clinical features are believed to arise from cholinergic dysfunction by reduced activity of enzyme choline acetyltransferase (which synthesizes acetylcholine [Ach]) and neuronal transfer of choline.

Etiology

Hallmarks of AD are accumulation of β-amyloid and formation of neurofibrillary tangles. Amyloid is a general term for protein fragments the body produces normally. Beta-amyloid is a fragment snipped from amyloid precursor protein (APP). In a healthy brain,

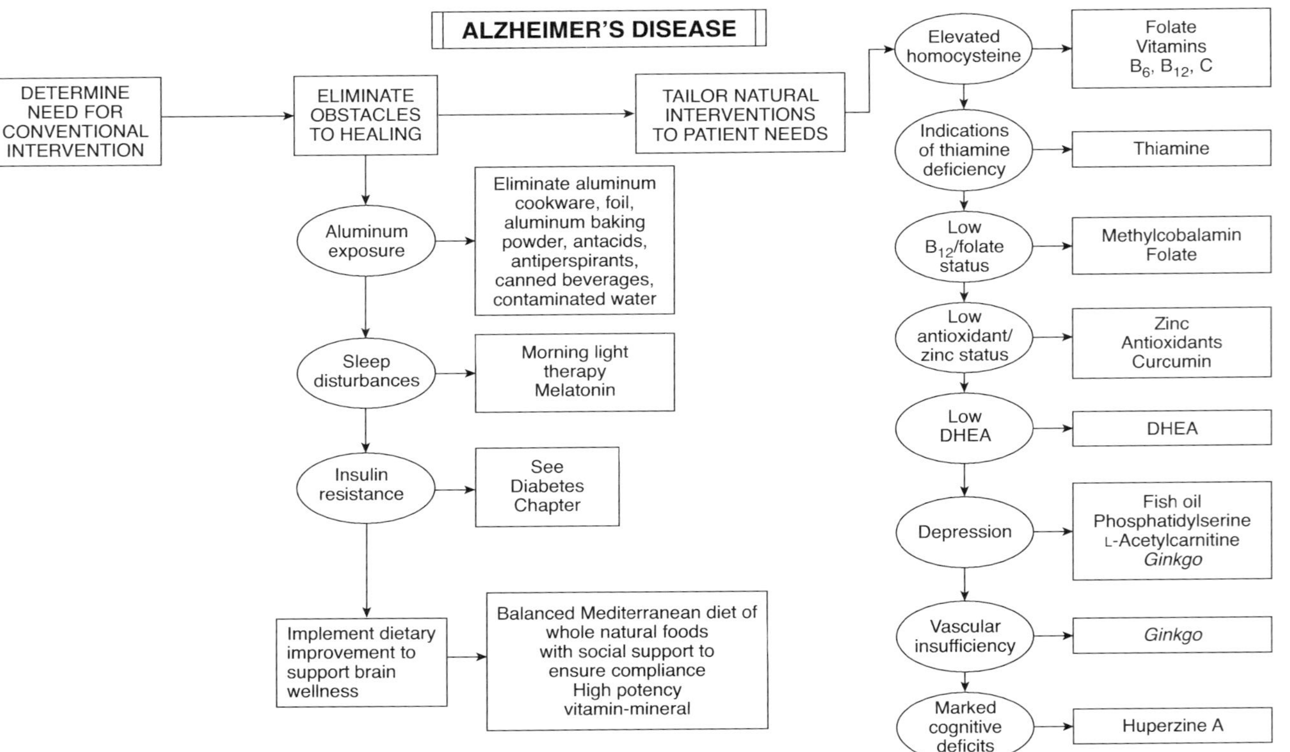
ALZHEIMER'S DISEASE
DETERMINE NEED FOR CONVENTIONAL INTERVENTION
ELIMINATE OBSTACLES TO HEALING
TAILOR NATURAL INTERVENTIONS TO PATIENT NEEDS
Aluminum exposure
Eliminate aluminum cookware, foil, aluminum baking powder, antacids, antiperspirants, canned beverages, contaminated water
Sleep disturbances
Morning light therapy Melatonin
Insulin resistance
See Diabetes Chapter
Implement dietary improvement to support brain wellness
Balanced Mediterranean diet of whole natural foods with social support to ensure compliance High potency vitamin-mineral
Elevated homocysteine
Folate Vitamins B_6, B_{12}, C
Indications of thiamine deficiency
Thiamine
Low B_{12}/folate status
Methylcobalamin Folate
Low antioxidant/zinc status
Zinc Antioxidants Curcumin
Low DHEA
DHEA
Depression
Fish oil Phosphatidylserine L-Acetylcarnitine *Ginkgo*
Vascular insufficiency
Ginkgo
Marked cognitive deficits
Huperzine A

these fragments are broken down and eliminated. In AD, beta-amyloid protein fragments accumulate into hard plaques between neurons, blocking transmission of messages and leading to death of brain cells, neurofibrillary tangles, and dementia. Tau, a microtubule-associated protein, is the major constituent of neurofibrillary tangles and is produced in soluble hyperphosphorylated form when beta-amyloid levels become toxic.

Genetic factors play a major role: amyloid precursor gene on chromosome 21 (close association between Down's syndrome and AD); presenilin genes on 14 and 1; apolipoprotein E gene *(APOE)* on 19; mutations on 21, 14, and 1—rare and associated with symptoms before age 50. The most significant genetic finding is the link with *APOE; APOE* of e4 type is linked to much greater risk; e2 type is linked to greater protection.

Genetically linked aberrant immune system regulation of inflammation may contribute. Innate immune function in brain normally removes plaque. Long-term excessive reaction to immune protofibrils of amyloid proteins can promote AD. Immunotherapeutic trials resulted in both beneficial and adverse effects. Antioxidants protect against untoward immune processes; consider natural anti-inflammatories used for cardiovascular disease.

- **Lifestyle factors:** diet—excess saturated or *trans* fatty acids may predispose neurons to aluminum (Al)-induced toxicity. Sleep—abnormal sleep-wake cycles and decreased morning light exposure (see melatonin, later).
- **Other factors:** traumatic head injury; long-term exposure to Al, silicon, environmental neurotoxins, and free radicals; increased oxidative damage.
- **Homocysteine:** increased plasma (and perhaps urine) homocysteine is a strong, independent risk factor for dementia and AD, just as it is for atherosclerosis. Plasma level greater than 14 μmol/L nearly doubles risk of AD. Control homocysteine with folate and vitamins B_{12}, B_6, and C.

The tremendous increase in AD parallels rise in type 2 diabetes and insulin resistance, suggesting a possible connection. It is well established that individuals with type 2 diabetes have a 1.5- to 4-fold higher-than-normal risk for AD as well as vascular dementia. Impaired insulin signaling and insulin resistance in the brain or the decrease in cerebral insulin receptors associated with aging may be another important factor in the pathogenesis of AD. Furthermore, hyperglycemia induces increased peripheral use of insulin, resulting in reduced insulin transport into the brain.

Insufficient insulin signaling makes neurons energy deficient and vulnerable to oxidizing or other metabolic insults, leading to the destruction of mitochondria and ultimately the neuron. Cerebral hypoinsulinemia (as well as hyperinsulinemia) leads to beta-amyloid accumulation and increased tau phosphorylation. Measures to improve glycemic control and improve both peripheral and brain insulin sensitivity appear to be important steps in the prevention of AD.

- Al: concentrated in neurofibrillary tangles and significantly contributes to AD; strong affinity for and cofactor with paired helical filament tau (PHFt) involved in forming neurofibrillary tangles. Al selectively binds to PHFt, induces PHFt aggregation, and retards brain's ability to break down PHFt. Long-term exposure of animals to ecologic doses of Al induces ghostlike neurons with cytoplasmic and nuclear vacuolations, with Al deposits; neuritic plaques in hippocampus; amyloid deposits in cerebrovasculature; behavioral changes reminiscent of AD. Brain and serum Al levels increase with age as AD incidence increases with age. Patients with AD have much higher Al levels than unaffected people and patients with other dementias (ethyl alcohol, atherosclerosis, stroke). Efforts to remove Al help but probably are too late, after disease is well established. Even in those without mental disease, elevated Al is linked with poorer mental function. Sources of Al are water supply (immediately enters brain tissue), food, antacids, antiperspirants.

DIAGNOSTIC CONSIDERATIONS

Only 50% of patients with dementia have AD; comprehensive diagnostic workup paramount. Rule out conditions that can mimic dementia (e.g., depression can mimic dementia in the elderly). The most common reversible cause of dementia is drug toxicity. Other causes are metabolic and nutritional disorders such as hypoglycemia; thyroid disturbances; and vitamin B_{12}, folate, and thiamine deficiencies. Diagnosis depends on clinical judgment. Workup: detailed history; neurologic and physical examination; psychological evaluation with particular attention to depression; general medical evaluation revealing subtle metabolic, toxic, or cardiopulmonary disorders inducing confusion in elderly; neurophysiologic tests to document the type and severity of cognitive impairment; social worker mobilization of community resources; laboratory tests (electrocardiography [ECG], EEG, computed tomography [CT] scan, magnetic resonance imaging [MRI]).

- **Diagnostic process:** exclude other possible diagnoses.
  — *Step 1:* diagnose dementia accurately (10% to 50% error rate when diagnosis is based only on first evaluation). Avoid misdiagnosing pseudodementia functional illness. Depression mimics dementia in the elderly.

Causes of and Mechanisms in the Development of Senile Dementia.

ETIOLOGY	PATHOGENESIS
Degenerative etiology	Disturbances of gene expression and thus of protein metabolism
Altered genetic code	Disturbance of the synthesis of specific proteins
Alzheimer's disease	Reduction in acetylcholine synthesis resulting from decreased choline acetyltransferase activity
Huntington's chorea	Disturbance of the GABA-nergic system
Idiopathic dementia	
Localized form	Decline in cognitive function
Parkinson's disease	Reduction in dopamine turnover
Pick's disease	Reduction in cholinergic activity
Loss of neuronal redundancy	Disturbance of cerebral metabolism following infection or trauma Reduction in cholinergic activity caused by loss of neurons and synapses
Cerebrovascular disease	
Chronic meningitis	
Tuberculous, mycotic	
Encephalomyelitis	
Encephalopathy following head injury (boxers)	
Epileptic dementia	
Virus encephalopathy	
Nutritive etiology	

ETIOLOGY	PATHOGENESIS
Chronic alcoholism	
Diabetes mellitus	
Disturbances of electrolyte metabolism	
Hypoglycemia	Insulin, starvation
Hyponatremia	Diuretics
Hypothyroidism	
Korsakoff's syndrome	Thiamine trasketolase deficiency
Nicotinamide deficiency	
Vitamin B deficiency	Disturbances of energy formation
Toxic etiology	
Addiction to barbiturates, psychotropic drugs, etc.	
Chronic carbon monoxide intoxication	
Chronic cesium intoxication	
Mycotoxins	
Renal/hepatic encephalopathy	
Vincristine intoxication	

— *Step 2:* do careful neurologic examination to reveal (1) focal, circumscribed brain disease; (2) diffuse, bilateral brain dysfunction; or (3) no evidence of neurologic dysfunction. Routine neurologic examination recognizes (1) and (3) but not diffuse brain dysfunction displaying subtle indications: patient's level of consciousness, attentiveness to examiner, comprehension, performance of tasks, facial expressions, quality of speech, posture, respiratory rhythm, and gait.
A comprehensive evaluation includes:
- Detailed history
- Neurologic and physical examinations
- Psychological evaluation with particular attention to depression
- General medical evaluation to detect subtle metabolic, toxic, or cardiopulmonary disorders that can precipitate confusion in the elderly
- Series of standardized neurophysiology tests—Mini-Mental State Examination or Folstein test—to document type and severity of cognitive impairment

- **Recommended tests for appropriate laboratory assessment:**

Recommended Laboratory Tests Used in the Diagnosis of Dementia

TEST	RATIONALE
CBC	Anemia, infection
VDRL	Syphilis
Electrolytes	Metabolic dysfunction
Liver function tests	Hepatic dysfunction
BUN	Renal dysfunction
TSH, T_4, T_3, T_3U	Thyroid dysfunction
Serum B_{12} and RBC folate	Deficiency
Urinalysis	Renal/hepatic dysfunction
Hair mineral analysis	Heavy metal intoxication
ECG	Heart function
EEG	Focal vs. diffuse
CT scan	Atrophy, intracranial mass

- **EEG:** an important tool in differentiating dementias. Normal electroencephalogram does not rule out dementia, particularly in early stages, but provides valuable information. AD has characteristic symmetric diffuse slowing on electroencephalogram. EEG differentiates focal (e.g., intracranial mass or vascular disease) and diffuse (e.g., metabolic disorders or normal pressure hydrocephalus) dysfunction.
- **MRI:** useful diagnostic information in minutes; noninvasive; characterizes neuronal markers and neurotransmitters (glutamate, gamma-aminobutyric acid [GABA]).
- **CT, MRI, single-photon emission computed tomography (SPECT), or positron emission tomography (PET):** can help to exclude other cerebral pathology or subtypes of dementia.
- **Pittsburgh Compound B (PiB)–PET:** new procedure for directly and clearly imaging beta-amyloid deposits in vivo using a chemical tracer that binds selectively to A-beta deposits.
- **Fingerprint patterns:** abnormal in Alzheimer's disease and Down's syndrome; increased number of ulnar loops on fingertips, with concomitant decrease in whorls, radial loops, and arches. Ulnar loops (pointing toward ulnar bone, away from

thumb) frequently are found on all 10 fingertips. Radial loops (pointing toward thumb), when they occur, are shifted away from index and middle fingers—where they most commonly occur—to ring and little fingers. Appearance of Alzheimer's fingerprint pattern warrants immediate aggressive preventive approach.

THERAPEUTIC CONSIDERATIONS

Prevention by (1) addressing suspected pathophysiology and (2) using natural measures to improve mental function in early stages; in advanced stages natural measures are of only limited benefit.

Diet

- A diet high in saturated fat and *trans* fatty acids and low in antioxidants may lead to increased serum and brain concentrations of Al and transition metal ions.
- Poor-quality diets may elicit cerebral inflammation, causing neurologic damage that results in AD. Dietary risk factors for AD are shared with those for atherosclerosis.
- Mediterranean-type diet slows cognitive decline, reduces risk of progression from mild cognitive impairment (MCI) to AD, reduces risk of AD, and decreases all-cause mortality in AD patients. It also lowers predementia syndromes and their progression to overt dementia.
- Key dietary factors: higher fish consumption (and omega-3 fatty acids), monounsaturated fatty acids (olive oil), light to moderate alcohol use (red wine), and increased nonstarchy vegetable and fruit consumption.
- Lower risk of AD with Mediterranean diet may not be mediated by C-reactive protein, fasting insulin, or adiponectin levels. Dietary components may work directly on reducing beta-amyloid formation or deposition. Polyphenols in grapes, grapeseed extract, and red wine prevent beta-amyloid formation and promote tau disassembly. They are absorbed into the brain after oral administration.
- Celery *(Apium graveolens)* consumption may offer protection against AD. Celery and celery seed extracts contain 3-n-butylphthalide (3nB), responsible for characteristic odor of celery and its health benefits. In animals, 3nB improved learning deficits and long-term spatial memory. Treatment with 3nB reduced total cerebral beta-amyloid plaque deposition and

lowered brain beta-amyloid levels; 3nB markedly directed APP processing toward a pathway that precludes beta-amyloid formation.

Estrogen

Estrogen has been promoted to offer protective and possibly therapeutic benefits in AD. However, evidence is contradictory. Women on hormone replacement therapy (HRT) had a lower rate of AD; but women taking HRT were healthier before taking hormones compared with controls (i.e., women prescribed HRT were less likely to have hypertension, diabetes, and history of stroke than nonusers). However, Women's Health Initiative Memory Study suggested an increase in dementia risk for women using HRT compared with controls, especially when given after menopause. Clinical trials in women with AD have concluded that estrogen therapy does not improve dementia symptoms in women with AD and should definitely be avoided postmenopause. Given the cloud of uncertainty about benefits of HRT, risks of conventional estrogen therapy to prevent AD outweigh benefits.

Aluminum

Avoid all known sources of Al—antacids, antiperspirants, Al-containing baking powder, cookware, foil food wrap, canned beverages, nondairy creamers, table salt additives. Citric acid and calcium citrate supplements increase absorption of Al (but not lead [Pb]) from water and food. Al absorption is decreased by magnesium (Mg) (competes for absorption at intestinal mucosa and blood-brain barrier). Recommend Mg-rich diet: unprocessed whole foods (avoid milk and dairy), vegetables, whole grains, nuts, and seeds.

Nutrition

Directly related to cognition in the elderly; nutrient deficiency common.

- **Antioxidants:** Oxidative damage plays a major role in AD. Antioxidant nutrients offer significant protection. Studies have focused on vitamins C and E and beta-carotene. As with other chronic degenerative diseases, better results may be achieved with a broader range of supplemental nutrients. It is entirely possible (and likely probable) that vitamins E and C and beta-carotene may simply be markers of increased "phytochemical antioxidant" intake rather than playing a significant role on their own. Fruits and vegetables contain an array of antioxidant compounds beyond nutritional antioxidants. Some of these may exert specific effects of considerable benefit against the pathophysiology of AD. Often researchers make the mistake of thinking that the antioxidant activity of a particular fruit or vegetable is solely a result of its vitamin C or E or beta-carotene content. However, these nutrient antioxidants often account for only a small fraction of a food's antioxidant effect. The overwhelming antioxidant activity of fruits and vegetables comes from phytochemicals—flavonoids, phenols, and other carotenoids.

- **Thiamin (vitamin B_1):** deficiency rather uncommon (except in alcoholics), but many elderly do not get even recommended daily allowance (RDA) (1.5 mg). B_1 potentiates and mimics brain neurotransmitter of memory, Ach. B_1 (3 to 8 g/day) improves mental function in AD and age-related impaired mental function (senility) without side effects.
- **Vitamin B_{12}:** deficiency induces impaired nerve function, causing numbness, paresthesias, or burning feeling in feet, and impaired mental function that mimics AD in the elderly. B_{12} deficiency is common in the elderly and a major cause of depression in this age group. Best test is serum cobalamin or urine methylmalonic acid; plasma homocysteine indicates B_{12} and folate status. B_{12} declines with age, and deficiency is found in 3% to 42% of persons aged 65 and older. Untreated deficiency affects neurologic and cognitive function. Vitamin B_{12} screening tests are indicated in elderly given positive cost/benefit ratio. Urinary methylmalonic acid assay is the best: sensitive, noninvasive, and relatively convenient for patient. Correcting B_{12} deficiency improves mental function and quality of life. Low B_{12} levels are common in patients with AD. High homocysteine levels increase AD risk. B_{12} and/or folate supplements may completely reverse symptoms in some patients, but in general there is little improvement in patients with AD symptoms longer than 6 months because of irreversible changes. Active forms in body: methylcobalamin and adenosylcobalamin.
- **Zinc (Zn):** common nutrient deficiency in the elderly and possible major factor in AD development. Enzymes involved in DNA replication, repair, and transcription are Zn dependent. Long-term Zn deficiency may cause cascading effects of error-prone or

ineffective DNA-handling enzymes in nerve cells. Zn is required by antioxidant enzymes (superoxide dismutase). Levels of Zn in brain and cerebrospinal fluid in patients with AD are markedly decreased. There is a strong inverse correlation between serum Zn and senile plaque count. Supplementation is beneficial in AD. "The zinc paradox": Zn is neurotoxic at high concentrations and accumulates at sites of degeneration. Total tissue Zn is markedly reduced in brains of patients with AD. Much higher concentration of copper-zinc superoxide dismutase in and around damaged brain tissue of patients with AD suggests increased Zn in damaged areas from body's efforts to neutralize free radicals by increasing local production of dismutases. Possible corollary: higher focal Zn results in increased amyloid formation when free radical scavenging is inadequate.

- **Phosphatidylcholine (PC):** dietary PC can increase brain Ach in normal patients. AD is characterized by decreased cholinergic transmission. PC supplementation would seem beneficial in AD, but basic defect in cholinergic transmission in AD results in impaired enzyme Ach transferase, which combines choline (provided by PC) with acetyl moiety to form neurotransmitter Ach. Providing more choline (by PC) will not increase enzyme activity. Mild to moderate dementia may be helped by high-quality PC (15 to 25 g q.d.); discontinue if no noticeable improvement within 2 weeks.
- **Phosphatidylserine (PS):** the major phospholipid in the brain; helps determine integrity and fluidity of cell membranes. Deficiency of methyl donors (*S*-adenosylmethionine [SAM], folate, B_{12}) or essential fatty acids may inhibit production of PS. Low brain PS is linked to impaired mental function and depression in the elderly. PS is useful in treating depression and/or impaired mental function in the elderly, including AD (100 mg t.i.d.).
- **L-Acetylcarnitine (LAC):** thought to be much more active than other forms of carnitine in brain disorders; close structural similarity to Ach; mimics Ach and benefits patients with early-stage AD and elderly with depression or impaired memory; powerful antioxidant within neurons; stabilizes cell membranes; improves energy production within neurons; delays progression of AD (2 g b.i.d.); also beneficial for non-AD mild mental deterioration in the elderly (1500 mg q.d.); enhances effect of acetylcholinesterase inhibitors in patients with AD unresponsive to drugs alone (2 g q.d.).

Other Therapies

- **DHEA (dehydroepiandrosterone):** the most abundant steroid hormone in the bloodstream, with extremely high brain levels. Levels decline dramatically with aging—symptomatic, including impaired mentality. DHEA itself has no known function but is a source for all endogenous steroids (e.g., sex hormones and corticosteroids). Declining DHEA is linked to diabetes, obesity, hypercholesterolemia, heart disease, and arthritis. DHEA may enhance memory and cognition. Doses: men older than 50 years, 25 to 50 mg q.d.; women, 15 to 25 mg; men and women aged 70 years and older, 50 to 100 mg q.d. Excessive doses cause acne and, in women, menstrual irregularities. Use laboratory assessment before prescribing and as tool to monitor and modulate therapy.
- **Melatonin:** synthesized from serotonin, released by pineal gland. Master hormone normalizes circadian rhythms and sleep cycles; powerful antioxidant for cancer therapies; protects neurons from heavy metal cobalt (Co) damage (Co found in high levels in patients with AD). Melatonin inhibits induction of oxidative damage and beta-amyloid release; may be preventive treatment because Co is essential nutrient, as in B_{12}. Dose of 3 mg at 8 PM increased sleeping time, decreased nighttime activity, improved cognitive and noncognitive functions. Morning light therapy induces greater improvement.

Botanical Medicines

- ***Ginkgo biloba* extract (GBE):** standardized to 24% *Ginkgo* flavon glycosides/6% terpenoids; great benefit in senility and AD; increases brain functional capacity; normalizes Ach receptors in hippocampus of aged animals, increasing cholinergic transmission (*Textbook, "Ginkgo biloba* [Ginkgo Tree]"). GBE (240 mg q.d.) helps reverse or delay mental deterioration only in early stages of AD; may help patient maintain normal life, avoid nursing home; improves Clinical Global Impressions score (120 mg q.d.), stabilizes AD, and significantly improves mental function without side effects; equally as effective as second-generation cholinesterase inhibitors (tacrine, donepezil, rivastigmine, metrifonate) in treating mild to moderate AD and with lower dropout rate among patients; reverses mental deficits caused by vascular insufficiency or depression; must be taken consistently for at least 12 weeks to determine efficacy.

- **Huperzine A (HupA):** alkaloid isolated from moss *Huperzia serrata,* long used in China for fever and inflammation, but no antipyretic or anti-inflammatory properties in experimental models; potent inhibitor of acetylcholinesterase; more selective and much less toxic than conventional drugs (physostigmine, tacrine, donepezil); used by more than 100,000 people since early 1990s with no serious adverse effects; considerable benefit for dementia; 200 mcg b.i.d. improves memory, cognition, and behavior in AD. In the most recent study, Huperzine A at 400 mcg b.i.d. for at least 16 weeks showed a 2.27-point improvement in the Alzheimer's Disease Assessment Scale–Cognitive Subscale (ADAS-Cog). Clinical global impression of change and activities of daily living were not significant.
- ***Bacopa monnieri* (BM):** Ayurvedic botanical used for memory enhancement, epilepsy, insomnia; mild sedative; reduces memory dysfunction in rat models of AD; inhibits in vitro formation of reactive species and DNA damage from toxins, mimicking effect of excess nitric oxide exposure on neurons.
- ***Curcuma longa* (turmeric):** curcumin protects against age-related brain damage and AD in particular. Elderly (aged 70 to 79) residents of rural India who eat large amounts of turmeric have the lowest incidence of AD in the world: 4.4 times lower than that of Americans. Curcumin inhibits amyloid-beta protein (Aβ) aggregation, and Aβ-induced inflammation and the activities of beta-secretase and acetylcholinesterase. Oral curcumin therapy inhibits Aβ deposition, Aβ oligomerization, and tau phosphorylation in the brains of AD animal models and improves behavioral impairment in animal models. Unfortunately, the two clinical trials conducted to date failed to show any benefit. Failure to produce positive results may be a result of poor pharmacokinetic profile of the curcumin used. There remains the possibility that curcumin might be one of the most promising compounds for AD therapies. Studies in stroke suggest a neuroprotective role of curcumin and the ability to reduce plaque burden in models of AD. Curcumin decreases naphthalene and 4-hydroxy-2-nonenal–induced cataract formation on the lens by decreasing rate of apoptosis and subsequent opacification resistance of the lens. Postulated mechanism: induction of glutathione *S*-transferase, which decreases lipid peroxidation. This may explain cataractogenesis-inhibiting effects.

THERAPEUTIC APPROACH

Goal is prevention or starting therapy as soon as dementia is noted.

- **Dietary and lifestyle recommendations:**
  - — Avoid Al (antiperspirants, antacids, beverage cans, cookware).
  - — Follow general healthful dietary and lifestyle plan.
  - — Achieve ideal body weight and take measures to improve insulin sensitivity.
  - — Increase whole foods: wild small ocean fish, cereals, vegetables, and monounsaturated fats.
  - — Employ the principles of the Mediterranean diet.
  - — Decrease total calories and unhealthy fats.
  - — Use morning light therapy.
- **Supplements:**
  - — High-potency multiple vitamin-mineral supplement
  - — Vitamin C: 500 to 1000 mg t.i.d.
  - — Vitamin E: 100 to 200 international units (IU) q.d.(mixed tocopherols)
  - — Thiamin: 3 to 8 g q.d.
  - — Fish oils: 1000 to 3000 mg EPA plus DHA q.d.
  - — PS: 100 mg t.i.d.
  - — L-Acetylcarnitine: 500 mg t.i.d.
  - — Methylcobalamin: 1000 mcg b.i.d.
- **Botanical medicine:**
  - — GBE (24% *Ginkgo* flavon glycosides/6% terpenoids): 240 to 320 mg q.d.
  - — HupA: 400 mcg b.i.d.

Angina Pectoris

DIAGNOSTIC SUMMARY

- Squeezing pain or pressure in the chest appearing immediately after exertion. Other precipitating factors include emotional tension, cold weather, or a large meal. Pain may radiate to the left shoulder blade, left arm, or jaw. The pain typically lasts for only 1 to 20 minutes.
- Stress, anxiety, and high blood pressure typically are present.
- The majority of patients demonstrate an abnormal electrocardiographic reading (transient ST-segment depression) in response to light exercise (stress test).

GENERAL CONSIDERATIONS

Angina pectoris results when oxygen supply and occasionally other nutrients are inadequate for metabolic needs of heart muscle. Primary cause is atherosclerosis; also platelet aggregation, coronary artery spasm, nonvascular mechanisms (e.g., hypoglycemia), and increased metabolic need (e.g., hyperthyroidism). Primary lesion of atherosclerosis is atheromatous plaque blocking coronary arteries; symptomatic after major coronary artery is more than 50% blocked, transient platelet aggregation (*Textbook,* "Atherosclerosis"), and coronary artery spasm.

- **Prinzmetal's variant angina:** most common form of coronary artery spasm, not caused by plaque, occurs at rest or at odd times during day or night; more common in women younger than 50.
- **Magnesium (Mg) insufficiency–induced coronary artery spasm:** more common in men than in women; important cause of myocardial infarction (MI) and significant in angina pectoris.

DIAGNOSTIC CONSIDERATIONS

Diagnosis frequently made by history alone. Workup: 12-lead electrocardiogram (ECG) at rest, chest radiograph, ECG stress test or

- DETERMINE NEED FOR CONVENTIONAL INTERVENTION
  - Unstable angina → Refer for hospitalization
  - Severe vascular occlusion → IV EDTA chelation therapy
- MINIMIZE OBSTACLES TO HEALING
  - Lifestyle indiscretions → Eliminate smoking, ETOH, caffeine
  - Stress → Stress management: relaxation, meditation, guided imagery
  - Eliminate harmful food components → Minimize saturated fats, cholesterol, fried foods, simple carbohydrates, food allergens
  - Sedentary lifestyle → Carefully–graded progressive exercise
  - Decreased NO production → Arginine
- TAILOR NATURAL INTERVENTIONS TO PATIENT NEEDS
  - Add food components that support cardiovascular wellness → Increase gel-forming fiber, garlic, onions, vegetables, fish High-potency vitamin-mineral
  - Minimize oxidative stress → Antioxidants
  - Coronary vasospasm. Prinzmetal; hypertension → Magnesium Potassium CoQ10 Crataegus P5P
  - Hyperlipidemia → Pantethine
  - Poor exercise tolerance → CoQ10 L-carnitine L-arginine Crataegus Ammi visnaga

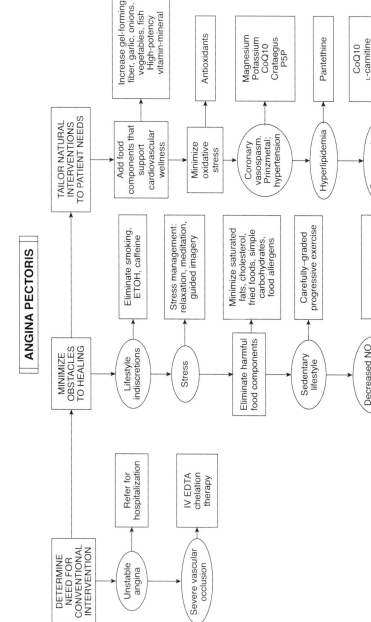

24-hour Holter monitor (ambulatory ECG). Electrocardiographic changes seen with angina provide evidence of previous MI, and ST-segment and T-wave changes occurring during attacks of pain—displacement of ST segment with or without T-wave inversion. Hypoglycemia-induced angina does not manifest with rate or ST-segment abnormalities.

THERAPEUTIC CONSIDERATIONS

Angina pectoris is a serious condition requiring careful treatment and monitoring. Prescription medications may be necessary; condition controllable with help of natural measures. Significant blockage of coronary artery: intravenous (IV) ethylenediaminetetraacetic acid (EDTA) chelation, angioplasty, or coronary artery bypass may be appropriate. Two primary therapeutic goals: improve energy metabolism within heart and improve blood supply to heart. Heart uses fats as major metabolic fuel; defects in fat metabolism in heart greatly increase risk of atherosclerosis, MI, and angina attacks. Impaired use of fatty acids by heart results in accumulation of fatty acids within heart muscle, causing extreme susceptibility to cellular damage and MI. Carnitine (Crn), pantethine, and coenzyme Q10 (CoQ10) are essential to fat metabolism and extremely beneficial in angina; prevent accumulation of fatty acids within heart muscle by improving conversion of fatty acids into energy.

Nutritional Supplements

- **Antioxidant supplements:** plasma level of antioxidants is more predictive of unstable angina than is severity of atherosclerosis. They prevent tolerance to oral nitrate treatment for angina. Nitrate tolerance is linked to increased vascular superoxide that degrades nitric oxide formed from nitroglycerine, lowering cyclic guanosine monophosphate (cGMP) (intracellular regulator and vasorelaxant). Vitamin C is main aqueous antioxidant and scavenger of superoxide; vitamin E is main lipid-phase antioxidant. High-dose vitamins C and E can prevent nitrate tolerance.
- **Carnitine:** vitamin-like compound that transports fatty acids across mitochondrial membrane and stimulates metabolism of long-chain fatty acids by mitochondria. Crn deficiency decreases mitochondrial fatty acid levels and energy production. Normal heart function depends on adequate Crn. The normal heart stores more Crn than it needs; heart ischemia induces decreased

Crn and energy production in heart and increased risk for angina and heart disease. Crn (900 mg q.d.) improves angina and heart disease, allows heart muscle to use limited oxygen more efficiently, improves exercise tolerance and heart function. Crn is an effective alternative to drugs (beta-blockers, calcium channel antagonists, and nitrates), especially in patients with chronic stable angina pectoris. Crn (40 mg/kg/day) may prevent production of toxic fatty acid metabolites that activate phospholipases, disrupt cell membranes, impair heart contractility and compliance, and increase susceptibility to irregular beats and eventual death of heart tissue.

- **Pantethine:** stable form of pantethine is active form of pantothenic acid, a fundamental component of coenzyme A (CoA). CoA transports fatty acids within cell cytoplasm and mitochondria. Pantethine reduces hyperlipidemia (pantothenic acid does not); 900 mg pantethine q.d. reduces serum triglyceride and cholesterol and increases high-density lipoprotein (HDL) with no toxicity; inhibits cholesterol synthesis and accelerates fatty acid breakdown in mitochondria. Heart pantethine decreases during ischemia.
- **CoQ10 (ubiquinone):** essential component of mitochondrial energy production; synthesized within body; synthesis impaired by nutritional deficiencies, genetic or acquired defect, or increased tissue need. Angina, hypertension, mitral valve prolapse, and congestive heart failure require increased tissue levels of CoQ10; elderly have increased CoQ10 needs. CoQ10 decline with age contributes to age-related decline in immunity. CoQ10 deficiency is common in patients with heart disease. High metabolic activity of heart tissue causes unusual susceptibility to CoQ10 deficiency. CoQ10 reduces frequency of anginal attacks by 53% in stable patients and increases treadmill exercise tolerance.
- **Mg:** deficiency may play a major role in angina, including Prinzmetal's. Deficiency produces coronary vasospasms; may be cause of nonocclusive MI. Sudden MI in death of men is linked to much lower heart Mg^{2+} and Potassium than that of matched controls. Researchers recommend Mg as treatment of choice for angina because of coronary vasospasm; helps manage arrhythmias and angina from atherosclerosis. IV Mg during first hour after acute MI reduces immediate and long-term complications and death rates. Beneficial effects of Mg in acute MI: improves energy production within the heart; dilates coronary arteries,

improves heart oxygenation; reduces peripheral vascular resistance (decreasing demand on heart); inhibits platelet aggregation; reduces size of infarct; and improves heart rate and arrhythmias.

- **Arginine:** beneficial in a number of cardiovascular diseases via increasing nitric oxide levels, thereby dilating blood vessels, improving blood flow, reducing thrombosis, and improving rheology. Degree of improvement can be quite significant. It is especially effective in increasing exercise tolerance. Dose: 6 g/day in divided dosages. At 3 g/day for 15 days, arginine increased activity of free radical scavenging enzyme superoxide dismutase and increased total thiols and ascorbic acid, with a concomitant decrease in lipid peroxidation, carbonyl content, serum cholesterol, and activity of pro-oxidant enzyme xanthine oxidase. These effects constitute additional mechanisms for use of arginine in angina and cardiac ischemia. Caution: in survivors of MI, arginine supplementation (9 g/day for 6 months) was associated with increase in mortality compared with placebo. This effect may be an aberration or result of use of higher doses of arginine.

Botanical Medicines

- ***Crataegus* species (hawthorn):** Berry and flowering tops extracts reduce angina attacks, lower blood pressure and serum cholesterol levels; improve blood and oxygen supply of heart by dilation of coronary vessels; improve metabolic processes in heart; improve cardiac energy metabolism, enhancing myocardial function with more-efficient use of oxygen; interact with key enzymes to enhance myocardial contractility (*Textbook, "Crataegus oxyacantha* [Hawthorn]").
- ***Ammi visnaga* (khella):** ancient Mediterranean medicinal plant used historically to treat angina and other heart ailments. Constituents dilate coronary arteries; mechanism of action similar to calcium channel blocking drugs. Constituent khellin is extremely effective in relieving angina symptoms, improving exercise tolerance, and normalizing ECGs. Higher doses (120 to 150 mg q.d.) of pure khellin are linked to mild side effects (anorexia, nausea, dizziness). Most clinical studies used high doses; several studies used only 30 mg khellin q.d., which offered good results with fewer side effects. Khella extracts standardized for khellin content (12%) are preferred at dose of 250 to 300 mg q.d. Khella works synergistically with hawthorn.

Other Therapies

- **Acupuncture:** improves angina, reducing nitroglycerin use, decreasing number of angina attacks, and improving exercise tolerance and ECGs.
- **Relaxation and breathing exercises:** improve angina symptoms when anxiety is significant contributor. In cardiac syndrome X, a form of angina in human beings with otherwise normal coronary arteries, transcendental meditation (20 minutes b.i.d. silently chanting mantra with eyes closed) reduces angina-like chest pain and normalizes ECGs.
- **IV EDTA chelation therapy:** alternative to bypass surgery or angioplasty; may be more effective and is definitely safer and less expensive. EDTA is amino acid–like molecule that binds with minerals (e.g., calcium [Ca], iron [Fe], copper [Cu], and lead [Pb]) and carries them to kidneys for excretion; commonly used for Pb poisoning but found to help atherosclerosis in late 1950s; Dr Norman Clarke treated patients with angina, cerebral vascular insufficiency, and occlusive peripheral vascular disease; 87% showed symptomatic improvement. Patients with blocked leg arteries, particularly diabetics, avoided amputation. EDTA chelates out excess Fe and Cu that stimulate free radicals in presence of oxygen. Free radicals damage endothelium, causing atherosclerosis. Giving too much EDTA or giving it too fast is dangerous, possibly resulting in kidney failure; but no deaths or significant adverse reactions in more than 500,000 patients treated under controlled protocols; improves blood flow throughout body—recommended for angina, peripheral vascular disease, and cerebral vascular disease; substantiated by numerous U.S. Food and Drug Administration (FDA)–approved studies. Insufficient evidence to ascertain efficacy or lack thereof for improving clinical outcomes of patients with atherosclerotic cardiovascular disease. (Contact American College for Advancement in Medicine [ACAM], 23121 Verdugo Drive, Suite 204, Laguna Hills, CA 92653; 1-800-532-3688 [outside California] or 1-800-435-6199 [inside California].)

THERAPEUTIC APPROACH

Primary therapy is prevention because angina usually is secondary to atherosclerosis. Once developed, restore proper blood supply to heart and enhance energy production within heart. Unstable angina (progressive increase in frequency and severity of pain over several days, increased sensitivity to precipitating factors, and prolonged coronary pain) mandates hospitalization.

- **Diet:** increase fiber, especially gel-forming and mucilaginous fibers (ground flaxseed, oat bran, pectin). Increase onions, garlic, vegetables, small wild ocean fish. Decrease saturated and *trans* fats, cholesterol, sugar, animal proteins. Avoid fried foods and food allergens. Patients with reactive hypoglycemia: eat small, frequent regular meals and avoid simple carbohydrates (e.g., sugar, honey, dried fruit, fruit juice).
- **Lifestyle:** stop smoking, alcohol use, coffee intake. Decrease stress by progressive relaxation, meditation, or guided imagery. Carefully follow graded, progressive, aerobic exercise (30 minutes three times weekly); start with walking.
- **Nutritional supplements:**
  - — Vitamin C: 500 to 1500 mg q.d.
  - — Vitamin E: 200 to 400 international units (IU) q.d. (prefer mixed tocopherols emphasizing gamma-tocopherol)
  - — CoQ10: 150 to 300 mg q.d. (CoQ10 blood levels must reach greater than 2.5 mcg/mL for efficacy.)
  - — L-Carnitine: 500 mg t.i.d.
  - — Pantethine: 300 mg t.i.d.
  - — Magnesium (aspartate, citrate, or other Krebs cycle intermediates): 200 to 400 mg t.i.d.
  - — L-Arginine: 1000 to 2000 mg t.i.d.
- **Botanical medicines:**
- *C. oxyacantha* (t.i.d.):
  - — Berries or flowers (dried): 3 to 5 g or as a tea
  - — Fluid extract (1:1): 1 to 2 mL (0.25 to 0.5 tsp)
  - — Solid extract (10% procyanidins or 1.8% vitexin-4′-rhamnoside): 100 to 250 mg
- *A. visnaga* (t.i.d.):
  - — Dried powdered extract (12% khellin content): 100 mg

Aphthous Stomatitis (Aphthous Ulcer/Canker Sore/Ulcerative Stomatitis)

DIAGNOSTIC SUMMARY

- Single or several discrete, shallow, painful ulcers found anywhere on mucosa: labial and buccal mucosa, maxillary and mandibular sulci, gingiva, soft palate, tonsillar fauces, floor of the mouth, ventral surface of the tongue.
- Lesions are from 1 to 15 mm in diameter, have fairly even borders, are surrounded by an erythematous border, and are often covered by a pseudomembrane.
- Lesions usually resolve in 7 to 10 days but are often recurrent; larger ulcers may last several weeks to months and can leave a scar.

GENERAL CONSIDERATIONS

Aphthous stomatitis, recurrent aphthous ulcers (RAUs), or canker sores constitute a common condition affecting 20% of the population. RAU is an idiopathic multifactorial disorder that can cause significant morbidity. Although usually self-limited, recurrence can be almost continuous. Inflammatory bowel disease, systemic lupus erythematosus, and Behçet's syndrome are systemic disorders associated with RAUs. Many people mistakenly identify RAUs as herpes simplex, although there is an uncommon form—herpetiform RAU—clusters of aphthae less than 1 mm in diameter. No consistent genetic associations have been demonstrated. Etiology: food sensitivities (e.g., gluten), stress, and/or nutrient deficiency. Lesions are mucosal ulcerations with mixed inflammatory cell infiltrates; T-helper cells predominate in preulcerative and healing phases; T-suppressor cells predominate in ulcerative phase. Lesions are mucosal ulcerations with mixed inflammatory cell infiltrates; T-helper cells predominate in preulcerative and healing phases;

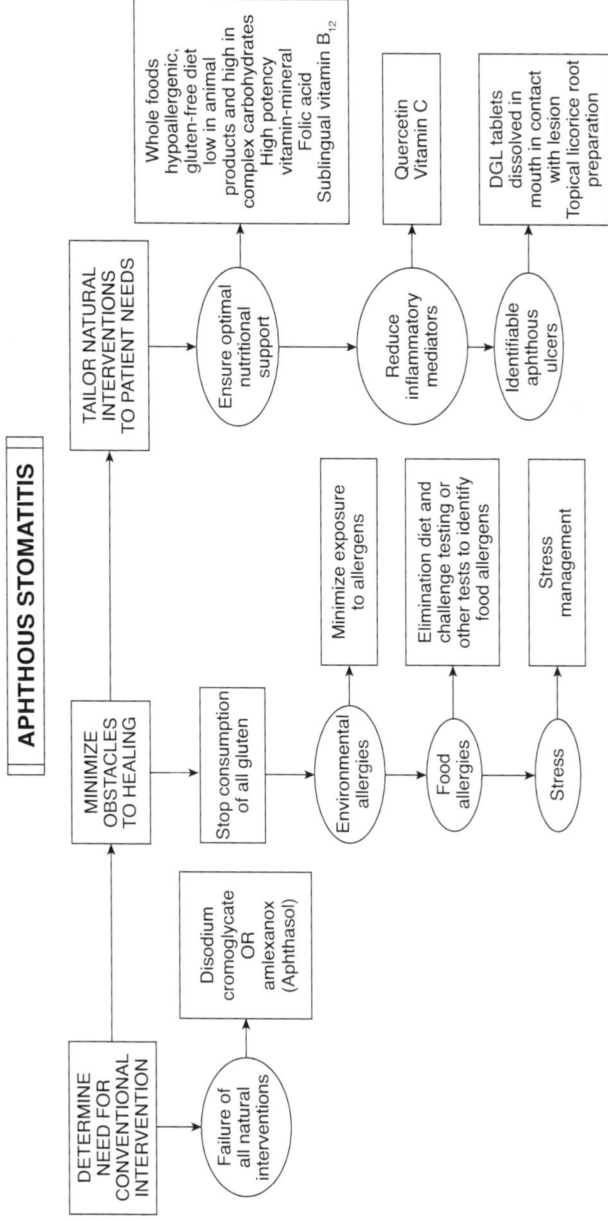
APHTHOUS STOMATITIS
DETERMINE NEED FOR CONVENTIONAL INTERVENTION
Failure of all natural interventions
Disodium cromoglycate OR amlexanox (Aphthasol)
MINIMIZE OBSTACLES TO HEALING
Stop consumption of all gluten
Environmental allergies
Minimize exposure to allergens
Food allergies
Elimination diet and challenge testing or other tests to identify food allergens
Stress
Stress management
TAILOR NATURAL INTERVENTIONS TO PATIENT NEEDS
Ensure optimal nutritional support
Whole foods hypoallergenic, gluten-free diet low in animal products and high in complex carbohydrates
High potency vitamin-mineral
Folic acid
Sublingual vitamin B_{12}
Reduce inflammatory mediators
Quercetin
Vitamin C
Identifiable aphthous ulcers
DGL tablets dissolved in mouth in contact with lesion
Topical licorice root preparation

T-suppressor cells predominate in ulcerative phase. Cause: dysregulation of immune system in the oral mucosa. Key features of immune dysfunction: lymphomononuclear infiltrate and hemagglutination antibodies against oral mucosa; reduced response of lymphocytes to mitogens; circulating immune complexes; alterations in natural killer cell activity; increased adherence of neutrophils; release of tumor necrosis factor-alpha; mast cell involvement.

THERAPEUTIC CONSIDERATIONS

- **Food and environmental allergens:** association of RAU with increased serum antibodies to food antigens and atopy strongly suggests that allergic reaction is involved. Immunoglobulin E (IgE)–bearing lymphocytes are increased in aphthous lesions; mast cells are increased in tissue from prodromal stages of recurrent ulcers. Mast cell degranulation is important in producing lesion. Elimination diet gives good results. Allergen does not have to be food; frequent allergens inducing RAU are benzoic acid, cinnamaldehyde, nickel, parabens, dichromate, sorbic acid; allergen elimination usually brings complete resolution or significant improvement.
- **Gluten sensitivity:** gluten sensitivity is the primary cause of RAU in many cases. Incidence of RAU is increased in patients with celiac disease. Jejunal biopsy of patients with RAU reveals villous atrophy typical of celiac disease plus signs of immunologic reactions to food antigens. Gluten may act directly on oral mucosa or produce functional changes in small intestine distinct from those of celiac disease. Gluten-sensitive enteropathy induces nutritional deficiencies. Withdrawing gluten causes complete remission of RAU in patients with celiac disease and some improvement in other patients. Even without villous atrophy, gluten sensitivity can produce RAU. Measure alpha-gliadin antibodies in any patient with RAU.
- **Stress:** precipitating factor in RAU, suggesting breakdown in host protective factors.
- **Nutrient deficiency:** oral cavity often is the first place where nutritional deficiency is visible—high turnover of mucosal epithelium. Thiamin (B_1) deficiency is the most significant. Low levels of transketolase (B_1-dependent enzyme) found in RAU compared with controls. Nutrient deficiencies are much more common in those with RAU: 14.2% deficient in iron (Fe), folate, B_{12}, or combination of these nutrients; 28.2% deficient in B_1, B_2, or B_6;

when deficiencies are corrected, majority are completely remitted. Lower dietary intake of folate and vitamin B_{12} is common in persons with RAU, and treatment with 1000 mcg/day has shown benefit regardless of serum B_{12} levels. Zinc (50 mg elemental) daily for 1 month has reduced aphthae and prevented reappearance for 3 months. In adolescents, a reduction in incidence of RAU and associated pain was induced from 2000 mg/day of ascorbate. Low nutrient status may explain why patients with RAU have increased oxidant/antioxidant status: decreased catalase and glutathione peroxidase activities and antioxidant potential levels in the erythrocytes and decreased antioxidant potential and increased malondialdehyde in plasma. Enzymatic and nonenzymatic antioxidant defense systems are impaired in patients with RAU.

- **Quercetin:** inhibits mast cell degranulation, basophil histamine release, and formation of other mediators of inflammation. Antiallergy drug disodium cromoglycate has similar structure and function and is effective in treating RAU. Quercetin increased number of ulcer-free days with mild symptomatic relief. Other flavonoids (acacetin, apigenin, chrysin, and phloretin, but not catechin, flavone, morin, rutin, or taxifolin) have antiallergy effects similar to the drug.
- **Deglycyrrhizinated licorice (DGL):** may be effective in promoting healing of RAU lesions. Solution of DGL used as mouthwash (200 mg powdered DGL dissolved in 200 mL warm water q.i.d.)—75% of patients had 50% to 75% improvement within 1 day, followed by complete healing of ulcers by third day; DGL tablets may be more convenient and effective. Let them melt in the mouth directly adjacent to the lesions. Topical preparations containing solid extract of licorice root are also available (e.g., Canker Goo, from Wise Woman Herbals, Creswell, OR; Canker-Melts from OraHealth, Bellevue, WA).
- ***Myrtus communis* (myrtle):** a paste containing *M. communis* (myrtle) for RAU applied four times daily for 6 days has proven clinically effective.

THERAPEUTIC APPROACH

No single factor is solely responsible for initiating aphthous lesions, but underlying tendency to ulceration may be facilitated in expression by these factors. The underlying problem may be gluten sensitivity plus nutrient deficiencies. Use anti-inflammatory nutrients. Also beneficial is individualized homeopathic treatment, where the medicine is administered in 6C potency as oral liquid for two doses only. For symptom relief, amlexanox (Aphthasol) is the first FDA-approved topical prescription for RAU. It is an immunomodulator that accelerates healing of aphthous ulcers. It inhibits inflammatory mediators (histamine and leukotrienes) from mast cells, neutrophils, and mononuclear cells in vitro, and clinical studies have shown 75% faster healing and 90% faster pain resolution.

- **Diet:** low in animal products, high in complex carbohydrates, free of known allergens and all gluten sources (i.e., grains)
- **Supplements**:
  — High-potency multiple vitamin-mineral
  — Calcium ascorbate: 2000 mg q.d.
  — Sublingual vitamin B_{12}: 1000 mcg q.d.
- **Botanical medicines:**
  — DGL: one or two 380-mg chewable tablets held in direct contact with the lesion
  — Topical licorice root preparations (e.g., Canker Goo, Canker-Melts) applied as needed

Asthma

DIAGNOSTIC SUMMARY

- Recurrent attacks of dyspnea, cough, and expectoration of tenacious mucoid sputum
- Prolonged expiration phase with generalized wheezing and musical rales
- Eosinophilia, increased serum immunoglobulin E (IgE), positive food and/or inhalant allergy test results

GENERAL CONSIDERATIONS

Bronchial asthma is a hypersensitivity disorder characterized by bronchospasm, mucosal edema, and excessive excretion of a viscous mucus that can lead to ventilatory insufficiency. Its prevalence is approximately 3% of the U.S. population, and although it occurs at all ages, it is most common in children younger than 10. There is a 2:1 male/female ratio in children that equalizes by the age of 30.

- **Major factors:** hypersensitivity of airways; beta-adrenergic blockade; cyclic nucleotide imbalance in airway smooth muscle; release of inflammatory mediators from mast cells. Rate in United States is rising rapidly, especially in children; reasons for this are increased stress on immune system (greater chemical pollution in air, water, and food; insect allergens from mites and cockroaches; earlier weaning of and introduction of solid foods to infants; food additives; higher incidence of obesity; genetic manipulation of plants—food components with greater allergenic tendencies).
- **Multiple genetic variables increasing susceptibility:** deficiency in glutathione *S*-transferase M1 (gene responding to oxidative stress) increases susceptibility; this suggests need for antioxidants. *ADAM33* gene on chromosome 20p13 is linked to airway remodeling (see later discussion of mediators) and corticosteroid resistance. Genes on chromosomes 7 and 12 are also implicated.
- Major categories:
  - — Extrinsic or atopic: immunologically mediated with increased serum IgE

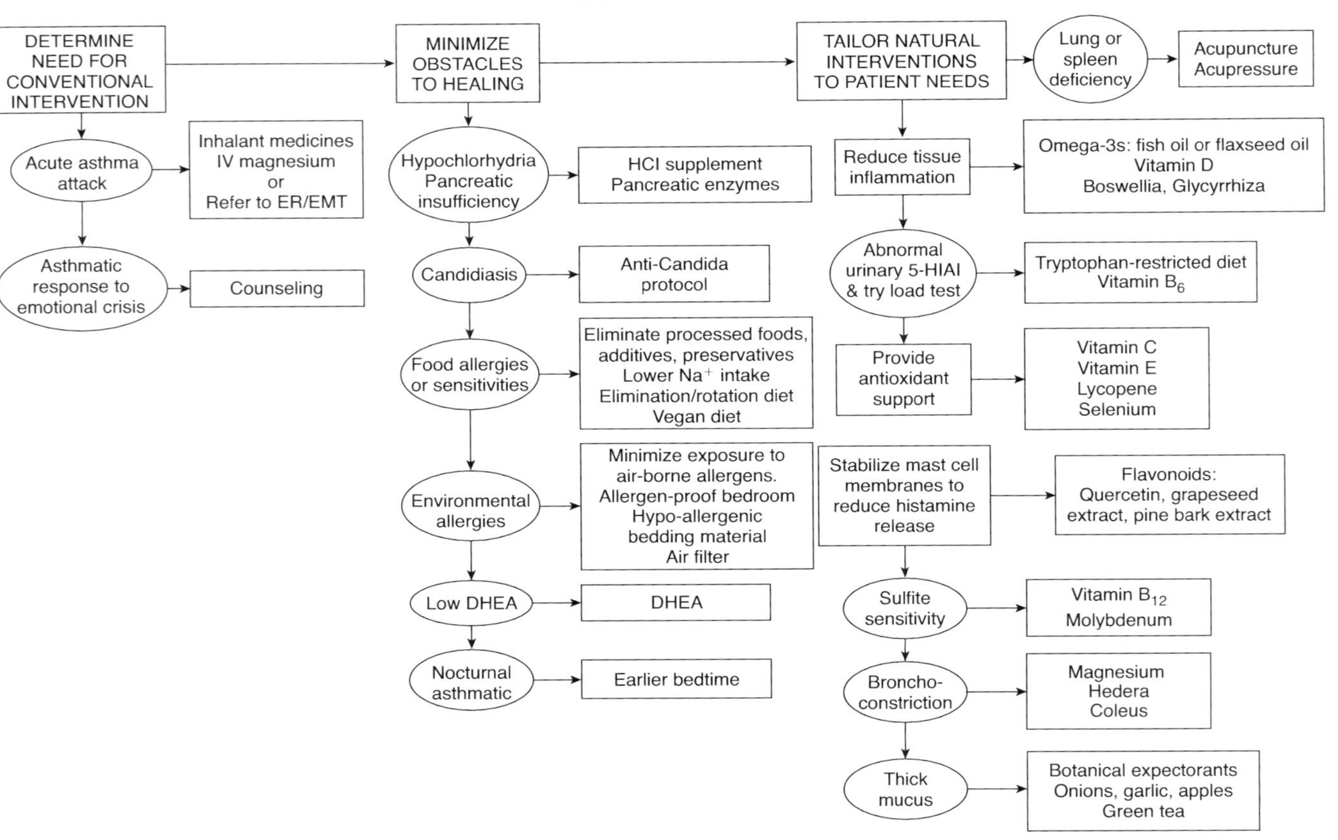
DETERMINE NEED FOR CONVENTIONAL INTERVENTION
Acute asthma attack
Inhalant medicines
IV magnesium
or
Refer to ER/EMT
Asthmatic response to emotional crisis
Counseling
MINIMIZE OBSTACLES TO HEALING
Hypochlorhydria
Pancreatic insufficiency
HCl supplement
Pancreatic enzymes
Candidiasis
Anti-Candida protocol
Food allergies or sensitivities
Eliminate processed foods, additives, preservatives
Lower Na+ intake
Elimination/rotation diet
Vegan diet
Environmental allergies
Minimize exposure to air-borne allergens.
Allergen-proof bedroom
Hypo-allergenic bedding material
Air filter
Low DHEA
DHEA
Nocturnal asthmatic
Earlier bedtime
TAILOR NATURAL INTERVENTIONS TO PATIENT NEEDS
Lung or spleen deficiency
Acupuncture
Acupressure
Reduce tissue inflammation
Omega-3s: fish oil or flaxseed oil
Vitamin D
Boswellia, Glycyrrhiza
Abnormal urinary 5-HIAI & try load test
Tryptophan-restricted diet
Vitamin B6
Provide antioxidant support
Vitamin C
Vitamin E
Lycopene
Selenium
Stabilize mast cell membranes to reduce histamine release
Flavonoids:
Quercetin, grapeseed extract, pine bark extract
Sulfite sensitivity
Vitamin B12
Molybdenum
Broncho-constriction
Magnesium
Hedera
Coleus
Thick mucus
Botanical expectorants
Onions, garlic, apples
Green tea

— Intrinsic: bronchial reaction caused not by antigen-antibody stimulation but by factors such as chemicals, cold air, exercise, infection, agents that activate alternative complement pathway, and emotional upset

Asthma is often clinically classified according to frequency of symptoms, forced expiratory volume in 1 second (FEV_1), and peak expiratory flow rate.

DIAGNOSTIC CONSIDERATIONS

U.S. National Asthma Education and Prevention Program (NAEPP) guidelines for diagnosis and management of asthma state that diagnosis of asthma begins by assessing whether any of the indicators listed here is present.

National Asthma Education and Prevention Program (NEAPP) Classification of Asthma Severity Before Treatment in Adults and Youths 12 Years and Older*

Component of Severity	Intermittent	PERSISTENT		
		Mild	Moderate	Severe
Symptoms	≤2 days/week	>2 days per week but not daily	Daily	Throughout the day
Nighttime awakenings	≤2x/month	3–4x/month	>1x/week but not nightly	Often 7x/week
Short-acting β-agonist use for symptoms	≤days/week	>2 days per week but not >1x/day	Daily	Several times per day
Interference with normal activity	None	Minor limitation	Some limitation	Extremely limited
Pulmonary function	Normal FEV_1 between exacerbations; FEV_1 ≥80% predicted; FEV_1/FVC normal	FEV_1 <80% predicted; FEV_1/FVC normal	FEV_1 ≥60% but <80% predicted; FEV_1/FVC reduced ≥5%	FEV_1 <60%; FEV_1/FVC reduced >5%
Exacerbations (consider frequency and severity)	0–1 per year	-	≥2 per year	-

*Severity level is determined in accordance with the worst impairment category

Data from Expert panel report 3: guidelines for the diagnosis and management of asthma National Asthma Education and Prevention Program, Third Expert Panel on the Diagnosis and Management of Asthma, National Heart, Lung, and Blood Institute, Bethesda, MD, 2007.

- Wheezing—high-pitched whistling sounds on expiration—especially in children. (Lack of wheezing and normal chest examination findings do not exclude asthma.)
- History of any of the following:
  - — Cough, worse particularly at night
  - — Recurrent wheeze
  - — Recurrent difficulty in breathing
  - — Recurrent chest tightness
- Symptoms occur or worsen in the presence of the following:
  - — Exercise
  - — Viral infection
  - — Animals with fur or hair
  - — House dust mites (in mattresses, pillows, upholstered furniture, carpets)
  - — Mold
  - — Smoke (tobacco, wood)
  - — Pollen
  - — Changes in weather
  - — Strong emotional expression (laughing or crying hard)
  - — Airborne chemicals or dusts
  - — Menstrual cycles
- Symptoms occur or worsen at night, awakening the patient

Spirometry: perform at time of initial diagnosis, after treatment is initiated and symptoms are stabilized, whenever control of symptoms deteriorates, and every 1 or 2 years on a regular basis.

Causes

- Complex interaction of environmental and genetic factors.
- Strongest risk factor: history of atopic disease. Presence of atopic dermatitis increases risk of asthma by threefold to fourfold.
- Allergies and response of the immune system are involved.

Inflammation and T-helper cell (Th1/Th2) balances: imbalances in T-helper cell immune responses comprise mechanism of immune system–mediated airway inflammation. $CD4^+$ T-helper cell categories: Th1 and Th2. Th1 cells release interferons and interleukin-2 (IL-2), increasing immune response of cancer, multiple sclerosis (MS), viruses, and type IV hypersensitivity. Th2 cells facilitate release of IL-4, IL-6, IL-9, IL-13, and IgE; eosinophilia; and activated B-cell humoral immunity. Related disorders: asthma, atopic syndromes, and allergies. Asthmatics have normal Th1 gene expression but upregulated Th2 genes, causing Th2 dominance. Genetics, fungi, heavy metals, nutrition, viruses, and pollution are factors in this upregulation.

"Hygiene hypothesis"—minimizing exposure to infectious agents by hygienic lifestyle choices favors Th2 dominance of immune responses to allergens, encouraging asthma and atopic diseases.

- **Mediators:** extrinsic and intrinsic factors involving Th2 imbalances trigger cytokine-activated release of mast cell mediators of bronchoconstriction and mucus secretion. Preformed mediators are histamine, chemotactic peptides (eosinophil chemotactic factor [ECF] and high-molecular-weight neutrophil chemotactic factor [NCF]), proteases, glycosidases, and heparin proteoglycan. Membrane-derived agents are lipoxygenase products (leukotrienes [LTs] and slow-reacting substance of anaphylaxis [SRS-A]), prostaglandins (PGs), thromboxanes (TXs), and platelet-activating factor (PAF). Effects of mediators are bronchoconstriction (histamine, LTC_4, LTD_4, LTE_4, PGF_{2alpha}, PGD_2, PAF), mucosal edema (histamine, LTC_4, LTD_4, PAF), vasodilation (PGD_2, PGE_2), mucous plugging (histamine, hydroxyeicosatetraenoic acid [HETE], LTC_4), inflammatory cell infiltrate (NCF, ECF-A, HETE, LTB_4, PAF), and epithelial desquamation (proteases, glycosidases, lysosomal enzymes, and basic proteins from neutrophils and eosinophils). Mediators cause airway remodeling in chronic asthma, affecting epithelium and mesenchymal tissues. Induced growth factors encourage fibroblasts, smooth muscle proliferation, and matrix protein deposits, thickening the wall.
- **Mild episodic asthma versus moderate to severe sustained asthma:** latter has subacute and chronic bronchial inflammation with infiltration of eosinophils, neutrophils, and mononuclear cells. Episodic asthma is caused by bronchial smooth muscle contraction.
- **Lipoxygenase products:** LTs are most potent chemical mediators in asthma. SRS-A (LTC_4, LTD_4, LTE_4) is 1000 times more potent a bronchoconstrictor than histamine. Asthmatics have imbalance in arachidonic acid metabolism, causing relative increase in lipoxygenase products; platelets from asthmatics show 40% decrease in cyclooxygenase metabolites and 70% increase in lipoxygenase products. Imbalance is aggravated in "aspirin-induced asthma"—aspirin and nonsteroidal anti-inflammatory drugs (NSAIDs) inhibit cyclooxygenase while promoting lipoxygenase, shunting arachidonic acid to lipoxygenase pathway and excessive LTs. Tartrazine (yellow dye No. 5) is cyclooxygenase inhibitor and induces asthma, especially in children. Tartrazine is antimetabolite of vitamin B_6.

- **Autonomic nervous system** (parasympathetic versus sympathetic innervation): $beta_2$ adrenergic receptors are localized in lung tissue and react to catecholamines. Parasympathetic vagus nerve stimulation releases acetylcholine (Ach), which binds to receptors on smooth muscle, forming cyclic guanosine monophosphate (cGMP). Increased cGMP and/or relative deficiency in cyclic adenosine monophosphate (cAMP) causes bronchoconstriction and degranulation of mast cells and basophils. Decreased sympathetic activity or diminished $beta_2$-receptor numbers or sensitivity also promotes the cyclic nucleotide imbalance. Some mediators block $beta_2$ receptors and elevate cGMP.
- **Adrenal gland:** cortisol activates beta receptors. Epinephrine (Epi) is the prime stimulator of beta receptors. Asthmatic attacks may be induced by relative deficiency of cortisol and Epi (which stimulate $beta_2$ receptors to catalyze formation of cAMP from AMP), leading to decreased cAMP/cGMP ratio and bronchial constriction.
- **Pertussis vaccine:** among children breastfed from first day of life, fed exclusively breast milk for first 6 months, and weaned after 1 year, the relative risk of developing asthma is 1% in children receiving no immunizations, 3% in those receiving vaccinations other than pertussis, and 11% in those receiving pertussis vaccine. In a group of 203 not immunized to pertussis, 16 developed whooping cough compared with only 1 of 243 in the immunized group.
- **Influenza vaccine:** although the relatively new cold-adapted trivalent intranasal influenza virus vaccine was deemed safe for children and adolescents, increased relative risk of 4.06 for asthma and reactive airway disease arose in children age 18 to 35 months.

THERAPEUTIC CONSIDERATIONS

General

- **Hypochlorhydria:** 80% of tested asthmatic children had inadequate gastric acid secretion; hypochlorhydria and food allergies are predisposing factors for asthma.
- **Increased intestinal permeability:** "leaky gut" permits increased food antigen load, overwhelming immune system, increasing risk of additional allergies and exposure to bronchoconstrictive compounds.

- Identify offending foods:
  - *Candida albicans:* gastrointestinal (GI) overgrowth implicated as causative factor in allergic conditions, including asthma. Acid protease produced by *C. albicans* is the responsible allergen.
  - Food additives: must be eliminated: coloring agents, azo dyes (tartrazine [orange], sunset yellow, amaranth and new coccine [both red]), and non–azo dye pate blue. Most common preservatives are sodium benzoate, 4-hydroxybenzoate esters, and sulfur dioxide. Sulfite sources are salads, vegetables (particularly potatoes), avocado dip served in restaurants, wine, and beer. Molybdenum deficiency may cause sulfite sensitivity; sulfite oxidase is the enzyme that neutralizes sulfites and is molybdenum dependent.
  - Salt: Increased intake worsens bronchial reactivity and mortality from asthma. Bronchial reactivity to histamine is positively correlated with 24-hour urinary sodium (Na) and rises with increased dietary Na.
- **Estrogen and progesterone:** for women with severe asthma, consider decreasing hormonal fluctuations. Estrogen and progesterone are smooth muscle relaxants. Airways of premenopausal and postmenopausal women may respond differently to exogenous hormone replacement therapy (HRT) and need assessment independent of this intervention. During premenstrual and menstrual phases, when hormones are low, asthmatic women have episodes and are hospitalized with decreased pulmonary function. Stabilizing hormone fluctuations (by pregnancy or oral contraceptives) improves pulmonary function and reduces need for medication. Liver detoxification and botanicals are safer methods to balance hormones. If these fail, natural HRT may be less risky (*Textbook,* "Asthma" and "Menopause").
- **DHEA (dehydroepiandrosterone):** decreased levels are common in postmenopausal women with asthma compared with matched controls. Transdermal 17 beta-estradiol (E2) and medroxyprogesterone acetate increase serum DHEAs in asthmatics, with no change in controls. Therapeutic benefit of DHEA in asthma is undemonstrated, but its importance to immune function suggests possible positive effects.
- **Melatonin:** concern exists that elevated melatonin may contribute to airway inflammation in nocturnal asthmatics and inflammation in rheumatoid arthritis (RA). In nocturnal asthmatics, peak serum melatonin is inversely correlated with overnight change

in FEV but not in non-nocturnal asthmatics or healthy controls. Release of melatonin is delayed in nocturnal asthmatics. Supplementation plus earlier bedtime may regulate late melatonin peaking and mitigate symptoms. Avoid giving melatonin to asthmatics, especially nocturnal type, until further study is completed.

Diet

- **Beneficial foods:** antioxidants in fruit and vegetables lower risk of poor respiratory health. Fruit high in vitamin C lowers prevalence of asthma symptoms and improves lung function in children. Even small increases in fruit intake are beneficial. Fish lowers airway hyperreactivity in children and increases lung function in adults. Fruit decreases phlegm. Fruit (>180 g/day), whole grains (>45 g/day), and moderate alcohol (1 to 3 glasses/day) have increased FEV by 139 mL and lowered by 50% the prevalence of chronic obstructive pulmonary disease (COPD) symptoms. Apples and red wine (moderate intake) antioxidants decrease asthma severity. Dietary intake of soy foods may be helpful: soy isoflavone genistein is associated with reduced severity of asthma. This effect may be a result of antioxidant action; but genistein is able to block eosinophil LTC_4 synthesis and inhibit the pathway of nuclear factor kappa B (NF-κB) and tumor necrosis factor-alpha (TNF-α) in asthma patients.
- **Food allergy** (*Textbook,* "Food Allergy Testing"): immediate-onset sensitivities can be caused by (decreasing order of frequency) egg, fish, shellfish, nuts, peanuts. Delayed onset can arise from (decreasing order of frequency) milk, chocolate, wheat, citrus, food colorings. Elimination diets identify allergens and treat asthma, especially in infants. Avoiding common allergens during infancy (first 2 years) reduces allergic tendencies in high-risk children (strong familial history).
- **Breastfeeding:** can prevent asthma. Children not breastfed are more likely to become asthmatic. Vitamin C in breast milk correlates with maternal intake; low maternal intake results in low infant intake, increasing susceptibility to oxidative stress. Applying preventive interventions (house dust control; avoidance of pets, tobacco smoke, day care during first year; breastfeeding exclusively or using partially hydrolyzed whey formula until age 4 months) for infants with atopic family history lowers risk for asthma at ages 1 and 2 years. A 90% reduction in recurrent wheezing has also been noted.
- **Antibiotics, probiotics, and mucosal IgA:** patients prescribed antibiotics before their first birthday are more than twice as

likely as untreated children to develop asthma. With multiple courses of antibiotics, risk is even higher—16% for every course of drugs taken before age 1. Explanations: (1) Antibiotics contribute to a state of "excess hygiene," leading to reduced exposure to microbes. This creates an oversensitive immune system, mounting an over-the-top allergic reaction to pollen and dust mites, resulting in asthma. (2) Antibiotics have negative effect on normal flora of GI tract and respiratory passages. Giving probiotics (active cultures of *Lactobacillus* and *Bifidobacterium* species) lowers risk of atopic allergic diseases like asthma and eczema. Some of this protective effect may be mediated by mucosal IgA, which participates in antigen elimination. Supplementing probiotics increases fecal IgA and calprotectin and reduces inflammatory markers (e.g., alpha$_1$-antitrypsin and TNF-α). In infants with high fecal IgA concentration at age 6 months, risk of having any allergic disease or any IgE-associated (atopic) disease before age of 2 years is cut by nearly 50%. High intestinal IgA in early life is associated with minimal intestinal inflammation and indicates reduced risk for IgE-associated allergic diseases.

- **Vegan diet:** long-term trial (eliminating all animal products) significantly improved 92% of 25 patients who completed the study (nine dropped out) based on vital capacity, FEV_1, physical working capacity, haptoglobin, IgM, IgE, cholesterol, and triglycerides. Vegan diet also reduces tendency for infectious disease. Seventy-one percent of patients responded in 4 months; 1 year was required for 92%. Diet excludes all meat, fish, eggs, dairy products, chlorinated tap water (drink spring water only), coffee, ordinary tea, chocolate, sugar, and salt. Herbal spices are allowed; water and herbal teas allowed up to 1.5 L q.d. Vegetables used freely are lettuce, carrots, beets, onions, celery, cabbage, cauliflower, broccoli, nettles, cucumber, radishes, Jerusalem artichokes, all beans except soya, and green peas. Potatoes are allowed in restricted amounts. Fruits used freely: blueberries, cloudberries, raspberries, strawberries, black currants, gooseberries, plums, pears. Apples and citrus fruits are not allowed. Grains are restricted or eliminated. Beneficial effects of vegan diet are elimination of food allergens, altered PG metabolism, increased intake of antioxidants and magnesium (Mg). Avoid dietary sources of arachidonic acid (animal products). Inflammatory PGs and LTs made from arachidonic acid intensify asthmatic reactions. Vegan diet reduces health care costs (corticosteroids, other drugs, therapies) and increases patients' sense of responsibility for their own health.

Nutrition

- **Omega-3 essential fatty acids (n-3 EFAs)**: children who eat fish more than once a week have one third the asthma risk of those who do not. Fish oil supplements with eicosapentaenoic acid (EPA) and docosahexaenoic acid (DHA) improve airway hyperresponsiveness to allergens and respiratory function. Benefits are from increasing ratio of n-3 to n-6 EFAs in cell membranes, reducing arachidonic acid. n-3 EFAs shift LT synthesis from inflammatory 4-series to less-inflammatory 5-series, improving asthma symptoms. Benefits may take as long as 1 year before apparent from turnover of cellular membranes toward n-3s.
- **Tryptophan metabolism and pyridoxine (vitamin B_6)** supplementation: asthmatic children have metabolic defect in tryptophan metabolism and reduced platelet transport for serotonin. Tryptophan is converted to serotonin (bronchoconstrictor in asthmatics). Serotonin is high in blood and sputum of asthmatics, causing elevated urinary 5-hydroxyindoleacetic acid (5-HIAI), the breakdown product of serotonin. Urinary 5-HIAI correlates well with symptom severity. Patients benefit from tryptophan-restricted diet or B_6 supplements. Plasma and red blood cell (RBC) pyridoxal phosphate in asthmatics is much lower than in controls. Fifty to 100 mg oral B_6 b.i.d. greatly decreases frequency and severity of wheezing and attacks and dosages of bronchodilators and corticosteroids. B_6 fails to improve well patients dependent on steroids, but B_6 is indicated in patients on theophylline. Theophylline depresses pyridoxal-5-phosphate (P5P); B_6 supplements reduce side effects of theophylline (headache, nausea, irritability, sleep disorders). Tryptophan load test (*Textbook*, "5-Hydroxytryptophan") may determine appropriateness and level of B_6 supplementation needed. Urinary excretion of kynurenic and xanthurenic acids increases in patients responding to B_6.
- **Antioxidants:** increased prevalence of asthma is explained by reduced intake of antioxidants. Patients in acute asthmatic distress have lowered serum total antioxidants. Genetics may influence antioxidant need. Use of 50 mg of vitamin E per day and 250 mg of vitamin C per day can protect children against ozone diminishing of pulmonary function. Antioxidants help maintain lung redox state that prevents oxidants from stimulating bronchoconstriction and increasing hyperreactivity to other agents. Analgesics (e.g., acetaminophen, which depletes antioxidant glutathione) must be used cautiously in asthmatics.

- **Vitamin C:** the major antioxidant in extracellular fluid lining airway surfaces. Children of smokers have a higher rate of asthma (smoke depletes respiratory vitamins C and E), and symptoms in adults appear increased by exposure to environmental pro-oxidants and decreased by vitamin C supplements. Nitrogen oxides are oxidants from endogenous and exogenous sources. Vitamin C protects against nitrogen oxide lung damage in laboratory animals. Asthmatics have much lower serum and white blood cell (WBC) ascorbate. Clinically, asthmatics have higher need for vitamin C. Seven of 11 studies showed significant improvements in respiratory measures and symptoms using 1 to 2 g vitamin C q.d. High-dose vitamin C therapy may lower histamine; histamine initially amplifies immune response by increasing capillary permeability and smooth muscle contraction, then suppresses accumulated WBCs to contain inflammation. Vitamin C prevents histamine secretion by WBCs and increases histamine detox. Vitamin C will lower blood histamine only if taken over time.
- **Flavonoids:** key antioxidants that inhibit histamine release from mast cells and basophils stimulated by antigens, phospholipase A_2 in neutrophils, lipoxygenase, anaphylactic contraction of smooth muscle, phosphodiesterase in lung (increasing cAMP), biosynthesis of SRS-A, and Ca influx. Standard quercetin or more bioavailable forms of quercetin spares vitamin C and stabilizes mast cell membranes. Sources are quercetin supplements, grapeseed, pine bark, green tea, or *Ginkgo biloba.* Proanthocyanidins from grapeseed or pine bark have affinity for lungs. In patients age 6 to 18 years, a proprietary pine bark extract (pycnogenol) improved pulmonary function and asthma symptoms compared with placebo. The pycnogenol group reduced or discontinued rescue inhalers, with concurrent reduction of urinary LTs. In another study, flavonoid preparation from purple passion fruit peel (PFP) at 150 mg daily given to asthma patients over 4 weeks reduced wheeze, cough, and shortness of breath. PFP extract also induced marked increase in FEV_1 (*Textbook,* "Flavonoids—Quercetin, Citrus Flavonoids, and Hydroxyethylrutosides").
- **Carotenes:** powerful antioxidants that increase integrity of respiratory epithelium; act as substrates for lipoxygenase, possibly competing with arachidonic acid, decreasing inflammatory LT formation. Asthmatics may have reduced plasma antioxidant potential because of low whole-blood carotenoids (beta-carotene, lycopene, alpha-carotene, beta-cryptoxanthin, lutein/

zeaxanthin), especially low lycopene, increasing susceptibility to damaging effects of oxidative stress. Lycopene may emerge as the most useful supplemental carotenoid. In animals, lycopene suppressed Th2 responses and reduced eosinophilic infiltrates in bronchoalveolar lavage fluid, lung tissue and blood, and the number of mucus-secreting cells in airways. Antioxidant status of carotenoids modifies some parameters in asthma. In two studies of lycopene (30 mg/day) in exercise-induced asthma, one failed to show benefit, whereas the other showed that in some patients it prevented airway constriction and reduced FEV_1.

- **Vitamin E:** antioxidant inhibitor of lipoxygenase and phospholipase.
- **Selenium (Se):** Reduced Se levels are found in asthmatics. Glutathione peroxidase (Se-dependent metalloenzyme) reduces hydroperoxyeicosatetraenoic acid (HPETE) to HETE, thereby reducing LT formation. Decreased glutathione peroxidase is common in asthmatics.
- **Vitamin B_{12}:** mainstay in childhood asthma for Jonathan Wright, MD. Weekly 1000-mcg intramuscular injections improve symptoms—less shortness of breath on exertion and improved appetite, sleep, and general condition. B_{12} is especially effective in sulfite-sensitive patients; offers best protection when given orally (1 to 4 mg) before challenge; forms sulfite-cobalamin complex, blocking sulfite effect.
- **Mg:** intravenous (IV) Mg (2 g of Mg sulfate infused every hour up to total of 24.6 g) is well proven and clinically accepted to halt acute asthma attack as well as acute exacerbations of COPD. IV Mg is necessary only in emergency: acute myocardial infarction (MI) or asthma. Oral Mg is effective to optimize body Mg stores—6 weeks needed to elevate tissue Mg. Supplementation is warranted because dietary Mg intake is independently related to lung function and asthma severity. Low levels of plasma Mg occur in asthmatics. Mg improves respiratory function and antioxidant status (i.e., increased glutathione), reduces reactivity to chemical challenge to methacholine, and improves measures of asthma control and quality of life. Doses: 300 mg q.d. in children to 340 mg q.d. in adults, usually in divided doses.
- **Vitamin D:** vitamin D deficiency is linked to increased airway reactivity, poorer lung function, and worse asthma control. Among children studied, 35% were vitamin D insufficient (30 ng/mL or less of 25-hydroxyvitamin D). Insufficient vitamin D

status was associated with higher odds of hospitalization or emergency department visits. Vitamin D supplementation may improve asthma control by blocking cascade of inflammation-causing proteins in the lung and by increasing production of IL-10, which has anti-inflammatory effects. Preliminary clinical evidence is encouraging, in prevention of childhood asthma, at dose of 1200 international units (IU) vitamin D_3 daily. If vitamin D levels do not increase as expected, measure 1,25-$(OH)_2$ vitamin D for overconversion.

Botanical Medicines

Misuse of botanicals in asthma can exacerbate symptoms, leading to hospitalization. Historical herbals for asthma are *Ephedra sinica* (ma huang) in combination with herbal expectorants, such as *Glycyrrhiza glabra* (licorice), *Grindelia camporum* (grindelia), *Euphorbia hirta* (euphorbia), *Drosera rotundifolia* (sundew), and *Polygala senega* (senega). *Ephedra* alkaloids are effective bronchodilators for mild to moderate asthma and hay fever. Peak bronchodilation occurs in 1 hour and lasts 5 hours after administration. This approach appears to have considerable merit, because *Ephedra* and its alkaloids have proven to be effective as bronchodilators in treating mild to moderate asthma and hay fever. However, *Ephedra* preparations are no longer sold in the United States owing to safety concerns.

- ***Hedera helix* (ivy):** In Europe, herbal preparations containing extracts from leaves of ivy enjoy great popularity for treating cough and asthma. More than 80% of herbal expectorants prescribed in Germany contain ivy extract. Ivy leaf contains saponins that show expectorant, mucolytic, spasmolytic, bronchodilatory, and antibacterial effects. Mucolytic and expectorant action is based on indirect $beta_2$ adrenergic effects; this action is a result of saponins alpha-hederin and hederacoside C, the latter of which is metabolized to alpha-hederin when ingested. The alpha-hederin inhibits intracellular uptake of $beta_2$ receptors and leads to increased $beta_2$ adrenergic response of the cell. Ivy leaf extract preparations are proven effective for improving respiratory function in children with chronic bronchial asthma.
- ***G. glabra* (licorice root):** documented anti-inflammatory and antiallergic (*Textbook, "Glycyrrhiza glabra* [Licorice]"). Primary active constituent is glycyrrhetinic acid; inhibits phospholipase A_2, which cleaves arachidonic acid from membrane phospholipid, initiating eicosanoid synthesis. Licorice is also an expectorant.

- ***Lobelia inflata* (Indian tobacco):** alkaloid lobeline is an efficient expectorant. *Lobelia* has a long history of use in asthma but promotes bronchoconstriction and is respiratory stimulant in vitro. It binds to nicotine Ach receptors in ganglia, promoting release of Epi and norepinephrine (NE) that provide therapeutic effects. It is effective alone but traditionally is used in combination with other botanical agents (*Capsicum frutescens* and *Symphlocarpus factida*).
- ***C. frutescens* (cayenne):** capsaicin induces long-lasting desensitization of airway mucosa to mechanical and chemical irritants. Capsaicin depletes substance P (which increases vascular permeability and flow) in respiratory nerves. Substance P is an undecapeptide linked to neurogenic inflammation by direct effect and synergy with histamine on peripheral nervous system. Respiratory and GI tracts have many substance P–containing neurons, believed to contribute to atopy (asthma and atopic dermatitis).
- ***Zizyphi fructus* (jujube plum):** traditional Chinese herb for treatment of asthma and allergic rhinitis that contains 100 to 500 nmol cAMP per gram of dry weight, a concentration 10 times more than that of any other plant or animal tissue reported. It contains beta adrenergic receptor stimulator that also raises cAMP.
- ***Thea sinensis* (green tea):** adjunctive in asthma containing methylxanthine and antioxidant constituents (*Textbook,* "Asthma").
- ***Allium*:** onions and garlic may block biosynthesis of arachidonic acid metabolites by inhibiting cyclooxygenase pathways, which generate thromboxane A_2 (TXA_2), PGD_2, and PGE_2. Onion contains quercetin plus benzyl and other isothiocyanates (mustard oils).
- ***Tylophora asthmatica:*** Ayurvedic medicine for asthma and other respiratory disorders whose mode of action is unknown but thought to be attributable to alkaloids (e.g., tylophorine), which have antihistamine, antispasmodic activity and inhibit mast cell degranulation. Good results: a dose of 200 mg *Tylophora* leaves b.i.d. for 6 days improved symptoms and respiratory function during treatment and for 2 weeks thereafter. Incidence of side effects (nausea, partial diminution of taste for salt, slight mouth soreness) 16.3% in *Tylophora* group and 6.6% in placebo group. Benefits of *Tylophora* are short-lived.
- ***G. biloba:*** unique terpenes (ginkgolides) antagonize PAF; key mediator in asthma, inflammation, and allergies. Ginkgolides compete with PAF for binding sites and inhibit events induced

by PAF. *Ginkgo* improves respiratory function and reduces bronchial reactivity. Dose: 120 mg pure ginkgolides q.d.; dose very expensive using 24% *Ginkgo* flavon glycoside and 6% terpenoid *G. biloba* extract.

- ***Aloe vera:*** may be effective for patients not dependent on corticosteroids. The extract is produced from supernatant of fresh leaves stored in dark at 4°C for 7 days to increase polysaccharide fraction. One gram of this extract produces 400 mg neutral polysaccharides versus 30 mg produced from leaves not subjected to cold or dark. At 5 mL of 20% solution of Aloe *vera* extract in saline b.i.d. for 24 weeks: 40% of patients without steroid dependence felt much better. Mechanism of action may be restoring protective mechanisms, with augmentation of immune system.
- ***Coleus forskohlii:*** forskolin increases intracellular cAMP, relaxing bronchial muscles and relieving respiratory symptoms (*Textbook, "Coleus forskohlii"*). Studies used inhaled doses of pure *forskolin;* efficacy of oral *C. forskohlii* extract has yet to be determined. Historical use and additional mechanisms of action recommend its use.
- ***Boswellia:*** Ayurvedic botanical that inhibits LT biosynthesis. It has reduced bronchial asthma 70% in 40 patients treated with gum resin at 300 mg t.i.d. for 6 weeks compared with improvement in 27% of controls. Effects—disappearance of dyspnea and rhonchi; reduced number of attacks; increased FEV, vital capacity, and peak expiratory flow rates; and decreased eosinophilia and sedimentation rates.

Acupuncture and Acupressure

Chronic asthma is linked to lung or spleen deficiency. Acute symptoms arise from environmental invasion by cold wind or internal condition of lung heat (inflammation and eosinophilia). Chronic asthma indicates lung weakness, or weakness of spleen, which nourishes lung qi. Grief weakens lung qi. As adjuncts to standard care for chronic asthma, acupuncture (20 treatments) induces 18.5-fold improvement (St. George's Respiratory Questionnaire); daily self-administered acupressure for 8 weeks induces 6.57-fold improvement with 11.8-fold improvement in irritability domain score.

THERAPEUTIC APPROACH

Underlying defects and initiating factors must be determined and resolved: (1) defect allowing sensitization; (2) metabolic defect causing excessive inflammatory response; (3) triggering allergens with lifestyle, diet, and environment changes to avoid them; (4) modulating inflammatory process to limit severity; (5) effective treatment for bronchoconstriction of acute attack.

- **Environment:** minimize exposure to airborne allergens (pollen, dander, dust mites). Avoid dogs, cats, carpets, rugs, upholstered furniture, surfaces where allergens can collect. Ensure bedroom is allergen proof; encase mattress in allergen-proof plastic; wash sheets, blankets, pillowcases, and mattress pads weekly. Consider Ventflex (hypoallergenic synthetic) bedding material. Install air purifier, such as HEPA (high-efficiency particulate air), attachable to central heating and air-conditioning system.
- **Diet:** eliminate all food allergens, additives, and bananas if they aggravate condition. Patient with many food allergies may need 4-day rotation diet (*Textbook,* "Rotation Diet Master Chart, Plans I and II"). Mild tryptophan reduction is helpful—essential if there is a metabolic defect in the tryptophan metabolism. Use garlic and onions liberally unless patient reacts to them. If patient willing, or asthma unresponsive, try vegan diet (for 4+ months), with possible exception of small wild cold-water ocean fish. Encourage moderate fruit consumption, especially apples.
- **Supplements** (adult doses; rule out potential allergens in supplements):
  - — Vitamin B_6: 25 to 50 mg b.i.d.
  - — Vitamin B_{12}: 1000 mcg q.d. (oral) or weekly intramuscularly; evaluate for efficacy after 6 weeks.
  - — Vitamin C: 10 to 30 mg/kg body weight in divided doses.
  - — Vitamin D: 1000 to 8000 IU q.d. Monitor blood levels to determine needed dose, as there is wide variability. Those whose blood levels do not rise in response to supplementation should have their $1,25(OH)_2D_3$ checked. (The higher doses should not be used for teenaged girls.)
  - — Vitamin E (mixed tocopherols): 100 to 200 IU q.d.
  - — Mg: 200 to 400 mg t.i.d.
  - — Quercetin: 400 mg 20 minutes before meals or enzymatically modified isoquercitrin (EMIQ) 100 mg q.d.
  - — Grapeseed extract (95% procyanidolic oligomers (PCO) content) or pine bark extract (e.g., pycnogenol): 150 to 300 mg q.d.
  - — Lycopene: 30 to 45 mg q.d.
  - — Se: 200 mcg q.d.

- Botanical medicines:
  — Choose one or more of the following:
    - *H. helix:* Ivy leaf is available primarily in tincture and fluid extract; dry powdered extract comes in capsules and tablets. Based on clinical studies, daily doses should deliver the following equivalent to dried herbal substance: 1 to 5 years, 150 mg; 6 to 12 years, 210 mg; older than 12 years, 420 mg. The typical dose of a 4:1 powdered extract for adults and children older than 12 years is 100 mg daily.
    - *G. glabra:* powdered root (1 to 2 g); fluid extract (1:1), 2 to 4 mL; solid (dry powdered) extract (4:1), 250 to 500 mg.
    - *Camellia sinensis:* liberal use (green tea only).
    - *T. asthmatica:* 200 mg leaves or 40 mg dry alcohol extract b.i.d.
    - *C. forskohlii* (standardized to 18% forskolin): 50 mg (9 mg forskolin) b.i.d. or t.i.d.
- **Counseling:** important for patients who respond to emotional crisis with asthmatic attacks and children with moderate to severe asthma, who may develop behavioral problems.
- **Acupuncture or acupressure:** regular acupuncture and home acupressure treatments.
- **Acute attack:** medical emergency; IV Mg or refer patient to emergency room or emergency medical services immediately.

Atherosclerosis

DIAGNOSTIC SUMMARY

- Associated with high blood pressure, weak pulse, and wide pulse pressure
- Symptoms and signs depend on arteries involved and degree of obstruction: angina, leg cramps (intermittent claudication), gradual mental deterioration, weakness or dizziness
- May be asymptomatic
- Diagonal earlobe crease

GENERAL CONSIDERATIONS

- Atherosclerosis: underlying pathogenesis in a group of disorders collectively termed *cardiovascular disease* (CVD)—heart disease or coronary artery disease (CAD), and myocardial, pulmonary, and cerebral infarction.
- CVD is number one cause of death in United States.

Understanding Atherosclerosis

Structure of an Artery

Three major layers:

- **Intima:** endothelium or internal lining of the artery; consists of layer of endothelial cells. Glycosaminoglycans (GAGs) line exposed endothelial cells to protect from damage and to promote repair. Beneath surface cells is internal elastic membrane—a layer of GAGs and other ground substance compounds, supporting endothelial cells.
- **Media:** smooth muscle cells. Interposed among the cells are GAGs and other ground substance structures that provide support and elasticity.
- **Adventitia:** external elastic membrane of connective tissue including GAGs; provides structural support and elasticity.

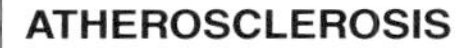

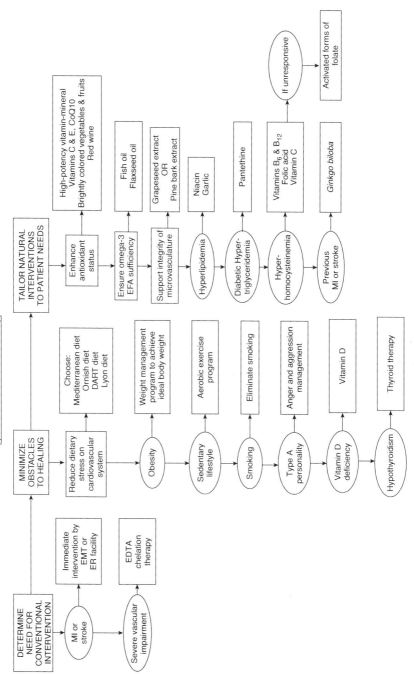

- DETERMINE NEED FOR CONVENTIONAL INTERVENTION
  - MI or stroke → Immediate intervention by EMT or ER facility
  - Severe vascular impairment → EDTA chelation therapy
- MINIMIZE OBSTACLES TO HEALING
  - Reduce dietary stress on cardiovascular system → Choose: Mediterranean diet, Ornish diet, DART diet, Lyon diet
  - Obesity → Weight management program to achieve ideal body weight
  - Sedentary lifestyle → Aerobic exercise program
  - Smoking → Eliminate smoking
  - Type A personality → Anger and aggression management
  - Vitamin D deficiency → Vitamin D
  - Hypothyroidism → Thyroid therapy
- TAILOR NATURAL INTERVENTIONS TO PATIENT NEEDS
  - Enhance antioxidant status → High-potency vitamin-mineral; Vitamins C & E, CoQ10; Brightly colored vegetables & fruits; Red wine
  - Ensure omega-3 EFA sufficiency → Fish oil; Flaxseed oil
  - Support integrity of microvasculature → Grapeseed extract OR Pine bark extract
  - Hyperlipidemia → Niacin; Garlic
  - Diabetic Hypertriglyceridemia → Pantethine
  - Hyperhomocysteinemia → Vitamins B_6 & B_{12}; Folic acid; Vitamin C → If unresponsive → Activated forms of folate
  - Previous MI or stroke → *Ginkgo biloba*

Process of Atherosclerosis

Lesions are initiated in response to injury to or disruption of normal functioning of arterial endothelium. Progression:

1. Damage or dysfunction of vascular endothelium from weakening of GAG layer as a result of insulin resistance, reactive oxygen and nitrogen species, impaired repair processes, heavy metal toxicity, hyperhomocysteinemia, and inhibition of either nitric oxide production or availability.
2. Sites of injury become more permeable to plasma constituents—lipoproteins. Binding of lipoproteins to GAGs disintegrates integrity of ground substance matrix and causes increased affinity for cholesterol. Simultaneously, monocytes, T lymphocytes, and platelets adhere to damaged area, releasing growth factors that stimulate smooth muscle cells to migrate from media into intima and replicate.
3. Smooth muscle cells dump cellular debris into intima, leading to further development of plaque.
4. Fibrous cap (collagen, elastin, and GAGs) forms over intimal surface. Fat and cholesterol deposits accumulate.
5. Plaque grows until it either blocks artery directly or ruptures to form a clot that travels through general circulation until it occludes a blood vessel. Plaque instability poses greater risk for myocardial infarction (MI) or stroke. Targeting plaque stabilization appears to be more clinically important than simply enlarging the lumen.

Causative Factors

- Risk factors are divided into two categories: major and other risk factors. The accompanying box lists the major risk factors. Risk for a heart attack increases with number of major risk factors.

Major Risk Factors for Atherosclerosis

- Smoking
- Elevated blood cholesterol levels
- High blood pressure
- Diabetes
- Physical inactivity
- Other risk factors

Association of Risk Factors with the Incidence of Atherosclerosis

Major Risk Factors	Increase in Incidence
Presence of one of the major risk factors	30%
High cholesterol and high blood pressure	300%
High cholesterol and a smoker	350%
High blood pressure and a smoker	350%
Smoker, high blood cholesterol, and high blood pressure	720%

- Others may be more significant. See box that lists these additional factors.
- Develop strategic approach to plaque stabilization by addressing endothelial dysfunction, local and systemic inflammation, reactive oxygen species, activation of mast cells, and infiltration and activation of macrophages.

Other Risk Factors for Atherosclerosis

- Insulin resistance
- Low thyroid function (*Textbook,* Hypothyroidism)
- Low antioxidant status
- Elevations of C-reactive protein (CRP)
- Low levels of essential fatty acids
- Increased platelet aggregation
- Increased fibrinogen formation
- Low levels of magnesium and potassium
- Elevated levels of homocysteine
- "Type A" personality

Determining a Patient's Risk

To help determine a patient's overall risk for heart attack or stroke, try the risk-determination scale. Although it does not address several other factors—CRP, lipoprotein(a) [Lp(a)], fibrinogen, and coping style—the score provides good indication of patient's risk for heart attack or stroke.

Risk-Determination Scale for Heart Disease and Stroke

	SCALE OF RISK				
	1	**2**	**3**	**4**	**5**
Blood pressure (systolic)	<125	125-134	135-149	150-164	≥165
Blood pressure (diastolic)	<90	90-94	95-104	105-114	≥115
Smoking (cigarettes per day)	None	1-9	10-19	20-29	≥30
Heredity I*	None	>65	50-64	35-49	<35
Heredity II†	0	1	2	4	≥4
Diabetes duration (years)	0	1-5	6-10	11-15	>15
Total cholesterol (mg/dL)	<200	200-224	225-249	250-274	≥275
HDL-C (mg/dL)	≥75	65-74	55-64	35-54	<35
Total cholesterol/ HDL-C ratio‡	<3	3-3.9	4-4.9	5-6.4	≥6.5
Exercise (hours per week)	>4	3-4	2-3	1-2	0.1
Supplemental EPA/DHA (mg) intake	>600	400–599	200-399	100-199	<100
Supplemental vitamin C (mg) and vitamin E (IU) intake	>400	251-499	250	125-249	0-124
Average daily servings of fruits and vegetables	>5	4-5	3	1-2	0
Age	<35	36-45	46-55	56-65	>65
Subtotals					

*Age of patient when he or she had a heart attack or stroke.
†Number of immediate family members having had a heart attack before the age of 50.
‡The value of the total cholesterol is to be divided by the value of the HDL-C.
Risk = sum of all five columns; 14-20 = very low risk; 21-30 = low risk; 31-40 = average risk; 41-50 = high risk; ≥51 = very high risk.
DHA, docosahexaenoic acid; EPA, eicosapentaenoic acid; HDL-C, high-density–lipoprotein cholesterol; IU, international units.

Clinical Evaluation

Complete cardiovascular assessment can include tests listed in the accompanying box.

Assessment of the Cardiovascular System

- Laboratory tests
- Total cholesterol
- Low-density–lipoprotein cholesterol
- High-density–lipoprotein cholesterol
- C-reactive protein
- Lipoprotein(a)
- Fibrinogen
- Homocysteine
- Ferritin (an iron-binding protein)
- Lipid peroxides
- Exercise stress test
- Electrocardiography
- Echocardiography

Risk Factors

Smoking

- Most important risk factor for CVD; smokers have 70% greater risk of death from CVD than nonsmokers. The more cigarettes smoked and the longer the period of years smoking, the greater the risk of dying from a heart attack or stroke.
- Average smoker dies 7 to 8 years sooner than nonsmoker.
- Tobacco smoke contains 4000 chemicals; more than 50 are carcinogens extremely damaging to cardiovascular system. These toxins are carried in bloodstream on low-density–lipoprotein cholesterol (LDL-C). They either damage lining of arteries directly or damage LDL-C molecule, which then damages arteries.
- Elevated LDL-C worsens effect of smoking on cardiovascular system: more toxins travel through it.
- Smoking elevates cholesterol, presumably by damaging liver feedback mechanisms, which control cholesterol synthesis.
- Smoking promotes platelet aggregation and elevated fibrinogen, independent risk factors for CVD.
- Smoking elevates blood pressure.
- Even passive exposure to cigarette smoke is damaging to cardiovascular health.
- There is a 36% reduction in relative risk of mortality for patients with CAD who quit compared with those who continued smoking.

- Encouragement to stop smoking by physicians during routine office call results in 2% cessation rate after 1 year. Supplementary measures—follow-up letters or visits—have additional effect. Behavioral modification in group or individual sessions led by psychologists has no greater effect than 2% rate from simple advice from a physician. Acupuncture has overall efficacy of 3%. Hypnosis has been judged ineffective because no biomedical marker has been used, even though it has a success rate of 23%. Nicotine replacement therapy (gum or patch) is effective in 13% of smokers. Collectively, these results are not encouraging. It appears that the best results occur when people quit "cold turkey."

Tips to Help Patients Stop Smoking

- List all the reasons why you want to quit smoking and review them daily.
- Set a specific day to quit, tell at least 10 friends that you are going to quit smoking, and then ... DO IT!
- Throw away all cigarettes, butts, matches, and ashtrays.
- Use substitutes. Instead of smoking, chew on raw vegetables, fruits, or gum. If your fingers seem empty, play with a pencil.
- Take one day at a time.
- Realize that 40 million Americans have quit. If they can do it, so can you!
- Visualize yourself as a nonsmoker with a fatter pocketbook, pleasant breath, unstained teeth, and the satisfaction that comes from being in control of your life.
- Join a support group. Call the local branch of the American Cancer Society and ask for referrals. You are not alone.
- When you need to relax, perform deep breathing exercises rather than reaching for a cigarette.
- Avoid situations that you associate with smoking.
- Each day, reward yourself in a positive way. Buy yourself something with the money you have saved or plan a special reward as a celebration for quitting.

Elevated Blood Cholesterol Levels

- Elevated cholesterol greatly increases risk of death from CVD. Recommendations: total cholesterol (TC) below 200 mg/dL; LDL-C below 130 mg/dL; high-density–lipoprotein cholesterol (HDL-C) above 40 mg/dL in men and 50 mg/dL in women; triglycerides (TGs) below 150 mg/dL.
- Cholesterol is transported in the blood by lipoproteins. Major categories of lipoproteins are very-low-density lipoprotein (VLDL), LDL, and HDL.
- VLDL and LDL transport fats (TGs and cholesterol) from liver to body cells. HDL returns fats to the liver. Elevations of either VLDL or LDL are linked to increased risk for atherosclerosis.

- Elevations of HDL-C are associated with low risk of heart attacks.
- Ratios of TC to HDL-C and of LDL-C to HDL-C are cardiac risk factor ratios; they reflect whether cholesterol is being deposited into tissues or broken down and excreted. Recommended ratio of TC to HDL-C is below 4.2; ratio of LDL-C to HDL-C is above 2.5.
- Lower LDL-C and raise HDL-C: for every 1% drop in LDL-C, risk of heart attack drops by 2%. For every 1% increase in HDL-C, risk for heart attack drops 3% to 4%.

Further Refinement of Determining Risk

- LDL-C is termed "bad cholesterol," but some forms are worse than others. Oxidized LDL-C is proinflammatory trigger for progression of atherosclerosis and plaque rupture.
- Smaller LDL-C molecules of higher density are linked to greater risk than larger, less-dense molecules. Small, dense LDL-C contains more apolipoprotein CIII (ApoCIII). ApoB particles are more atherogenic than larger, less-dense LDL-Cs and are markers for CVD risk. Smaller particles are more heavily and preferentially glycated than larger, more buoyant LDL-C particles, suggesting importance of avoiding hyperglycemia and excessive glycation.
- Lp(a) is a plasma lipoprotein whose structure and composition resemble LDL-C but with additional adhesive protein called *apolipoprotein(a).* Elevated Lp(a) is independent risk factor for CHD, particularly with elevated LDL-C. High Lp(a) is associated with 10 times greater risk for heart disease than elevated LDL-C. That is because LDL-C on its own lacks adhesive apolipoprotein(a). LDL-C does not easily stick to artery walls. High LDL-C carries less risk than normal or low LDL-C with high Lp(a). Lp(a) below 20 mg/dL poses low risk; levels between 20 and 40 mg/dL pose moderate risk; levels above 40 mg/dL pose high risk.

Elevations of Triglycerides

- Hypertriglyceridemia (HTG) is independent risk factor for CVD. HTG combined with elevated LDL-C and high LDL-C/HDL-C ratio (>5) increases risk sixfold. An 88-mg/dL (1.0-mmol/L) increase in plasma TG increases relative risk of CVD by 30% in men and 75% in women.
- Metabolic interrelationships among TG levels and other risk factors—atherogenic lipid profile: low HDL-C and elevated

small, dense LDL; insulin resistance; prothrombotic propensity; and low grade systemic inflammation.
- Plan and execute TG-lowering strategy.

Inherited Elevations of Cholesterol and Triglycerides

- Elevations of blood lipids can be caused by genetic factors—familial hypercholesterolemia (FH), familial combined hyperlipidemia (FCH), and familial hypertriglyceridemia (FHTG).
- Among the most common inherited diseases, affecting 1 in 500 people.
- Problem: defect in receptor protein for LDL-C in the liver. Normally, the liver LDL-C receptor removes cholesterol from the blood by facilitating binding and absorption of LDL-C by the liver cell. The receptor signals the liver cell to stop making cholesterol. In FH, defective LDL-C receptors fail to send that message.
- Damage to LDL-C receptors occurs with normal aging and in disease states; diabetes is prominent owing to glycosylation of receptor proteins.
- Cholesterol tends to rise with age.
- Diet high in saturated fat and cholesterol decreases number of LDL-C receptors, reducing negative feedback mechanism to liver cells.
- Lifestyle and dietary changes can increase function or number of LDL-C receptors or both. The most dramatic effects are in people without inherited causes, but even people with FH can benefit.
- FCH, FHTG, and FH have similar defects. In FCH, there is accelerated liver production of VLDL. Patients may have only high blood TGs, only high cholesterol, or both. In FHTG, there is only elevated TGs, and HDL-C tend to be low. In FHTG, VLDL particles made by the liver are larger than normal and carry more TGs. FHTG is worsened by diabetes, gout, and obesity.
- Recommendations given later under "Therapeutic Considerations" for lowering lipids are helpful for FCH and FHTG, although these conditions require more-aggressive support.

Diabetes

- Atherosclerosis is a key factor in chronic complications of diabetes.
- Diabetics have twofold to threefold higher risk of dying prematurely of heart disease or stroke than nondiabetics; 55% of deaths in diabetics are caused by CVD.
- Even mild insulin resistance and poor glucose control increase incidence and progression of CVD. See chapter on diabetes.

High Blood Pressure

Elevated blood pressure is often a sign of considerable atherosclerosis and a major risk factor for heart attack or stroke. Presence of hypertension is the most significant risk factor for stroke.

Physical Inactivity

- Sedentary lifestyle is major risk factor for CVD.
- Physical activity protects against development of CVD and favorably modifies other CVD risk factors—high blood pressure, blood lipids, insulin resistance, and obesity.
- Physical activity treats and manages CVD or increased risk—hypertension, stable angina, prior MI, peripheral vascular disease, heart failure, or recovering from cardiovascular event.

Other Risk Factors

- More significant than so-called major risk factors. More than 300 risk factors have been identified.
- Inflammatory mediators influence stages of atheroma development.
- CRP, an acute-phase reactant reflecting degrees of inflammation, is an independent risk factor for CAD. CRP level is a stronger predictor of cardiovascular events than LDL-C level; screening for both biomarkers is more prognostic. Elevated CRP is linked to insulin resistance and metabolic syndrome.
- Diagnostic criteria for metabolic syndrome include at least three of the following metabolic risk factors in one person:
  - Central obesity (waist-to-hip ratio >1 for men; >0.8 for women)
  - Atherogenic dyslipidemia (TGs >150 mg/dL; low HDL-C [<40 mg/dL in men and <50 mg/dL in women])
  - Hypertension (≥130/85 mm Hg)
  - Insulin resistance or glucose intolerance (fasting blood sugar >101 mg/dL)
  - Prothrombotic state (e.g., high fibrinogen or plasminogen activator inhibitor in the blood)
  - Proinflammatory state (e.g., elevated high-sensitivity CRP in the blood)

THERAPEUTIC CONSIDERATIONS—GENERAL GUIDELINES

- Reduce risk factors: smoking, obesity, physical inactivity, diabetes, and hypertension. Healthy diet and lifestyle dramatically reduce CVD-related mortality.

- Improve blood cholesterol levels.
- Address additional risk factors: antioxidant status, elevated CRP, fibrinogen levels.

Diet—General Guidelines

- Reduce saturated fat and *trans* fatty acids.
- Increase vegetables, fruit, dietary fiber, monounsaturated fats, and omega-3 fatty acids.
- Improve structure and composition of cell membranes with essential structural components—monounsaturated and omega-3 fatty acids.
- Prevent oxidative and free radical damage with antioxidants.
- Mediterranean diet:
  - Olive oil: principal source of fat.
  - Centers on abundance of plant food (fruits; potatoes, beans, other vegetables; breads; pasta; nuts; seeds).
  - Foods are minimally processed, and people focus on seasonally fresh and locally grown.
  - Fresh fruit: daily dessert; sweets containing concentrated sugars or honey consumed only a few times a week.
  - Dairy products (cheese and yogurt) consumed daily in low to moderate amounts.
  - Fish consumed regularly.
  - Poultry and eggs in moderate amounts (up to four times a week) or not at all.
  - Red meat in low amounts.
  - Wine in low to moderate amounts, normally with meals.
- Total benefit of this diet reflects interplay among many beneficial compounds rather than any single factor.
- Follow low glycemic diet. Consumption of foods with high glycemic load increases risk of CHD in women by 68%; women in highest glycemic-load quartile have relative risk of 2.2 for CHD compared with those in lowest quartile.

Olive Oil and Omega-3 Fatty Acids

- Olive oil consists not only of monounsaturated fatty acid (oleic acid) but also several antioxidants.
- Olive oil mildly lowers LDL-C and TGs, increases HDL-C, and helps prevent LDL-C oxidation.
- Longer-chain omega-3 fatty acids eicosapentaenoic acid (EPA) and docosahexaenoic acid (DHA) have little effect on cholesterol levels; but they lower TGs significantly, reduce platelet aggregation; improve endothelial function and arterial flexibility;

improve blood and oxygen supply to the heart; and mildly lower blood pressure by vasodilation and promoting sodium excretion.

- Levels of EPA and DHA within red blood cells are good predictors of heart disease. These laboratory values is termed the **omega-3 index.** An omega-3 index of 8% is linked to greatest protection; index of 4% is linked to the least.
- Omega-3 index may be the best predictor of CAD compared with CRP; TC, LDL-C, or HDL-C; and homocysteine.
- Combined 1000 mg of EPA and DHA daily achieves or surpasses the 8% target of omega-3 index.
- Raising omega-3s through diet or supplements may reduce overall cardiovascular mortality by 45%.
- Dose recommendation: 1000 mg EPA plus DHA a day.
- To lower TGs: 3000 mg EPA plus DHA q.d.
- Although longer-chain omega-3s exert more-pronounced effects than alpha-linolenic acid (ALA) from vegetable sources, populations with lowest rates of heart attack have relatively high intake of ALA: Japanese on Kohama Island and people of Crete. Intake of ALA is viewed as more a protective factor than oleic acid.

Nuts and Seeds

- Higher consumption of nuts and seeds reduces risk of CVD.
- Substituting nuts for equivalent amount of carbohydrates reduces heart disease risk by 30%.
- More impressive 45% risk reduction arises when fat from nuts is substituted for saturated fats (meat and dairy).
- Nuts have cholesterol-lowering effect.
- Nuts are rich source of L-arginine, precursor of nitric oxide. By increasing nitric oxide, arginine may improve blood flow, reduce blood clotting, and improve blood fluidity (less viscous).
- Walnuts are rich source of both antioxidants and ALA. In comparing a cholesterol-lowering Mediterranean diet with a diet in which walnuts replace 32% of energy from monounsaturated fat (olive oil) for 4 weeks, the walnut diet improved endothelial cell function (increased endothelium-dependent vasodilation and reduced vascular cell adhesion molecule 1). The walnut diet also reduced TC (−4.4%) and LDL-C (−6.4%).

Vegetables, Fruits, and Red Wine

- Mediterranean diet focuses on carotene- and flavonoid-rich fruits, vegetables, and beverages (e.g., red wine).

- Dietary antioxidants reduce risk of heart disease and stroke. Higher blood levels of antioxidants are linked to lower levels of CRP.
- Sources of antioxidants in Mediterranean diet: tomato products and red wine.
- **Tomatoes** contain the carotene lycopene. Lycopene exerts greater antioxidant activity compared with beta-carotene in general but specifically against LDL-C oxidation.
- **Red wine "French paradox"** may arise from flavonoids and other polyphenols in red wine that protect against oxidative damage to LDL-C and reduce inflammatory mediators. Yet moderate alcohol consumption alone is protective by improving ratios of HDL-C to LDL-C and CRP and levels of fibrinogen. Red wine exerts greatest effects.
- Effects of alcohol on CVD risk, morbidity, and total mortality are counterbalanced by alcohol's addictive and psychological effects.
- Major benefits of red wine polyphenols improve endothelial cell function. Grape polyphenol extract (600 mg) causes an increase in flow-mediated dilation, peaking at 60 minutes.
- **Green tea** reduces risk for CVD. Mechanism: improves endothelial cell function. Green tea polyphenols (catechins) decrease oxidation of LDL-C, lower LDL-C levels, and improve LDL-C/HDL-C ratio. A dose-dependent response with green tea polyphenols reduces several biomarkers of atherosclerosis and ischemia (e.g., inhibition of endothelial cell–derived vascular cell adhesion molecule 1, angiotensin II, platelet-derived growth factor BB, ApoE, and inducible nitric oxide synthase).
- Another mechanism of action for red wine and green tea polyphenols: inhibiting formation of new blood vessels within the vascular lesion. Angiogenesis is controlled by two major proangiogenic factors: matrix metalloproteinases (MMPs), which degrade extracellular matrices, and vascular endothelial growth factor (VEGF), which stimulates endothelial cell migration and proliferation and the formation of new blood vessels. Both red wine and green tea polyphenols inhibit this process in vitro.
- **Foods and beverages rich in antioxidants. Pomegranate *(Punica granatum)* juice:** remarkably rich in antioxidants—soluble polyphenols, tannins, and anthocyanins. Components of pomegranate juice can retard atherosclerosis, reduce plaque formation, and improve arterial health. In patients with CHD and myocardial ischemia, pomegranate juice (240 mL/day for 3 months) reduced stress-induced ischemia, without changes in

cardiac medications, blood sugar, hemoglobin A_{1c}, weight, or blood pressure. In a study of progression of carotid lesions and changes in oxidative stress and blood pressure, pomegranate juice (50 mL daily for 1 to 3 years) induced reduction in common carotid intima-media thickness (IMT), by up to 30%, after 1 year. Pomegranate juice increased serum paraoxonase 1 (PON1) activity by 83%, reduced serum LDL-C basal oxidative state and LDL-C susceptibility. It decreased antibodies against oxidized LDL-C and increased serum total antioxidant status, reduced systolic blood pressure. Maximal effects were observed after 1 year of pomegranate juice consumption.

THERAPEUTIC CONSIDERATIONS—LOWERING CHOLESTEROL

- Conventional medicine lowers TC, LDL-C, and TGs using HMG-CoA (3-hydroxy-3-methylglutaryl-coenzyme A) reductase inhibitors, called **statin drugs.** Statins originated with red yeast *(Monascus purpureus)* fermented on rice, a traditional Chinese medicine used for 2000 years. Red yeast rice provides compounds termed **monacolins** (e.g., lovastatin, also called monacolin K). The U.S. Food and Drug Administration (FDA) has ruled that red yeast rice products can be sold only if free of monacolin. Debate remains whether statins constitute optimal primary prevention of CAD in patients with only elevated LDL-C, especially relative to CRP and role of nutrition. Diversifying cholesterol-lowering components in the same dietary portfolio, efficacy of dietary treatment of hypercholesterolemia is increased. Results are comparable with those of statins (with similar lipid-lowering effects for LDL-C and size of LDL-C).
- Best clinical approach: incorporate broad-spectrum array of dietary components with positive impact on lipids.

Importance of Soluble Dietary Fiber in Lowering Cholesterol

- Soluble dietary fiber found in legumes, fruits, and vegetables lowers cholesterol.
- The greater the degree of viscosity or gel-forming nature, the greater the effect on lowering cholesterol.
- New, highly viscous, soluble fiber blends are showing greater effect than previously used fiber sources.
- Patients with high cholesterol levels see significant reductions with frequent oatmeal or oat bran consumption.

- In individuals with high cholesterol levels above 200 mg/dL, consuming 3 g of soluble oat fiber lowers TC by 8% to 23%.
- Polyunsaturated fatty acids contribute as much to cholesterol-lowering effects of oats as fiber content. Although oat bran has higher fiber content, oatmeal is higher in polyunsaturated fatty acids.
- Encourage patients to eat 35 g of fiber daily from fiber-rich foods.
- Achieving higher fiber intake is also associated with lower inflammatory mediators such as CRP.

Impact of Various Sources of Fiber on Serum Cholesterol Levels

Fiber	Dose (g)	Typical Reduction in Total Cholesterol
Oat bran (dry)	50-100	20%
Guar gum	9-15	10%
Pectin	6-10	5%
Psyllium	10-20	10% to 20%
Vegetable fiber	27	10%

Natural Products to Lower Cholesterol Levels

In many cases, dietary therapy, although important, is not sufficient alone to normalize lipid levels.

Niacin

- Niacin is the only proven cholesterol-lowering agent that actually reduces overall mortality.
- Niacin lowers LDL-C by 16% to 23% and raises HDL-C by 20% to 33%. These effects compare quite favorably with conventional drugs.
- Niacin lowers LDL-C, Lp(a), TGs, CRP, and fibrinogen levels and concurrently raises HDL-C.
- Niacin has advantages over statin drugs. Although lovastatin produces greater reduction in LDL-C, niacin provides better overall results despite the fact that fewer patients are able to tolerate full dose of niacin because of skin flushing. Percentage increase in HDL-C, a better indicator for CHD, is dramatically in favor of niacin (33% versus 7%). Although niacin produces a 35% reduction in Lp(a), lovastatin did not produce any effect. Niacin reduces Lp(a) even in diabetics.

- In patients with normal TCs but low HDL-C, niacin at 4.5 g/day, increased HDL-C by 6% to 10%; niacin, by 30%.
- In patients with abnormal, atherogenic, small, dense LDL-C particles and low levels of specific fraction of HDL-C with greater protective effect, niacin at 3000 mg daily increased LDL-C particle size and raised HDL-C and HDL-2C better than statins.
- Niacin at higher doses (≥3000 mg q.d.) can impair glucose tolerance and has been avoided in diabetic patients. Newer studies with slightly lower doses (1000 to 2000 mg) show no adverse effect on blood sugar regulation. Other studies actually show reduced hemoglobin A_{1c}, indicating improved blood sugar control.
- The most common blood lipid abnormalities in patients with type 2 diabetes are elevated TGs; decreased HDL-C; and preponderance of small, dense LDL-C particles. Niacin addresses all these areas better than lipid-lowering drugs.
- Niacin produces beneficial lipid-altering effects on particle distribution in patients with CAD that are not well reflected in typical lipoprotein analysis.
- Systemic markers of inflammation decrease in patients receiving niacin. Niacin decreases lipoprotein-associated phospholipase A_2 and CRP levels (20% and 15%, respectively).
- The addition of niacin to existing medical regimens for patients with CAD and already well-controlled lipid levels improves distribution of lipoprotein particle sizes and inflammatory markers in a manner expected to improve protection against a cardiovascular event.
- Niacin does not appear to enhance benefits of statins in patients with well-controlled lipid levels. Other studies are under way to determine effect of niacin combined with statins in patients with very low HDL-C and/or poorly controlled LDL-C.

Side Effects of Niacin

- Skin flushing that typically occurs 20 to 30 minutes after ingestion.
- Other occasional side effects: gastric irritation, nausea, liver damage.
- To combat skin flushing, sustained-release, timed-release, and slow-release niacin products are available. However, earlier timed-release preparations were more toxic to the liver than regular niacin.
- Newer timed-released preparations—intermediate-release products—are well tolerated even when combined with statin drugs.

- The safety and tolerability of intermediate-release niacin preparation have been evaluated. Most adverse reactions were mild or moderate in severity. Researchers concluded that intermediate-release nicotinic acid is well tolerated.
- Inositol hexaniacinate has long been used in Europe to lower cholesterol and improve blood flow in intermittent claudication. It yields slightly better clinical results than standard niacin but is much better tolerated with fewer side effects.
- Regardless of form used, periodic checking (at least every 3 months) of cholesterol and liver function is indicated.
- Avoid niacin in patients with preexisting liver disease or elevations in liver enzymes. Alternatives: policosanol, garlic, or pantethine.
- For best results, niacin should be taken at night, because most cholesterol synthesis occurs during sleep. If pure crystalline niacin is used, begin with 100 mg a day and increase over 4 to 6 weeks to full therapeutic dose of 1.5 to 3 g/day. If a timed-released preparation or inositol hexaniacinate is used, give 500-mg dose at night and increase to 1500 mg after 2 weeks. If after 1 month of therapy the dose of 1500 mg/day fails to lower LDL-C, increase dose to 3000 mg.

Plant Sterols and Stanols

- Phytosterols and phytostanols are structurally similar to cholesterol and can act in the intestine to lower cholesterol absorption by displacing cholesterol from intestinal micelles. Because phytosterols and phytostanols are poorly absorbed themselves, blood cholesterol drops owing to increased excretion. These compounds are in functional foods (e.g., margarine and other spreads, orange juice) and in supplements.
- Phytosterols and phytostanols lower LDL-C in some people. Daily intake of 2 g of stanols or sterols reduces LDL-C by 10%. Higher doses produce little additional benefit. Effects of phytosterols and phytostanols are additive with diet or drug interventions; eating foods low in saturated fat and cholesterol and high in stanols or sterols can reduce LDL-C by 20%; adding sterols or stanols to statins is more effective than doubling statin dose alone. Individuals most likely to respond have high cholesterol absorption and low cholesterol biosynthesis. Phytosterols and phytostanols have antiplatelet and antioxidant effects as well.
- Phytosterol or phytostanol intake at higher doses may reduce carotenoid absorption. However, this effect is partially reversed by increasing fruit and vegetable intake.

Pantethine

- Pantethine is stable form of pantetheine, active form of vitamin B_5 or pantothenic acid. Pantothenic acid is most important component of coenzyme A (CoA), key to transport of fats within cells and energy-producing mitochondria. Without CoA, fats could not be metabolized to energy.
- Pantethine has lipid-lowering activity; pantothenic acid has little owing to pantethine's ability to be converted to cysteamine. Pantethine therapy (900 mg/day) reduces serum TG (−32%), TC (-19%) and LDL-C (−21%) and increases HDL-C (+23%). It appears to be especially useful in lowering blood lipids in diabetic patients.
- Lipid-lowering effects of pantethine are most impressive when its toxicity (virtually none) is compared with drugs.
- Mechanism of action: inhibition of cholesterol synthesis and acceleration of fat metabolism as an energy source.

Garlic (*Allium sativum*) and Onion (*Allium cepa*)

- Garlic affects process of atherosclerosis at many steps.
- Garlic lowers blood cholesterol even in apparently healthy persons. Commercial preparations providing daily dose of at least 10 mg of alliin or a total allicin potential of 4000 mg can lower total serum cholesterol by about 10% to 12% and LDL-C by 15%; HDL-C usually increases by 10% and TGs drop by 15%.
- Although effects are modest, the combination of lowering LDL-C and raising HDL-C can greatly improve HDL-C/LDL-C ratio.
- Garlic preparations reduce elevated blood pressure, inhibit platelet aggregation, reduce plasma viscosity, promote fibrinolysis, prevent LDL-C oxidation, and exert positive effects on endothelial function, vascular reactivity, and peripheral blood flow.

Comparing Natural Cholesterol-Lowering Agents

Comparative Effects on Blood Lipids of Several Natural Compounds

	Niacin	Garlic	Policosanol	Pantethine
TC (% decrease)	18	10	24	19
LDL-C (% decrease)	23	15	25	21
HDL-C (% increase)	32	31	15	23
TGs (% decrease)	26	13	5	32

HDL-C, high-density–lipoprotein cholesterol; LDL-C, low-density–lipoprotein cholesterol; TC, total cholesterol; TGs, triglycerides.

Niacin produces best overall effect. Niacin (1500 to 3000 mg at night) reduces TC by 50 to 75 mg/dL within first 2 months in patients with initial TC higher than 250 mg/dL. In patients with initial cholesterol higher than 300 mg/dL, it may take 4 to 6 months before levels begin to normalize. Once cholesterol is below 200 mg/dL, reduce niacin by 500 mg for 2 months. If cholesterol creeps up above 200 mg/dL, increase niacin dose to previous levels. If cholesterol remains below 200 mg/dL, drop niacin by another 500 mg and recheck cholesterol levels in 2 months. Continue with this reduction in dose until niacin can be stopped entirely and cholesterol levels remain below 200 mg/dL.

- Pantethine is recommended primarily for HTG, especially in diabetics. It not only improves cholesterol and TG levels but also normalizes platelet lipid composition and function and blood viscosity.
- For high Lp(a), both niacin and vitamin C reduce Lp(a) dramatically (−35% and −27%, respectively).
- **Rule out hypothyroidism** in all patients with elevated blood lipids, especially elevated Lp(a). Patients with overt hypothyroidism are prone to CAD because of increased LDL-C and decreased HDL-C.
- **"Subclinical" hypothyroidism:** Patients with subclinical hypothyroidism (normal T_3 and free thyroxine index with a raised thyroid-stimulating hormone [TSH] level) have not only elevated levels of LDL-C but also elevated Lp(a). See chapter on hypothyroidism.

THERAPEUTIC CONSIDERATIONS—ANTIOXIDANT STATUS

- Dietary antioxidant nutrients protect against development of CVD. Fats and cholesterol are susceptible to free radical damage. Damaged fats and cholesterol form lipid peroxides and oxidized cholesterol, which damage artery walls and accelerate progression of atherosclerosis. Antioxidants block formation of damaging compounds.
- Human antioxidant system is a complex scenario of interacting components. No single antioxidant can be effective, especially in absence of supporting cast. Most antioxidants require "partner" antioxidants, allowing them to work more efficiently (e.g., vitamins C and E, selenium, and coenzyme Q10 [CoQ10]).
- Phytochemicals and plant-derived antioxidants potentiate activities of vitamin and mineral antioxidants. Phytochemicals such as carotenes (lycopene and lutein) and flavonoids prevent free radical damage. Beta-carotene is of little importance in protecting

against LDL-C oxidation. (Unlike lycopene and lutein, beta-carotene does not become incorporated into LDL-C effectively, although it may help protect the endothelium.)

- Lutein may be the most effective carotene against atherosclerosis. Lycopene, beta-carotene, and cryptoxanthin are mainly located in larger, less-dense LDL-C particles; lutein and zeaxanthin are found preferentially in most easily oxidized, smaller, denser LDL-C particles.
- Support of nonantioxidant vitamins and minerals may also be important. Multivitamin-multimineral supplements are appropriate. Serum vitamin B_6 and vitamin C levels are inversely associated with CRP level.

Vitamin E, Coenzyme Q10, and Selenium

- Vitamin E protects against oxidation of LDL-C because it is easily incorporated into LDL-C molecule.

Effect of Increasing Doses of Vitamin E on Oxidation Parameters

Dose (mg/day)	Lag Time*	Propagation Rate†
0	94	7.8
25	99	8
50	100	7.9
100	106	7.7
200	111	7.5
400	116	6.8
800	120	6.5

*The time before oxidation occurs after the addition of an oxidizing agent. The higher the number, the greater the beneficial effect.

†The rate at which lipid peroxidation progresses. The lower the number, the greater the beneficial effect.

- The higher the dose of vitamin E, the greater the degree of protection against oxidative damage to LDL-C. Doses above 400 IU produce clinically significant effects.
- Vitamin E improves insulin sensitivity and plasma lipids in non–insulin-dependent diabetics.
- Vitamin E levels may be more predictive of incipient heart attack or stroke than TC levels.
- French paradox may arise from higher vitamin E levels, as well as red wine.

Vitamin E protects against heart disease and strokes by its ability to do the following:

- Reduce LDL-C peroxidation and increase plasma LDL-C breakdown
- Inhibit excessive platelet aggregation
- Increase HDL-C
- Increase fibrinolytic activity
- Reduce CRP
- Improve endothelial cell function
- Improve insulin sensitivity

Large-scale studies of vitamin E and CVD have resulted in conflicting and inconsistent outcomes. Some disappointing results may have arisen from the choice of synthetic vitamin E (D,L-alpha-tocopherol) versus the more-active natural form (D-alpha tocopherol). There is also the problem of the interference by statin drugs in vitamin E and CoQ10 metabolism, thereby increasing needs for both compounds.

- Vitamin E and CoQ10 work synergistically; each is required for regeneration of the other. Blood CoQ10 is in both oxidized (inactive) and reduced (active) forms. During increased oxidative stress or low vitamin E, more CoQ10 is converted to its oxidized (inactive form). With provision of higher vitamin E, biologic activity of CoQ10 is enhanced, and vice versa.
- Combination of vitamin E and CoQ10 works better than either alone.
- In addition to CoQ10, vitamin E also requires adequate selenium for optimal antioxidant effects. Selenium is a component of antioxidant enzyme glutathione peroxidase. This enzyme works with vitamin E to prevent free radical damage to cell membranes. Studies of vitamin E in cancer and heart disease are often faulty because they fail to encompass partnership among selenium, vitamin E, and CoQ10.
- Low selenium status is associated with CAD.

Intervention Trials with Vitamin E for Secondary Prevention

Study	Number of Subjects	Dose	Duration	Outcome
HOPE (2000)	9541	400 IU (D-alpha)	4.5 years	No effect
SPACE (2000)	196	800 IU (D-alpha)	1.4 years	−70%
GISSI (1999)	11,324	300 IU (synthetic)	3.5 years	−35% (vs. placebo)
CHAOS (1996)	9541	400-800 IU (D-alpha)	1.4 years	−47%

Vitamin C

- Vitamin C is an antioxidant in aqueous (water) environments in outside and inside cells. It is first line of antioxidant protection in the body. Its primary antioxidant partner is fat-soluble vitamin E.
- Along with CoQ10, vitamin C regenerates oxidized vitamin E.
- Vitamin C works with antioxidant enzymes (e.g., glutathione peroxidase, catalase, and superoxide dismutase).
- Vitamin C helps prevent LDL-C oxidation, even in smokers.
- High dietary intake of vitamin C reduces risk of death from heart attacks and strokes, and other causes including cancer. Reductions in disease risk correspond to increased longevity of 5 to 7 years for men and 1 to 3 years for women.
- Vitamin C levels correspond to TC and HDL-C. The higher the vitamin C content of blood, the lower TC and TGs and the higher HDL-C. The benefits for HDL-C were particularly impressive.

In summary, vitamin C lowers risk of CVD by doing the following:

- Acting as an antioxidant
- Strengthening collagen structures of arteries
- Lowering TC, Lp(a), and blood pressure
- Raising HDL-C levels
- Inhibiting platelet aggregation
- Promoting fibrinolysis
- Reducing markers of inflammation

Grapeseed and Pine Bark Extracts

- Plant flavonoids are proanthocyanidins (procyanidins or procyanidonic oligomers [PCOs]).
- PCOs exist in many plants and in red wine.
- Commercial sources of PCOs include extracts from grapeseeds and bark of maritime (Landes) pine.
- Mechanisms of protection: antioxidant activity, effects on endothelial cells.

THERAPEUTIC CONSIDERATIONS—MISCELLANEOUS RISK FACTORS

Platelet Aggregation

- Once platelets aggregate, they release compounds that dramatically promote formation of atherosclerotic plaque, or they can form a clot.

- Adhesiveness of platelets is determined largely by types of dietary fats and level of antioxidants.
- Although saturated fats and cholesterol increase platelet aggregation, omega-3s (both short-chain and long-chain) and monounsaturated fats have the opposite effect.
- Adding **monounsaturated and omega-3 fatty acids,** antioxidant nutrients, and flavonoids, vitamin B_6 also inhibits platelet aggregation and lowers blood pressure and homocysteine levels.
- A significant inverse graded relationship exists between serum pyridoxal-5-phosphate (P5P) and both CRP and fibrinogen. CAD risk from low P5P is additive when considered in combination with elevated CRP concentrations or with an increased LDL-C/HDL-C ratio.
- **Vitamin B_6** supplementation may help reduce risk of atherosclerotic mortality.
- **Garlic** preparations standardized for alliin content and garlic oil inhibit platelet aggregation.

Fibrinogen

- Elevated fibrinogen levels are another clear risk factor for CVD. There is a stronger association between cardiovascular deaths and fibrinogen levels than for cholesterol.
- Natural therapies designed to promote fibrinolysis: exercise, omega-3s, niacin, garlic, and nattokinase.
- **Mediterranean diet** alone reduces fibrinogen and other markers of inflammation: 20% lower CRP, 17% lower interleukin-6, 15% lower homocysteine, and 6% lower fibrinogen.
- **Natto** is a traditional Japanese food prepared from fermented soybeans by *Bacillus subtilis.*
- **Nattokinase** is a serine proteinase isolated from natto with potent fibrinolytic and thrombolytic activity.
- In patients with cardiovascular risk factors and patients undergoing dialysis, two capsules of nattokinase (2000 fibrinolysis units per capsule) daily orally for 2 months decreased fibrinogen, factor VII, and factor VIII by 7%, 13%, and 19%, respectively, for the cardiovascular group; and 10%, 7%, and 19%, respectively, for the dialysis group.

Homocysteine

- Homocysteine is an intermediate in conversion of amino acid methionine to cysteine.

- Functionally deficiency in folic acid, vitamin B_6, or vitamin B_{12} causes homocysteine to rise.
- Elevated homocysteine is an independent risk factor for heart attack, stroke, or peripheral vascular disease. Elevations in homocysteine are found in 20% to 40% of patients with heart disease and are associated with CAD.
- For each increase of 5 μmol/L in homocysteine, risk of CHD increases by 20%, independently of traditional CHD risk factors.
- Interrelated atherogenic mechanisms arising from hyperhomocyteinemia: advanced thickening and smooth muscle cell proliferation of endothelial vessel wall intima, enhanced lipid deposition in vessel walls, forced detachment of endothelial cells, activation of leukocytes and thrombocytes, increased LDL-C oxidation, initiation of platelet thromboxane synthesis, enhanced oxidative stress induced by peroxide formation during homocysteine oxidation, and prothrombotic coagulation interference.
- Homocysteine promotes atherosclerosis by damaging the artery, reducing integrity of vessel walls, and interfering with formation of collagen.
- Folic acid (400 mcg daily) alone can reduce homocysteine in some subjects, but not all; importance of vitamins B_{12} and B_6 to homocysteine metabolism indicates all three should be used together.
- Folic acid will lower homocysteine only in the presence of adequate vitamins B_{12} and B_6.

"Type A" Personality

- Type A behavior: extreme sense of time urgency, competitiveness, impatience, and aggressiveness.
- Twofold increase in CHD risk.
- Damaging to cardiovascular system is regular expression of anger.
- Positive correlation exists between serum cholesterol level and aggression. The higher the aggression score, the higher the cholesterol level.
- A negative correlation exists between ratio of LDL-C to HDL-C and controlled affect score—the greater the ability to control anger, the lower this ratio. Those who learn to control anger experience reduction in risk for heart disease, whereas an unfavorable lipid profile is linked with aggressive (hostile) anger coping style.
- Anger expression plays a role in CRP levels. Greater anger and severity of depression, separately and in combination with hostility, are linked to elevations in CRP.

- Other mechanisms linking emotions, personality, and CVD: increased cortisol secretion, endothelial dysfunction, hypertension, and increased platelet aggregation and fibrinogen.

 Ten tips that help improve coping strategies:
 1. Do not starve your emotional life. Foster meaningful relationships. Provide time to give and receive love in your life.
 2. Learn to be a good listener. Allow the people in your life to really share their feelings and thoughts uninterruptedly. Empathize with them; put yourself in their shoes.
 3. Do not try to talk over somebody. If you find yourself being interrupted, relax; do not try to outtalk the other person. If you are courteous and allow someone else to speak, eventually (unless he or she is extremely rude) he or she will respond likewise. If not, explain that he or she is interrupting the communication process. You can do this only if you have been a good listener.
 4. Avoid aggressive or passive behavior. Be assertive, but express your thoughts and feelings in a kind way to help improve relationships at work and at home.
 5. Avoid excessive stress in your life as best you can by avoiding excessive work hours, poor nutrition, and inadequate rest. Get as much sleep as you can.
 6. Avoid stimulants such as caffeine and nicotine. Stimulants promote the fight-or-flight response and tend to make people more irritable in the process.
 7. Take time to build long-term health and success by performing stress-reduction techniques and deep breathing exercises.
 8. Accept gracefully those things over which you have no control. Save your energy for those things that you can do something about.
 9. Accept yourself. Remember that you are human and will make mistakes from which you can learn along the way.
 10. Be more patient and tolerant of other people. Follow the golden rule.

Other Nutritional Factors

Magnesium and Potassium

- Absolutely essential to proper functioning of entire cardiovascular system.
- Magnesium or potassium supplementation or both effectively treat a wide range of CVDs—angina, arrhythmias, congestive heart failure, and high blood pressure. Many of these applications have been used for more than 50 years.

- Best dietary sources of magnesium: tofu, legumes, seeds, nuts, whole grains, and green leafy vegetables.
- Low magnesium levels contribute to atherosclerosis and CVD via promotion of endothelial dysfunction by generating a proinflammatory, prothrombotic, proatherogenic environment.
- Intravenous magnesium therapy is valued treatment measure in acute MI. Intravenous magnesium during the first hour of admission to a hospital for acute MI produces a favorable effect in reducing immediate and long-term complications as well as death rates. The beneficial effects of magnesium in acute MI relate to its ability to do the following:
  - Improve energy production within the heart
  - Dilate the coronary arteries, resulting in improved delivery of oxygen to the heart
  - Reduce peripheral vascular resistance, resulting in reduced demand on the heart
  - Inhibit platelets from aggregating and forming blood clots
  - Reduce the size of the infarct (blockage)
  - Improve heart rate and arrhythmias

Vitamin D Deficiency

Individuals with vitamin D (25-OH-D) levels below 30 ng/mL are more likely to be at high risk for CVD, for CHD, and for both CHD and heart failure.

THERAPEUTIC CONSIDERATIONS—PREVENTING RECURRENT HEART ATTACK

- People who have experienced a heart attack or stroke and live through it are extremely likely to experience another.
- Primary prevention of subsequent cardiovascular events: control major risk factors.
- Most popular conventional "secondary" recommendation: low-dose aspirin (325 mg/day or every other day); but there may be effective alternatives, especially for those who cannot tolerate aspirin.
- Lower doses of aspirin (e.g., 50 to 150 mg/day or every other day) have not proven effective in reducing CVD mortality.

Aspirin

- Aspirin decreases risk of CVD events in both primary and secondary trials.

- Aspirin and other nonsteroidal anti-inflammatory drugs (NSAIDs) are associated with a significant risk of peptic ulcer. There is an increased risk of gastrointestinal bleeding from peptic ulcers at all dosage levels.
- However, dose of 75 mg/day was associated with a 40% reduction in ulcers compared with 300 mg/day and 30% compared with 150 mg/day.
- Because it is unknown whether 75 mg/day of aspirin is helpful in preventing a second heart attack, most physicians recommend at least 300 mg. To prevent stroke, the dose is 900 mg.
- These dosage recommendations carry significant risk for peptic ulcer but may be appropriate for high-risk patients unwilling to adopt the natural approach.

Dietary Alternatives to Aspirin

- Dietary modifications are not only more effective in preventing recurrent heart attack than aspirin but can also reverse blockage of clogged arteries.
- Mediterranean diet
- **Lifestyle Heart Trial conducted by Dean Ornish:** low-fat vegetarian diet for at least 1 year, including fruits, vegetables, grains, legumes, and soybean products. There were no limits on calories. No animal products were allowed except egg whites and 1 cup of nonfat milk or yogurt daily. The diet contained 10% fat; 15% to 20% protein; 70% to 75% predominantly complex carbohydrates from whole grains, legumes, and vegetables. Stress reduction techniques—breathing exercises, stretching, meditation, imagery, and other relaxation techniques—were practiced for an hour each day. Exercise for at least 3 hours each week was encouraged. At end of the year, experimental group showed significant overall regression of atherosclerosis of coronary blood vessels.
- Omega-3 fatty acids from either fish or vegetable sources reduce risk of heart disease.
- **Dietary and Reinfarction Trial (DART):** it was only when intake of omega-3s (from fish) was increased that future heart attacks were reduced.
- **Lyon Diet Heart Study:** increasing omega-3s from plant sources (ALA) offered the same degree of protection as increased fish intake.

Preventing a Subsequent Stroke

- To prevent a subsequent stroke and promote recovery from a stroke: *Ginkgo biloba* extract.

- Extract of *G. biloba* leaves standardized to contain 24% ginkgo flavon glycosides and 6% terpenoids has been studied in depth for decreased blood supply to the brain (cerebrovascular insufficiency).
- *G. biloba* extract enhances stroke recovery.

Other Considerations

Angiography, Coronary Artery Bypass Surgery, or Angioplasty

Angiography, coronary artery bypass surgery, and angioplasty are used far more frequently than is justified by objective evaluation of their appropriateness and efficacy. See chapter on angina for advice for patient care when these procedures are unavoidable.

Intravenous Chelation Therapy

Far less invasive is intravenous ethylenediaminetetraacetic acid (EDTA) chelation therapy. This useful yet controversial procedure is also discussed in the angina chapter.

Earlobe Crease

- Presence of a diagonal earlobe crease has been recognized as a sign of CVD since 1973.
- The earlobe is richly vascularized; decrease in blood flow over extended period of time collapses vascular bed, leading to diagonal crease.
- The crease is seen more commonly with advancing age, until age of 80, when incidence drops dramatically. Association with heart disease is independent of age.
- Although presence of an earlobe crease does not prove heart disease, it strongly suggests it. Examination of earlobe is easy screening procedure.
- Correlation does not hold with Asians, Native Americans, or children with Beckwith's syndrome.

THERAPEUTIC APPROACH

- Atherosclerosis is commonly and directly related to diet and lifestyle.
- Treatment and prevention: reduce all known risk factors.
- Any treatment plan must be individualized to ensure optimal results.

Dietary Recommendations

Mediterranean diet; table "Food Choices for Lowering Cholesterol" provides additional guidance; box "Foods Typically Containing Partially or Totally Hydrogenated Vegetable Oils and Trans Isomers" lists foods to avoid because of their *trans*-fatty acid content.

- Eat less saturated fat and cholesterol by reducing or eliminating animal products.
- Increase fiber-rich plant foods (fruits, vegetables, grains, legumes, and raw nuts and seeds).
- Increase monounsaturated fats and omega-3s.
- Follow a low-glycemic diet.

Foods Typically Containing Partially or Totally Hydrogenated Vegetable Oils and *Trans* Isomers

- Virtually all refined and processed foods
- Margarine
- Cakes
- Cookies
- Candies
- Doughnuts
- Bread
- Canned soups
- Crackers
- Processed cheese
- Canned foods
- Cereals
- Snack foods
- Salad oils, except olive oil, which is recommended

Food Choices for Lowering Cholesterol

Decrease Consumption of the Following:	Substitute with the Following:
Red meat	Fish and white-meat poultry
Hamburgers and hot dogs	Soy-based alternatives
Eggs	Egg Beaters and similar products, tofu
High-fat dairy products	Low-fat or nonfat dairy products
Butter, lard, and other saturated fats	Vegetable oils
Ice cream, pies, cake, cookies, and so on	Fruits

Decrease Consumption of the Following:	Substitute with the Following:
Refined cereals, white	Whole grains, whole wheat bread, and so on
Fried foods, fatty snack foods	Vegetables, fresh salads
Salt and salty foods	Low-sodium foods, light salt
Coffee and soft drinks	Herbal teas, fresh fruit, and vegetable juices

Lifestyle Recommendations

- Achieve ideal body weight.
- Exercise aerobically on a regular basis.
- Do not smoke.

Supplements

- High-potency multivitamin and mineral
- Vitamin C: 250 to 500 mg t.i.d.
- Vitamin E (mixed tocopherols): 100 to 400 IU q.d.
- Grapeseed or pine bark extract: 100 mg q.d.
- Fish oil: minimum 1000 mg of EPA plus DHA q.d.
- Vitamin D: 1000 to 4000 IU q.d.

Atopic Dermatitis (Eczema)

DIAGNOSTIC SUMMARY

- Chronic, pruritic, inflammatory skin
- Dry, hyperkeratotic skin
- Lesions: excoriations, papules, eczema (patches of erythema, exudation, and scaling with small vesicles formed within epidermis), and lichenification (hyperpigmented plaques of thickened skin with accentuated furrows)
- Scratching and rubbing lead to lichenification, most commonly in antecubital and popliteal flexures
- Personal or family history of atopy

GENERAL CONSIDERATIONS

Atopic dermatitis (AD; eczema) is a common condition. Etiopathogenesis of AD involves interplay of the following:

- Cutaneous barrier dysfunction and mutations in genes coding for skin proteins (filaggrin)
- Dysregulation of immune system and role of thymic stromal lymphopoietin (TSLP) in allergic inflammation
- Environmental factors

Filaggrin and Epidermal Barrier Dysfunction

- Genetic basis: family history of atopic disease is major risk factor. AD is a complex trait—interactions between genes and environmental factors and interplay among multiple genes.
- Gene encoding filaggrin *(FLG)* is most consistently replicated.
- Filaggrin is a protein that facilitates aggregation of keratin filaments; it is known as filament aggregating protein. It binds cytokeratin into tonofilaments and, when proteolyzed, forms small hygroscopic molecules—amino acids—which comprise natural moisturizing factor (NMF).
- NMF is responsible for hydration of stratum corneum.

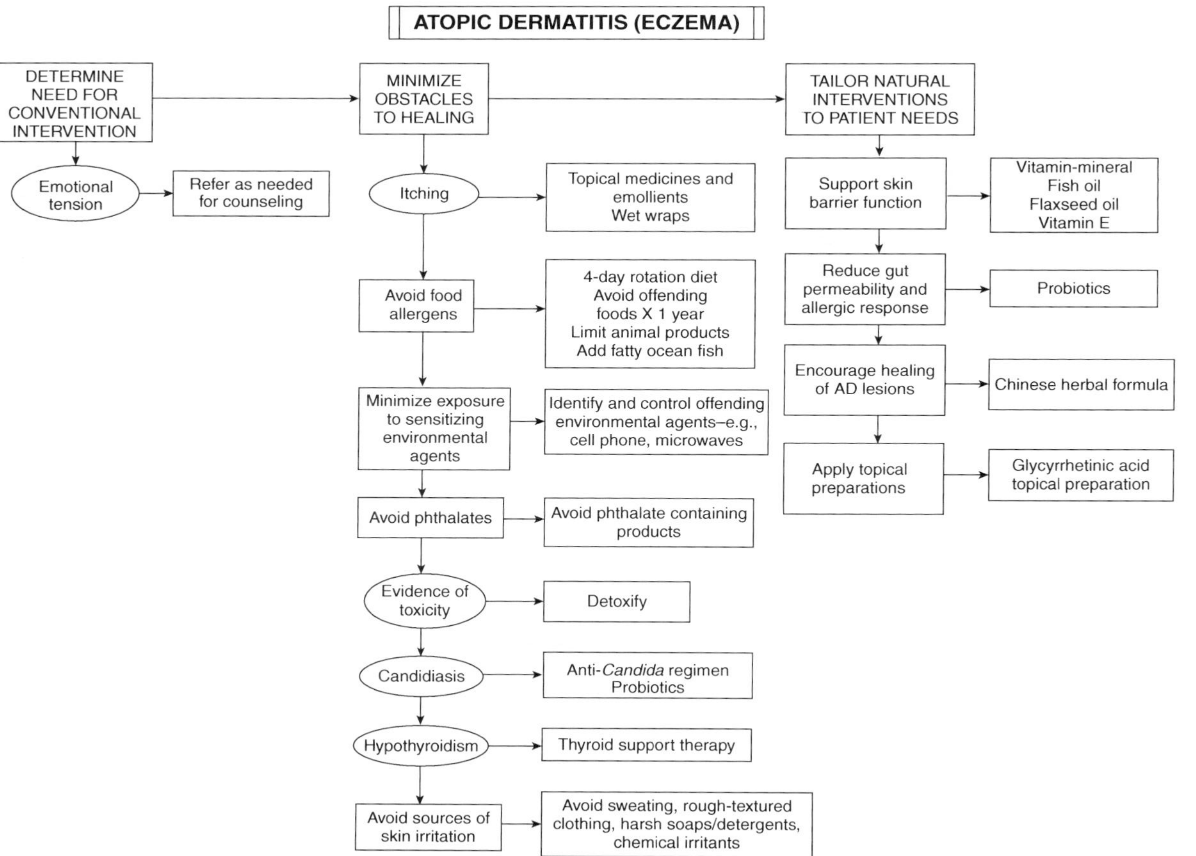
ATOPIC DERMATITIS (ECZEMA)
DETERMINE NEED FOR CONVENTIONAL INTERVENTION
Emotional tension
Refer as needed for counseling
MINIMIZE OBSTACLES TO HEALING
Itching
Topical medicines and emollients
Wet wraps
Avoid food allergens
4-day rotation diet
Avoid offending foods X 1 year
Limit animal products
Add fatty ocean fish
Minimize exposure to sensitizing environmental agents
Identify and control offending environmental agents–e.g., cell phone, microwaves
Avoid phthalates
Avoid phthalate containing products
Evidence of toxicity
Detoxify
Candidiasis
Anti-*Candida* regimen
Probiotics
Hypothyroidism
Thyroid support therapy
Avoid sources of skin irritation
Avoid sweating, rough-textured clothing, harsh soaps/detergents, chemical irritants
TAILOR NATURAL INTERVENTIONS TO PATIENT NEEDS
Support skin barrier function
Vitamin-mineral
Fish oil
Flaxseed oil
Vitamin E
Reduce gut permeability and allergic response
Probiotics
Encourage healing of AD lesions
Chinese herbal formula
Apply topical preparations
Glycyrrhetinic acid topical preparation

- Filaggrin mutations are linked to northern European ancestry; 15% of cases of AD are attributable to such mutations. If a person is born with one filaggrin mutation, risk of AD is 40%.
- Additional acquired stressors to skin barrier initiate inflammation.
- Sustained hapten access through a defective barrier stimulates a Th1-to-Th2 shift in immunophenotype, which further impairs the barrier.
- Secondary *Staphylococcus aureus* colonization not only amplifies inflammation but further stresses the barrier in AD.
- New "outside to inside, back to outside" paradigm for pathogenesis of AD now highlights "barrier repair" therapy.

Immune Dysregulation, Thymic Stromal Lymphopoietin, and Allergic Inflammation

- IgE is elevated in 80% of patients with AD. Activation of type 2 T-helper (Th2) cells in response to antigens plays major role in AD.
- TSLP is interleukin-7 (IL-7)–like cytokine secreted by barrier-defective skin and is elevated in skin biopsies from lesional AD patients. TSLP profoundly triggers Th2 commitment and rises when stimulated by phthalates.
- Phthalates are present in a vast array of products, in which they are typically used to solubilize and stabilize fragrances. Pervasive exposure to phthalates may play a role in pathogenesis of AD.
- TSLP sensitizes lungs to allergens and may help to explain frequently observed evolution of AD to asthma, known as the "atopic march."
- Gastric *Helicobacter pylori* directly stimulates epidermal cells to secrete TSLP, and *H. pylori* antibody is positive in 70% of AD patients. Treatment of infection, proven by reduced C-urea breath test and anti–*H. pylori* antibody titers, resulted in partial improvement in AD.

Environmental Factors: Atopic Dermatitis and Allergy

- Sensitization to foods triggers isolated skin symptoms in 30% of children. Symptoms: immediate reactions within minutes after ingesting food without exacerbation of AD and early and late exacerbations of AD.
- Identify clinically relevant sensitizations to foods using skin-prick tests, specific immunoglobulin E (IgE) and IgG_4 blood tests, and food challenges to initiate dietary interventions and avoid unnecessary dietary restrictions.

- Defective skin barrier and increased intestinal permeability facilitate allergen sensitization. Skin care to maintain skin barrier function and avoidance of allergenic foods during infancy may prevent allergen sensitization, reducing severity of AD and food allergies.

Predictors of Severity

- Children with AD whose eczema started during first year of life were more likely to have severe disease than were those whose eczema started later.
- History of atopy (asthma, hay fever, or both) in children is associated with severe AD.
- Children with eczema living in urban areas are at increased risk of severe disease compared with counterparts in rural environment. Urban environmental risk is independent of ethnicity.
- Other factors—breastfeeding, family size, gender, birth weight, gestational age, child's age, atopy (hay fever, asthma, or eczema) in parents and siblings have little association with disease severity.
- Lack of protective effect from breastfeeding is not consistent with other studies (see later).

THERAPEUTIC CONSIDERATIONS

- None of the myriad prescription and over-the-counter medicines commonly used to treat AD has shown effective long-term ability to cure AD. Side effects—growth retardation, cutaneous complications, sedation, and allergic reactions—are a major concern. Some of these medicines can result in rebound flare-up usually worse than primary lesions.
- Naturopathic medicine attempts to understand underlying causes of AD, attending to additional factors: those affecting digestive system—food allergies and candidal overgrowth. Although no one treatment option is universally effective, patient-specific combination therapeutics acting in synergy are encouraged for optimal efficacy.

Food Allergy, Gut Permeability, and Candidal Overgrowth

- Food allergy plays a major role in AD.
- Breastfeeding offers prophylaxis against AD and allergies in general. Breastfeeding helps prevent allergy. Yet breastfed infants with allergies should be treated by allergen avoidance; in some cases breastfeeding cessation is recommended to avoid traces of food antigens in breast milk. Development of AD in breastfed infants is usually result of transfer of allergic antigens

in breast milk; mothers should avoid common food allergens (milk, eggs, peanuts; fish, soy, wheat, citrus, and chocolate). Maternal avoidance of these common allergens is associated with complete resolution in majority of cases.

- In older or formula-fed infants, cow's milk, eggs, and peanuts are most common food allergens inducing AD. Other allergens: fish, wheat, soybean. Egg-free diet has induced improvement in severity of AD, with greatest effect in those most severely affected.
- Virtually any food can be offending agent.
- Diagnosis of food allergy in childhood eczema is best achieved via elimination diet and challenge method.
- Elimination of wheat, milk products, eggs, peanuts, tomatoes, and artificial colors and preservatives results in significant improvement in 75% of cases.
- If laboratory methods are used, most useful method might be enzyme-linked immunosorbent assay (ELISA) IgE and IgG_4.
- Presence of food allergies is responsible for children with AD having "leaky gut"—increased gut permeability, increased antigen load, overwhelming the immune system and increasing likelihood of developing additional allergies.
- Hypoallergenic diets decrease gut permeability and improve atopic eczema.
- Identify offending foods promptly to avoid increasing gut permeability. Dealing with multiple food allergies is difficult for the patient: diet is often unrealistically restrictive.
- Elimination of allergenic foods and restoration of normal intestinal permeability can stop development of new allergies.
- Encourage patients to find out whether, if they can avoid offending foods for 6 to 12 months, their antibody to allergens will decrease to point that they can tolerate the reintroduction of some foods at least twice a week.
- Loss rate of food allergy in patients with AD after 1 year was 26% for five major allergens (egg, milk, wheat, soy, peanut) and 66% for other food allergens.

Candida albicans

- Overgrowth of common yeast *C. albicans* in gastrointestinal tract is causative factor in allergic conditions such as AD.
- Elevated anticandidal antibodies are common in atopic persons. Severity of lesions correlates with level of IgE antibodies in relation to candidal antigens. Appropriate anticandidal therapy (see *Candida* chapter) may cause clinical improvement in AD.

Nutritional Supplements

Probiotics

- Intestinal flora play major role in AD; probiotic therapy is indicated. Probiotic *Lactobacillus rhamnosus* strain GG alone or in conjunction with *Lactobacillus reuteri* given to infants with AD and cow's milk allergy reduced severity of eczema.
- Positive therapeutic effect of probiotics may be more pronounced in patients with allergic constitution, as evidenced by positive responses to skin prick test and increased IgE levels. These tests may be useful in forecasting who may be most responsive to probiotics.

Essential Fatty Acids

- Evening primrose oil (EPO) (dose: at least 3000 mg q.d., providing 270 mg gamma-linolenic acid) shows benefit.
- Omega-6 oils support skin barrier function. However, overall therapeutic results appear more favorable with omega-3 oils than with EPO. Several EPO studies failed to demonstrate any therapeutic benefit over a placebo.
- Fish oil supplements providing eicosapentaenoic acid (EPA) and docosahexaenoic acid (DHA) or simply eating more small wild fatty fish (e.g., mackerel, herring, salmon) causes incorporation of omega-3s into membrane phospholipid pools. Degree of clinical improvement correlates with increase in concentration of DHA in serum phospholipids.
- Epidemiologic studies have found protective associations between fish intake in pregnancy, lactation, infancy, and childhood and atopic outcomes. Similar studies of fish oil supplements have also found protective and therapeutic effects.

Vitamin E

In one study, at a dose of 400 IU q.d. for 8 months, vitamin E was superior to placebo in treating AD.

Botanical Medicines

Two categories for AD: internal and external

- Licorice *(Glycyrrhiza glabra):* useful in either application. Internally, licorice preparations exert anti-inflammatory and antiallergic effects. Licorice-containing Chinese herbal formula:
  - *Ledebouriealla seseloides*
  - *Potentilla chinensis*
  - *Clematis chinensis*

— *Clematis armandii*
— *Rehmania glutinosa*
— *Paeonia lactiflora*
— *Lophatherum gracile*
— *Dictamnus dasycarpus*
— *Tribulus terrestris*
— *Schizonepeta tenuifolia*

- Several double-blind studies have confirmed the benefit of this Chinese formula.
- Licorice plays a major role in the efficacy of the Chinese herbal formula. Base dosage on level of delivered licorice.
- Licorice applied topically: use commercial preparations featuring pure glycyrrhetinic acid. Glycyrrhetinic acid exerts effects similar to topical hydrocortisone in treatment of eczema, contact and allergic dermatitis, and psoriasis.

Other Therapeutic Considerations

Endocrine Factors

Hypothyroid patients with eczema respond well to thyroid hormone therapy.

Scratching Cessation

- Scratching is extremely detrimental in AD: it breaks skin, aiding bacterial ingress, and promoting barrier dysfunction and lichenification. Factors that limit itching promote healing and prevent recurrence.
- Wet wraps block scratching, increase hydration, potentiate medicine and emollients, and promote restful sleep. After applying medicine and emollient, wrap affected area in warm, wet gauze or, alternatively, 100% cotton socks with toe portion cut off. Apply dry layer over wet layer, and leave it on overnight. Use wet wraps 5 to 14 days.

Psychological Approach

Emotional tension can provoke and aggravate itching of AD. AD patients show higher anxiety, hostility, and neurosis than matched controls. Psychotherapeutics may reduce use of corticosteroids for up to 2 years.

Environmental Considerations

Dust Mite Exposure

In patients with dust mite sensitization and eczema, sublingual immunotherapy is beneficial. Paradoxically, lower levels of eczema can be found in children with higher dust mite exposure; reducing house dust in early infancy could increase risk of AD.

Microwave Exposure

Cell phone use continuously for an hour increases allergic response to dust and pollen in adults with eczema. Microwave radiation exposure also increases plasma levels of substance P and vasoactive intestinal peptide in AD. Microwave radiation emitted from cell phones may actually increase sensitivity to specific allergens in some patients.

THERAPEUTIC APPROACH

- Relieve and prevent itching.
- Address barrier dysfunction.
- Control food allergens.
- Avoid phthalates.
- Detoxify.
- Rule out presence of *H. pylori;* treat accordingly.

Diet

- Four-day rotation diet; eliminate all major allergens (wheat, milk, eggs, peanuts in 81% of cases). As patient improves, slowly reintroduce allergens; stringent rotation diet can be modified.
- Include cold-water fish—wild salmon, mackerel, herring, sardine, and halibut; limit other animal products.

Supplements

- High-potency multiple vitamin-mineral formula
- Vitamin E: 400 international units (IU) daily (mixed tocopherols)
- Fish oil: 1000 to 3000 mg EPA and DHA daily
- Probiotics: 5 to 10 billion viable *Lactobacillus acidophilus* and *Bifidobacterium bifidum* cells daily

Topical Treatments

- Ceramide-containing emollients reduce transepidermal water loss (e.g., CeraVe, Nature Pure's Hippophae-Ceramide Cream, sea buckthorn oil, ceramides, squalane, olive oil, beeswax, extracts of St. John's wort, *Gingko biloba, Calendula,* and chamomile).
- Glycyrrhetinic acid–containing treatments: chamomile, feverfew, oatmeal, and *Cardiospermum* preparations

- Atopiclair Rx contains glycyrrhetinic acid, shea butter, bisabolol (chamomile), vitamin E, *Aloe vera,* and grapeseed.
- One percent feverfew (parthenolide-free extract: Aveeno Daily Moisturizer, Ultra-Calming)
- Colloidal oatmeal contains starches and beta-glucans that have protective and water-holding functions; polyphenols (avenanthramides) are antioxidants, anti-inflammatories, and ultraviolet absorbers.
- Saponins have cleansing activity (Aveeno Overnight Itch Relief Cream).

Patients should take the following measures:

- Avoid sweating and rough-textured clothing.
- Wash clothing with mild soaps only and rinse thoroughly.
- Avoid exposure to chemical irritants and any other agent that might cause skin irritation.

Psychological Approach

- Rule out high levels of anxiety, hostility, or neurosis.
- Refer, if necessary, for psychotherapy.

Attention Deficit Hyperactivity Disorder

DIAGNOSTIC SUMMARY

- Neurobehavioral disorder that begins in early childhood with persistence into adolescence and adulthood
- One or more symptoms of disabling inattentiveness, hyperactivity, and impulsivity
- Commonly accompanied by comorbid conditions—mood disorders or learning disabilities

GENERAL CONSIDERATIONS

Attention-deficit/hyperactivity disorder (ADHD) is defined by the *Diagnostic and Statistical Manual, Fifth Edition* as developmentally inappropriate inattention and impulsivity with or without hyperactivity. ADHD has three subtypes:

- Predominantly hyperactive-impulsive
  - Most symptoms (six or more) are in hyperactivity-impulsivity categories.
  - Fewer than six symptoms of inattention are present, although inattention may be present to some degree.
- Predominantly inattentive
  - Majority of symptoms (six or more) are in inattention category and fewer than six symptoms of hyperactivity-impulsivity are present, although hyperactivity-impulsivity may still be present to some degree.
  - Children with this subtype are less likely to act out or have difficulties getting along with other children. They may sit quietly, but they are not paying attention to what they are doing. Therefore the child may be overlooked, and parents and teachers may not notice that he or she has ADHD.
- Combined hyperactive-impulsive and inattentive
  - Six or more symptoms of inattention and six or more symptoms of hyperactivity-impulsivity are present.

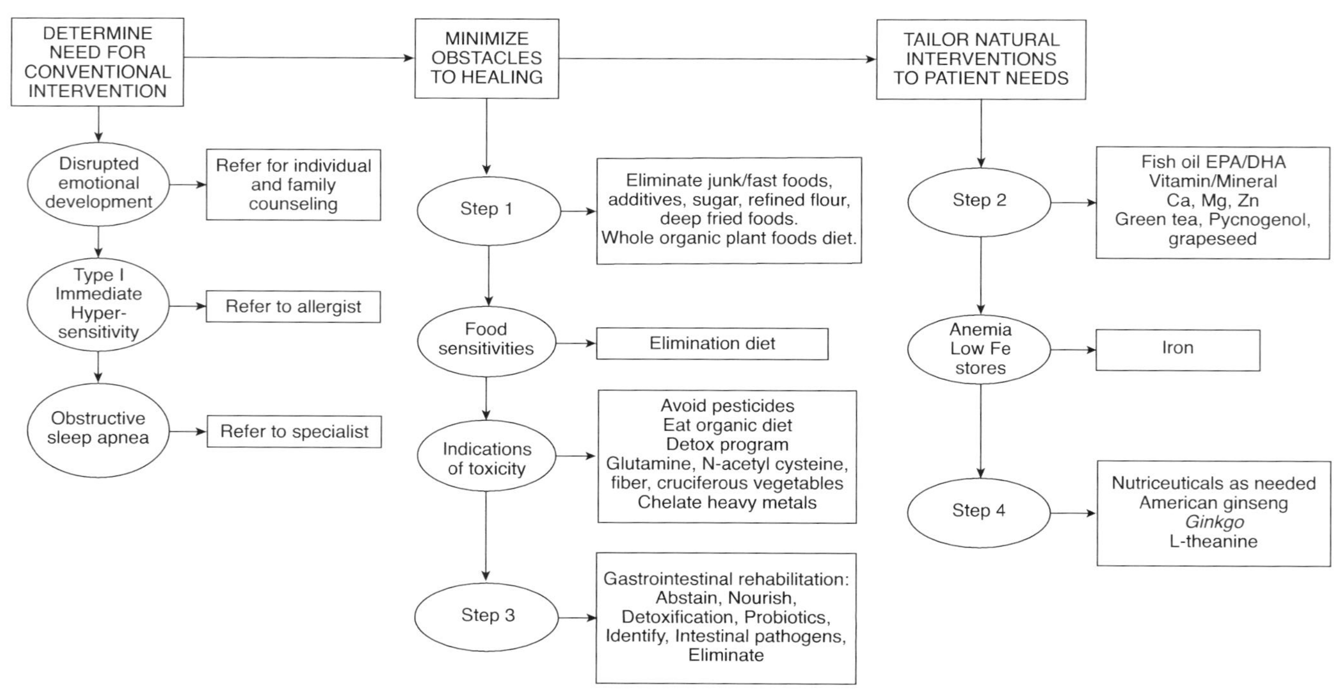
ATTENTION DEFICIT HYPERACTIVITY DISORDER
DETERMINE NEED FOR CONVENTIONAL INTERVENTION
Disrupted emotional development
Refer for individual and family counseling
Type I Immediate Hyper-sensitivity
Refer to allergist
Obstructive sleep apnea
Refer to specialist
MINIMIZE OBSTACLES TO HEALING
Step 1
Eliminate junk/fast foods, additives, sugar, refined flour, deep fried foods. Whole organic plant foods diet.
Food sensitivities
Elimination diet
Indications of toxicity
Avoid pesticides
Eat organic diet
Detox program
Glutamine, N-acetyl cysteine, fiber, cruciferous vegetables
Chelate heavy metals
Step 3
Gastrointestinal rehabilitation: Abstain, Nourish, Detoxification, Probiotics, Identify, Intestinal pathogens, Eliminate
TAILOR NATURAL INTERVENTIONS TO PATIENT NEEDS
Step 2
Fish oil EPA/DHA
Vitamin/Mineral
Ca, Mg, Zn
Green tea, Pycnogenol, grapeseed
Anemia Low Fe stores
Iron
Step 4
Nutriceuticals as needed
American ginseng
Ginkgo
L-theanine

To be diagnosed with ADHD, a child must have symptoms for 6 or more months and to a degree that is greater than other children of the same age.

Children who have symptoms of inattention may:

- Be easily distracted, miss details, forget things, and frequently switch from one activity to another
- Have difficulty focusing on one thing
- Become bored with a task after only a few minutes, unless they are doing something enjoyable
- Have difficulty focusing attention on organizing and completing a task or learning something new
- Have trouble completing or turning in homework assignments, often losing things (e.g., pencils, toys, assignments) needed to complete tasks or activities
- Not seem to listen when spoken to
- Daydream, become easily confused, and move slowly
- Have difficulty processing information as quickly and accurately as others
- Struggle to follow instructions

Children who have symptoms of hyperactivity may:

- Fidget and squirm in their seats
- Talk nonstop
- Dash around, touching or playing with anything and everything in sight
- Have trouble sitting still during dinner, school, and story time
- Be constantly in motion
- Have difficulty doing quiet tasks or activities

Children who have symptoms of impulsivity may:

- Be very impatient
- Blurt out inappropriate comments, show their emotions without restraint, and act without regard for consequences
- Have difficulty waiting for things they want or waiting their turn in games
- Often interrupt conversations or others' activities

ADHD is linked to difficulties in school—learning and behavior. If not intensively managed, a child with ADHD experiences academic impairment, increased risk of injuries, and problems with self-esteem and socialization. In adolescence and adulthood, there is high risk of depression or anxiety, substance abuse and addictions, traffic accidents, financial problems, vocational underachievement, and social problems. Nevertheless, ADHD can be transcended; many with ADHD achieve personal success. There is a greater incidence in boys than in girls (2:1). Onset is usually by 3 years of age, although diagnosis is often not made until later when the child is in school.

Etiology

- Diminished function of polysynaptic dopaminergic circuits belonging to executive centers within the brain's prefrontal cortex. Executive centers are inhibitory and are responsible for impulse control and ability to maintain sustained attention.
- Brains of those with ADHD exhibit differences morphologically and metabolically from normal controls with regard to prefrontal executive centers.
- Other neurotransmitters (norepinephrine) are also incriminated. Decreased sensitivity of dopaminergic (D4) receptors and heightened dopamine reuptake by presynaptic dopamine transporter are both suggested to result in diminished dopaminergic activity within executive centers.
- However, these defects are not necessarily permanent, because as children with ADHD grow up, the brain develops normal dopamine activity, and anatomic variations lessen; ADHD symptoms also tend to improve.
- Genetic factors: There are differences in the genes encoding for both D2 and D4 dopamine receptors in ADHD. Genetic polymorphisms are linked to increased activity of presynaptic dopamine transporter (which would result in increased uptake of dopamine).
- Other genetic factors: inherited tendencies toward allergic states, decreased immune competence, and various genetic polymorphisms, resulting in diminished capacity to detoxify drugs, heavy metals, and xenobiotics. Thus, environmental and dietary factors influence how and whether genetic factors manifest as ADHD.

THERAPEUTIC CONSIDERATIONS

- The prevailing conventional approach to ADHD is use of amphetamine drugs for purely symptomatic relief. Examples include methylphenidate (Ritalin), amphetamine and dextroamphetamine (Adderall), methylphenidate (Concerta), and lisdexamfetamine dimesylate (Vyvanse). They improve ADHD symptoms by potentiating neurotransmitter dopamine within all brain regions, including those affected in ADHD. Although these drugs improve behavior and cognitive functioning in 75% of children in formal placebo-controlled trials, in actual clinical practice they provide

little long-term benefit with a high prevalence of adverse effects—decreased appetite, sleep problems, anxiety, and irritability.
- Nonstimulant drugs such as atomoxetine (Strattera) promote suicidal thoughts.
- ADHD may be treated without long-term reliance on drugs.
- The primary goal in many cases is enhancement of cognitive function. Fifty percent of people with ADHD have learning disabilities, and most have cognitive deficits with diminished nonverbal working memory. This results in a diminished sense of time and a decreased ability to hold events or tasks in mind. Tardiness, missed appointments, procrastination, poor task planning, and failure to meet deadlines exemplify diminished working memory.

Environmental Neurotoxins

Environmental factors affecting development of ADHD may begin at or before conception.
- Maternal-to-fetal transport of neurotoxins during pregnancy may occur. Examples include heavy metals such as lead and mercury; solvents; pesticides; polychlorinated biphenyls (PCBs); alcohol; or other drugs of abuse.
- The mother may herself exhibit ADHD and give birth to child with ADHD. This is acquired ADHD.
- Children remain susceptible to neurotoxins after birth.
- Maternal tobacco and drug use increase risk of ADHD. Up to 25% of all behavioral disorders in children are linked to exposure to cigarette smoking during pregnancy.
- The incidence of long-term, low-level lead intoxication in North American children is alarmingly high. Cognitive deficits and behavioral disturbances are linked to whole blood lead levels above 10 mg/dL. Low-level lead intoxication is associated with addictive behaviors and impulsivity, suggesting neurologic changes consistent with the reward deficiency syndrome, as described earlier. Improvement in ADHD has occurred in some children with moderate lead elevations who were treated with intravenous ethylenediaminetetraacetic acid (EDTA) chelation.
- In addition to lead, other heavy metals (mercury, cadmium, and aluminum), pesticides, and PCBs are nearly ubiquitous contaminants.

Food Additives, Sugar, and the Feingold Hypothesis

- Benjamin Feingold, MD—the "Feingold hypothesis": many hyperactive children are sensitive to artificial food colorings, flavors, and preservatives.

- Virtually every study (both negative and positive) has demonstrated that some hyperactive children consistently react with behavioral problems when challenged with specific food additives.
- Some children definitely react quite strongly to food additives, warranting exclusion of these compounds for at least 10 days to judge their significance in all cases of ADHD.
- There appears to be an interrelationship between sugar intake and artificial food dyes. Destructive-aggressive and restless behavior correlates with amount of sugar consumed. The higher the sugar intake, the worse the behavior. Amazingly, 74% of children tested displayed abnormal glucose tolerance or hypoglycemia.

Essential Fatty Acids

- Children with ADHD have measurable reduction in tissue levels of the omega-3 fatty acids eicosapentaenoic acid (EPA) and docosahexaenoic acid (DHA) compared with age-matched controls.
- Omega-3 (EPA and DHA) supplementation in ADHD is considered a sensible intervention even by many mainstream physicians. Omega-3 fatty acids improve many symptoms of ADHD—impulsive-oppositional behavior—not typically helped by pharmaceuticals.
- Nerve endings in areas of the brain affected in ADHD should be rich in DHA because they are highly fluid and should be composed of 80% DHA. DHA deficiency increases permeability of the blood-brain barrier in animals and may protect the brain from influx of neurotoxins.
- Human breast milk is rich in DHA. Children who are formula fed are at twice the risk of developing ADHD as those who are breastfed. The role of DHA in brain development, intelligence, and possible protection against ADHD finally led to its inclusion in many infant formulas and other foods.

Individual Nutrients and Attention Deficit Hyperactivity Disorder

Children with ADHD show multiple nutrient deficiencies, highlighting the importance of broad-spectrum nutritional support. The following minerals are critical in ADHD:

- **Magnesium:** Magnesium levels in serum, red blood cells, and hair are low in most children with ADHD. These children improve in behavior when given magnesium supplements.

- **Zinc:** Both hair and serum zinc deficits often accompany ADHD. Children with low serum zinc levels also often have lower free fatty acids, suggesting that abnormalities in fatty acid metabolism are linked partly to zinc deficiency. Lower hair zinc levels correlate with poorer response to treatment with amphetamines. Positive effects of zinc therapy are seen in hyperactive children.
- **Iron:** Anemia from iron deficiency affects 20% of infants; many more have milder iron deficiencies without anemia, leaving them at risk for impairment of brain development. Iron deficiency is much more common in children with ADHD. Iron therapy in nonanemic children with ADHD has been found to result in diminished ADHD symptoms within 30 days.

Food Allergy

- There is a very strong relationship between allergies and ADHD, including food allergies. Brainwave electroencephalographic changes occur immediately after ingestion of a known food allergen.
- Food and other allergies are linked to a higher incidence of recurrent ear infections (otitis media). Recurrent otitis media is associated with increased risk of ADHD.
- Both food allergy and ADHD are associated with sleep disturbances, which can contribute to worsening of ADHD.
- Heavy snoring and sleep apnea are prevalent in allergic children and may worsen ADHD. Sleep improves in children with ADHD who eat a low–allergy potential (oligoantigenic) diet.
- Food allergy elimination or desensitization can be as effective as drug therapy in reducing ADHD symptoms.

Obstructive Sleep Apnea

- Attention deficits are common (95%) in children and adults with obstructive sleep apnea (OSA). OSA is found in 30% of children diagnosed with ADHD and may be central to the etiology of ADHD.
- In children, chronic nasal or tonsillar or pharyngeal congestion is the most common causative factor leading to OSA. Childhood obesity is becoming a leading cause. OSA should be considered in all childhood ADHD; be familiar with OSA signs and symptoms and local resources for diagnosis and treatment.
- Diagnostic clues to OSA: nocturnal mouth breathing, snoring, enuresis, daytime urinary incontinence, and daytime

drowsiness. Refer patient for nocturnal oximetry testing or polysomnography.

- Questionnaires and physical examination are relatively insensitive for picking up OSA in children; be watchful. OSA fragments sleep with frequent hypoxic episodes, reducing a child's intellectual capacity, attentional performance, and quality of life.
- Reduce nasal congestion and decrease recurrent upper respiratory infections.
- In children with OSA who do not respond to conservative measures, tonsilloadenoidectomy may benefit ADHD and comorbidities. Inform parents of risks of untreated OSA versus risks and/or benefits of this surgery.

Dysbiosis, Gastrointestinal Permeability, and Intestinal Parasites

Probiotics with bifidobacteria and lactobacilli may help. These organisms are part of the first-line defense in gut immunity and restore gut permeability that has been altered by food allergies. Stool analysis may rule out parasitic infection or altered bacterial flora leading to disturbances in gut mucosal immunity (discussed in the following section).

Immune System Impairment

- Subtle immune dysfunction may be prominent in ADHD. Both cellular and humoral immunity are abnormal in children with ADHD. Plasma complement is lower. Immune dysfunction in ADHD may be either directly inherited or a result of nutritional, toxicologic, or atopic factors.
- ADHD may be, in part, an autoimmune disorder. Antineural antibodies have been found in blood and cerebrospinal fluid in patients with ADHD.
- Gut mucosal immunity might be impaired in ADHD, leading to increased susceptibility to gut pathogens and food allergies.

Cognitive Behavioral Therapies

- All children with ADHD symptoms should undergo thorough neurobehavioral and cognitive assessment. Many features associated with gifted children can be mistaken for ADHD.
- Children with mood disorders or learning disabilities and those from abusive environments or who have sustained serious trauma may benefit from specific psychological or cognitive behavioral interventions and may not respond to ADHD-specific drugs.

- Cognitive behavioral therapies implemented in schools and in the home are efficacious in treating ADHD.

Neurofeedback (Electroencephalographic Biofeedback)

- Provides real-time feedback about brainwave activity through electronic instrumentation.
- Helps the patient learn self-regulation of brainwave intensity and frequency.
- Effects: cortical slowing and diminished brainwave intensity in prefrontal region and frontal lobes.
- Designed to train patients to increase production of brainwave patterns that reduce or eliminate cortical slowing and many associated ADHD symptoms.
- Studies show cessation of methylphenidate (Ritalin) in children without loss of treatment effect.
- Rapid transcranial magnetic stimulation, used as safer alternative to electroconvulsive therapy, shows promise in treating a variety of neuropsychiatric conditions, including ADHD, particularly in children who have more severe forms of ADHD or serious comorbidities and those who are resistant to treatment.

Botanical Medicines

Procyanidolic Oligomers

- Extracts from grapeseed skin and bark of maritime pine (pycnogenol) are rich sources of procyanidolic oligomers—plant flavonoids.
- Have broad-spectrum antioxidant effects; increased oxidative damage is a central factor in ADHD.
- Pycnogenol (1 mg/kg body weight per day) improved antioxidant status in ADHD children. It also improved hyperactivity and improved attention and visual-motor coordination and concentration of children with ADHD.

Ginkgo biloba Extract

G. biloba extract induces improvements in inattentiveness, hyperactivity, and socialization in adults and children with ADHD.

L-Theanine

- Amino acid found in green tea that may improve sleep quality in children with ADHD.
- Reduces anxiety, increases concentration, improves sleep quality, and stabilizes mood without sedation. It also improves cerebral dopaminergic activity.

- Research dose for boys with ADHD: 400 mg L-theanine q.d.

THERAPEUTIC APPROACH

- Reasonable approach with high probability of success: multimodal, addressing as many factors as is practical.
- Basic workup: rule out common disorders that may manifest as ADHD to design specific treatments—for example, celiac disease, depression, lead poisoning, sleep apnea, and visual or auditory problems
- Assess by laboratory testing other contributory factors—increased intestinal permeability; food allergies or intolerances; and iron, magnesium, zinc, and omega-3 fatty acid deficiencies.
- Treat empirically if financial constraints prevent ordering noninsured tests.

Step 1

- Eliminate junk foods, fast foods, and food additives, sugary foods and beverages, white flour products, and deep-fried foods.
- Increase whole organic plant foods. In some cases, converting to whole-foods diet can result in marked improvements in behavior and cognitive performance.

Step 2

- Nutritional supplementation: pharmaceutic grade fish oil DHA and EPA concentrate; high-potency multivitamin and trace mineral supplement; additional calcium, magnesium, and zinc (additional iron is beneficial in children and adolescents if anemia or low iron stores are documented); potent antioxidants (e.g., pine bark [pycnogenol] or grapeseed extract).

Step 3

- Gastrointestinal rehabilitation: reduce intestinal permeability, improve nutrient absorption, and increase immune response to gut pathogens while diminishing hypersensitivities.
- Mnemonic *ANT PIE* (*a*bstain, *n*ourish, *t*oxins and detoxification, *p*robiotics, *i*dentify, *e*liminate).
  - **Abstain** from junk foods, deep-fried foods, sugary drinks, and other foods that harm or irritate the gut, unnecessary drugs, and excessive alcohol.

— **Nourish** digestive tract with nutrients that support gut healing; functional foods that combine low allergy potential protein and nutrients.
— **Toxins and detoxification**: avoid pesticides by eating organic foods and consuming nutrients that improve efficiency of detoxification processes—for example, L-glutamine, *N*-acetylcysteine, dietary fiber, and cruciferous vegetables. Regular exercise and stress reduction.
— **Probiotics:** therapeutic bacteria (and some yeasts) that improve gastrointestinal microecology, improve immune response toward gut pathogens, reduce immune hypersensitivities, and stimulate gut repair.
— **Identify** allergenic or intolerant foods and gut pathogens. Food allergies (type I or immediate hypersensitivity food reactions) can be identified by skin prick testing, radioallergosorbent testing, or enzyme-linked immunosorbent assay testing for immunoglobulin E (IgE) anti-food antibodies. Refer patients with evidence of type I hypersensitivity food allergies (e.g., postprandial swelling of the lips, urticaria, wheezing) to allergists; anaphylaxis could occur with inadvertent exposure. Delayed hypersensitivity reactions (usually type III mediated) are best identified with elimination test diet, followed by carefully observed reintroductions of individual foods eliminated in test diet. IgG anti-food antibodies may be tested, but only before any dietary manipulation occurs.
— **Intestinal parasites, yeast, and pathogenic bacteria:** identify by stool testing, *Candida* and *Helicobacter pylori* serology, breath testing, and urinary organic acids.
— **Eliminate** foods to which patient is allergic or intolerant with elimination test diet or laboratory testing. Gut pathogens, parasites, and *Candida* overgrowth may be treated.

Step 4

- **Nutraceuticals:** improve behavior and cognition; may be necessary earlier if parents are pressured to submit their child to a drug regimen. For example, *G. biloba* extract and/or L-theanine may provide some benefit.

Bacterial Sinusitis

DIAGNOSTIC SUMMARY

- History of acute viral respiratory infection, dental infection, or nasal allergy
- Nasal congestion and purulent discharge
- Fever, chills, and frontal headache
- Pain, tenderness, redness, and swelling over the involved sinus
- Transillumination shows opaque sinus
- Chronic infection may produce no symptoms other than mild postnasal discharge, a musty odor, or a nonproductive cough.

GENERAL CONSIDERATIONS

The primary predisposing factor is a viral upper respiratory infection (common cold). Allergic rhinitis and other factors interfering with normal protective mechanisms may precede viral infection and are also predisposing factors. Any factor inducing mucous membrane edema may obstruct meatal drainage. Transudate serves as a medium for bacteria. Streptococci, pneumococci, staphylococci, and *Haemophilus influenzae* are the most common. Allergy is common in chronic sinusitis; 25% of chronic maxillary sinusitis involves underlying dental infection. Vasoconstrictors and antihistamines give transient relief, but prolonged use is contraindicated—reflex reaction after long-term administration.

THERAPEUTIC CONSIDERATIONS

- **Antibiotics:** their value is limited. Analysis of clinical trials: antibiotic treatment in acute maxillary sinusitis in the general practice population is not sufficiently based on evidence. Antibiotics are warranted in severe or unresponsive cases. Although 80% of patients treated without antibiotics improve within 2 weeks, antibiotics have a small treatment effect in the primary care setting in patients with uncomplicated acute sinusitis with symptoms for more than 7 days. Newer, more potent

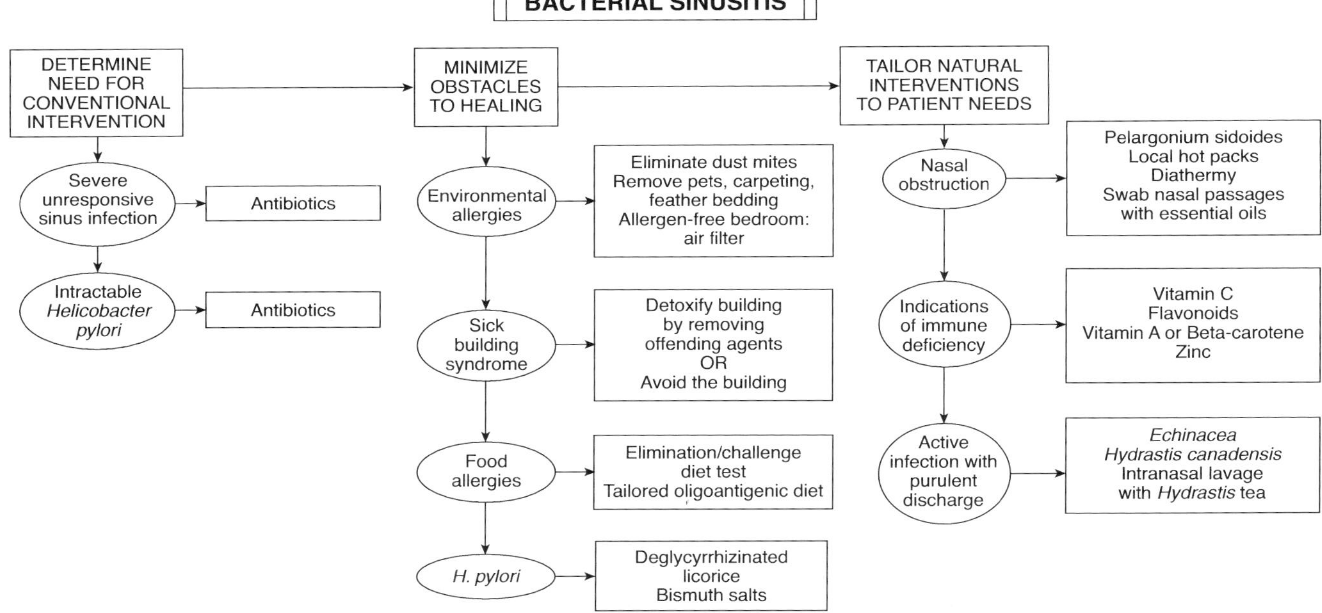
BACTERIAL SINUSITIS
DETERMINE NEED FOR CONVENTIONAL INTERVENTION
Severe unresponsive sinus infection
Antibiotics
Intractable *Helicobacter pylori*
Antibiotics
MINIMIZE OBSTACLES TO HEALING
Environmental allergies
Eliminate dust mites
Remove pets, carpeting, feather bedding
Allergen-free bedroom: air filter
Sick building syndrome
Detoxify building by removing offending agents
OR
Avoid the building
Food allergies
Elimination/challenge diet test
Tailored oligoantigenic diet
H. pylori
Deglycyrrhizinated licorice
Bismuth salts
TAILOR NATURAL INTERVENTIONS TO PATIENT NEEDS
Nasal obstruction
Pelargonium sidoides
Local hot packs
Diathermy
Swab nasal passages with essential oils
Indications of immune deficiency
Vitamin C
Flavonoids
Vitamin A or Beta-carotene
Zinc
Active infection with purulent discharge
Echinacea
Hydrastis canadensis
Intranasal lavage with *Hydrastis* tea

antibiotics (lactam antibiotics) are more effective than penicillin, amoxicillin, and other less-potent antibiotics. Overuse of antibiotics in children with sinusitis or otitis media can generate antibiotic-resistant bacterial pathogens. In chronic sinusitis, antibiotics are of little or no benefit. Addressing the underlying cause (respiratory or food allergens) and providing supportive therapy (saline nasal sprays, immune-enhancing herbs, and natural decongestants) is the most rational approach.

- **Allergy:** approximately 84% of those with chronic sinusitis have allergies.
- **Screen chronic sinusitis patients** aggressively for environmental and food allergies. Control the patient's environment. Eliminate dust mites by washing at temperature of at least 58°C, using an air-filtering vacuum cleaner and air cleaner with a high-efficiency particulate air filter, and keeping humidity below 50%. Remove all pets, carpeting, and feather bedding, if necessary.
- **Mucolytics:** mucociliary clearance depends on properties and volume of mucus, ciliary function, and mucociliary interactions. In chronic sinusitis, viscoelasticity of mucus is higher than optimal for mucociliary clearance. Mucolytics (*N*-acetylcysteine [NAC], proteolytic enzymes) can reduce viscoelasticity. NAC is a commonly used agent. The free NAC sulfhydryl group interacts with disulfide bonds of mucus glycoproteins, breaking the protein network into less-viscous strands. Use nasal NAC 10% solution diluted with saline, sodium bicarbonate, and sterile water or use an oral supplement. Enzymes (trypsin, chymotrypsin, *Serratia* peptidase, bromelain, streptokinase) may break down proteins at the inflammation site, exert antimicrobial effects, or act on the peptide region of mucus glycoproteins when administered topically. The ratio of viscosity to elasticity influences mucociliary transport. *Serratia* peptidase is rapidly effective for a variety of acute or chronic ear, nose, and throat disorders, including sinusitis. Oral bromelain also is beneficial for chronic sinusitis.
- **Sick building syndrome:** environmental chemicals within buildings can induce lethargy, headache, and blocked or runny nose—symptoms of chronic sinusitis.
- ***Helicobacter pylori:*** in atopic patients with symptoms of peptic ulcer, urticaria, sinusitis, and exercise-induced anaphylaxis increased when patients were positive for *H. pylori. H. pylori*–specific immunoglobulin E (IgE) and IgG reactivity was identified, with endoscopy confirming *H. pylori* in stomachs or sinuses of those

with *H. pylori* antibodies. Antibiotic therapy for *H. pylori*–induced ulcers resolves allergy symptoms in a significant number of such patients.

Pelargonium Sidoides (South African Geranium)

- Extracts from rhizomes and tubers of *P. sidoides* exert effects beneficial in upper respiratory infections (e.g., acute bronchitis); P. sidoides is an approved drug in Germany for this indication (see chapter on Bronchitis and Pneumonia).
- *P. sidoides* has immune-enhancing effects, antibacterial and antiviral effects, and ability to prevent adhesion of bacteria to epithelial cells.
- For acute rhinosinusitis of presumably bacterial origin, patients are given ethanolic extract of *P. sidoides* (EPs 7630) at 3 mL t.i.d. for a maximum of 22 days. The extract induced significant decrease in Sinusitis Severity Score compared with placebo. This result was confirmed by all secondary parameters, indicating a more favorable course and a faster recovery with EPs 7630.

THERAPEUTIC APPROACH

- **Therapeutic goals:** in acute sinusitis, reestablish drainage and clear acute infection.
- **Methods:** local heat application, local use of volatile oils, antibacterial botanicals, and immune system support (*Textbook,* "Bacterial Sinusitis")
  - — Isolate and eliminate food or airborne allergens and correct underlying problem allowing allergy to develop (*Textbook,* "Food Reactions").
  - — Acute phase: eliminate common food allergens (milk, wheat, eggs, citrus, corn, and peanut butter) pending definitive diagnosis.
  - — Local applications of heat may alleviate short- and long-term symptoms of allergic rhinitis.
- Supplements
  - — Vitamin C: 500 mg t.i.d.
  - — Bioflavonoids: 1000 mg q.d.
  - — Vitamin A: 5000 IU q.d. (or beta-carotene 25,000 IU q.d. if patient has genetics allowing conversion to vitamin A)
  - — Zinc: 30 mg q.d.
  - — *N*-acetylcysteine: 200 mg t.i.d.

— Serratia peptidase or bromelain:
  - Bromelain (1200 to 1800 milk clotting units [MCU]): 250 mg t.i.d. between meals
  - *Serratia* peptidase (enteric coated): 50 mg t.i.d. between meals
- Botanicals
  — *Echinacea* species (t.i.d.): dried root (or as tea), 0.5 to 1 g; freeze-dried plant, 325 to 650 mg; juice of aerial portion of *Echinacea purpurea* stabilized in 22% ethanol, 2 to 3 mL; tincture (1:5), 2 to 4 mL; fluid extract (1:1), 2 to 4 mL; solid (dry powdered) extract (6.5:1 or 3.5% echinacoside), 150 to 300 mg
  — *Hydrastis canadensis:* dose based on berberine content, preferably standardized extracts: dried root or as infusion (tea), 2 to 4 g; tincture (1:5): 6 to 12 mL (1.5 to 3 tsp); fluid extract (1:1), 2 to 4 mL (0.5 to 1 tsp); solid (powdered dry) extract (4:1 or 8% to 12% alkaloid content), 250 to 500 mg
  — *P. sidoides:* Dose recommendations for EPs 7630 or equivalent preparation:
  - Adults: 3 mL t.i.d. or 2 20-mg tablets t.i.d. for up to 14 days
  - Children: ages 7 to 12 years, 30 drops (1.5 mL) t.i.d.; age 6 years or younger, 10 drops (0.5 mL) t.i.d.
- Local treatment
  — Intranasal douche with *Hydrastis* tea
  — Swab passages with oil of bitter orange, menthol, or eucalyptus packs over sinuses (care should be taken to avoid irritation)
- Physical therapy
  — Hot packs
  — Diathermy: 30 minutes (discontinue if pain increases without drainage)

Benign Prostatic Hyperplasia

DIAGNOSTIC SUMMARY

- Symptoms of bladder outlet obstruction: progressive urinary frequency, urgency, and nocturia; hesitancy and intermittency with reduced force and caliber of urine
- Enlarged nontender prostate
- Uremia with prolonged obstruction

GENERAL CONSIDERATIONS

- BPH is the fourth most common diagnosis in older men; 50% of men over age 50 are affected, and 90% of men will have an enlarged prostate by age 80.
- Progression involves urinary retention, risk of recurrent urinary tract infections, bladder calculi, and occasionally renal insufficiency.
- Management options include exercise, low-fat diet, supplementary medications, minimally invasive therapies, and prostate surgery.
- The most common symptoms are lower urinary tract symptoms (LUTS)—frequent urination, urgency, nocturia, weak urinary stream, incomplete bladder emptying, straining to void, and intermittent stream.
- Prostate cancer, bladder cancer, overactive bladder, urinary tract infections, prostatitis, urethral stricture, and bladder stones can also cause LUTS and must be ruled out before BPH is diagnosed.
- The main risk factors are abdominal obesity and genetic factors or family history.
- Increased waist size, increased body mass index, and body weight elevation increase the volume of the prostate gland.

Hormones and Benign Prostatic Hyperplasia

- BPH is linked to androgens; BPH does not develop in men who were castrated before puberty and who have depleted

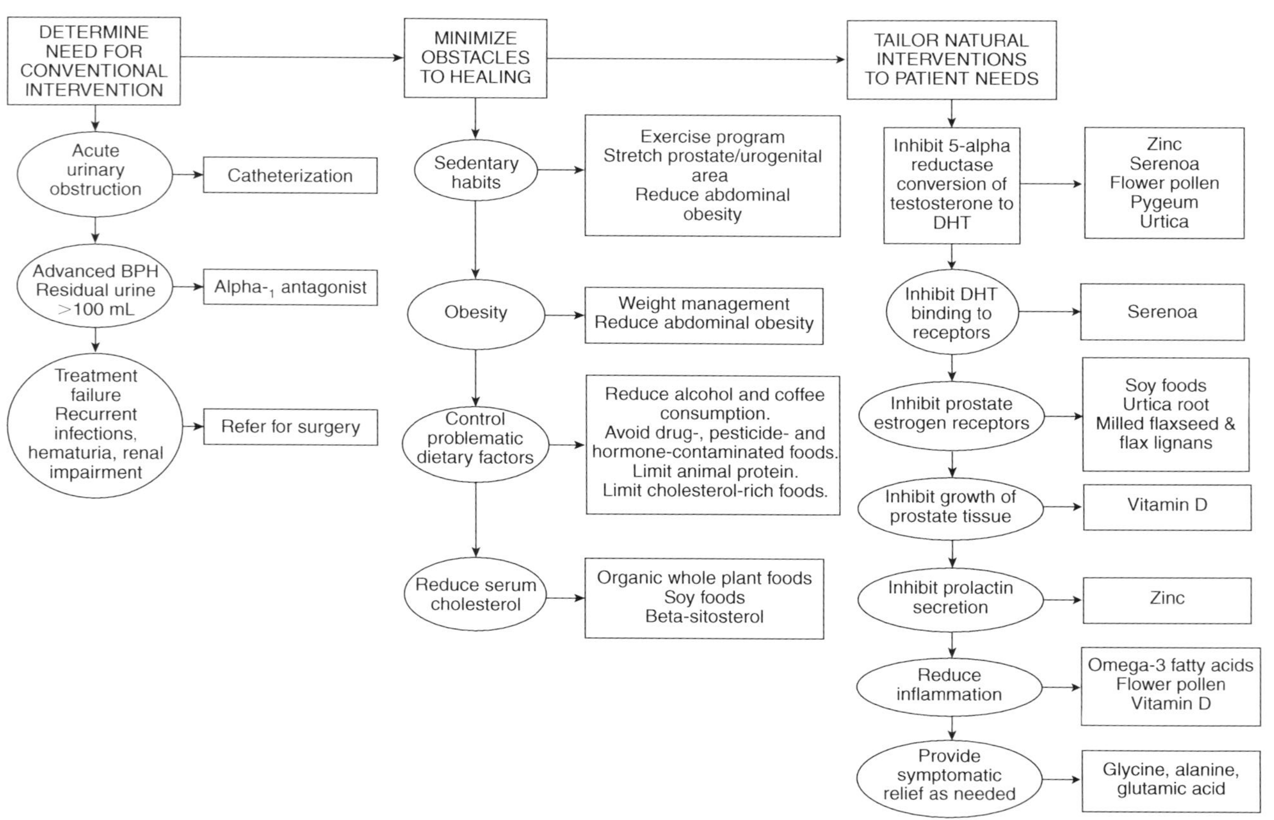
BENIGN PROSTATIC HYPERPLASIA
DETERMINE NEED FOR CONVENTIONAL INTERVENTION
Acute urinary obstruction
Catheterization
Advanced BPH Residual urine >100 mL
Alpha-$_1$ antagonist
Treatment failure Recurrent infections, hematuria, renal impairment
Refer for surgery
MINIMIZE OBSTACLES TO HEALING
Sedentary habits
Exercise program Stretch prostate/urogenital area Reduce abdominal obesity
Obesity
Weight management Reduce abdominal obesity
Control problematic dietary factors
Reduce alcohol and coffee consumption. Avoid drug-, pesticide- and hormone-contaminated foods. Limit animal protein. Limit cholesterol-rich foods.
Reduce serum cholesterol
Organic whole plant foods Soy foods Beta-sitosterol
TAILOR NATURAL INTERVENTIONS TO PATIENT NEEDS
Inhibit 5-alpha reductase conversion of testosterone to DHT
Zinc Serenoa Flower pollen Pygeum Urtica
Inhibit DHT binding to receptors
Serenoa
Inhibit prostate estrogen receptors
Soy foods Urtica root Milled flaxseed & flax lignans
Inhibit growth of prostate tissue
Vitamin D
Inhibit prolactin secretion
Zinc
Reduce inflammation
Omega-3 fatty acids Flower pollen Vitamin D
Provide symptomatic relief as needed
Glycine, alanine, glutamic acid

circulating androgens. In men with BPH, medical or surgical castration reduces prostate volume.

- For testosterone to affect the prostate, it must be converted to dihydrotestosterone (DHT) by enzyme 5-alpha-reductase. DHT has twice the effect on the prostate as testosterone. Although testosterone levels decline with age, DHT levels in the prostate remain similar to those in young men even if serum levels are low. Circulating DHT, at low serum plasma levels and tightly bound to plasma proteins, has limited effect on prostate growth.
- Estrogens in men are predominantly products of peripheral aromatization of testicular and adrenal androgens. Testicular and adrenal androgens decline with aging, but total plasma estradiol does not decline. Estradiol remains constant or even increases with age in men because of increased aromatase activity in the aging male with increased body fat. Fat cells contain aromatase, which converts certain androgens to estrogen.
- Limiting aromatase or inhibiting the binding of estrogen to prostate cells may reduce the incidence of BPH or slow its progression.

DIAGNOSTIC CONSIDERATIONS

International Prostate Symptom Score

- The International Prostate Symptom Score (IPSS) is a useful subjective assessment tool for BPH patients; it is a modification of the American Urological Association (AUA) Symptom Index.
- The questionnaire assesses degree of LUTS and quality of life.
- Patients can fill out the IPSS form before examinations, but minimal interference from health care providers must be ensured.
- A score of 7 or less is mildly symptomatic, 8 to 19 is moderately symptomatic, and 20 to 35 is severely symptomatic.
- Both the AUA index and the IPSS questionnaire are sensitive enough to be used in evaluating symptoms and selecting treatment.

Physical Examination

- Digital rectal examination (DRE) is used to determine the consistency and shape of the prostate and abnormalities suggestive of prostate cancer, BPH, or prostatitis.

- An approximate size can be determined with DRE, but inadvertent misestimation can be made even by physicians who are highly experienced. Prostate size can be determined most accurately by a transrectal ultrasound scan.

Urine and Blood Tests

- Dipstick urinalysis testing or microscopic urinalysis is used to screen for infection and hematuria, proteinuria, pyuria, glycosuria, and ketonuria.
- If the urine dipstick result is positive, urine culture may be necessary to determine whether LUTS is independent of BPH.

Prostate-Specific Antigen

- Symptoms of BPH and prostate cancer can be similar
- Prostate-specific antigen (PSA) may differentiate BPH from prostate cancer. False-positive and false-negative PSA test results are common; therefore the benefits and risks of such testing should be considered carefully.
- PSA testing is used to screen for prostate cancer and its severity, along with imaging, PSA density (PSAD), staging, and Gleason score.
- PSA is a controversial test owing to lack of specificity, which can lead to overdiagnosis and overtreatment of indolent prostate cancers.

Prostate-Specific Antigen and Benign Prostatic Hyperplasia

- PSA is a glycoprotein secreted by glands of the prostate, released in serum by disruption of normal prostatic tissue—cancer, inflammation, BPH, or trauma.
- The drugs finasteride (5-mg) and dutasteride (0.5-mg) inhibit 5-alpha-reductase and used to treat BPH and male-pattern baldness (1-g dose of finasteride).They typically lower PSA by 50%.
- Ejaculation and DRE may increase PSA levels, but effects are variable or insignificant.
- Prostate biopsy causes elevation of PSA. After biopsy, PSA testing should be postponed for 3 to 6 weeks.
- Elevated PSA indicates prostate cancer in 90% of patients; but midrange elevations can be caused by BPH, and there can be prostate cancer without elevation of PSA.
- To distinguish diseases when PSA is elevated, the free-to-total PSA ratio is measured; more free PSA than complexed PSA

suggests BPH rather than cancer. A ratio of 20% or greater for free PSA suggests BPH.

- **PSAD** can differentiate cancer and BPH in men with PSA levels of 4 to 10 ng/mL and normal DRE results. PSAD should be higher in men with prostate cancer than in those with benign disease, because cancer causes greater elevation in PSA per prostate volume. To determine PSAD, PSA level is divided by prostate volume (measured via transrectal ultrasound). PSAD greater than 0.15 suggests higher risk of prostate cancer. Lower PSAD suggests BPH. This method is not conclusive, but it can be one piece of the puzzle.

THERAPEUTIC CONSIDERATIONS

Surgery may be indicated in patients in whom medical therapy has failed or who have recurrent infections, hematuria, or renal insufficiency. In the past, medical treatment involved a transurethral resection of the prostate, which carries a risk of morbidity (sexual dysfunction, incontinence, bleeding); this procedure should be avoided unless absolutely necessary. Thermal microwave and laser therapies to reduce hyperplastic tissue are available. These newer procedures are less expensive and have fewer complications, although subsequent therapies are often required.

Lifestyle and Exercise

- There is an inverse association between physical activity and BPH and a positive one between abdominal obesity and BPH.
- Sympathetic nervous system activity increases risk of BPH. The fight-or-flight arm of the autonomic nervous system may cause prostate smooth muscle to contract, worsening LUTS. Higher caloric intake does not seem to increase BPH risk when accompanied by increased physical activity.
- Physical activity may do the following:
  1. Increase blood flow to the area, removing wastes efficiently
  2. Decrease sympathetic stress responses, relaxing prostatic tissue
  3. Reduce excess abdominal weight and lower body pressure, thus relaxing the prostate and rectal region and improving blood flow

Dietary and Nutritional Factors

- Diets high in total fat (not specific with regard to type of fat) and/or high in red meat (the impact of conventional versus grass feeding is unknown) are linked to higher BPH risk.

- Diets high in protein and vegetables are associated with a decreased risk.
- Avoid pesticides, increase fruit, increase zinc and essential fatty acids, decrease coffee, decrease butter, avoid margarine, and keep serum cholesterol below 200 mg/dL. Moderate intake of alcohol may benefit BPH but make LUTS worse.

High-Protein Diet

- Research evaluating protein intake and BPH is mixed. Theoretically, a high protein intake may not help because of a greater osmolar load, which may influence urinary output, and because protein imposes an extra burden on the urinary system.
- Ingestion of excess animal protein as a means to increase total protein intake should be avoided. High-quality, plant-derived protein and cold-water fish in moderate amounts are preferred.

Zinc

- Zinc supplementation reduces the size of the prostate and symptoms of BPH in the majority of patients.
- Zinc may be protective against BPH. Higher zinc intake is associated with reduced risk of BPH.
- Mechanism: zinc can inhibit 5-alpha reductase and inhibit prolactin. Prolactin increases uptake of testosterone by the prostate, leading to increased DHT by providing additional substrate.

Alcohol

- Only beer raises prolactin; a higher alcohol intake may be associated with BPH. Alcohol intake of at least 25 ounces per month is directly correlated with diagnosis of BPH.
- Association is most significant for beer, wine, and sake, and less so for distilled spirits. Alcohol may be protective with regard to BPH but not LUTS.

Amino Acids

- A combination of glycine, alanine, and glutamic acid (in 2 375 mg capsules administered t.i.d. for 2 weeks and 1 capsule t.i.d. thereafter) relieves many BPH symptoms.
- The mechanism is unknown but is likely related to amino acids acting as inhibitory neurotransmitters and reducing the feeling of bladder fullness. Thus amino acid therapy is only palliative.

Cholesterol

- Association among cholesterol, BPH, and LUTS has been mixed. In the case of BPH, no positive association has been shown for cholesterol.

Beta-Sitosterol

- Beta-sitosterol is a plant sterol (cholesterol is the main animal sterol). Sources include rice bran, wheat germ, corn oil, soybeans, peanuts and their products, *Serenoa repens,* avocados, pumpkin seed, *Pygeum africanum,* and cashew fruit.
- Beta-sitosterol improves BPH. On average, urinary flow increases by 4.5 mL/s; residual urinary volumes decreases by 33.5 mL. The IPSS shows statistically significant improvement.

Vitamin D

- Vitamin D supplementation is associated with reduced risk of BPH. The association was observed only among men who used both multivitamins and single vitamin D supplements. There were no associations between supplement use and BPH risk with the exception of a trend toward decreased BPH risk with increased intake of supplemental vitamin D.
- Vitamin D_3 may have protective effects against prostate cancer.
- The mechanism in BPH involves attachment of this molecule to vitamin D receptors on prostate and bladder cells and inhibition of prostate growth, lowering excessive contractility and reducing inflammation.

Cadmium

- Although cadmium is an antagonist of zinc and increases activity of 5-alpha-reductase, its concentration in the prostate and its effects are unclear. Several studies have produced conflicting results.

Botanical Medicines

The chance of clinical success with botanical treatments appears to be determined by degree of obstruction, as indicated by volume of residual urine. For levels less than 50 mL, results are usually excellent. For levels between 50 and 100 mL, results are quite good. With residual urine between 100 and 150 mL, it will be tougher to produce significant improvement within the customary 4- to 6-week period. If volume of residual urine is below 150 mL, saw palmetto extract and other botanicals alone are unlikely to produce significant improvement.

Serenoa Repens (Saw Palmetto)

- Liposterolic extract of fruit of the saw palmetto palm tree (also called *Sabal serrulata*), native to Florida, improves signs and symptoms of BPH.
- The mechanism involves inhibition of DHT binding to both cytosolic and nuclear androgen receptors, inhibition of 5-alpha-reductase, and interference with intraprostatic estrogen receptors.
- Results have been excellent, comparing quite favorably with those with finasteride (Proscar) and tamsulosin (Flomax) in terms of efficacy but with a better side effect profile.
- The effect of *Serenoa* extract is most obvious in early stages of BPH (i.e., mild to moderate hypertrophy). Roughly 90% of men with mild to moderate BPH experience improvement in symptoms during first 4 to 6 weeks after starting *Serenoa* (320 mg of liposterolic extract per day). *Serenoa* extract may show little clinical benefit in more-advanced cases.
- Although *Serenoa* is often very effective on its own, better results may be achieved by combining *Urtica dioica* root extract (discussed later) with *Serenoa* extract. This combination produces clinical benefit equal to that of finasteride. Like extract of *Serenoa, Urtica* extract appears to interact with binding of DHT to cytosolic and nuclear receptors.
- Lignans in *Urtica* may modulate hormonal effects owing to their affinity for sex hormone–binding globulin.

Cernilton

- Cernilton, an extract of rye grass flower pollen, has been used to treat prostatitis and BPH in Europe for more than 40 years. The overall success rate is 70%.
- Patients who respond experience less nocturia and diurnal frequency (reduction of 70%) and reductions in residual urine volume.
- Cernilton exerts some anti-inflammatory action, produces a contractile effect on the bladder, and relaxes the urethra.
- Cernilton contains constituents that inhibit growth of prostate cells.
- Although Cernilton does not improve urinary flow rates, residual volume, or prostate size compared with placebo or comparative study agents, it improves self-rated urinary symptom scores and reduces nocturia compared with placebo and an amino acid mixture.

- Combinations of Cernilton, saw palmetto, beta-sitosterol, and vitamin E have reduced nocturia, frequency, and overall BPH symptoms without causing any adverse side effects.

Pygeum Africanum

- Bark of *P. africanum*, an evergreen tree native to Africa, used traditionally for urinary tract disorders, contains fat-soluble sterols and fatty acids.
- Virtually all research on *Pygeum* has featured extract standardized to 14% triterpenes, including beta-sitosterol and 0.5% *N*-docosanol.
- The in vitro therapeutic effect of *Pygeum* may result in part from inhibition of epidermal growth factor (EGF), basic fibroblast growth factor (bFGF), and insulin-like growth factor 1 (IGF-I).
- *Pygeum* extract reduces symptoms and clinical signs of BPH, especially in early cases. However, saw palmetto produces comparatively greater reduction of symptoms and is better tolerated. Effects on urine flow rate and residual urine content are better in clinical studies with saw palmetto.
- However, there may be circumstances in which *Pygeum* is more effective than saw palmetto. Saw palmetto seems not to produce the effects of *Pygeum* on prostate secretion, but the two extracts have overlapping mechanisms of action and can be used in combination.

Urtica Dioica (Stinging Nettle)

- Extracts of root of *U. dioica* have also been shown to be effective in the treatment of BPH.
- *Urtica* given over a treatment period of 18 months is superior to placebo with no side effects.

THERAPEUTIC APPROACH

Therapeutic Goals for Benign Prostatic Hyperplasia

- Normalize prostate nutrient levels
- Restore normal steroid hormone levels
- Inhibit excessive conversion of testosterone to DHT
- Inhibit DHT-receptor binding
- Reduce inflammation
- Eliminate excess estradiol production
- Limit promoters of hyperplastic process (e.g., prolactin)

Severe BPH resulting in significant acute urinary retention may require catheterization; a sufficiently advanced case may not respond rapidly enough to therapy and may require short-term $alpha_1$ antagonist by itself or combined with 5-alpha-reductase medication or surgical intervention.

Lifestyle

- Increase exercise to four to six times a week.
- Properly stretch prostate and urogenital area to increase blood flow.

Diet

- Initially, higher in vegetable protein, low in carbohydrate, low in animal fats, and high in unsaturated oils.
- After patient responds, less-strict, whole-foods, balanced approach.
- Limit alcohol and coffee. Avoid drug-, pesticide-, and hormone-contaminated foods. Limit cholesterol-rich foods. Soy foods should be used regularly.

Supplements

- Zinc: 30 to 45 mg elemental zinc q.d. (picolinate preferred) for maximum of 6 months. Reduce dose to 15 to 30 mg/day after 6 months and consider monitoring copper status in long-term therapy.
- Glycine: 250 mg q.d.
- Glutamic acid: 250 mg q.d.
- Alanine: 250 mg q.d.
- Vitamin D_3: 2000 to 5000 international units (IU) q.d.

Botanicals

- Liposterolic extract of saw palmetto *(S. repens)* (standardized at 85% to 95% fatty acids and sterols): 160-320 mg b.i.d.
- Flower pollen extract (e.g., Cernilton): 63 mg b.i.d. to t.i.d.
- *P. africanum* extract (14% triterpene content): 50 to 100 mg q.d.
- *U. dioica* extract: 120 to 150 mg b.i.d.
- Beta-sitosterol: 60 to 130 mg q.d.

Bronchitis and Pneumonia

DIAGNOSTIC SUMMARY: BRONCHITIS

- Diagnosis of acute bronchitis: rule out other causes of acute cough—pneumonia, common cold, acute asthma, exacerbation of chronic obstructive pulmonary disease.
- For presumed diagnosis of acute bronchitis, viral cultures, serologic assays, and sputum analyses should not be routinely performed; responsible organism is rarely identified.
- With acute cough and sputum suggestive of acute bronchitis, absence of the following findings reduces likelihood of pneumonia sufficiently to eliminate need for chest radiograph: (1) heart rate above 100 beats per minute; (2) respiratory rate above 24 breaths per minute; (3) oral body temperature higher than 38°C; and (4) chest examination findings of focal consolidation, egophony, or fremitus.

DIAGNOSTIC SUMMARY: PNEUMONIA

Diagnosis of pneumonia is usually made by physical examination and confirmed by chest radiographs. Common physical examination findings include the following:

- **Rales:** bubbling or crackling sound. Rales on one side of chest and rales heard while patient is lying down are strongly suggestive of pneumonia.
- **Rhonchi:** abnormal rumblings indicating presence of thick fluid.
- **Percussion:** dull thud instead of healthy hollow-drum–like sound; indicates conditions suggesting pneumonia:
  1. Consolidation (lung becomes firm and inelastic)
  2. Pleural effusion (fluid buildup in space between lungs and lining around it)
- **Sputum** suggestive of infection: bloody; thick, opaque; yellow, green, or brown; positive Gram stain. Sputum culture and sensitivity are not always helpful in identifying cause of pneumonia owing to contamination with throat or mouth bacteria.

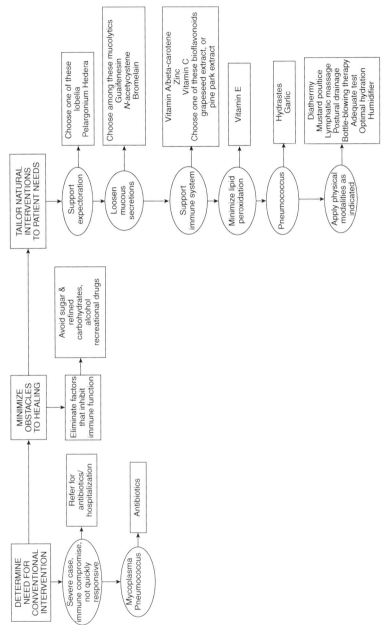

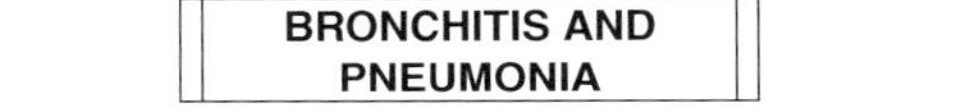

DETERMINE NEED FOR CONVENTIONAL INTERVENTION

- Severe case, immune compromise, not quickly responsive → Refer for antibiotics/ hospitalization
- Mycoplasma Pneumococcus → Antibiotics

MINIMIZE OBSTACLES TO HEALING

- Eliminate factors that inhibit immune function → Avoid sugar & refined carbohydrates, alcohol recreational drugs

TAILOR NATURAL INTERVENTIONS TO PATIENT NEEDS

- Support expectoration → Choose one of these lobelia Pelargonium Hedera
- Loosen mucous secretions → Choose among these mucolytics Guaifenesin *N*-acetycystene Bromelain
- Support immune system → Vitamin A/beta-carotene Zinc Vitamin C Choose one of these bioflavonoids grapeseed extract, or pine park extract
- Minimize lipid peroxidation → Vitamin E
- Pneumococcus → Hydrastes Garlic
- Apply physical modalities as indicated → Diathermy Mustard poultice Lymphatic massage Postural drainage Bottle-blowing therapy Adequate test Optimal hydration Humidifier

- **Urine test** (Alere BinaxNOW, Alere, Scarborough, ME) can detect *Streptococcus pneumoniae* or *Legionella pneumophila* antigens within 15 minutes. It may identify 77% of pneumonia cases and may rule out infection in 98% of patients who do not have *S. pneumoniae.* However, the test is not useful diagnosing *S. pneumoniae* pneumonia in children because the organism is common in this population whether or not they have pneumonia. *L. pneumophila* causes legionnaires' disease and sometimes pneumonia.
- **Chest x-ray study:** to confirm diagnosis of pneumonia, but it need not be positive for clinical diagnosis to be made. Positive chest radiograph for pneumonia may reveal lung infiltrates or complications (e.g., pleural effusions).

SPECIAL CONSIDERATIONS WITH PNEUMONIA

More than 100 types of bacteria, viruses, and fungi cause bronchitis or pneumonia. The three most common forms of pneumonia are viral, mycoplasmal, and pneumococcal types.

Viral Pneumonia

- Most often caused by adenovirus, influenza, parainfluenza, and respiratory syncytial virus
- Develops as complication of viral upper respiratory infection

Clinical Summary for Viral Pneumonia

- People at risk for more-serious viral pneumonia are often immunocompromised.
- Antibiotics are of no value.
- Symptoms often begin slowly and may not be severe at first.
- Most common symptoms:
  1. Cough (may cough up mucus or even bloody mucus)
  2. Fever: mild or high
  3. Shaking chills
  4. Shortness of breath (may occur only when climbing stairs)

Mycoplasmal Pneumonia

- Caused by *Mycoplasma pneumoniae. Mycoplasma* is a genus of bacteria lacking cell walls.
- "Walking pneumonia."
- Antibiotics are usually not necessary but may speed recovery. Effective classes of antibiotics: macrolides, quinolones, and tetracyclines.

Clinical Summary for Mycoplasmal Pneumonia

- Most commonly occurs in children or young adults
- Insidious onset over several days
- Nonproductive cough, minimal physical findings, temperature below 102°F
- Headache and malaise: common early symptoms
- White blood cell count: normal or slightly elevated
- X-ray pattern: patchy or inhomogeneous

Pneumococcal Pneumonia

- Pneumococcal pneumonia *(S. pneumoniae):* most common bacterial pneumonia and most common cause of pneumonia hospitalization.
- Careful clinical judgment must be used to determine severity of disease and status of patient's immune system. Antibiotics or hospitalization is often necessary, especially for the elderly or immunocompromised.
- Resistance rates to antibiotics and resistant strains are increasing.
- Consider natural treatments in cases resistant to antibiotics or as adjunct to strengthen immune response and increase therapeutic effect.

Clinical Summary for Pneumococcal Pneumonia

- Preceded by upper respiratory infection.
- Sudden onset of shaking, chills, fever, chest pain.
- Sputum: pinkish or blood-specked at first, then rusty at height of infection; finally yellow and mucopurulent during resolution.
- Gram-positive diplococci in sputum smear.
- Rapid urine test (BinaxNOW) for *S. pneumoniae* antigens is positive.
- Initially, chest excursion is diminished on involved side; breath sounds are suppressed; fine inspiratory rales.
- Later, classic signs of consolidation: bronchial breathing, crepitant rales, dullness.
- Leukocytosis,
- Radiograph: lobar or segmental consolidation.

GENERAL CONSIDERATIONS

- **Bronchitis:** inflammation of mucous membranes of bronchi, airways carrying airflow from trachea into lungs.
- **Pneumonia:** inflammation of lungs.

- Both are characterized by cough with or without sputum.
- Acute bronchitis often occurs during acute viral illness—common cold or influenza. Viruses cause 90% of cases of acute bronchitis.
- Pneumonia is usually seen in immunocompromised individuals—for example, drug and alcohol abusers—leading to nosocomial and opportunistic pneumonias with high mortality rates. Acute pneumonia is the seventh leading cause of death in United States and is particularly dangerous in the elderly.
- In healthy people, pneumonia follows an insult to host defenses: viral infection (influenza), exposure to cigarette smoke or other noxious fumes, impairment of consciousness (which depresses the gag reflex, allowing aspiration), neoplasms, and hospitalization (*Textbook,* Bronchitis and Pneumonia).
- In immunocompetent, nonelderly adults, cigarette smoking is the strongest independent risk factor for invasive pneumococcal disease.
- The airway distal to the larynx is normally sterile. Mucus-covered ciliated epithelium that lines the lower respiratory tract propels sputum to larger bronchi and trachea, evoking the cough reflex. Respiratory secretions contain substances that exert nonspecific antimicrobial actions: alpha$_1$-antitrypsin, lysozyme, and lactoferrin. Potent alveolar defense mechanisms include alveolar macrophages, rich vasculature for rapidly delivering lymphocytes and granulocytes, and efficient lymphatic drainage network.

THERAPEUTIC CONSIDERATIONS

Regardless of the form of bronchitis or pneumonia the basic approach involves use of (1) **expectorants,** (2) **mucolytics,** and (3) **immunosupportive nutrients**. Antibiotics are of limited value in acute bronchitis, but they are useful in pneumonia.

Expectorants

Impaired cough reflexes are thought to contribute to recurrent bronchitis and pneumonia. Botanical expectorants increase quantity, decrease viscosity, and promote expulsion of secretions of respiratory mucous membranes. Many have antibacterial and antiviral activity. Some expectorants are antitussives; however, *Lobelia inflata* promotes cough reflex. Thus *Lobelia* clears lungs better than other expectorants when cough is productive. Other expectorants include *Glycyrrhiza glabra* (licorice), *Pelargonium sidoides* (South African geranium), *Hedera helix* (ivy), and wild cherry bark.

Pelargonium Sidoides (South African Geranium)

P. sidoides is a medicinal plant in the geranium family native to South Africa. The common name, *umckaloabo,* is close to the Zulu word for "severe cough." Intricate groupings of thick dark-red rhizomes and tubers underground withstand grass fires in its habitat. An extract from rhizomes and tubers—ethanolic extract EPs 7630 (Umcka) is an approved drug for acute bronchitis in Germany. Primary active ingredients include highly oxygenated coumarins (e.g., umckalin) and polyphenolic compounds. Umcka uses a three-pronged approach in acute bronchitis: it (1) enhances immune function; (2) is antimicrobial—antimycobacterial and antiviral—and inhibits attachment of bacteria and viruses to mucous membranes of respiratory tract; and (3) acts as an expectorant. EPs 7630 at 100 mcg/mL interferes with replication of seasonal influenza A virus strains (H1N1, H3N2), respiratory syncytial virus, human coronavirus, parainfluenza virus, and coxsackievirus, but not highly pathogenic avian influenza A virus (H5N1), adenovirus, or rhinovirus. EPs 7630 induces reduction in Bronchitis Severity Score (BSS), which includes coughing, expectoration, chest pain, dyspnea, and wheezing from baseline versus after 7 days of treatment. In clinical studies with Umcka in 2500 adults and children, adverse events occurred on par with placebo and involved mild gastrointestinal complaints and skin rashes. There were no known drug interactions.

Hedera Helix (Ivy)

Extracts from leaves of ivy relieve cough and asthma. More than 80% of herbal expectorants prescribed in Germany consist of ivy extracts. Ivy leaf contains saponins that show expectorant, mucolytic, spasmolytic, bronchodilatory, and antibacterial effects. Mucolytic and expectorant action is based on indirect $beta_2$ adrenergic effects, as a result of the saponins alpha-hederin and hederacoside C, the latter being metabolized to alpha-hederin when ingested. An indirect effect is that alpha-hederin inhibits intracellular uptake of $beta_2$ receptors and leads to increased $beta_2$ adrenergic response of the cell. Ivy is often a monopreparation with good safety, compliance, and efficacy in acute and chronic bronchitis. A combination of ivy and thyme *(Thymus vulgaris)* for acute bronchitis induced a 50% reduction in coughing fits from baseline 2 days earlier than placebo. Treatment was well tolerated with no difference in frequency or severity of side effects between thyme-ivy combination and placebo.

Mucolytics

Mucolytics are used to improve quality of mucous secretions to promote expectoration. Guaifenesin (glycerol guaiacolate) is a derivative of a compound isolated from beech wood. Guaifenesin is an approved over-the-counter expectorant and mucolytic. Alternatives include *N*-acetylcysteine (NAC) and bromelain.

N-Acetylcysteine (NAC)

NAC has an extensive history as a mucolytic for acute and chronic lung conditions. It directly splits sulfur linkages of mucoproteins, reducing viscosity of bronchial and lung secretions. NAC improves bronchial and lung function, reduces cough, and improves oxygen saturation in the blood. NAC is helpful in all lung and respiratory disorders (e.g., chronic bronchitis and chronic obstructive pulmonary disease). Oral NAC reduces risk of exacerbations and improves symptoms in patients with chronic bronchitis compared with placebo. NAC can increase manufacture of glutathione, a major antioxidant for the entire respiratory tract and lungs. The dose is 200 mg t.i.d.

Bromelain

Bromelain is used as adjunctive therapy for bronchitis and pneumonia because of its fibrinolytic, anti-inflammatory, and mucolytic actions and its enhancement of antibiotic absorption. Its mucolytic activity provides efficacy in pneumonia, bronchitis, and sinusitis.

Vitamin C

- Before the advent of pharmaceutical antibiotics, many controlled and uncontrolled studies demonstrated efficacy of large doses of vitamin C in bronchitis and pneumonia, but only when they were started on the first or second day of infection. If administered later, it only lessens severity of disease.
- In pneumonia, white blood cells take up large amounts of vitamin C.
- Vitamin C therapy in elderly patients with pneumonia leads to better clinical outcomes. The benefit of vitamin C is most obvious in patients with the most severe illness, many of whom

tend to have low initial plasma and white blood cell levels of vitamin C.

Vitamin A

- Vitamin A is especially valuable in children with measles, perhaps owing to the increased rate of excretion of vitamin A during severe infections.
- Patients with fever excrete more retinol than those without fever. A remarkable 34% of patients studied excreted a quantity of retinol equivalent to 50% of the U.S. recommended daily allowance.
- This may be particularly important for children. In children with measles (average age 10 months), providing 400,000 international units (IU) (120 mg of retinyl palmitate), one half on admission and one half a day later, reduced death rate by 50% and duration of pneumonia, diarrhea, and hospital stay by 33%.
- **Zinc and vitamin A:** In children aged 6 months to 3 years, those given initial high doses of vitamin A followed by 4 months of elemental zinc (10 mg/day for infants and 20 mg/day for children older than 1 year) exhibited reduced incidence of pneumonia, not seen in with vitamin A alone.

Vitamin E

Patients with influenza complicated by pneumonia experience a sharp rise in lipid peroxidation (LPO) products, especially those who are seriously ill. Administrating alpha-tocopherol decreases LPO products and results in a more-benign clinical course.

Garlic (Allium Sativum)

- Garlic has broad-spectrum antibiotic activity against both gram-positive and gram-negative bacteria.
- Garlic is an effective antibacterial agent against *S. pneumoniae;* consider it in cases of antibiotic resistance or as adjunct to antibiotic therapy.
- Alternatively, berberine-containing plants (e.g., *Hydrastis canadensis* [goldenseal]) may be helpful.

Bottle Blowing and Salt Pipes

- In adults hospitalized for community-acquired pneumonia, patients instructed to sit up and take 20 deep breaths 10 times daily or to sit up and blow bubbles in a bottle containing 10 mL of water through a plastic tube 20 times on 10 occasions daily

experienced a significantly reduced length of hospitalization. The number of days with fever was lowest with bottle-blowing.
- Early mobilization itself decreases hospital stay in pneumonia patients.
- Despite positive clinical results, C-reactive protein levels, peak expiratory flow, and vital capacity were not affected.
- Changes in respiratory pressure associated with bottle blowing may provide an environment for more-efficient bacterial clearance.
- Decreased impairment of pulmonary function and increased total lung capacity manifests in patients who have undergone coronary artery bypass. This modality or a similar activity (e.g., playing a wind instrument) may decrease frequency and duration of respiratory events in patients vulnerable to respiratory infections.
- An alternative to bubble blowing is use of a salt pipe. These inhaler-type devices contain tiny salt particles said to ease breathing. The practice originated in central Europe, where respiratory patients spent time in salt caves or mines to relieve breathing problems.

THERAPEUTIC APPROACH

The basic approach involves expectorants, mucolytics, and immunosupportive nutrients. Helpful general physical modalities and measures are as follows:
- Diathermy to chest and back: 30 minutes q.d.
- Mustard poultice: once q.d.
- Lymphatic massage: t.i.d.
- Postural drainage: t.i.d.
- Bottle-blowing therapy: blowing bubbles in a bottle containing 10 mL water through a plastic tube 20 times on 10 occasions a day
- Plenty of rest
- Optimal hydration
- Humidifier

Expectorants

Choose one or more of the expectorants listed here.

Lobelia Inflata

- Dried herb: 0.2 to 0.6 g t.i.d.
- Tincture: 15 to 30 drops t.i.d.
- Fluid extract: 8 to 10 drops t.i.d.

Glycyrrhiza Glabra

- Powdered root: 1 to 2 g
- Fluid extract (1:1): 2 to 4 mL (0.5 to 1 tsp)
- Solid (dry-powdered) extract (4:1): 250 to 500 mg

Pelargonium Sidoides

Dosage for EPs 7630 or equivalent preparation:

- Adults: 1.5 mL t.i.d. or 20-mg tablets t.i.d. for up to 14 days.
- Children: age 7 to 12 years, 20 drops (1 mL) t.i.d.; age 6 years or younger, 10 drops (0.5 mL) t.i.d.

Hedera Helix

Ivy leaf is available primarily in tincture and fluid extract and dry powdered extract in capsules and tablets. Daily doses of dried herbal substance should deliver an amount equal to the following:

- 1 to 5 years: 150 mg; 6 to 12 years: 210 mg; older than 12 years: 420 mg
- Typical dose for adults and children older than 12 years for a 4:1 dried powdered extract: 100 mg q.d.

Mucolytics

Choose one or more of the mucolytics listed here.

Guaifenesin

- Adults and children age 12 years and older: 200 to 400 mg every 4 hours. Avoid taking more than 2400 mg in a 24-hour period.
- Children age 6 to 11 years: 100 to 200 mg every 4 hours; no more than 1200 mg in a 24-hour period.
- Children age 2 to 5 years: 50 to 100 mg every 4 hours; no more than 600 mg in 24 hours.
- Not recommended for children under age 2 years.

N-Acetylcysteine

- 200 mg t.i.d.

Bromelain

- 1200 to 1800 milk clotting units [MCU]
- 500 to 750 mg t.i.d. between meals

Supplements

- Vitamin A: 50,000 IU/day for 1 week *or* beta-carotene 200,000 IU/day (vitamin A should not be used in women of childbearing age owing to possible teratogenic effects)
- Vitamin C: 500 mg every 2 hours
- Vitamin E (mixed tocopherols): 200 IU q.d.
- Choose one of the following:
  - — Bioflavonoids (mixed citrus): 1000 mg q.d.
  - — Grapeseed *(Vitis vinifera)* extract (95% procyanidolic oligomers) 150 to 300 mg q.d.
  - — Pine bark extract *(Pinus pinaster)* 150 to 300 mg q.d.
- Zinc: 30 mg elemental zinc q.d.

ADDITIONAL RECOMMENDATIONS FOR PNEUMOCOCCAL PNEUMONIA

Choose garlic, *H. canadensis,* or both.

Garlic

Daily dose is equal to at least 4000 mg of fresh garlic, which translates to at least 10 mg allicin or a total allicin potential of 4000 mcg.

Hydrastis Canadensis

Standardized extracts are recommended. The following doses are given t.i.d.:

- Dried root or as infusion (tea): 2 to 4 g
- Tincture (1:5): 6 to 12 mL (1.5 to 3 tsp)
- Fluid extract (1:1): 2 to 4 mL (0.5 to 1 tsp)
- Solid (powdered dry) extract (4:1 or 8% to 12% alkaloid content): 250 to 500 mg

Cancer: Integrated Naturopathic Support

DIAGNOSTIC SUMMARY

Cancer is a group of more than 200 individual diseases characterized by uncontrolled growth, proliferation, and spread of abnormal cells. Diagnosis and treatment vary depending on type of cancer cells and location, extent of total tumor burden, health and performance status of the patient, prior treatments administered, and which conventional treatment regimens are currently considered standard of care.

GENERAL CONSIDERATIONS

The Role of Naturopathic Medicine

1. Primary prevention and risk reduction
2. Screening and early diagnosis
3. Integrative co-treatment during active cancer therapies
4. Posttreatment recovery support
5. Long-term secondary prevention

Prevention should take precedence over treatment. Occurrence involves two compounding factors: genetic susceptibility and environmental exposure to carcinogens. Environmental factors contribute more than half the risk for the 11 most common cancers. Naturopathy reduces lifestyle-based risk factors and counteracts some genetic factors. Cancer has long latency period; reducing risk factors—diet, lifestyle, and environmental toxins—can either delay or prevent progression from preclinical cancer to clinical cancer. Women who have less-frequent mammography screening actually have 20% less breast cancer; lower diagnosis rates reflect spontaneous resolution of 20% of cancers. Newer genetic tests and metabolic tests can identify risk factors for cancers. Many of these reflect metabolic aberrations

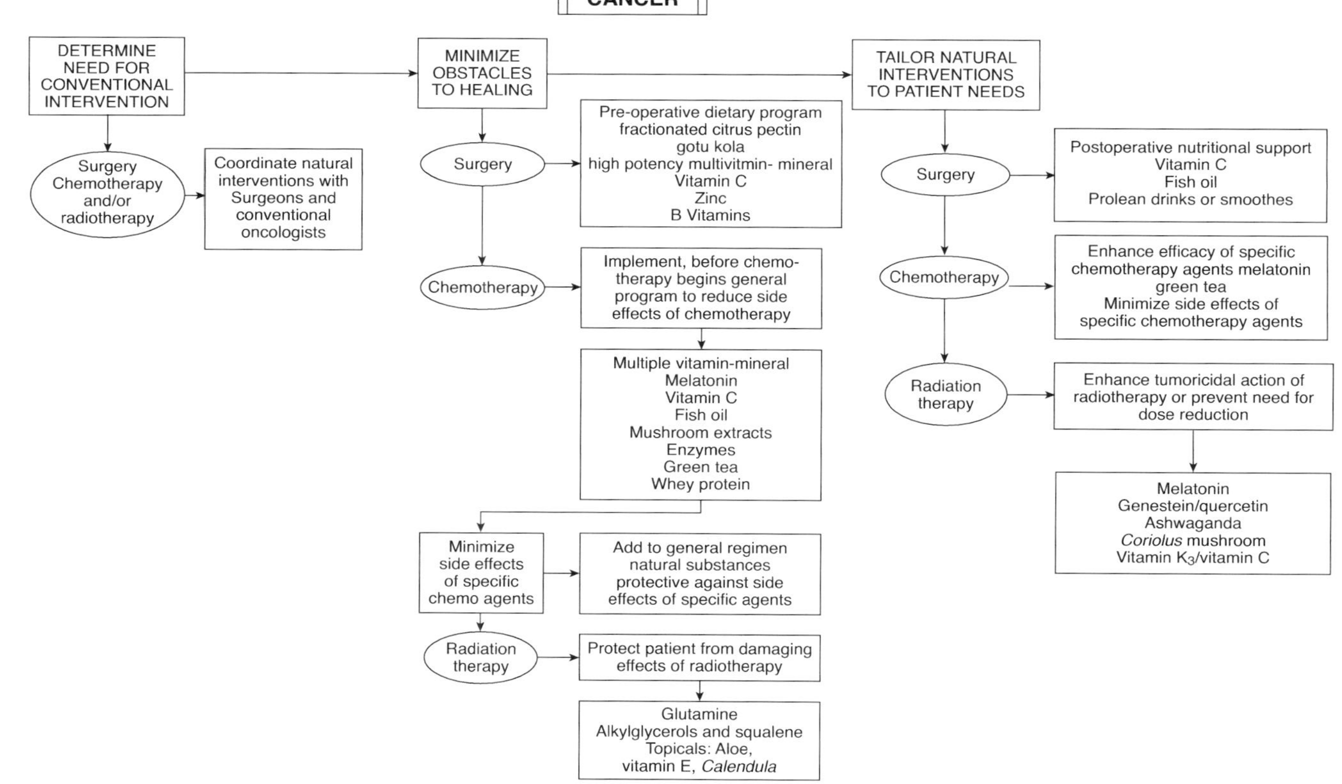
CANCER
DETERMINE NEED FOR CONVENTIONAL INTERVENTION
Surgery Chemotherapy and/or radiotherapy
Coordinate natural interventions with Surgeons and conventional oncologists
MINIMIZE OBSTACLES TO HEALING
Surgery
Pre-operative dietary program fractionated citrus pectin gotu kola high potency multivitmin- mineral Vitamin C Zinc B Vitamins
Chemotherapy
Implement, before chemo-therapy begins general program to reduce side effects of chemotherapy
Multiple vitamin-mineral Melatonin Vitamin C Fish oil Mushroom extracts Enzymes Green tea Whey protein
Minimize side effects of specific chemo agents
Add to general regimen natural substances protective against side effects of specific agents
Radiation therapy
Protect patient from damaging effects of radiotherapy
Glutamine Alkylglycerols and squalene Topicals: Aloe, vitamin E, Calendula
TAILOR NATURAL INTERVENTIONS TO PATIENT NEEDS
Surgery
Postoperative nutritional support Vitamin C Fish oil Prolean drinks or smoothes
Chemotherapy
Enhance efficacy of specific chemotherapy agents melatonin green tea Minimize side effects of specific chemotherapy agents
Radiation therapy
Enhance tumoricidal action of radiotherapy or prevent need for dose reduction
Melatonin Genestein/quercetin Ashwaganda Coriolus mushroom Vitamin K3/vitamin C

that reduce DNA repair or increase abnormal cell signaling. Early identification allows for correction or amelioration of these risk factors with dietary, lifestyle, and supplemental modification. For example, with regard to the link between hyperinsulinemia and breast cancer, early identification of hyperinsulinemia can reverse predisposition and reduce risk of ever developing breast cancer. Even genetic factors are at least partially responsive to modification—for example, the incidence of breast cancer in carriers of the *BRCA* gene. Women who lost 10 or more pounds between ages 18 and 30 years had up to a 65% lower risk of developing breast cancer between ages 30 and 40 years.

Sensitive screening and diagnostic testing are needed to diagnose cancer at early, more-curable stages. Roles of naturopathy include the following:

- Helping guide patients in selecting the best oncology care team and facility
- Reducing side effects of conventional therapies
- Improving tumoricidal activity of conventional therapies
- Improving the environment factors that allowed malignancy (e.g., removing tumor promoting factors—hyperinsulinemia, nutrient deficiencies, exogenous hormones, smoking)
- Supporting patients metabolically while starving tumor
- Slowing or stopping abnormal cell division
- Promoting normal cell differentiation and apoptosis
- Reducing metastasis and angiogenesis
- Enhancing cell-to-cell communication and intracellular signaling
- Using natural antitumor, proapoptotic agents
- Blocking hormonal stimulation of tumors by normalizing hepatic clearance of hormones
- Supporting a healthy immune response
- Supporting secondary prevention for patients after completion of active treatment
- Dealing with death and dying when indicated
- Encouraging prevention and screening for family members of patients

Stages of Cancer Development

- **Initiation:** damage to cellular DNA leading to mutations and resulting in development of cancerous cell.

- **Promotion:** factors in cellular environment (free radicals, xenobiotic chemicals, hormones) "feed" cancerous cell growth into a tumor.
- **Progression:** tumor metastasizes to other parts of body.

Cell Cycle

The cell cycle is usually divided into the following phases:

- **G0 phase:** resting state, or gap phase. Many cells spend most of their time in this phase either at rest or performing assigned duties. Generally resistant to chemotherapy.
- **G1 phase:** gap 1 phase, or interphase. Cells synthesize DNA and prepare for cell division.
- **S phase:** synthesis phase. Cells duplicate DNA to create daughter cells.
- **G2 phase:** gap 2 phase. DNA synthesis completed. Microtubules of mitotic spindles produced.
- **M phase:** mitosis. Division of DNA and cellular proteins into two daughter cells. Return to G0 or resting phase.

Chemotherapy Agent Efficacy According to Cell Cycle Phase

Certain chemotherapeutic agents work best in particular phases of cell cycle:

- **G1:** asparaginase
- **S phase:** antimetabolites, procarbazine, topotecan, topoisomerase I inhibitors
- **G2 phase:** etoposide, bleomycin, paclitaxel, and topoisomerase II inhibitors
- **M phase:** vinca alkaloids

Types of Cancer

- **Sarcomas:** cells of mesenchymal origin (e.g., bone, muscle, fibrous tissue)
  - — Bone (e.g., osteosarcoma)
  - — Soft tissues (e.g., leiomyosarcoma)
- **Leukemia:** white blood cell–producing tissues (bone marrow)
  - — Chronic lymphocytic leukemia
  - — Chronic myelogenous leukemia
  - — Acute lymphocytic leukemia
  - — Acute myelogenous leukemia
- **Lymphoma:** lymphatic system, especially lymph nodes
  - — Hodgkin's disease
  - — Non-Hodgkin's lymphoma

- **Cell type:** T cell or B cell
  - Physical form: follicular, diffuse
  - Degree of indolence or aggressiveness

Staging

Staging expresses extent of spread to make treatment decisions, evaluate responses, and make survival prognoses. Usually staging is based on anatomic spread, but certain cancers have other pertinent characteristics (e.g., any breast cancer of inflammatory subtype is stage IV regardless of spread; in colon cancer, depth of penetration through colon wall is critical).

Complete Staging Description

- Origin of tumor
- Histologic type and grade
- Extent of spread of tumor and locations of metastatic lesions
- Functional status of patient
- TNM score includes size of tumor *(T)*, number of involved lymph nodes *(N)*, and presence or absence of distant metastasis *(M)*. For example, breast cancer with primary tumor 2.5 cm, positive lymph nodes in ipsilateral axilla, and no metastasis would be T2, N1, M0.
- Staging designation
  - **Stage 0:** in situ or noninvasive
  - **Stage I:** small localized disease
  - **Stage II:** larger disease but localized; may involve small number of local lymph nodes
  - **Stage III:** regionally advanced
  - **Stage IV:** advanced metastasis

Tumor Markers

Tumor markers are tissue proteins in blood whose elevation indirectly reveals cancer progression. Caveats include the following:

- Most are not useful as screening tests. Noncancerous tissue can also secrete higher amounts of these markers in conditions such as inflammation and infection.
- Tumor may express different marker than typical for that tumor type.
- Tumor markers are most useful for monitoring response to treatment or disease progression.
- Raw number is less important than direction of change.

Common Tumor Markers

Tumor Marker	Typical Tumor Types
Carcinoembryonic antigen	Colorectal, breast, small cell lung
Prostate-specific antigen	Prostate, some breast
CA 15-3	Breast
CA 19-9	Pancreas, hepatic, biliary, gastric, colon
CA 27-29	Breast
CA 125	Ovarian
Beta-HCG	Testis, trophoblastic neoplasia
$Beta_2$ microglobulin	Multiple myeloma, lymphoma
Thyroglobulin	Thyroid

HCG, human chorionic gonadotropin.

Performance Indexes

Performance indexes indicate level of health of patient. Most commonly used are the Karnofsky score and the Eastern Cooperative Oncology Group (ECOG) score. Performance indexes are based on the patient's ability to perform daily activities, need for assistance, and need for medical treatment; they reflect patient vitality and ability to withstand and respond to further treatment. Patients with similar stages of disease but radically different performance index scores may have quite different outcomes.

Tumor Response Criteria and Terminology

Tumor response does not always mean cure or even an improvement in survivability. Cytotoxic therapy selects for resistant clones of tumor cells, which will over time no longer respond to treatment. A newer theory is that chemotherapy may kill tumor stromal cells without destroying tumor stem cells, which can trigger a relapse.

- **Cure:** treatment that allows patient to live as long as an age-matched cohort or die of other causes, even if some disease remains.
- **Remission:** complete disappearance of all detectable tumors. Millions of tumor cells may remain. Remission is a better term than *cure.*
- **Complete response:** complete disappearance of all evidence of disease for at least 2 measurement periods at least 4 weeks apart.

- **Partial response:** decrease of at least 50% in diameter of all measurable lesions with no new lesions for at least 4 weeks.
- **Stable disease:** less than 50% up to an increase of 25% in measurable lesions.
- **Progression:** increase of more than 25% or appearance of new lesions.
- **Palliation:** treatment not aimed at cure, simply reduction of symptoms or transient extension of life for brief period.

THERAPEUTIC CONSIDERATIONS

Based on current understanding, judiciously combining naturopathic therapies with conventional treatments can improve success, survival, and quality of life. An integrated approach also reduces the need for patients to make the difficult choice of either natural therapy or declining conventional treatments or vice versa. In making therapeutic decisions, results must be at least as good as those of conventional therapies to justify declining those therapies. This advice may determine whether a patient lives or dies. Make recommendations based on hard data, not on theory, anecdote, or opinion.

Goals of Naturopathic Oncology Support during Active Treatment

- Improve nutrition
- Selectively starve tumor
- Inhibit metastasis
- Reduce side effects of conventional treatment
- Maximize tumor kill from conventional therapies
- Support normal cell division and cellular signaling
- Remove tumor promoters—for example, inflammatory signals, hormones
- Use appropriate, effective antitumor herbs and nutrients (avoid waste of money on worthless products)
- Support healthy, balanced immune function
- Support positive attitude and healthy lifestyle
- Encourage regular secondary cancer screening after completion of treatment

Stages of Clinical Care

The typical clinical pattern in most cancer cases is as follows:

1. Detection of abnormality suggestive of cancer—for example, a mass, lymphadenopathy, pain, bleeding, unexplained weight loss.

2. Evaluation of suspicious finding with imaging studies; biopsy of questionable lesion; diagnosis of malignancy; staging. Biopsy allows for histologic grading of tumor and assessment of receptors and molecular markers that may affect diagnosis and treatment decisions.
3. Surgery to remove or debulk tumor. If inoperable, neoadjuvant chemotherapy before surgery to shrink tumor and make more-conservative surgery less invasive.
4. Chemotherapy, radiation, hormones, or biologic response modifiers.
5. Monitor for recurrence. Biologic response modifiers based on type of cancer—for example, antiestrogen therapies after surgery, chemotherapy, and radiation to reduce risk of recurrence of estrogen receptor (ER)–positive breast cancer.

Goals of Natural Therapies

- Reduce surgical complications
- Improve healing and recovery
- Support formation of healthy scar and connective tissue

Patients may be debilitated by disease or previous treatments and may need more-aggressive support. Surgery may allow spread of tumor cells during the perioperative period.

Natural Medicine Support for Surgery

General preoperative guidelines (begin 2 weeks before surgery) are as follows:

- **Avoid:** alcohol, recreational drugs, tobacco, coffee (taper slowly to minimize withdrawal headaches), sugar, fried foods, anything capable of causing increased bleeding (e.g., aspirin, *Ginkgo biloba,* garlic, fish oil). Discontinue any drugs or herbs that may react with anesthesia (e.g., kava, *Hypericum,* valerian) at least 5 days before surgery.
- **Increase:** fiber, protein (1 to 2 g/kg body weight), vegetables, fresh fruit, fluids, essential fatty acids (EFAs), probiotics, vitamin C with bioflavonoids.

Preoperative Nutritional Support

- Fractionated citrus pectin (FCP; 6 g b.i.d.) to inhibit micrometastases. Fractionation breaks down pectin into correct size to specifically bind to galectin-3 receptors. Whole pectins are less efficient owing to large molecular size. Advise all cancer patients to use FCP preoperatively and postoperatively.

- Increase: fiber, protein (1 to 2 g/kg body weight), vegetables, fresh fruit, fluids, probiotic agents, vitamin C with bioflavonoids

  See list of preoperative nutrients at the end of this chapter.

Postoperative Nutrition

Resume nutritional support as soon as patient can consume solid foods. Do not start vitamins or herbs if patient is NPO. If the patient is able to consume liquids, add herbal teas and homeopathic remedies. When solid food is allowed without restriction, resume all indicated medications. Be aware of all pharmaceuticals being used, to ensure no adverse interactions with nutraceuticals. Consult *A–Z Guide to Drug-Herb-Vitamin Interactions* (Alan R Gaby, editor) or Indiana University Department of Medicine's online resource "Drug Interactions," available at http://medicine.iupui.edu/CLINPHARM/DDIS. Continue all presurgical support for at least 2 weeks after surgery or until patient is fully recovered. Particularly important at this time is modified citrus pectin or FCP to inhibit aggregation and attachment of dislodged circulating tumor cells. Continue pectin for 3 to 6 months.

Additional postoperative nutrients include the following:

- **Vitamin E:** reduces risk of thromboses and adhesions
- **Bromelain and other proteolytic enzymes:** reduce inflammation, pain, and risk of thrombophlebitis
- **Protein drinks and smoothies:** amino acids for tissue collagen repair

Patient must do the following:

- **Ambulate** as soon as possible to prevent blood clots, constipation, muscle atrophy
- **Return home** as soon as possible to prevent nosocomial infection, sleep disruptions, medication errors
- **Not leave hospital** if patient feels something is wrong

Instruct patients to report unusual symptoms—fever, swelling, and excessive pain. Although hospital stays are generally limited according to diagnostic codes, attending doctors can override guidelines for medical reasons or complications.

Newer timing schedules—"metronomic chemotherapy," using smaller doses more frequently—are better tolerated and, at times, more effective than conventional timing. Other modifications—intrahepatic chemotherapy and chemoembolization procedures—enable treatment of tumors previously untreatable.

Chemotherapy and Targeted Biologic Response Agents

Clinical uses of chemotherapy treatment include the following:

- **Neoadjuvant:** before other treatments; shrinks tumor for easier treatment by surgery or radiation; used in breast cancers, some rectal cancers, bladder cancer, esophageal cancer.
- **Adjuvant:** after control of visible tumor with surgery or radiation; destroys undetectable cancer cells; reduces likelihood of recurrence; used in breast cancer, colon cancer. Types of adjuvant chemotherapy: (1) induction chemotherapy—first-line treatment; (2) consolidation therapy—another agent combination is used to further "consolidate" improvements from first treatment.
- **Second-line chemotherapy:** tumor recurrence; to put the patient into remission; agents different from first treatment (may be resistance cells).
- **Palliative:** to reduce symptoms, such as pain, by temporarily shrinking tumor pressing on vital organ or nerve; not intended to cure; may extend life for short period.
- **High-dose chemotherapy:** to kill all cancer cells; side effect is loss or complete destruction of bone marrow capacity; patient needs "rescue" therapy—bone marrow or stem cell transplant; used in hematologic malignancies (e.g., leukemia, multiple myeloma) or in aggressive cancers (e.g., advanced breast cancer).

Actions of Chemotherapeutic Drugs

- **Cytotoxic:** kill all rapidly dividing cells
- **Cytostatic:** slow cell division, allowing reestablishment of check point regulation, but does not cause cell death
- **Secondary effects:** antiangiogenic in lower doses

Drugs are given in combinations of agents to take advantage of differences in actions for specific activities against particular tumor types. Chemotherapy is given in cycles: specific number of infusions followed by rest period.

Families of Chemotherapy Drugs

- **Alkylating agents and platinum compounds:** substitute alkyl group for hydrogen to produce defects in DNA. Examples: cisplatin, carboplatin, cyclophosphamide. Platinum drugs work similarly by causing DNA cross-linking.
- **Antitumor antibiotics:** bind between DNA base pairs, interfere with normal mitosis, generate free radicals. Examples: doxorubicin (DOX), mitomycin, bleomycin.

- **Antimetabolites:** substitute structural analogues of normal metabolites, interfere with DNA replication. Examples: methotrexate (MTX), fluorouracil (5-FU), hydroxyurea.
- **Microtubule and chromatin inhibitors:** interfere with normal intracellular mechanisms necessary for mitosis. Block either topoisomerase enzymes used in DNA replication or bind to tubulin and block assembly or disassembly of microtubules. Microtubule inhibitors: vinblastine, vinorelbine, paclitaxel, docetaxel. Topoisomerase inhibitors: irinotecan and etoposide.

Targeted Biologic Agents

- **Antiangiogenic agents:** inhibit the growth of new blood vessels. Many of these agents block growth signals by inhibiting epidermal growth factor receptors. Examples: thalidomide, angiostatin, endostatin, cetuximab, bevacizumab, matrix metalloproteinase inhibitors, taxane-based agents at low doses.
- **Immune modulators, vaccines, monoclonal antibodies:** increase immune response. Examples: interferon, interleukins, trastuzumab. Bone marrow–stimulating agents: filgrastim, epoetin alfa, sargramostim. Monoclonal antibodies— Herceptin and Rituxan; also work via targeting immune system against specific markers on tumor cell surfaces.
- **Hormones and hormone inhibitors:** manipulate signals that regulate cell growth. Estrogen inhibitor: tamoxifen. Testosterone inhibitor: leuprolide. Therapeutic hormone: prednisone. Appetite stimulant: megestrol. Newer antiestrogen agents, aromatase inhibitors, work by blocking synthesis of estrogen in fat cells, rather than blocking ERs on tumors. Similar agents—Casodex—inhibit binding of testosterone in prostate cancer.
- **Gonadotropin-releasing hormones:** Agonists—for example, Lupron—are commonly used in prostate cancer to inhibit production of testosterone. Examples: prednisone in chemotherapy combination cyclophosphamide; Doxorubicin (DOX); Oncovin; prednisone, used for hematologic malignancies; Megace, used to stimulate appetites in advanced cancer patients.

Side Effects of Chemotherapy

Side effects vary depending on agent, timing, dosage, and protective measures used to reduce side effects. Individual factors include general health, efficiency of liver enzymes, amount of prior treatment (bone marrow suppression). Side effects are specific to agent. Acquire several references and review them regularly.

- **Short-term side effects:** nausea and vomiting, mucositis, diarrhea, fatigue, hair loss, anemia, leukopenia, thrombocytopenia, bruising, cardiac damage, neuropathy, pneumonitis, nephropathy, tinnitus, infections, "chemo brain," hand-foot syndrome, alterations of taste and smell, anorexia
- **Long-term side effects:**
  — Development of tumor resistance to chemotherapy
  — Increased risk of secondary cancers
  — Increased risk of leukemia and lymphoma
  — Infertility and premature menopause
  — Persistent unexplained fatigue
  — Persistent bone marrow suppression or myelodysplasia
  — Persistent "chemo brain" or short-term memory dysfunction

Chemotherapy Resistance Testing

- Testing of tumor tissue for resistance to chemotherapeutic agents. Small amount of fresh, unpreserved tumor tissue is taken during biopsy or surgery. Cell cultures are grown and tested for resistance to agents. The test costs $3000 to $4000. Requires fresh living tumor tissue shipped via overnight express service on dry ice. This test is most useful for later cases wherein first-line therapies failed to deliver expected results.
- Genetic testing of tumor tissue for characteristics indicating best agents and recurrence risk.

General Recommendations for Chemotherapy

To Improve Effectiveness

Specific nutrients can enhance specific chemotherapy agents. Addition of appropriate nutrients increases therapeutic efficacy. Nutrients are taken for at least 2 weeks before chemotherapy until completion of treatment. Actions: normalize cell division, increase apoptosis, increase cancer cell uptake of chemotherapy drugs, reduce drug resistance, stimulate normal cell differentiation. Match nutrients to planned chemotherapy agents for best effects and to minimize negative interactions with chemotherapy.

- **Melatonin:** 20 mg of melatonin nightly may double response rates and rates of survival at 1 year in a variety of stage IV cancer types. Reduces toxicity: thrombocytopenia, neurotoxicity, cardiotoxicity.
- **Green tea:** enhances inhibitory effects of DOX against Ehrlich ascites tumors 2.5-fold in mice. Effect only seen in tumor cells, not healthy cells.

To Reduce Side Effects of Chemotherapy

Variations in mode of action and path of elimination for each chemotherapy agent cause damage to certain organs. Minimize side effects with nutritional support throughout treatment; drug damage may be irreversible. General measures for all cases: optimal hydration, healthy diet, high-potency multiple vitamin. Excessive side effects may cause reduction in dose of therapeutic agents, potentially reducing therapeutic effectiveness.

Know each agent being used and relevant nutrient interactions and contraindications, especially when combinations of drugs are used. Selection of appropriate nutrients and botanicals is complex and based on many factors. General recommendations are safe for all types of chemotherapy.

- **Multiple vitamin:**
  - — Vitamin A: 5000 international units (IU)
  - — Mixed natural carotenoids: 10,000 to 25,000 IU
  - — B complex: 25 to 50 mg
  - — Folic acid: 400 to 800 mcg
  - — Vitamin B_{12}: 200 to 1000 mcg
  - — Vitamin E succinate: 400 IU
  - — Vitamin C: 500 to 1000 mg
  - — Vitamin D: 400 to 800 IU
  - — Trace minerals: full complement
- **Melatonin:** 20 mg at bedtime.
- **Vitamin C:** 3000 to 10,000 mg q.d. in divided doses according to bowel tolerance. Although not a replacement for conventional therapy, ascorbate may extend periods of remission and promote healing and recovery after treatment. Intravenous (IV) infusions of 30 to 100 g may show some benefit but have not been shown to be a replacement for conventional therapy. Rather, vitamin C may extend periods of remission and promote healing and recovery after treatment.
- **Fish oils:** provide 2 g total combined eicosapentaenoic acid (EPA) and docosahexaenoic acid (DHA) daily.
- **Mushroom extracts, immune support:** use a variety of immune modulators, switching them regularly to avoid downregulation of receptors. Standard doses for *Coriolis versicolor* mushroom is 3 g of the extract daily. Suggested dose for maitake D fraction is 0.5 to 1.0 mg of extract per kilogram body weight. Other botanical immune modulators may be used as desired.
- **Enzymes:** use pancreatic enzymes with meals and mixed enteric-coated enzymes between meals.

- **Green tea:** capsules and beverages to total the equivalent of 5 to 10 cups daily. Caffeinated form is preferred if patient tolerates caffeine. Green tea in high doses reduces effectiveness of bortezomib (Velcade); avoid green tea when patients are using this agent until new information clarifies this issue.
- **Whey protein shake:** administer with fruit daily as a source of easily assimilated protein and amino acids, particularly glutamine.

Recommendations for Specific Individual Chemotherapy Agents

Individual agents are discussed in the following paragraphs, with nutrients considered in addition to basic protocol described earlier. Unless larger doses are indicated for an agent already mentioned, it is not discussed in this section. For more on chemotherapy agents, consult *Physicians' Cancer Chemotherapy Drug Manual 2015* by Edward Chu and Vincent DeVita, Jr.

- **Doxorubicin (DOX; Adriamycin):** inhibits DNA synthesis, RNA polymerases, topoisomerase. Side effects: hair loss, leukopenia, nausea and vomiting, cardiotoxicity, increased risk of secondary leukemia. Major concern: irreversible cardiotoxicity caused by free radical injury to mitochondria. When symptoms manifest clinically, damage may be already irreversible. Protective nutrients: vitamin C, vitamin E, L-carnitine, coenzyme Q10 (CoQ10). Several of these agents increase beneficial effects of DOX. Green tea enhances 2.5-fold inhibitory effects of DOX on tumor growth by increasing concentration of DOX in tumor cells but not in healthy cells. Genistein also increases antitumor effects of DOX and is effective in both ER-positive and ER-negative breast cancer cells.
- **Cyclophosphamide (Cytoxan):** alkylating agent inactive until transformed by p450 enzyme system into cytotoxic metabolites active in all phases of cell cycle. It is orally active, does not require IV infusion, and is used in combinations for breast and ovarian cancers, leukemias, lymphomas, and sarcomas. Side effects: myelosuppression, nausea and vomiting, bladder toxicity, alopecia, increased risk of bladder cancer, long-term side effects of acute leukemia; cardiac toxicity synergistic when combined with DOX. Protective natural agents: fish oils, folic acid, vitamin E, *Withania somnifera* (ashwagandha), and mushroom extracts. Fish oils enhance antitumor efficacy of Cytoxan and protect against side effects, possibly via liver p450 enzymes. Folic acid

decreases side effects and increases antitumor response. Vitamin E combined with Cytoxan may produce stronger antitumor response than chemotherapy alone. Mushroom extracts from *C. versicolor* help partially reverse immunosuppression induced by Cytoxan. Because of tendency to cause cystitis, keep patients taking Cytoxan well hydrated—at least 2 quarts of pure water daily.

- **Cisplatin and carboplatin:** platinum-based agents cross-link DNA strands to inhibit DNA synthesis and cell replication. Cisplatin is used for ovarian and testicular cancer and is limited by side effects and higher degree of nephrotoxicity, neurotoxicity, and myelosuppression. Carboplatin is better tolerated when given in lower weekly doses. Protective agent: concurrent glutathione. Administration of IV glutathione immediately before giving cisplatin reduces side effects and slightly increases chemotherapy efficacy. Chemotherapy dose reductions because of side effects have not been found to be required. Similar results arise for newer platinum compound oxaliplatin. Concurrent administration of selenium with cisplatin allows for higher doses with less toxicity and higher therapeutic index. Milk thistle extracts reduce toxicity of cisplatin, but avoid them on day of treatment to prevent overly rapid clearance of chemotherapeutic agents. Vitamin A has a synergistic effect when combined with cisplatin for head and neck cancers. Beta-carotene is not recommended except in dietary sources because it may increase death rates in cancer patients who smoke. Vitamin C improves antineoplastic activity of cisplatin, as does vitamin E. Spleen extracts in combination with cisplatin stabilize white blood cells, body weight, and fatigue. PSK enhances cytotoxicity of cisplatin against ovarian cancer cells but not normal cells.
- **Fluorouracil (5-FU), capecitabine (Xeloda), and floxuridine (FUDR):** pyrimidine analogue antimetabolites. 5-FU is used for colorectal cancers and is combined with Cytoxan and MTX for breast cancers. It treats pancreatic, ovarian, head and neck, and skin basal cell cancers. Toxicity and side effects: mucositis (mouth sores), diarrhea, bone marrow depression. Unusual symptom: hand-foot syndrome, characterized by redness, swelling, and numbness in hands and feet. Neurologic symptoms: confusion and seizures. 5-FU can cause inflammation and blockage of tear ducts and chronic conjunctivitis, cardiac changes that are less frequent and less severe than with Adriamycin. Vitamin E increases antitumor activity of 5-FU against colorectal cancer

by upregulating proapoptotic enzyme p21. Augmentation of proapoptotic protein Bax arises from vitamin E combined with 5-FU. Vitamin B_6 at 100 mg q.d. to t.i.d. may reduce incidence and severity of hand-foot syndrome.

- **Methotrexate (MTX):** antifolate analogue that inhibits enzyme dihydrofolate reductase, blocking conversion of folic acid into active metabolite folinic acid. Without folinic acid, cells cannot duplicate their DNA. Folic acid at levels in multivitamins does not interfere with this drug, but avoid higher doses. Toxicity: myelosuppression, mucositis severe enough to limit dose, and dose-dependent nausea and vomiting, acute renal failure. Monitor liver enzymes and kidney functions regularly during treatment. Other side effects: pneumonitis, severe headaches, skin rashes, itching, photosensitivity, and hyperpigmentation. "Radiation recall" can occur: areas previously irradiated again develop redness and pain. Both men and women can experience gonadal failure after treatment with MTX. Avoid interactions with penicillin, aspirin, and antiinflammatories, which reduce renal elimination of MTX. The amino acid glutamine may increase intratumoral MTX: glutamine decreases intratumoral glutathione, making tumors more susceptible to MTX. Glutamine is a primary nutrient for gastrointestinal (GI) enterocytes lining the GI tract, reducing incidence of mucositis and diarrhea caused by MTX. Vitamin A may limit GI damage from MTX without reducing antitumor benefit.
- **Paclitaxel (Taxol) and docetaxel (Taxotere):** Taxanes are semisynthetic isolates from yew species (Pacific yew for paclitaxel [Taxol] and European yew for docetaxel [Taxotere]). They bind tubulin, polymerizing microtubule and inhibiting mitosis and cell division. Applications: ovarian, breast, lung, gastric, bladder, prostate, esophageal, and head and neck cancers. Taxanes are radiosensitizers, sensitizing tumors to radiotherapies. Side effects: hypersensitivity reactions, neuropathy, arthralgia, myalgias, mucositis, onycholysis, and myelosuppression. Taxol causes greater arthralgia and myalgia; Taxotere causes greater myelosuppression. Helpful nutrients: vitamin C, glutamine, and EFAs. Vitamin C improves response to Taxol synergistically. Glutamine 10 g t.i.d. helps reduce myalgias and neuropathy linked to taxanes. The EFAs gamma-linolenic acid, alpha-linolenic acid, EPA, and DHA enhance cytotoxic activity of Taxol against human breast cancer cells in an in vitro model.

Gamma-linolenic acid is most active; linoleic acid offers no benefit.

Radiation Therapy

Effect: damages ionization of DNA of localized cells, leading to apoptosis during next mitosis cycle.

Types of Radiation Therapy

This section deals only with ionizing radiation.

- **Machine-generated sources:** several forms—two-dimensional (2D) external beam therapy, three-dimensional (3D) conformal therapy, intensity-modulated radiation therapy (IMRT), and tomotherapy. Degree of sophistication and control of field shape increase with each listed type. The 2D external beam is oldest and causes most collateral damage. The 3D conformal therapy and IMRT types use more angles of treatment and field-shaping collimators to reduce radiation exposure of healthy tissues. The newest and most sophisticated is tomotherapy; the field and dose are administered according to results of simultaneous computed tomography (CT) scan, permitting greater targeting accuracy. Gamma Knife surgery, used for intracranial neurologic lesions, is also highly targeted.
  - Photon radiation: no mass and no charge.
  - Particle radiation, including neutron therapy and proton therapy. Effective even in low-oxygen environments.
    - Neutrons have mass but no charge.
    - Protons have mass and positive charge.
- **Brachytherapy:** use of localized radiation sources placed within a tumor. Precise targeting spares healthy tissue. Options: permanent seeds (prostate cancer) or temporary high-intensity source within a tumor or operative site. Examples: high-dose brachytherapy for prostate—radioactive seeds are placed within prostate for short periods; brachytherapy within lumpectomy site immediately after surgery. Advantages: precise dose to areas of greatest concern; less radiation reaches healthy tissue.
  - Permanent placement of seeds now common for prostate cancer.
  - Temporary placement of high-intensity source within tumor.
- **Radioimmunotherapy:** radioactive moieties linked to monoclonal antibodies injected into bloodstream. Antibodies target abnormal tissue marker and deliver bulk of radiation to specific tumor tissues, sparing other tissues.

Side Effects of Radiation Therapy

Radiation therapy is more tolerable than chemotherapy. Factors influencing side effects include the following:

- Location of tumor
- Size of treatment field
- Organs or tissues within treatment field
- Prior or concurrent chemotherapy (radiosensitizing)
- Presence or absence of radioprotective agents

Early side effects: localized superficial burning; discoloration and desquamation; fatigue; reduced blood counts; and collateral damage to localized nerves, organs, and tissues within treatment field.

Long-term side effects: secondary cancers, scarring or tissue fibrosis, and impaired organ function.

Use newest and most sophisticated machinery available with ability to limit radiation exposure to uninvolved tissues. Ascertain type of radiation planned, treatment field, and adjacent organs. Examples: radiation only to the abdomen will cause nausea; radiation to prostate causes either proctitis or cystitis depending on the field; head and neck radiation induces severe mucositis and pain, leading to dehydration and inability to eat, then dry mouth because of damage to salivary glands. Radiation to lateral breast areas may not damage heart, lungs, or esophagus; but treating medial breast areas may damage these tissues.

Naturopathic Support during Radiation Therapy

Goals

- Assist patient in deciding if radiation is appropriate by reviewing survival data.
- Identify most advanced equipment in region to maximize tumor kill while minimizing collateral damage to healthy tissues.
- Consider radiosensitizing support to maximize tumor kill.
- Consider and select appropriate radioprotective agents.

Radiopotentiation

Improving radiation tumor kill by use of the following:

- **Pharmaceuticals:** 5-FU, paclitaxel, cisplatin given concurrently with radiation to enhance tumor DNA damage.
- **Increase tissue oxygenation** (radiation is less effective in hypoxic tissues): hyperthermia (increases local circulation by vasodilation), carbogen gas inhalation, hemoglobin-inducing therapies (either erythropoietin or transfusions).

- **Natural therapies to potentiate radiation:** either enhance tumoricidal action or prevent need for dose reduction because of side effects (radioprotection). Natural radiopotentiators include the following:
  - — **Melatonin:** improves survival rates at 1 year and reduce side effects.
  - — **Flavonoids:** genistein (most active) and quercetin increase tumor cell death from radiotherapy.
  - — ***W. somnifera* (ashwagandha):** Ayurvedic plant that increases tumor tissue radiosensitivity by 50%.
  - — ***Coriolis* mushroom extract (PSK):** improves survival; enhances immunity.
  - — **Combined vitamin K_3** plus vitamin C: pretreatment for radiation therapy, reduces tumor volume.

Radioprotection

All antioxidants are helpful. Standard doses of antioxidants in a high-potency multiple vitamin-mineral will not reduce efficacy of radiation therapy but will protect normal cells. Antioxidants are crucial to apoptotic cascade; they trigger apoptosis after radiation therapy. CoQ10: at massive doses (1400 to 2800 mg daily) modestly reduces radiotherapy-induced tumor kills. However, at normal or mildly elevated doses (700 mg daily), no reduction in tumor kill occurs. Similar results occur with vitamins E and C. Typical doses given during or immediately before radiotherapy lead to normal or enhanced tumor responses to radiotherapy. Similar conclusions have been reached about other antioxidants—*N*-acetylcysteine (NAC) at normal clinical doses does not protect tumor cells. The safest conclusion: standard doses of antioxidants, as in high-potency multiple vitamin-minerals, do not reduce efficacy of radiotherapy, but protect normal cells. Because antioxidants are crucial in the apoptotic cascade, they may enhance secondary response to radiotherapy by triggering greater rates of apoptosis after treatment. Until effects of megadoses are ascertained, focus more on other botanicals with known benefits; limit antioxidant nutrients to doses in multivitamins to minimize conflicts with radiotherapy.

- **Glutamine:** given in combination with radiotherapy, it protects mucus membranes during radiotherapy; helps heal radiation-induced enteritis and proctitis. Glutamine increases selectivity of radiotherapy for tumor cells.
- **Alkylglycerols and squalene** maintain bone marrow function and white blood cell counts during radiation therapy. Squalene prolongs survival after lethal doses of whole-body radiation.

- **Topical agents** to reduce burning of skin surface during radiation therapy: aloe vera gel (fresh leaf most effective), vitamin E, methylsulfonylmethane creams, *Calendula* creams. Apply nightly throughout treatment, but must be completely washed off before treatment so as not to alter penetration or scattering of radiation therapy beams. A degree of redness and peeling is common, particularly in fair-skinned patients, but the agents mentioned here may help with healing and discomfort.

Antioxidants during Chemotherapy and Radiation

Use of antioxidants with chemotherapy is controversial. Most antioxidants reduce side effects and improve tumoricidal action. Radiation therapy and many chemotherapeutic drugs do not kill malignant cells directly by wreaking havoc in their DNA. They harm DNA to a minor extent, yet affected cells perceive inflicted damage as irreparable and actively self-destruct. Antioxidants enhance cancer cell apoptosis. Common chemotherapy agents induce tumoricide without lipid or protein oxidation. Oxidative stress actually *reduces* efficacy of chemotherapy agents. Antioxidants enhance tumor-killing action of chemotherapy agents. Oxidative byproducts of chemotherapy damage organs, increase risk of secondary cancers, and increase production of vascular endothelial growth factor, which is implicated in growth and invasiveness of tumors. Benefits of appropriately chosen and antioxidants at proper doses outweigh theoretical concerns.

- Many patients discontinue or delay chemotherapy because of side effects that can be reduced with nutrition.
- Others refuse chemotherapy because of the fear of side effects.
- Chemotherapy and radiation therapy are implicated in secondary cancers, which are theoretically preventable with nutrition.
- Approximately 50% of tumors have abnormal p53 enzymes involved in apoptosis, and thus are less responsive to chemotherapy. Antioxidants can partially reverse this abnormality.
- Chemotherapy alone for common cancers does not dramatically improve survival. Antioxidants allow higher, more-effective doses without dose-limiting toxicity.
- Antioxidants reduce negative side effects, increase tumor responses, and increase survival times. With a few specific exceptions, consider them essential to any naturopathic cancer protocol.

Drug-Nutrient Interactions

- Interference (or benefit) can occur at the levels of absorption, hepatic activation or clearance, or intracellular pathways within tumor cells.

- Assess all medicines—natural and conventional—that patients are using, to determine potential interactions. Example: common antidepressants given for reduction of hot flashes can interfere with therapeutic benefit of tamoxifen by inhibiting activity of cytochromes p450, 2C9, and 2D6, necessary for hepatic activation of tamoxifen into its active metabolite.

Diet for Cancer Patients

Approximately 30% to 40% of cancers are preventable with appropriate lifestyle and diet. High-fiber, nutrient-dense whole organic foods: fruits, vegetables, beans, seeds, small wild cold-water fish. Minimize high-calorie, low-nutrient foods: junk foods, candy, soft drinks. Incorporate allium (onions, garlic) and cruciferous vegetables (e.g., broccoli). See *How to Prevent and Treat Cancer with Natural Medicine* by Michael Murray.

Preoperative Nutritional Support

- Diet high in protein, fruits, vegetables; low in alcohol, caffeine, saturated fats, junk foods.
- Avoid blood-thinning herbs and nutrients.
- Avoid herbs that alter liver metabolism of anesthetic agents or preoperative and postoperative medicines.
- Stop smoking 3 weeks before surgery.
- FCP 8 g b.i.d. (to inhibit micrometastases).
- Gotu kola to reduce adhesions—three cups tea daily.
- High-potency multivitamin-mineral.
  - Vitamin C: 2000 to 5000 mg/day; promotes healing and immunity; helps to build strong collagen.
  - Zinc (60 mg/day) speeds healing, localizes to healing tissues; most active in second phase of healing.
  - B vitamins (20 to 100 mg): generally included in multivitamin formula.
- Immune support reduces probability of infection: hospital-acquired respiratory infections.
- Protein powder or free-form glutamine and arginine speed postoperative recovery and promote protein synthesis for collagen formation. Glutamine reduces total hospital costs, rates of infection, and nitrogen balance in bone marrow transplantation patients.
- Arnica and Traumeel are homeopathic remedies that have been traditionally used to speed recovery from injury or trauma.

Secondary Prevention

Natural medicine alone may be inadequate treatment for most cancers. Applying newer concepts of cancer biology can modify physiology to reduce tumor progression and enhance natural defenses against cancer.

Cancer is more than just accumulated genetic alterations. It entails breakdown in cellular signaling and regulation. Derangements in one or more of the following are involved in most cancers:

- Altered hormonal status (increased estrogen, altered estrogen clearance or ratios, or changes in testosterone).
- Hyperinsulinemia and metabolic syndrome.
- Chronic inflammation.
- Altered intracellular signaling.
- Altered signaling from the host environment. Differences in regulatory signaling from surrounding tissues can even affect behavior of cancer cells.
- Increased cell division.
- Decreased apoptotic signaling and caspases.
- Oxidative stress, hypoxia inducible factor, and angiogenesis.
- Mitochondrial dysfunction.
- Epigenetic changes leading to altered activity of DNA regardless of mutations.
- Nutrient deficiencies (e.g., vitamin D, antioxidants, EFAs).
- Differences in activity of tumor stem cells versus tumor stromal cells.

Applying these understandings helps at all stages of cancer treatment, but also extends remission or controls growth from microscopic disease to more-active disease. In prostate cancer, modifying these factors may be the only treatment needed. Active lifestyle modification can frequently control or even regress some early and nonaggressive prostate cancers. Developing long-term programs for secondary prevention involves identifying and modifying as many risk factors as possible. Some are determined by history (e.g., hormone replacement therapy, smoking, alcohol, exposure to radiation, xenobiotic chemicals). Others are noted on physical examination (e.g., obesity, abdominal adiposity, nodular prostate, lymphadenopathy), and most risk factors are identified on laboratory evaluation. Testing varies with type of cancer risk, family history, gender of patient, and so on, but in most cases should include complete blood count, comprehensive chemistry, 25-hydroxyvitamin D, markers for inflammation (e.g., C-reactive protein, cytokine), markers for hormonal and metabolic derangement (e.g., 2:16 estrogen ratios, insulin, hemoglobin A_{1c}, lipids), and individual risk factors (e.g., heavy metals, xenobiotics). The naturopathic concept of body as an integrated ecosystem fits well with this part of cancer therapy. It is not our goal to destroy every single cancer cell, but to upgrade internal ecology such that any stray cancer cells find it difficult or impossible to grow and spread.

Carpal Tunnel Syndrome

DIAGNOSTIC SUMMARY

- Insidious onset of numbness and tingling, primarily in first three fingers, often bilaterally
- Pain over palmar surface of wrist, which may extend proximally up to forearm or shoulder
- Pain often worse at night and may wake the patient
- Positive Tinel's and Phalen's signs
- Neurodiagnostic testing showing altered nerve conduction of median nerve at carpal tunnel

GENERAL CONSIDERATIONS

Carpal tunnel syndrome (CTS) involves compression of median nerve within carpal tunnel. Sensory impairment occurs in the first three digits and the lateral half of the fourth digit. Pain may be felt in the palm, anterior wrist, and forearm and proximally to the shoulder. Loss of fine motor skills and strength in abduction and opposition of the thumb may develop. Atrophy of the opponens pollicis muscle may occur.

Etiology

Most cases are idiopathic. Nonspecific flexor tenosynovitis is the most common identified cause. The most common histologic findings are noninflammatory synovial fibrosis and vascular proliferation. Consider factors that cause the canal to get smaller or factors that cause the contents to swell. Causes of CT include the following:

- Increased volume of canal contents or edema (nonspecific flexor tenosynovitis, obesity, pregnancy, oral contraceptives)
- Trauma (fracture, repetitive wrist flexion)
- Aberrant anatomy (cysts, lipomas, arthritic spurs)
- Infections (septic arthritis, Lyme disease)

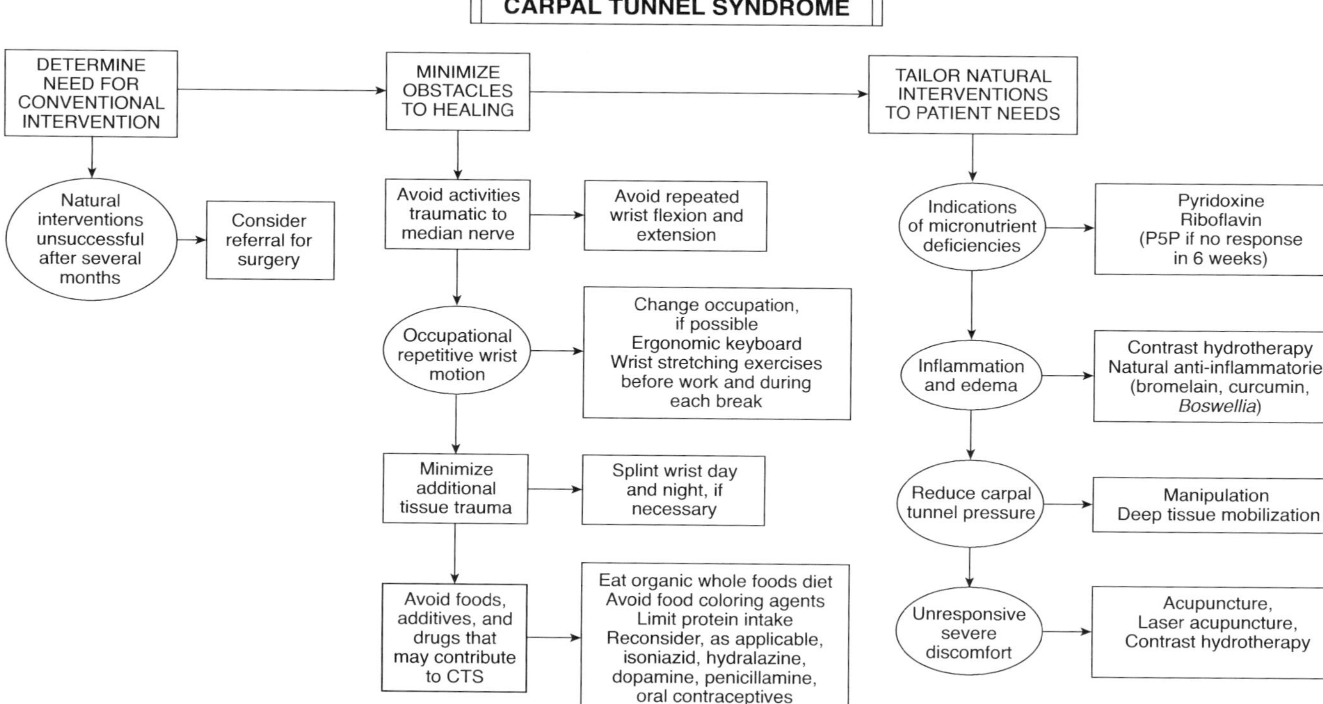
CARPAL TUNNEL SYNDROME
DETERMINE NEED FOR CONVENTIONAL INTERVENTION
Natural interventions unsuccessful after several months
Consider referral for surgery
MINIMIZE OBSTACLES TO HEALING
Avoid activities traumatic to median nerve
Avoid repeated wrist flexion and extension
Occupational repetitive wrist motion
Change occupation, if possible
Ergonomic keyboard
Wrist stretching exercises before work and during each break
Minimize additional tissue trauma
Splint wrist day and night, if necessary
Avoid foods, additives, and drugs that may contribute to CTS
Eat organic whole foods diet
Avoid food coloring agents
Limit protein intake
Reconsider, as applicable, isoniazid, hydralazine, dopamine, penicillamine, oral contraceptives
TAILOR NATURAL INTERVENTIONS TO PATIENT NEEDS
Indications of micronutrient deficiencies
Pyridoxine
Riboflavin
(P5P if no response in 6 weeks)
Inflammation and edema
Contrast hydrotherapy
Natural anti-inflammatories (bromelain, curcumin, *Boswellia*)
Reduce carpal tunnel pressure
Manipulation
Deep tissue mobilization
Unresponsive severe discomfort
Acupuncture,
Laser acupuncture,
Contrast hydrotherapy

- Metabolic conditions (diabetes, hypothyroidism)
- Inflammatory conditions (rheumatoid arthritis, gout, connective tissue disease)

Risk Factors and Frequency of Occurrence

CTS usually occurs after age 30; women are affected three times as often as men. Repetitive strain injury (RSI) as a cause of CTS is not well supported by current literature. Identified risk factors include repetitive activities with flexed or extended wrist; hysterectomy without oophorectomy; pregnancy; hypothyroidism; diabetes; and recent menopause (last menstrual period 6 to 12 months earlier).

DIAGNOSTIC CONSIDERATIONS

There is no single reference standard for diagnosis of the syndrome. A combination of symptoms, signs, and tests may characterize CTS.

History

- Insidious onset of intermittent tingling or numbness, often bilaterally, of first three fingers and lateral half of fourth digit.
- Symptoms often worse at night, waking the patient.
- Loss of fine motor skills; loss of grip strength with "things slipping from my fingers."
- Relief is gained from shaking affected hand or hands.
- Katz and Stirrat self-administered hand diagram test has 80% sensitivity and 90% specificity for CTS.
- Loss of finger dexterity and atrophy are late complaints.

Physical Examination

- Decreased sensation over distribution of median nerve to sharp, light touch and vibration (128-Hz tuning fork).
- Many patients are unable to localize symptoms to median distribution; they feel the whole hand is involved, perhaps because of autonomic nerve involvement.
- Tingling in distribution of median nerve produced by tapping on the wrist crease **(Tinel's sign);** tingling in distribution of median nerve produced by holding wrist in forced flexion for 60 to 90 seconds **(Phalen's test);** or tingling produced by forcibly extending the wrist and applying pressure over the median nerve **(reverse Phalen's test)** are signs of CTS. Early perceived loss of strength may be a result of loss of sensory feedback, not loss of strength.

- Manual muscle tests may elicit weakness of LOAF muscles (muscles innervated by median nerve in the hand; lubricals first and second, opponens pollicus, abductor pollicus, flexor pollicis brevis). As CTS advances, atrophy of the thenar eminence and weakness of the thumb abductor muscle may develop.

Other Diagnostic Tests

- **Carpal compression test:** examiner exerts direct compression with thumbs over patient's carpal tunnel for 30 seconds and reproduces symptoms; was reported to have 89% sensitivity and 96% specificity when performed with Durkan gauge.
- Other studies have reported that Tinel's, Phalen's, reverse Phalen's, and carpal tunnel compression tests are more sensitive and specific tests for diagnosis of tenosynovitis of flexor muscles of the hand, rather than being specific tests for CTS.
- Weakness of the thumb abductor muscle is a strong indication to order neurophysiologic testing (**nerve conduction studies** [NCSs] and/or electromyography). In CTS, NCSs may show motor and sensory latencies across the wrist.
- **Magnetic resonance imaging** (MRI) and **high-definition ultrasound** imaging can measure dimensions of carpal tunnel and size of median nerve, but these tests are expensive and not needed in uncomplicated CTS.

Differential Diagnosis

When the clinical picture is unclear, other sources of paresthesia should be considered—for example, compression of the brachial plexus in the thoracic outlet, impingement of the median nerve under the pronator teres muscle, or entrapment of radial or ulnar nerves. The initial presentation of complex regional pain syndrome (reflex sympathetic dystrophy) may appear to be CTS.

THERAPEUTIC CONSIDERATIONS

Many patients report spontaneous recovery from CTS. CTS from pregnancy most often is self-resolving. The presence of waxing and waning symptoms gives a false sense of success from conservative treatment. The cost of conservative care in persistent CTS may be greater than carpal tunnel release performed as an office procedure. For progressive neurologic deficit and pain, an open release procedure may be the best choice because of a high rate of success and low rate of complications. Unless the surgeon has good skills, more-expensive endoscopic procedures have poorer outcomes.

Physical Medicine

Splinting

- The most recommended treatment is 4 weeks in a neutral wrist splint full time; this provides better results than night-only splinting, but night-only splinting has higher compliance.
- Splinting is most effective when started within 3 months of onset of CTS. Specialized splints are not more effective than good-quality well-fitted off-the-shelf splints.
- Splinting should not be done after carpal tunnel release.

Therapeutic Ultrasound

Ultrasound therapy for 2 weeks is not beneficial, but ultrasound (1 MHz, 1.0 W/cm^2, pulse 1:4, 15 minutes per session) may help after 20 sessions over 7 weeks. The cost of 15 to 20 sessions of ultrasound may be prohibitive.

Yoga and Stretching

- Ten yoga postures held for 30 seconds each, followed by 10 to 15 minutes of relaxation have reduced pain and increased grip strength, with effects persisting for more than 8 weeks.
- Carpal tunnel pressure rises in pressure with wrist flexing, wrist extending, making a fist, holding objects, and performing isolated isometric flexion of a finger against resistance. However, after 1 minute of specific stretching-loading exercises, intratunnel pressures drops to normal and remains normal for more than 15 minutes.

Manual Manipulation

- Soft tissue and joint mobilization of forearm, wrist, and hand may be used, but not spinal manipulation alone.
- Myofascial release and self-stretching techniques may be performed three to five times daily. This treatment increases dimensions in the carpal tunnel and reduces distal latencies or increase in motor response amplitudes.
- Nerve and tendon gliding exercise has been found to produce no changes in Phalen's test, Tinel's test, or NCS results, but it reduced the number of reported surgeries.

Low-Level Laser Therapy

Low-level laser therapy (LLLT) combined with microcurrent transcutaneous electrical nerve stimulation, applied for 3 to 4 weeks to patients who failed to improve with standard medical or surgical treatment, induced significant improvement in scores on the McGill Pain Questionnaire; sensory and motor latency scores with electromyography; and Tinel's and Phalen's test results.

Hydrotherapy

An anecdotal naturopathic treatment to relieve CTS pain is immersing the wrist and hand in hot water for 3 minutes, then immersing in cold water for 30 seconds, repeated three to five times once or twice a day. It is important to ensure that the hot water immersion is deeper than the cold.

Acupuncture

A comparison of prednisolone (20 mg for 2 weeks, then 10 mg for 2 weeks) with eight sessions of acupuncture over 4 weeks showed acupuncture to be effective in symptom control. Acupuncture decreased distal motor latency and prednisolone did not.

Erognomics

There is insufficient epidemiologic evidence that computer work causes CTS. Work practices (other than high-force work, such as that done by meat packers) have a direct influence on CTS.

Nutrition

Vitamin B Supplementation

- Incidence of CTS has increased with the increased presence of pyridoxine (vitamin B_6) antimetabolites (hydrazine dyes, isoniazid, hydralazine, dopamine, penicillamine, and oral contraceptives) in the environment and the intake of excessive protein.
- **Vitamin B_6** supplementation for CTS with 50 mg initially and increased to 200 to 300 mg has been beneficial. Greater effect is seen when B_6 and B_2 are given together, perhaps as a result of B_2-dependent enzymes, which convert pyridoxine to the active form pyridoxal 5′-phosphate (P5P). Studies have been inconsistent. Therapeutic failure of B_6 therapy could be a result of lack of riboflavin or a genetic defect that disallows sufficient quantities of B_6 to be converted to active P5P form. If CTS is unresponsive to B_6, prescribe P5P.

Medications

- Steroid injection proximal to the carpal tunnel provides relief for up to 8 weeks, but 50% of recipients require surgery within a year.
- Oral prednisolone (20 mg for 2 weeks, then 10 mg for 2 weeks) provides short-term relief over 8 weeks. Nonsteroidal anti-inflammatory drugs and diuretics provide no relief and should *not* be used owing to side effects.
- No studies have been found evaluating the use of the "natural" anti-inflammatory medications (bromelain, curcumin, *Boswellia,* various oils). Remedies that address noninflammatory synovial fibrosis and vascular proliferation would theoretically be beneficial.

Surgery

- Surgery should not be considered before 6 months of more-conservative treatment.
- Indicated for persistent (not resolving after 1 year) or deteriorating (worsening clinically plus or minus deterioration on NCSs) CTS.
- Surgery should not be delayed beyond 3 years. Open carpal tunnel release is a common outpatient procedure, less expensive than endoscopy. There is no difference in long-term results, but pain is reduced during the first 2 weeks after endoscopy compared with open procedures.
- Surgery with early mobilization, surgery with oral homeopathic *Arnica* and topical *Arnica* ointment, and surgery with controlled cold therapy all have shown benefits over surgery alone.

Therapeutic Approach for Mild to Moderate Idiopathic Carpal Tunnel Syndrome

About 50% of patients improve spontaneously. Identify and reduce causes of strain and vibration, and prevent repeated trauma.

Physical Medicine

- **Regular wrist stretching, yoga, and exercises.** Key to these exercises: performing them several times daily and "breaking up" activities that are strenuous and repetitive. Nerve and tendon gliding may be helpful.
- **Splint.** For moderate persistent CTS, use full-time splinting in neutral. Splinting is less effective if not started within 3 months of onset or if splints are worn only at night.
- **Acupuncture.** Needle PC-7 and PC-6 on affected side. Consider laser acupuncture.

- **Manipulation or deep tissue mobilization.** Manipulation of fixated carpals or separation of distal radius and ulna may relieve pressure in carpal tunnel.
- **Contrast hydrotherapy**. Immerse affected area for 3 minutes in hot water followed by 30-second immersion in cold water three to five times daily. Heat alone is contraindicated.

Diet

- Avoid all sources of hydrazines and all foods containing yellow dyes.
- Limit daily protein intake to maximum of 0.75 g/kg body weight.

Supplements

- Pyridoxine: 50 to 200 mg q.d. in divided doses of 25 to 50 mg b.i.d. to q.i.d. If no response to pyridoxine, try P5P: 10 mg b.i.d. to q.i.d.
- Riboflavin: 5 to 10 mg q.d.

Celiac Disease

DIAGNOSTIC SUMMARY

- Chronic intestinal malabsorption caused by intolerance to gluten
- Bulky, pale, frothy, foul-smelling, greasy stools with increased fecal fat
- Weight loss and signs of multiple vitamin and mineral deficiencies
- Increased levels of serum antiendomysial and/or transglutaminase antibodies
- Diagnosis confirmed by jejunal biopsy

GENERAL CONSIDERATIONS

Celiac disease (CD) is also known as nontropical sprue, gluten-sensitive enteropathy, or celiac sprue. Characteristics include malabsorption and abnormal small intestine structure that reverts to normal on removal of dietary protein gluten. Gluten and polypeptide derivative, gliadin, are found in wheat, barley, and rye. Symptoms appear in the first 3 years of life, after cereals are introduced to the diet. The second peak is in the third decade. Although CD is thought of as diagnosed early in life, more diagnoses are made in adulthood than in childhood. Breastfeeding has prophylactic effect; breastfed babies have decreased risk. Early introduction of cow's milk is a major etiologic factor. Breastfeeding plus delay in introducing cow's milk and cereals are preventive steps.

- **Chemistry of grain proteins:** gluten is a major component of wheat endosperm, composed of gliadins and glutenins. Gliadin triggers CD. In rye, barley, and oats, the proteins triggering CD are secalins, hordeins, and avenins, respectively, and prolamins collectively. The cereal grain family is Gramineae; close taxonomic relation to wheat suggests ability to activate CD. Rice and corn do not activate CD and are further removed taxonomically from wheat. Gliadins are single polypeptide chains (molecular weight 30,000 to 75,000 mol) with high glutamine and

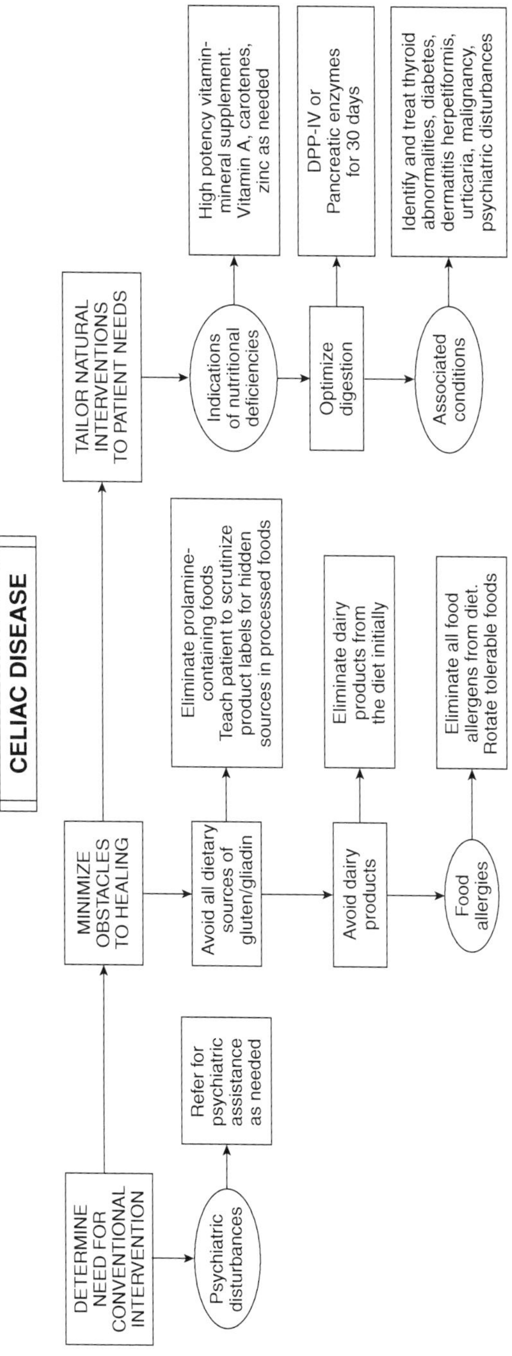
CELIAC DISEASE
DETERMINE NEED FOR CONVENTIONAL INTERVENTION
Psychiatric disturbances
Refer for psychiatric assistance as needed
MINIMIZE OBSTACLES TO HEALING
Avoid all dietary sources of gluten/gliadin
Eliminate prolamine-containing foods
Teach patient to scrutinize product labels for hidden sources in processed foods
Avoid dairy products
Eliminate dairy products from the diet initially
Food allergies
Eliminate all food allergens from diet.
Rotate tolerable foods
TAILOR NATURAL INTERVENTIONS TO PATIENT NEEDS
Indications of nutritional deficiencies
High potency vitamin-mineral supplement.
Vitamin A, carotenes, zinc as needed
Optimize digestion
DPP-IV or Pancreatic enzymes for 30 days
Associated conditions
Identify and treat thyroid abnormalities, diabetes, dermatitis herpetiformis, urticaria, malignancy, psychiatric disturbances

proline. Gliadin's four electrophoretic fractions are alpha-, beta-, gamma-, and omega-gliadin. Alpha-gliadin may be the fraction most capable of activating CD, but beta- and gamma-gliadin also are capable. Omega-gliadin is nonactivating but has the highest glutamine and proline. Hydrolyzed gliadin does not activate CD, suggesting deficient brush border peptidase or similar digestive defect.

- **Opioid activity:** pepsin hydrolysates of wheat gluten have opioid activity, the factor linking wheat ingestion to schizophrenia. Hypothesis: gluten is a pathogenic factor in schizophrenia (substantiated by studies).
- **Pathogenesis:** genetic cause linked to human leukocyte antigen (HLA) DQ2 in 95% of patients and DQ8 in the remainder. These gene loci relate to immunologic recognition of antigens and specific T-cell immune responses. Hypothesis: CD may arise from abnormalities in immune response, rather than gliadin "toxicity." Gliadin sensitizing is humoral and cell mediated; T-cell dysfunction is a key factor in enteropathy. Circulating antibodies are specific for CD (antiendomysial antibody [AEA]) and are used as serum markers to screen patients and estimate CD prevalence. Tissue transglutaminase (tTG) is the autoantigen for AEA; enzyme-linked assay using recombinant tTG is highly sensitive and specific for CD. Anti-tTG antibody titers fall and can become undetectable during gluten-free diet; tTG-gliadin complexes stimulate gluten-specific T cells to induce anti-tTG antibody production. T cells may react to smaller gliadin peptides, and B cells may respond to the larger tTG enzyme. CD risk is greater when large amounts of gluten are introduced during early childhood.
- **Clinical aspects:** CD lesions are often histologically indistinguishable from tropical sprue, food allergy, diffuse intestinal lymphoma, and viral gastroenteritis. CD can cause disaccharidase deficiency, leading to lactose intolerance. Increased intestinal permeability causes multiple food allergies. Cow's milk intolerance may precede CD. Improving nutritional status, even taking multiple B vitamin, produces improvement in quality of life.
- **Associated conditions:** Most significant condition associated with CD is early death. Compared with controls, there was a 39% increased risk of death in patients with CD, 72% increased risk in those with gut inflammation related to gluten, and 35% increased risk in those with gluten sensitivity but no CD. There

are 55 health conditions linked to CD and gluten sensitivity, including irritable bowel disease, inflammatory bowel disease, anemia, migraines, epilepsy, fatigue, canker sores, osteoporosis, rheumatoid arthritis, lupus, multiple sclerosis, and almost all other autoimmune diseases. Others: thyroid abnormalities, insulin-dependent diabetes mellitus, psychiatric disturbances (including schizophrenia), dermatitis herpetiformis, and urticaria are linked to gluten intolerance. Increased risk of malignant neoplasms exists (e.g., non-Hodgkin's lymphoma) in celiac patients, perhaps because of decreased micronutrient absorption of vitamin A and carotenoids (*Textbook,* "Beta-carotene and Other Carotenoids" and "Vitamin A") and gliadin-activated suppressor cell activity. Alpha-gliadin activates suppressor cells of celiac patients but not healthy control subjects or patients with Crohn's disease. Casein and beta-lactoglobulin do not activate suppressor cells. Depressed immunity increases susceptibility to infection and neoplasm. Gluten sensitivity is weakly linked to mood scores, cognitive impairment, and autism.

DIAGNOSIS

Endoscopy with jejunal biopsy was the old definitive diagnostic procedure. Of the new markers, the test for human anti-tTG antibodies (immunoglobulin A [IgA] anti-tTG) is emerging as most widely used, owing to lower cost compared with antiendomysial antibody (IgA EMA) and greater sensitivity compared with antigliadin antibody (AGA) testing. IgA EMA can detect CD with sensitivity and specificity of 90% and 99%, respectively. Anti-tTG also has high sensitivity (99%) and specificity (>90%) for identifying CD. An equivocal result on tTG testing should be followed by IgA EMA. With IgA EMA testing, it is recommended that total serum IgA level be checked in parallel, because celiac patients with IgA deficiency may be unable to produce antibodies on which these tests depend, leading to false-negative result. Endoscopy or gastroscopy and biopsy should still be performed if clinically warranted.

THERAPEUTIC CONSIDERATIONS

- **Diet**: gluten-free diet—no wheat, rye, barley, triticale, or oats. Buckwheat and millet also are excluded; they contain prolamins with antigenicity similar to alpha-gliadin. Rotate other foods.

Eliminate milk and milk products until patient redevelops normal intestinal structure and function.

- **Patient response:** clinical improvement is seen within a few days or weeks (30% respond within 3 days, another 50% within 1 month, and 10% within another month). Ten percent respond only after 24 to 36 months of gluten avoidance. Failure to respond suggests incorrect diagnosis; patient not adhering to diet or exposed to hidden sources of gliadin; or associated disease or complication, such as zinc deficiency. Multivitamin-mineral supplements treat underlying deficiency and provide cofactors for growth and repair.
- **Pancreatic enzymes:** Pancreatic insufficiency occurs in 8% to 30% of celiac patients. Pancreatic enzyme supplements (2 capsules per meal, with each containing lipase 5000 international units [IU], amylase 2900 IU, and protease 330 IU; total of 6 to 10 capsules daily) enhance clinical benefit of gluten-free diet during first 30 days but with no greater benefit after 60 days. Use pancreatic enzymes during first 30 days after diagnosis (*Textbook,* "Celiac Disease"). A better choice than pancreatic enzymes might be enzyme preparations containing dipeptidyl-peptidase IV (DPP-IV) from fungal sources. This enzyme targets both gliadin and casein (milk protein) and is resistant to breakdown by other digestive enzymes. DPP-IV is key enzyme responsible for digestion of these proteins and is found in lower amounts in intestinal mucosa of people with CD. It has an inverse correlation with level of mucosal damage among those with and without CD. The lower the DPP-IV, the higher the damage to the intestinal lining. Preparations containing DPP-IV are often recommended to safeguard against hidden sources of gluten.

THERAPEUTIC APPROACH

- Eliminate all sources of gliadin (primarily wheat, rye, and barley—be careful to check for gluten additives).
- Initially eliminate dairy products.
- Correct underlying nutritional deficiencies.
- Treat associated conditions.
- Identify and eliminate all food allergens.
- If no response within 1 month, reconsider diagnosis and search for hidden sources of gliadin.

A strict gluten-free diet is difficult in the United States because of the ubiquitous distribution of gliadin and other activators of CD in processed foods. Read labels carefully for hidden sources of gliadin (e.g., soy sauce, modified food starch, ice cream, soup, beer, wine, vodka, whisky, malt). Patients should consult resources for patient information on gluten-free recipes.

Patient Resources

Gluten Intolerance Group
31214 124th Ave. SE
Auburn, WA 98092
Website: www.gluten.net

Celiac Support Association
P.O. Box 31700
Omaha, NE 68131-0700
Website: www.csaceliacs.org

Celiac Disease Foundation
13251 Ventura Blvd., Suite 1
Studio City, CA 91604
Website: http://celiac.org

Cervical Dysplasia

DIAGNOSTIC SUMMARY

- Abnormal Pap smears (atypical cells of undetermined significance [ASC-US]; low-grade squamous intraepithelial lesions [LGSILs]; high-grade squamous intraepithelial lesions [HGSILs]),
- Human papillomavirus (HPV) testing for presence of high-risk strains.
- Colposcopy, endocervical curettage, cervical biopsies.

Current U.S. cervical disease management guidelines include algorithms for managing high-risk HPV strains, ASC-US, atypical cells for which high-grade lesions cannot be ruled out (ASC-H), LGSILs, and HGSILs. Guidelines continue to evolve. Recommendations for HPV testing and cytology testing and the combination of the two, colposcopy and biopsies, follow-up cytology testing, and colposcopy based on abnormal results are complex and often change. Guidelines differ depending on the patient's age, history of previous abnormal cytology testing, pregnancy status, previous exposure to diethylstilbestrol (DES), immunosuppression status (e.g., kidney transplant), human immunodeficiency virus (HIV) status, and hysterectomy for benign indications and prior history of cervical intraepithelial neoplasia (CIN). We recommend that the clinician consult the latest available guidelines for screening and evaluation with colposcopy, biopsy, and follow-up testing from the American College of Obstetricians and Gynecologists, the American Cancer Society, and/or the U.S. Preventive Services Task Force.

GENERAL CONSIDERATIONS

Cervical dysplasia (CD) is a precancerous lesion with risk factors similar to those of cervical cancer. Etiologic lifestyle factors include early age of first intercourse, multiple sexual partners (in heterosexual women without barrier contraception), other infectious agents (*Chlamydia,* herpes simplex virus), history of genital warts, immunosuppression (HIV, organ transplant), smoking, oral contraceptive (OC) use, pregnancy, and many nutritional factors. All risk factors are closely related.

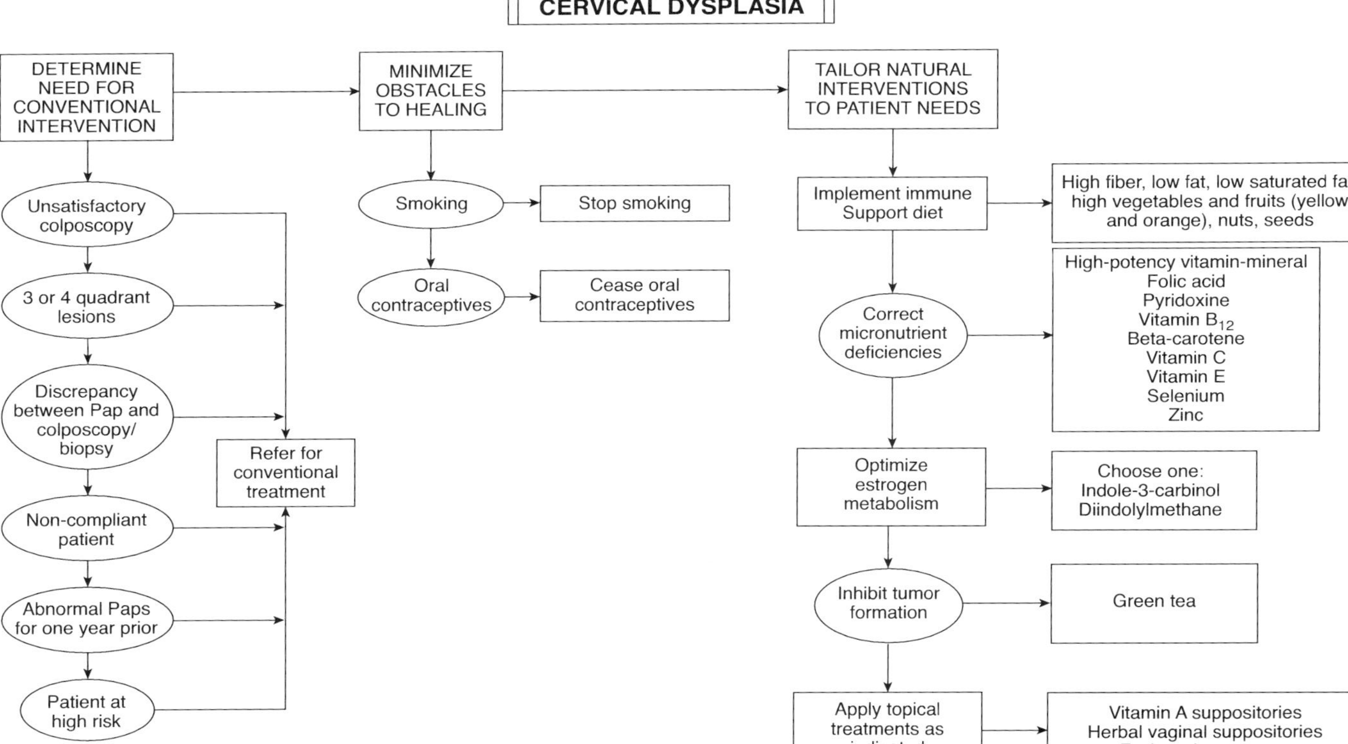
CERVICAL DYSPLASIA
DETERMINE NEED FOR CONVENTIONAL INTERVENTION
Unsatisfactory colposcopy
3 or 4 quadrant lesions
Discrepancy between Pap and colposcopy/ biopsy
Non-compliant patient
Abnormal Paps for one year prior
Patient at high risk
Refer for conventional treatment
MINIMIZE OBSTACLES TO HEALING
Smoking
Stop smoking
Oral contraceptives
Cease oral contraceptives
TAILOR NATURAL INTERVENTIONS TO PATIENT NEEDS
Implement immune Support diet
High fiber, low fat, low saturated fat, high vegetables and fruits (yellow and orange), nuts, seeds
Correct micronutrient deficiencies
High-potency vitamin-mineral
Folic acid
Pyridoxine
Vitamin B_{12}
Beta-carotene
Vitamin C
Vitamin E
Selenium
Zinc
Optimize estrogen metabolism
Choose one:
Indole-3-carbinol
Diindolylmethane
Inhibit tumor formation
Green tea
Apply topical treatments as indicated
Vitamin A suppositories
Herbal vaginal suppositories
Escharotic treatment

Human Papillomavirus

- **Epidemiology:** cervical cancer is linked to long-term persistent HPV infection, transmitted by genital-to-genital contact. Time from exposure to lesion or abnormal Pap smear can be a few weeks or decades. Approximately 80% of adults may be infected. Roughly 60% of young women are infected, but less than 10% develop cervical lesions. Host immunity defends against clinical disease. HPV infections often are transient, resulting only in ASC-US. Clinical disease can include flat or raised genital warts; cervical, vaginal, vulvar, or perianal dysplasias; or invasive cancers. HPV is detected in 50% to 80% of vaginal, 50% of vulvar, and nearly all penile and anal cancers.
- **Total of 120 HPV varieties:** 30 HPV types infect squamous epithelium of lower anogenital tracts of men and women. HPV types 6, 11, 42, 43, and 44 result in classic genital warts of cauliflower appearance or flat lesions. Types 16, 18, 31, 33, 35, 45, 51, 52, and 56 are high-risk types found in lower genital tract cancers and intraepithelial lesions. Lesions caused by low-risk and high-risk HPV types can regress to normal even without treatment, but prognosis cannot be predicted. Eighty percent of cervical cancers are linked to types 16, 18, 31, and 45; 15% are associated with types 31, 33, 35, 51, and 52. LGSILs can be caused by both low- and high-risk HPV types. High-risk types are seen in 75% to 85% of low-grade lesions; mixed low- and high-risk types in 15%; and low-risk types exclusively in only 2% to 25%.
- **Histology:** 95% of cervix cancers originate in the squamocolumnar junction of the cervical os. In adolescence, glandular epithelium covers much of exocervix, but as adolescence progresses columnar epithelium is replaced by squamous cells. This actively growing area is susceptible to multiple insults and HPV because of the metaplastic nature of the conversion process.
- **Development and progression:** HPV exposure commonly occurs during unprotected intercourse in heterosexual women. Approximately 60% of those in their teens and 20s test positive for HPV DNA by polymerase chain reaction. Three outcomes from HPV exposure are (1) permanent latency or only transient cytologic changes; (2) cytologic changes diagnostic of HPV (in 60% of affected women, atypia or LGSILs spontaneously regress, and in 20 to 30% they persist); and (3) development of HGSILs in 10%. A total of 70% of women clear the virus within the first year. Low-grade lesions can regress, persist, or progress. Progression peaks at ages 25 to 29 years, 4 to 7 years after peak incidence of

mild dysplasia. Most low-grade lesions do not progress to invasive cancer, even without treatment. Even HPV type 16, detected in 60% of cancers, tends to result in regression. Invasive cancer incidence plateaus in white American women 15 years after peak incidence of CIN III, between the ages of 40 and 45 years.

Risk Factors

- **Sexual activity:** early age at first intercourse and/or multiple sexual contacts without condom increase risk for CD or carcinoma. Cervical cancer may be a sexually transmitted disease linked to HPV. The variability in time from exposure to identified lesion prevents identification of sexual partners who transmitted HPV. Oral HPV lesions are rare. Nonsexual exposure may occur from examination tables, doorknobs, tanning beds, and so on. Other infections (herpes simplex, chlamydia, bacterial vaginosis) may be cofactors that alter cervical immunity, cause inflammation, facilitate HPV entry into basal cells, accelerate HPV replication in cell nuclei, and/or coexist with HPV.
- **Smoking:** smokers have three times the risk of nonsmokers, and 17 times the risk in women aged 20 to 29 years. Smoking may depress immunity and induce vitamin C deficiency. Cervical cells may concentrate nicotine. Smoking may be linked to risky sexual behavior.
- **Oral contraceptives:** OC use shows no overall change in risk of invasive cervical cancer, but there is a modestly increased risk in long-term OC users. OCs are linked to a rare cervical cancer, adenocarcinoma, with increased incidence over the past several decades; invasive squamous cancer has declined since "the Pill" was introduced. An increased risk of invasive adenocarcinoma may occur with OC use longer than 12 years. OCs potentiate the adverse effects of smoking and decrease levels of nutrients including vitamins C, B_6, and B_{12}; folic acid; riboflavin; and zinc.

THERAPEUTIC CONSIDERATIONS

Perform follow-up Pap test to determine what course of action is needed. Many cases of mild CD (ASC-US, LGSILs) resolve spontaneously. Median time required for progression from CD to carcinoma in situ ranges from 86 months for LGSILs to 12 months for HGSILs. With LGSILs, the natural approaches provided in this chapter can be followed with another Pap smear and colposcopy at 3 months. If colposcopy reveals abnormal tissue, endocervical curettage may be appropriate. Prescribing a patient diagnosed with HGSILs a colposcopy with endocervical curettage is recommended.

Dietary Factors

- **Multiple nutrient deficiencies:** cofactors for CD. Approximately 67% of CD patients have abnormal anthropometric or biochemical parameters: height/weight ratios, triceps skin fold thickness, mid-arm muscle circumference, serum albumin, total iron-binding capacity, hemoglobin, creatinine height index, prothrombin time, and lymphocyte count. Other patients have marginally "normal" nutritional status.
- **Vitamin assessment by biochemical evaluation:** plasma and red cell folate; serum beta-carotene; vitamins A, B_{12}, and C; erythrocyte transketolase for thiamine determination; erythrocyte glutathione reductase for riboflavin determination; and erythrocyte aspartate transaminase for pyridoxine determination. At least one abnormal vitamin level is found in 67% of cervical cancer patients. Approximately 38% display multiple abnormalities.
- **General dietary factors:** high fat intake increases risk for cervical cancer. A diet rich in fruits and vegetables (with fiber, carotenes, and vitamin C) protects against carcinogenesis. Increasing concentrations of serum lycopene are negatively associated with CIN I, CIN III, and cervical cancer. Increasing concentrations of serum alpha- and gamma-tocopherols and higher dietary intakes of dark green and deep yellow vegetables and fruits are associated with a 50% decreased risk of CIN III. Significant reductions in risk of cervical cancer of 40% to 60% are observed for women in the highest versus the lowest tertiles of dietary fiber, vitamin C, vitamin E, vitamin A, alpha-carotene, beta-carotene, lutein, and folate.

Nutritional Botanical Supplements

Combinations of products may work best. Multiple vitamins and mineral formulas, vitamins A and E, and calcium are linked to lower risk of cervical cancer and lower HPV viral load. Multiple vitamins and minerals, vitamins A and E, and calcium are associated with lower risk of CIN II or III. Patients who take multiple vitamins and minerals have lower HPV viral load and decreased frequency of CIN I.

- **Vitamin A and beta-carotene**: minor association between dietary retinoids and CD risk, but a strong inverse correlation between beta-carotene intake and CD risk. Only 6% of patients with untreated cervical cancer have less-than-normal serum vitamin A, but 38% have stage-related abnormal beta-carotene. Low serum beta-carotene is linked to a three-times increased risk for severe dysplasia. Serum vitamin A and beta-carotene are much lower in CD patients than in control subjects. Unfortunately, response rates to intervention with oral carotenoids have been inconsistent. Response rate is highest for women with no HPV detected, lower for those ranked at indeterminate or low risk, and lowest for those classified at high risk. In conclusion, beta-carotene may not enhance regression of high-grade CIN, especially in HPV-positive subjects. That said, mixed natural carotenoids have been a mainstay of comprehensive naturopathic treatment. Carotenes and retinols improve integrity and function of epithelial tissues, provide antioxidant properties, and enhance immune function (*Textbook,* "Beta-Carotene and Other Carotenoids"). Beta-carotene is more advantageous than retinoids; it has greater antioxidant properties, immune-enhancing effects, and tendency to be concentrated in epithelial tissues.

- **Topical vitamin A:** Four consecutive 24-hour applications of retinoic acid followed by two more applications at 3 and 6 months applied with a collagen sponge in a cervical cap may induce regression of moderate dysplasia.
- **Vitamin A suppositories:** part of multifactorial treatment using oral folic acid, vitamin C, and carotenes with topical vitamin A suppositories and herbal vitamin suppositories. For more-severe disease, topical "escharotic" treatment can be used for moderate, severe dysplasia and carcinoma in situ.
- **Vitamin C:** diminished intake and plasma levels of vitamin C in CD patients. Inadequate intake is an independent risk factor for premalignant cervical disease and carcinoma in situ. Ascorbate acts as an antioxidant, maintains normal epithelial integrity, improves wound healing, enhances immunity, and inhibits carcinogen formation.
- **Folic acid:** Low folic acid levels are implicated in many cases of CD, although this link is decreased now with widespread folic acid fortification of the food supply. When cervical cells lack folic acid, they become "macrocytic" in the same way that red blood cells (RBCs) do. Cervical cytologic abnormalities related to folate deficiency precede hematologic abnormalities. Folate is the most commonly deficient vitamin in the world, especially among women who are pregnant or taking OCs. Folate deficiency is the probable cause of many abnormal

cytologic smears, rather than "true" dysplasia. Even with food fortification, folic acid is still a factor in many cases of CD. OCs induce localized interference with folate metabolism—tissue levels at end-organ targets (cervix) are deficient. RBC folate is decreased (especially with CD), whereas serum levels are normal or increased. OCs induce synthesis of a macromolecule that inhibits folate uptake by cells. Folate supplements (10 mg q.d.) improve or normalize cytologic smears in CD patients. Regression rates for untreated CD are 1.3% for mild and 0% for moderate infection. Folate-induced regression-to-normal rates have been reported to be 20%, 63.7%, and 100% in different studies. The progression rate of untreated CD is 16% at 4 months. The folate-supplemented rate is 0% (even though women remained on OCs). Lower folic acid status enhances the effect of other risk factors for CD. For example, low RBC folate appears to be a major risk factor for HPV infection of the cervix. Higher circulating folate is independently associated with lower likelihood of becoming positive for high-risk human papillomaviruses (HR-HPVs) and of having persistent HR-HPV infection and greater risk for HGSILs.

- **Vitamin B_{12}:** use vitamin B_{12} with folate to avoid folate masking underlying B_{12} deficiency. Women with higher plasma folate who also have sufficient plasma vitamin B_{12} have 70% lower odds of being diagnosed with CD.
- **Pyridoxine:** vitamin B_6 (RBC transaminase test) is decreased in one third of CD patients. Decreased B_6 status affects metabolism of estrogens and tryptophan and impairs immunity.
- **Selenium:** serum, dietary, and soil selenium are inversely correlated with all epithelial cancers and are much lower in CD patients. Significantly lower selenium and zinc levels are found in both HGSIL and cervical cancer patients compared with controls. Activity of the selenium-containing antioxidant enzyme glutathione peroxidase is lower in patients with HGSILs or cancer than in controls, and total antioxidant ability decreases from control group to those with CIN to those with cancer. One anticarcinogenic effect is increased glutathione peroxidase activity. Toxic elements (lead, cadmium, mercury, gold) have selenium-antagonistic properties.
- **Copper/zinc ratio, zinc, and retinol:** increased serum copper/zinc ratio (Cu/Zn) is a nonspecific reaction to inflammation or malignancy. Serum Cu/Zn may be a tool to establish extent of cancer. A ratio greater than 1.95 indicated malignancy in 90% of patients

studied. Elevated ratios also are seen with OC use, pregnancy, acute and chronic infections, chronic liver disease, and inflammatory conditions. Serum Cu/Zn should not be used to predict malignancy in these patients. Decreased available Zn may cause retinol-binding protein to be absent or undetectable in 80% of dysplastic tissue versus 23.5% of normal tissue. There is an inverse relationship between serum retinol and Zn and incidence of CD.

- **Indole-3-carbinol (I3C) and diindolylmethane (DIM):** I3C is a phytochemical in cabbage family vegetables. It is converted in the stomach to DIM. I3C and DIM are antioxidants and potent stimulators of the body's natural detoxifying enzymes. Increasing intake of cabbage family vegetables or taking I3C or DIM as supplements increases conversion of estrogen from cancer-producing forms to nontoxic breakdown products. The body breaks down estrogen into two byproducts: 16α-hydroxyestrone, which promotes estrogen-dependent cancer; or 2-hydroxyestrone, which does not stimulate cancer cells. Women with HGSILs have altered estrogen metabolism, with higher 16α-hydroxyestrone and lower 2-hydroxyestrogen than normal. Half of women with HGSILs (biopsy-proved CIN II or III) who were given 200 or 400 mg of I3C for 12 weeks demonstrated complete regression of severe dysplasia, compared with none in the placebo group. HPV was detected in 7 of 10 placebo patients, in 7 of 8 in a 200-mg/day group, and in 8 of 9 in a 400-mg/day group. DIM (2 mg/kg/day) or placebo was given for 12 weeks to patients with HGSILs (biopsy-proved CIN II or III) who were scheduled for loop electrosurgical excision procedure (LEEP). Although there was no difference in outcomes between DIM and placebo groups, 49% of DIM patients showed improved Pap smear findings with either less-severe abnormality or a normal result. Colposcopy improved in 56% of DIM of subjects.
- **Green tea:** Constituents polyphenol E and epigallocatechin-3-gallate (EGCG) have been effective against HPV-infected cervical cells and lesions in both laboratory and clinical studies. Green tea appears to induce apoptosis of HPV-infected cervical cells and to arrest cell cycles, modify gene expression, and inhibit tumor formation. A study compared topical green tea polyphenol ointment and/or oral ingestion versus green tea polyphenol capsule or EGCG capsule. All treatment groups improved more than placebo group, but those given topical treatment improved most significantly.

Miscellaneous Considerations

- **Vaginal depletion pack (vag pack):** has a long history of efficacy for CD. The mechanism of action is not yet elucidated. It may promote sloughing of superficial abnormal cervical cells. It is effective as part of a multifaceted approach (*Textbook,* "Vaginal Depletion Pack").
- **Escharotic treatment:** topical herbal cryotherapy treatment of the cervix used to remove abnormal cells. Ingredients include zinc chloride mixed with *Sanguinaria canadensis,* a botanical. Full description of this protocol is in (*Textbook* Appendix 2). Escharotic treatment is indicated for CIN II and CIN III, both HGSILs, but only when a satisfactory colposcopy has been performed by a clinician. Use of escharotic treatment rather than LEEP or conization must fall within guidelines outlined under "Therapeutic Approach." The escharotic treatment is best implemented twice a week with 2 full days between treatments. The zinc chloride solution must be made by a compounding pharmacy as a prescription item.

THERAPEUTIC APPROACH

Treatment of CD requires proper monitoring and coordination of care if one practitioner is doing workup with colposcopy and biopsies and another implements natural or integrated treatment. The basic approach is to eliminate all factors associated with CD and optimize patient's nutritional status. End smoking and OC use; patient must follow supplementation program listed here.

Protocols for Natural Treatment

A. Criteria for naturopathic protocol
   1. ASC-US.
   2. ASC-US with documented HPV.
   3. ASC-H: endocervical curettage is negative or positive with a satisfactory colposcopy.
   4. Low-grade squamous intraepithelial neoplasia: endocervical curettage is negative with a satisfactory colposcopy.
   5. High-grade squamous intraepithelial neoplasia: endocervical curettage is negative with a satisfactory colposcopy.
   6. ASC-H: endocervical curettage is positive with a satisfactory colposcopy, but the patient is at low risk for more-serious disease or has a low-risk type of HPV or, even if she does not have low-risk HPV, the natural treatment protocol may be recommended at the discretion of the practitioner.

7. Low-grade squamous intraepithelial neoplasia: endocervical curettage is positive with a satisfactory colposcopy, but the patient is at low risk for more-serious disease or has a low-risk type of HPV, or the practitioner may recommend the natural treatment protocol at his or her discretion.
8. High-grade squamous intraepithelial neoplasia: endocervical curettage is positive, with a satisfactory colposcopy, but the patient is at low risk or, even if not, the natural treatment protocol may be recommended at the discretion of the practitioner and considered carefully after colposcopy, biopsies, and careful evaluation.
9. It is possible to treat carcinoma in situ in select cases, but this is definitely a judgment call and should be considered very carefully after colposcopy, biopsies, and careful follow-up.

B. Referrals for colposcopy with biopsies
1. ASC-US if HPV DNA testing is positive for high-risk HPV; if no HPV testing is done, then the Pap test should be repeated twice at 4- to 6-month intervals. If HPV typing is negative for high-risk types, then the Pap test should be repeated in 12 months.
2. ASC-H.
3. LGSILs.
4. HGSILs.
5. Atypical glandular cells of undetermined significance (AGUS); endometrial biopsy is needed as well.
6. Adenocarcinoma in situ (AIS): endometrial biopsy is needed as well.
7. Pap smear diagnosis of microinvasion or frank invasion.
8. Endometrial cells present in a postmenopausal woman; also calls for an endometrial biopsy even if the cells are benign.
9. A patient who may not follow through with the recommended follow-up Pap smear after an abnormal Pap result.
10. Visible unknown cervical lesion regardless of the Pap smear test result.
11. Initial examination of a DES daughter.
12. Unexplained or persistent cervical bleeding.
13. Vulvar condyloma with abnormal Pap test result.
14. To be used for follow-up after treatment plan is completed, especially in HGSILs.

C. Referrals for conization or LEEP
1. Pap test results show more than one grade of dysplasia different from that seen on colposcopy or reported on in the biopsy.

2. Biopsy shows squamous intraepithelial lesions with three or four quadrants involved.
3. Unsatisfactory colposcopy with any degree of squamous intraepithelial lesions on biopsy.
4. The patient may not be a good candidate for ongoing treatment and the closer follow-up required by alternative treatments.
5. No improvement in pathology with the initial naturopathic plan or repeated alternate plan.
6. If AGUS is found on the Pap test and no disease is detected on colposcopy, biopsies and endocervical curettage are indicated.
7. If AIS is found on the Pap test and no disease is detected on colposcopy, biopsies and endocervical curettage are indicated.

D. At the discretion of the practitioner and patient
   1. Positive endocervical curettage with any degree of squamous intraepithelial lesions. A more-assertive approach is recommended.
   2. High-risk patients: the last Pap test more than 1 year previously, a history of genital warts, a history of CD, smokers, multiple sex partners with lack of safe sex practices. In these cases, a more-proactive and assertive approach is recommended.

E. Referral for probable hysterectomy
   1. Microinvasive cervical cancer
   2. Frank invasive cervical cancer
   3. Adenocarcinoma
      - Diet: immune supportive diet: high fiber, low fat, low saturated fat, high vegetables and fruits (especially yellow and orange), raw organic nuts and seeds
      - Supplements:
        - High-potency multiple vitamin and mineral formula
        - Folic acid: 10 mg q.d. for 3 months, then 2.5 mg q.d.
        - Vitamin B_{12} (methylcobalamin): 1 mg q.d.
        - Beta-carotene: 150,000 international units (IU) q.d. for 3 months, then decrease to 25,000 IU q.d. for 1 year
        - Vitamin C: 1 to 3 g q.d. for 3 to 12 months
        - Vitamin E (mixed tocopherols): 200 IU q.i.d. for 3 to 12 months
        - Selenium: 200 to 400 mcg q.d. for 3 to 12 months
        - Zinc (elemental): 20 to 30 mg q.d. for 3 to 12 months

- **Choose one of the following:**
  - I3C: 200 to 400 mg q.d. for 3 months
  - DIM: 2.2 mg per kg body weight q.d.

Botanical Medicine

- Green tea extract (>90% total polyphenol content): 150 to 300 mg q.d. for 3 to 12 months

Sample Treatment Protocols

A typical Cells of Undetermined Significance

Topical

- Week 1: insert vitamin A suppository every night for 6 nights.
- Week 2: insert herbal vaginal suppository every night for 6 nights.
- Week 3: repeat vitamin A suppository.
- Week 4: repeat herbal suppository.
- Weeks 5 to 12: insert green tea suppository 2 nights a week.

Supplementation as previously noted for a minimum of 3 months

Low-Grade Squamous Intraepithelial Lesions

Topical

- Week 1: insert vitamin A suppository every night for 6 nights.
- Insert vag pack suppository on night 7.
- Week 2: insert herbal suppository every night for 6 nights.
- Insert vag pack suppository on night 7.
- Week 3: repeat vitamin A suppository.
- Insert vag pack suppository on night 7.
- Week 4: repeat herbal suppository.
- Insert vag pack suppository on night 7.
- Weeks 5 to 12: insert green tea suppository twice a week.

Supplementation as previously noted for a minimum of 3 months

High-Grade Squamous Intraepithelial Lesions

Topical

- Escharotic treatment twice a week for 5 weeks.
- The last treatment is followed by 1 month of suppository routine as for LGSILs, then a green tea suppository twice a week for weeks 5 through 12.

Supplementation as previously noted for a minimum of 3 months

Chronic Candidiasis

DIAGNOSTIC SUMMARY

- Chronic fatigue and malaise
- Gastrointestinal (GI) bloating and cramps
- Vaginal yeast infection
- Allergies and/or low immune function
- Carbohydrate craving
- History of broad-spectrum antibiotic use

GENERAL CONSIDERATIONS

Candida is normal in the GI tract and vagina. Overgrowth, depleted immunity, damaged GI mucosa allow absorption of yeast cells, particles, toxins; result is "yeast syndrome" or "feeling sick all over": fatigue, allergies, immune system malfunction, depression, chemical sensitivities, and digestive disturbances. Women are eight times more likely than men to have syndrome; contributors are estrogen, birth control pills, and greater antibiotic use.

- **Causal factors:** multifactorial; correct factors predisposing overgrowth; requires more than killing yeast with antifungals, synthetic or natural; prolonged antibiotic use is the key factor in most cases—suppresses normal intestinal bacteria that control yeast, suppresses immunity, generates antibiotic-resistant microbes, may contribute to Crohn's disease.
- **Related syndromes:** small intestinal bacterial overgrowth and leaky gut associated with *Candida* overgrowth; may produce identical symptoms to the yeast syndrome.

Predisposing Factors to *Candida albicans* Overgrowth

- Decreased digestive secretions
- Dietary factors
- Impaired immunity
- Nutrient deficiency
- Drugs (particularly antibiotics)
- Impaired liver function
- Underlying disease states
- Altered bowel flora
- Prolonged antibiotic use

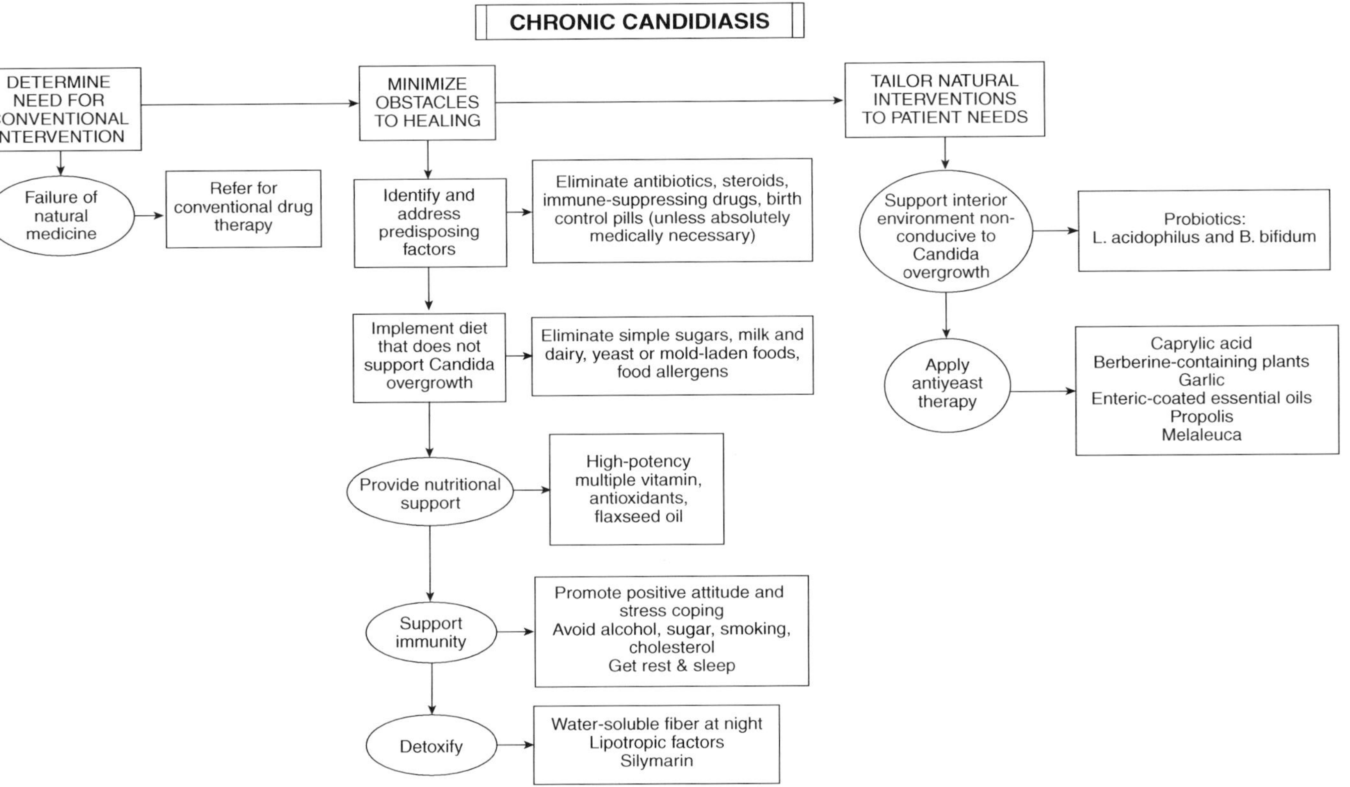
CHRONIC CANDIDIASIS
DETERMINE NEED FOR CONVENTIONAL INTERVENTION
Failure of natural medicine
Refer for conventional drug therapy
MINIMIZE OBSTACLES TO HEALING
Identify and address predisposing factors
Eliminate antibiotics, steroids, immune-suppressing drugs, birth control pills (unless absolutely medically necessary)
Implement diet that does not support Candida overgrowth
Eliminate simple sugars, milk and dairy, yeast or mold-laden foods, food allergens
Provide nutritional support
High-potency multiple vitamin, antioxidants, flaxseed oil
Support immunity
Promote positive attitude and stress coping
Avoid alcohol, sugar, smoking, cholesterol
Get rest & sleep
Detoxify
Water-soluble fiber at night
Lipotropic factors
Silymarin
TAILOR NATURAL INTERVENTIONS TO PATIENT NEEDS
Support interior environment non-conducive to Candida overgrowth
Probiotics:
L. acidophilus and B. bifidum
Apply antiyeast therapy
Caprylic acid
Berberine-containing plants
Garlic
Enteric-coated essential oils
Propolis
Melaleuca

DIAGNOSIS

- **Screening method:** comprehensive questionnaire (*Textbook*, "*Candida* Questionnaire")
- **Best method:** clinical evaluation—knowledge of yeast-related illness, detailed medical history, patient questionnaire
- **Comprehensive stool and digestive analysis (CSDA):** more clinically useful; evaluates digestion, intestinal environment, and absorption; indicates underlying digestive disturbance; may pinpoint other causes (e.g., small intestinal bacterial overgrowth, leaky gut syndrome)
- **Laboratory techniques (used only to confirm):** stool cultures for *Candida,* antibody to *Candida, Candida* antigens in the blood; rarely needed; confirm what history, physical examination, CSDA reveal; confirm *Candida* is factor, monitor therapy

Typical Chronic Candidiasis Patient Profile

Sex: Female
Age: 15 to 50 years

General Symptoms
- Chronic fatigue
- Loss of energy
- General malaise
- Decreased libido

Gastrointestinal Symptoms
- Thrush
- Bloating, gas
- Intestinal cramps
- Rectal itching
- Altered bowel function

Genitourinary Symptoms
- Vaginal yeast infection
- Frequent bladder infections

Endocrine Symptoms
- Primarily menstrual complaints

Nervous Symptoms
- Depression
- Irritability
- Inability to concentrate

Immune Symptoms
- Allergies
- Chemical sensitivities
- Low immune function

History
- Chronic vaginal yeast infections
- Chronic antibiotic use for infections or acne
- Oral birth control use
- Oral steroid hormone use

Associated Conditions
- Premenstrual syndrome
- Sensitivity to foods, chemicals, and other allergens
- Endocrine disturbances
- Eczema
- Psoriasis
- Irritable bowel syndrome

Other Symptoms
- Craving for foods rich in carbohydrates or yeast

THERAPEUTIC CONSIDERATIONS

Comprehensive approach more effective than simply killing yeast with drug or natural agent; address causes. Eradicate *Candida* with natural therapies; follow-up stool culture and analysis confirm *Candida* eliminated. If symptoms remain after yeast is eliminated, condition is unrelated to *Candida;* consider small intestinal bacterial overgrowth, pancreatic enzymes, and berberine-containing plants. Address predisposing factors, recommend *Candida* control diet, support organ systems as needed.

Triggers to Impaired Immunity in Candidiasis

- Antibiotic use
- Corticosteroid use
- Other drugs that suppress the immune system
- Nutrient deficiency
- Food allergies
- High-sugar diet
- Stress

Diet

- **Sugar:** chief nutrient of *Candida;* restrict sugar, honey, maple syrup, and fruit juice.
- **Milk and dairy products:** high lactose content promotes *Candida;* contain food allergens; may contain trace levels of antibiotics, disrupting GI bacteria and promoting *Candida.*
- **Mold- and yeast-containing foods:** avoid foods with high yeast or mold levels: alcohol, cheese, dried fruits, peanuts.
- **Food allergies:** common in patients with yeast syndrome; enzyme-linked immunosorbent assay (ELISA) tests for immunoglobulin E (IgE)– and IgG-mediated food allergies.

Hypochlorhydria

Gastric hydrochloric acid (HCl), pancreatic enzymes, and bile inhibit *Candida* and prevent its penetration into intestinal mucosa; decreased secretion allows yeast overgrowth; antiulcer and antacid drugs induce *Candida* overgrowth in the stomach; pancreatic enzymes—proteases keep small intestine free from parasites. Supplement as needed: HCl, pancreatic enzymes, substances promoting bile flow; use CSDA as guide.

Enhancing Immunity

- **Immune function:** essential; rule out other chronic infections caused by depressed immunity.
- **Decreased thymus function:** major factor in depressed cell-mediated immunity; history of repeated viral infections (e.g., acute rhinitis, herpes, prostatic or vaginal infections).
- **Vicious cycle:** triggering event (e.g., antibiotic, nutrient deficiency) induces immune suppression, allowing yeast overgrowth, competition for nutrients, secretion of mycotoxins and antigens that tax immune system.
- **Restore immunity:** improve thymus function; prevent thymic involution with antioxidants (carotenes, vitamins C and E, zinc, selenium), nutrients for synthesis or action of thymic hormones, and concentrates of calf thymus tissue.

Promoting Detoxification

Liver damage is the underlying factor; nonviral liver damage reduces immunity, allowing *Candida* overgrowth. Liver support: healthy lifestyle, avoidance of alcohol, regular exercise, vitamin-mineral supplement, lipotropic formula, silymarin, 3-day fast at change of each season.

- **Lipotropic factors:** promote flow of fat and bile through liver for a "decongesting" effect; increase intrahepatic levels of *S*-adenosylmethionine, a major lipotropic compound, and glutathione, a major detoxifying compound. Daily dose: 1000 mg choline and 1000 mg of either L-methionine and/or L-cysteine.
- **Promote elimination:** high-fiber plant foods; fiber formulas as needed.

Indications of the Need for Detoxification

- More than 20 lb overweight
- Diabetes
- Presence of gallstones
- History of heavy alcohol use
- Psoriasis
- Natural and synthetic steroid hormone use
- Anabolic steroids
- Estrogens
- Oral contraceptives
- High exposure to certain chemicals or drugs
- Cleaning solvents
- Pesticides
- Antibiotics
- Diuretics
- Nonsteroidal anti-inflammatory drugs
- Thyroid hormone
- History of viral hepatitis

Probiotics

Colon microflora affect immunity, cholesterol metabolism, carcinogenesis, aging. Species: *Lactobacillus acidophilus, Bifidobacterium bifidum* (dose of 1 to 10 billion viable organisms). Application: to promote proper intestinal environment after antibiotic therapy, vaginal yeast infections, and urinary tract infections.

Natural Antiyeast Agents

- **Herxheimer ("die off") reaction:** worsening symptoms; caused by rapid killing of *Candida* and absorption of yeast toxins, particles, and antigens; to minimize, follow dietary recommendations for 2 weeks before antiyeast agent; support liver; start antiyeast medication at a low dose and gradually increase over 1 month to full level.
- **Caprylic acid:** natural fatty acid antifungal; readily absorbed by intestines; use timed-release or enteric-coated formula for release throughout GI tract; dose for delayed release—1000 to 2000 mg with meals.
- **Berberine-containing plants** (Hydrastis canadensis, Berberis vulgaris, Berberis aquifolium, Coptis chinensis): berberine alkaloids are broad-spectrum antibiotics against bacteria, protozoa, and fungi, including *Candida;* dose based on berberine content—solid extract (4:1 or 8% to 12% alkaloids), 250 to 500 mg t.i.d.
- ***Allium sativum* (garlic):** significant antifungal activity and inhibition of *Candida;* dose based on allicin content—at least 10 mg allicin or a total allicin potential of 4000 mcg or one clove (4 g) fresh garlic.
- **Enteric-coated essential oils (oregano, thyme, peppermint, rosemary):** antifungal agents; oregano oil is 100 times more potent than caprylic acid; enteric coating ensures delivery to small and large intestines; dose—0.2-0.4 mL b.i.d. between meals.
- **Propolis:** rich in flavonoids, phenolics, terpenes, and other compounds found to be antifungal; mechanism of action unknown; dose depends on product.
- Melaleuca alternifolia (tea tree oil): topical application.

THERAPEUTIC APPROACH

- **Step 1:** identify and address predisposing factors—antibiotics, steroids, immune-suppressing drugs, birth control pills (unless absolutely medically necessary); CSDA; dietary factors, impaired immunity, impaired liver function, or an underlying disease state.

- **Step 2:** *Candida* control diet—eliminate simple sugars, milk and dairy, yeast- or mold-laden foods, food allergens.
- **Step 3:** nutritional support—high-potency multiple vitamin, antioxidants, 1 tbsp flaxseed oil daily.
- **Step 4:** support immunity—promote positive attitude and stress coping; avoid alcohol, sugar, smoking, cholesterol; get rest and sleep.
- **Step 5:** detoxification and elimination—3 to 5 g water-soluble fiber (guar, psyllium, pectin) at night; lipotropic factors, silymarin.
- **Step 6:** probiotics—1 to 10 billion viable *L. acidophilus* and *B. bifidum* cells daily.
- **Step 7:** antiyeast therapy—nutritional and/or herbal supplements; antiyeast drug if needed.
- Repeat stool cultures and antigen levels to monitor progress; take stronger prescription antiyeast agents if needed.

Chronic Fatigue Syndrome

DIAGNOSTIC SUMMARY

- Mild fever
- Recurrent sore throat
- Painful lymph nodes
- Muscle weakness
- Muscle pain
- Prolonged fatigue after exercise
- Recurrent headache
- Migratory joint pain
- Depression
- Sleep disturbance (hypersomnia or insomnia)

Chronic fatigue syndrome (CFS) is not a new disease; medical literature references to a similar condition appeared in the 1860s. Old names for CFS included chronic mononucleosis-like syndrome, chronic Epstein-Barr virus (EBV) syndrome, yuppie flu, postviral fatigue syndrome, postinfectious neuromyasthenia, chronic fatigue and immune dysfunction syndrome, Iceland disease, and Royal Free Hospital disease. The Centers for Disease Control and Prevention (CDC) criteria are controversial and restrictive; British and Australian criteria are less strict. CDC criteria allow a U.S. prevalence estimate of 11.5%; British criteria suggest 15%, and Australian criteria 38%.

Etiology

- **Infectious agents:** Owing in part to the similarity of CFS to acute or chronic infection, it was initially thought to be caused by virus (i.e., EBV mononucleosis). However, CFS is not caused by any single infectious agent. There is no CDC-ascertained association between CFS and infection. No one pathogen seems to cause CFS. However, CFS may have multiple causes leading to a common end point; thus some infectious agents may play contributing roles.

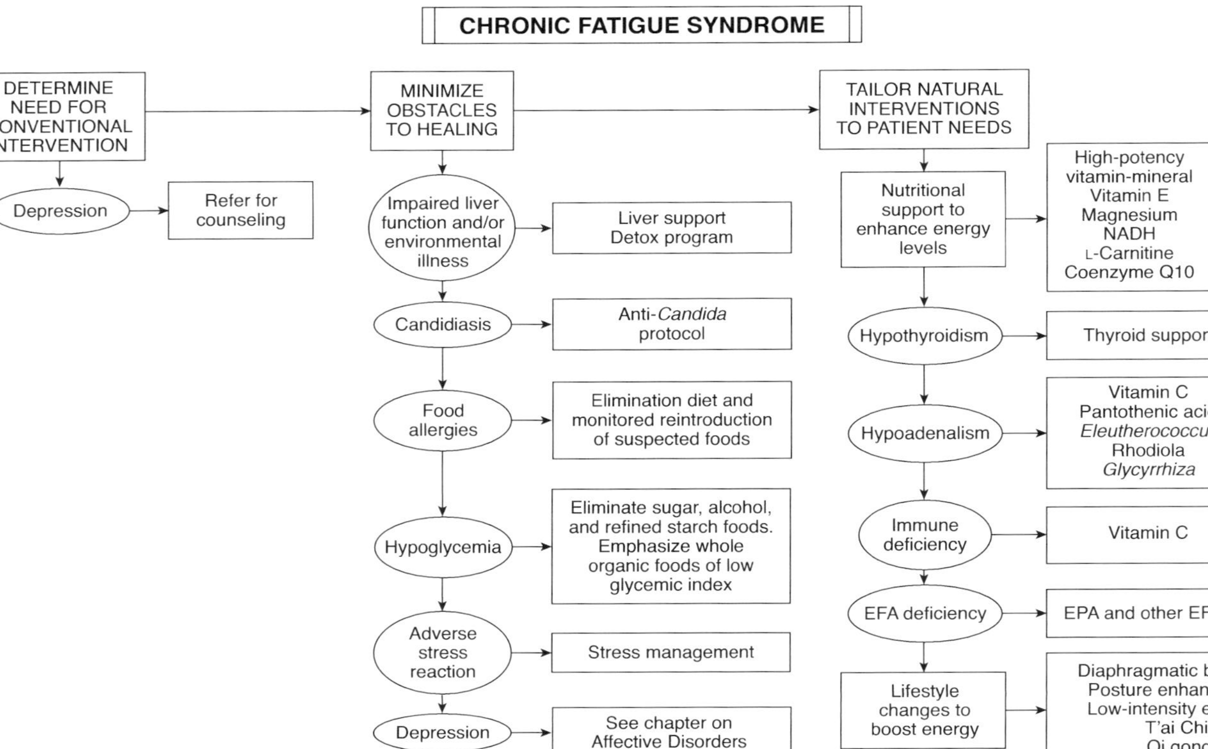
CHRONIC FATIGUE SYNDROME
DETERMINE NEED FOR CONVENTIONAL INTERVENTION
Depression
Refer for counseling
MINIMIZE OBSTACLES TO HEALING
Impaired liver function and/or environmental illness
Liver support Detox program
Candidiasis
Anti-*Candida* protocol
Food allergies
Elimination diet and monitored reintroduction of suspected foods
Hypoglycemia
Eliminate sugar, alcohol, and refined starch foods. Emphasize whole organic foods of low glycemic index
Adverse stress reaction
Stress management
Depression
See chapter on Affective Disorders
TAILOR NATURAL INTERVENTIONS TO PATIENT NEEDS
Nutritional support to enhance energy levels
High-potency vitamin-mineral Vitamin E Magnesium NADH L-Carnitine Coenzyme Q10
Hypothyroidism
Thyroid support
Hypoadenalism
Vitamin C Pantothenic acid *Eleutherococcus* Rhodiola *Glycyrrhiza*
Immune deficiency
Vitamin C
EFA deficiency
EPA and other EFAs
Lifestyle changes to boost energy
Diaphragmatic breathing Posture enhancement Low-intensity exercise T'ai Chi Qi gong

Causes of Chronic Fatigue

- Preexisting physical condition
- Diabetes
- Heart disease
- Lung disease
- Rheumatoid arthritis
- Chronic inflammation
- Chronic pain
- Cancer
- Liver disease
- Multiple sclerosis
- Prescription drugs
- Antihypertensives
- Anti-inflammatory agents
- Birth control pills
- Antihistamines
- Corticosteroids
- Tranquilizers and sedatives
- Depression
- Stress and/or low adrenal function
- Impaired liver function, environmental illness, or both
- Impaired immune function
- Chronic *Candida* infection
- Other chronic infections
- Food allergies
- Hypothyroidism
- Hypoglycemia
- Anemia and nutritional deficiencies
- Sleep disturbances
- Unknown cause

- **Immune system abnormalities:** elevated antibodies to viral proteins; decreased natural killer (NK) cell activity; low or elevated antibody levels; increased or decreased levels of circulating immune complexes; increased cytokines (e.g., interleukin-2); increased or decreased interferon levels; altered helper/suppressor T-cell ratio. No specific immunodysfunction pattern has been recognized, but the most consistent abnormality is decreased number or activity of NK cells. NK cells destroy cancerous or virus-infected cells. (CFS was at one time called low NK cell syndrome.) Reduced lymphocyte response to stimuli is perhaps caused by reduced activity or production of interferon, found in most cases. Low interferon permits reactivation of latent viruses. High interferon and interleukin-1 may cause CFS symptoms from physiologic effects, as seen during interferon therapy for cancer and viral hepatitis.
- **Fibromyalgia (FM) and multiple chemical sensitivities (MCSs):** the only difference in diagnostic criteria for FM and CFS is musculoskeletal pain in FM and fatigue in CFS. Diagnosis of FM or CFS depends on type of physician consulted. Approximately 70% of patients with FM and 30% with multiple chemical sensitivities (MCSs) meet CDC criteria for CFS; 80% of both FM and MCS patients meet the CFS criterion of fatigue for more than 6 months with 50% reduction in activity. More than 50% of CFS and FM patients have adverse reactions to various chemicals.

Diagnostic Criteria for Fibromyalgia

Major Criteria
- Generalized aches or stiffness of at least three anatomic sites for at least 3 months
- Six or more typical reproducible tender points
- Exclusion of other disorders that can cause similar symptoms

Minor Criteria
- Generalized fatigue
- Chronic headache
- Sleep disturbance
- Neurologic and psychological complaints
- Joint swelling
- Numbness or tingling sensations
- Irritable bowel syndrome
- Variation of symptoms in relation to activity, stress, and weather changes

- **Other causes of CFS:** preexisting physical condition (diabetes, heart disease, lung disease, rheumatoid arthritis, chronic inflammation, chronic pain, cancer, liver disease, multiple sclerosis); prescription drugs (antihypertensives, anti-inflammatory agents, birth control pills, antihistamines, corticosteroids, tranquilizers, and sedatives); depression; stress or low adrenal function; impaired liver function and/or environmental illness; impaired immune function; chronic candidiasis; other chronic infections; food allergies; hypothyroidism; hypoglycemia; anemia and nutritional deficiencies; and sleep disturbances.

Diagnosis

- **Identify as many factors as possible** contributing to fatigue.
- **Complete physical examination:** swollen lymph nodes (chronic infection), diagonal crease in both earlobes (impaired blood flow).
- **Laboratory:** avoid expensive tests unless absolutely necessary. Plasma neuropeptide Y (PNY) might be a potential biomarker for symptom severity in CFS. Clinical research has demonstrated a significant correlation of PNY with stress, negative mood, general health, depression, and impaired cognitive function. Obtain complete blood count and chemistry panel (including serum ferritin for menstruating women). Avoid tests to confirm diagnosis that will not affect treatment. Assess thyroid function, liver detoxification function, bowel dysbiosis, and gastrointestinal permeability (*Textbook*, "Chronic Fatigue Syndrome," "Comprehensive Stool Analysis 2.0," and "Intestinal Permeability Assessment").

Centers for Disease Control and Prevention Diagnostic Criteria for Chronic Fatigue Syndrome

Major Criteria

- New onset of fatigue causing 50% reduction in activity for at least 6 months
- Exclusion of other illnesses that can cause fatigue

Minor Criteria

- Presence of 8 of the 11 symptoms listed, or 6 of the 11 symptoms and 2 of the 3 signs

Symptoms

1. Mild fever
2. Recurrent sore throat
3. Painful lymph nodes
4. Muscle weakness
5. Muscle pain
6. Prolonged fatigue after exercise
7. Recurrent headache
8. Migratory joint pain
9. Neurologic or psychological complaints
   a. Sensitivity to bright light
   b. Forgetfulness
   c. Confusion
   d. Inability to concentrate
   e. Excessive irritability
   f. Depression
10. Sleep disturbance (hypersomnia or insomnia)
11. Sudden onset of symptom complex

Signs

1. Low-grade fever
2. Nonexudative pharyngitis
3. Palpable or tender lymph nodes

THERAPEUTIC CONSIDERATIONS

- **Multifactorial conditions** require tailored multiple therapies.
- **Energy level and emotional state:** determined by internal focus and physiology. The mental focus of CFS is on fatigue. Physiology is affected by chemicals, hormones, posture, and breathing (shallow). Address mind and body.
- **Depression:** a major cause of chronic fatigue and common in CFS. Depression is the most common cause of chronic fatigue in the absence of preexisting pathosis.
- **Stress:** underlying factor in a patient with depression, low immune function, or other cause of chronic fatigue (*Textbook,*

"Stress Management"). Evaluate stress effects with the Social Readjustment Rating Scale by Holmes and Rahe.

- **Impaired liver function and/or environmental illness:** exposure to toxins (food additives, solvents [e.g., cleaning materials, formaldehyde, toluene, benzene], pesticides, herbicides, heavy metals [e.g., lead, mercury, cadmium, arsenic, nickel, aluminum]) causes "congested" or "sluggish" liver and impaired hepatic detoxification, leading to diminished bile flow (cholestasis) and decreased phase I and/or phase II enzyme detoxification activity. Causes of cholestasis: dietary factors (saturated fat, refined sugar, low fiber intake), obesity, diabetes, gallstones, alcohol, endotoxins, hereditary disorders (Gilbert syndrome), pregnancy, steroid hormones (anabolic steroids, estrogens, oral contraceptives), chemicals (cleaning solvents, pesticides), or drugs (antibiotics, diuretics, nonsteroidal anti-inflammatory drugs, thyroid hormone), viral hepatitis. People with a sluggish liver may also complain of: depression, malaise, headaches, digestive disturbances, allergies and chemical sensitivities, premenstrual syndrome, constipation. People exposed to toxic chemicals often complain of the same symptoms.
- **Clinical judgment and laboratory tests:** serum bilirubin, aspartate aminotransferase, alanine aminotransferase, lactate dehydrogenase, glycoprotein 4-beta-galactosyl transferase, bile acid assay, clearance tests (*Textbook,* "Chronic Fatigue Syndrome"). Test results may be abnormal only after significant liver damage; many conditions in subclinical stages have normal laboratory values. Common patient symptoms: depression, general malaise, headaches, digestive disturbances, allergies and chemical sensitivities, premenstrual syndrome, constipation. Hair mineral analysis can screen for heavy metals; if inconclusive, use 8-hour lead mobilization test with chelating agent edetate calcium disodium, which measures lead excreted in urine for 8 hours after injection of ethylenediaminetetraacetic acid (EDTA).
- **Excessive gastrointestinal permeability:** common finding in CFS, measured by lactulose/mannitol absorption test (*Textbook,* "Intestinal Permeability Assessment"). Use food allergy control and nutrients to stimulate gastrointestinal regeneration. Support hepatic phase I and II detoxification and use oligoantigenic rice protein food replacement formula.
- **Impaired immune function, chronic infection, or both:** fatigue is the body's response to infection; the immune system works best when the body rests. Use immune function questionnaire

on page 176, and laboratory tests in *Textbook,* "Immune Function Assessment."

- **Chronic *Candida* infection:** impaired immunity allows *Candida* overgrowth in the intestines. Diagnosis is difficult; no single specific test exists. Stool cultures and elevated *Candida* antibody levels plus detailed history and patient questionnaire (*Textbook,* "Chronic Candidiasis").

Factors Predisposing to Candidal Overgrowth

- Impaired immune function
- Antiulcer drugs
- Broad-spectrum antibiotics
- Cellular immunodeficiency
- Corticosteroids
- Diabetes mellitus
- Excessive sugar in the diet
- Intravascular catheters
- Intravenous drug use
- Lack of digestive secretions
- Oral contraceptive agents

- **Patient profile:** female, 15 to 50 years old, chronic fatigue, lack of energy, malaise, decreased libido, thrush, bloating, gas, intestinal cramps, rectal itching, altered bowel function, vaginal yeast infection, frequent bladder infections, menstrual symptoms, depression, irritability, inability to concentrate, allergies, chemical sensitivities, low immunity, craving for foods rich in carbohydrates or yeast.
- **History:** chronic vaginal yeast infections, long-term antibiotic use for infections or acne, oral birth control use, oral steroid hormone use.
- **Associated conditions:** premenstrual syndrome; sensitivity to foods, chemicals, and other allergens; endocrine disturbances; psoriasis; irritable bowel syndrome.
- **Predisposing factors:** impaired immunity, antiulcer drugs, broad-spectrum antibiotics, cellular immunodeficiency, corticosteroids, diabetes mellitus, excess sugar intake, intravascular catheters, intravenous drug use, lack of digestive secretions, oral contraceptives.
- **Food allergies:** chronic fatigue is a key feature of food allergies, formerly known as allergic toxemia or allergic tension-fatigue syndrome. Symptoms include fatigue, muscle and joint aches, drowsiness, difficulty concentrating, nervousness, depression.

From 55% to 85% of people with CFS have allergies (*Textbook*, "Food Allergy Testing").

- **Hypothyroidism:** common cause of chronic fatigue that is often overlooked. Failure to treat reduces efficacy of other interventions (*Textbook*, "Hypothyroidism").
- **Hypoglycemia** must be ruled out because it contributes to depression. Depressed people have hypoglycemia, and depression is the most common cause of chronic fatigue.
- **Hypoadrenalism:** disruption of the hypothalamic-pituitary-adrenal (HPA) axis may be involved in CFS. Chronic fatigue patients have lower cortisol levels on wakening, reduced evening cortisol, and low 24-hour urinary-free cortisol, elevated basal adrenocorticotropic hormone (ACTH), and increased adrenal cortical sensitivity to ACTH but reduced maximal response and attenuated net integrated ACTH response to corticotropin-releasing hormone (CRH). This suggests a mild, central adrenal insufficiency resulting from either a deficiency of CRH or other central stimulus to the pituitary-adrenal axis. Hyperresponsiveness to ACTH may reflect a secondary adrenal insufficiency in which adrenal ACTH receptors are hypersensitive because of inadequate exposure to ACTH. Reduced response to large doses of ACTH suggests adrenal atrophy. Mild hypocortisolism reflects a defect at or above the hypothalamus, decreasing CRH and/or other secretagogues. HPA axis dysfunction may exacerbate symptoms. Glucocorticoid deficiency causes debilitating fatigue. A stressful event can induce fever, arthralgia, myalgia, adenopathy, postexertional fatigue, exacerbation of allergies, and disturbances of mood and sleep—symptoms typical of CFS and seen in partial or subclinical adrenal insufficiency. Endocrine testing, such as ACTH stimulation, is needed for accurate diagnosis. Glucocorticoids suppress immune function. Adrenal insufficiency may allow allergic responses, enhanced antibody titers to viral antigens, and increased cytokines. CFS may not be a discrete disease with a singular cause; it may be a clinical presentation with a variety of infectious and noninfectious antecedents and contributing factors. Pathophysiologic antecedents (acute infection, stress, preexisting or concurrent psychiatric illness) may converge in a final common clinical presentation. Reduced adrenal cortical secretion is a major feature.
- **Mind and attitude** affect immunity and energy. Many CFS patients are depressed or have no enthusiasm for life. They often lack social support. Cognitive therapy may help. Inform CFS

patients that they can get better. Positive mental attitude is critical to healing. Exercise or condition the attitude as conditioning the body. Prescribe mental exercises: visualizations, goal setting, affirmations, empowering questions.

Diet

Energy is related to quality of foods routinely ingested. Eliminate or restrict caffeine and refined sugar. Acute caffeine intake stimulates; regular caffeine intake induces chronic fatigue. Excessive caffeine intake is quite common in psychiatric disorders. The degree of fatigue correlates to the quantity of caffeine ingested. Abrupt cessation of coffee may trigger caffeine withdrawal—fatigue, headache, intense desire for coffee—that may last a few days.

Nutritional Supplements

- **High-potency vitamin/mineral combination:** deficiency of any nutrient can produce fatigue and susceptibility to infection.
- **Extra vitamin C:** 3000 mg/day in divided doses.
- **Magnesium (Mg):** subclinical Mg deficiency can result in chronic fatigue. Low red blood cell (RBC) Mg (a more-accurate measure of Mg status than routine blood analysis) is found in CFS. Cell Mg deficiency may not be caused by low intake, yet Mg supplements can alleviate fatigue. Oral Mg and potassium aspartate (1 g each) provide notable relief after 4 to 5 days; sometimes 10 days are required. Continue treatment for 4 to 6 weeks. Fatigue may not return. Mg is easily absorbed orally as aspartate or citrate, Krebs cycle intermediates that support cell adenosine triphosphate (ATP) production. Dose: 500 to 1200 mg/day in divided doses.
- **Essential fatty acids:** supplementation (combined linoleic acid, gamma-linolenic acid [GLA], eicosapentaenoic acid [EPA], docosahexaenoic acid [DHA]) given as 8 500-mg capsules q.d. for 3 months may improve clinical picture and RBC membrane phospholipid profile of patients with postviral fatigue. Brain lateral ventricular enlargement can occur in CFS. Cerebral magnetic resonance imaging at baseline and 16 weeks indicates that EPA markedly reduces lateral ventricular volume during treatment. CFS is associated with pathophysiologic brain changes (e.g., enlargement in cerebral ventricular volume).
- **Nicotinamide adenine dinucleotide** (NADH), the active coenzyme form of vitamin B_3, counters jet lag effects on cognition and

wakefulness and encourages ATP generation. NADH may improve quality of life in CFS. Dose: stabilized oral absorbable form at 10 mg daily for 1 month. In one small study, 31% responded favorably in contrast to 8% on placebo. No severe adverse effects are noted in human beings; no toxicity is noted in animals at megadoses.

- **L-Carnitine:** essential for transport of long-chain fatty acids across mitochondrial membrane. Two months of treatment gave statistically significant clinical improvement in 12 of 18 studied parameters after 8 weeks with no clinical deterioration. The greatest improvement occurs between 4 and 8 weeks. It is extremely safe, with no significant side effects. Use the L form; avoid the D form.
- **Coenzyme Q10 (CoQ10):** mitochondrial nutrient that acts as essential cofactor for production of ATP in mitochondria. Plasma CoQ10 is lower in CFS patients than in controls. Symptoms of fatigue and neurocognitive impairment may be related to CoQ10 depletion.

Other Therapies

- **Breathing, posture, and bodywork:** diaphragm breathing, good posture, bodywork (e.g., massage, spinal manipulation).
- **Exercise:** moderate level improves mood, ability to handle stress. Increases (up to 100%) NK activity and stimulates immune system. Intense exercise can have opposite effect. Tai chi exercises may enhance immunity. Graded exercise begins with mild walking and weight exercises, increasing time and intensity as is comfortable. This method is superior to relaxation and flexibility exercises.

Botanical Medicines

- ***Eleutherococcus senticosus*** **(Siberian ginseng):** supports adrenals, is a nonspecific adaptogen, increases T-helper cells and NK activity—valuable in treating CFS.
- ***Rhodiola rosea*** **(Artic root):** popular plant in traditional medical systems in Eastern Europe and Asia to help combat fatigue and restore energy. *Rhodiola* has an antifatigue effect that increases mental performance—the ability to concentrate—and decreases cortisol response to awakening stress.
- ***Glycyrrhiza glabra*** (licorice): antiviral and glucocorticoid-potentiating properties (*Textbook, "Glycyrrhiza glabra* [Licorice]") but is not well studied in CFS. Use whole root because glucocorticoid-potentiating glycyrrhizic and glycyrrhetinic acids are removed from deglycyrrhizinated licorice (DGL).

THERAPEUTIC APPROACH

- **Comprehensive diagnostic and therapeutic approach:** identify underlying factors affecting energy or immunity. Strong correlation among CFS, FM, and MCS suggests hepatic detoxification, food allergy control, and gut restoration diet. Support the immune system (*Textbook,* "Food Reactions").
- **Diet:** identify and control food allergies. Increase water, eliminate caffeine and alcohol. Eat whole organic foods. Control hypoglycemia; eliminate sugar and refined starch foods and take regular healthful small meals and snacks. Use medical food replacement for several weeks to speed detoxification.
- **Lifestyle:** diaphragmatic breathing, proper posture, regular low-intensity exercise.
- **Supplements:**
  - — High-potency vitamin/mineral combination (*Textbook,* "Nutritional Medicine")
  - — Vitamin C: 500 to 1000 mg t.i.d.
  - — Vitamin E: 100 to 200 international units (IU)/day (mixed tocopherols)
  - — Mg bound to citrate or Krebs intermediates: 200 to 300 mg t.i.d.
  - — Pantothenic acid: 250 mg q.d.
  - — NADH: 10 mg q.d. on an empty stomach
  - — L-Carnitine: 1500 to 2000 mg q.d. in divided doses (acetyl-L-carnitine may be more effective)
  - — Fish oil: 1,000 to 3,000 mg EPA + DHA q.d. for at least 3 to 4 months
  - — CoQ10: 200 to 300 mg q.d.
- Botanicals:
  - — *E. senticosus:* dried root, 2 to 4 g; tincture (1:5), 10 to 20 mL; fluid extract (1:1), 2.0-4.0 mL; solid (dry powdered) extract (20:1 or standardized to .1% eleutheroside E), 100 to 200 mg.
  - — *R. rosea:* therapeutic dose varies according to rosavin content. Typical dose is 200 to 300 mg q.d. of extract standardized to contain 3% rosavins and 0.8% to 1% salidroside.
  - — *G. glabra:* powdered root, 1 to 2 g; fluid extract (1:1), 2 to 4 mL; solid (dry powdered) extract (4:1), 250 to 500 mg.
- **Counseling:** direct counseling or referral to professional counselor to reinforce pattern of mental, emotional, and spiritual affirmations.

Questionnaire for recognition of impaired immune function:

- Do you get more than two colds per year?
- When you catch a cold, does it take more than 5 to 7 days to get rid of the symptoms?
- Have you ever had infectious mononucleosis?
- Do you have herpes?
- Do you have chronic infections of any kind?

Congestive Heart Failure

DIAGNOSTIC SUMMARY

- **Left ventricular failure:** exertional dyspnea, cough, fatigue, orthopnea, cardiac enlargement, rales, gallop rhythm, and pulmonary venous congestion.
- **Right ventricular failure:** elevated venous pressure, hepatomegaly, dependent edema.
- **Left and right ventricular failure:** combinations of the aforementioned.
- Diagnosis confirmed by echocardiography.

GENERAL CONSIDERATIONS

Congestive heart failure (CHF) is the inability of the heart to pump enough blood effectively. Contractile function of the heart is governed by five factors: (1) contractile state of myocardium, (2) preload of ventricle, (3) end-diastolic volume, (4) impedance to left ventricular ejection, and (5) heart rate (HR).

- **Causes of CHF:** long-term hypertension, previous myocardial infarction (MI), disorder of heart valve, cardiomyopathy, and chronic lung disease.

Precipitating or Exacerbating Factors in Congestive Heart Failure

- Low levels of essential fatty acids
- Increased platelet aggregation
- Increased demand
- Anemia
- Fever
- Infection
- Fluid overload
- Increased sodium intake
- High environmental temperature
- Renal failure
- Hepatic failure
- Thyrotoxicosis
- Arteriovenous shunt
- Respiratory insufficiency
- Arrhythmias
- Pulmonary embolism
- Ethanol ingestion
- Emotional stress
- Pregnancy
- Obesity
- Nutrient deficiency
- Uncontrolled hypertension
- Drugs
- Beta adrenergic blockers
- Antiarrhythmic drugs
- Sodium-retaining drugs
- Corticosteroids
- Nonsteroidal anti-inflammatory drugs

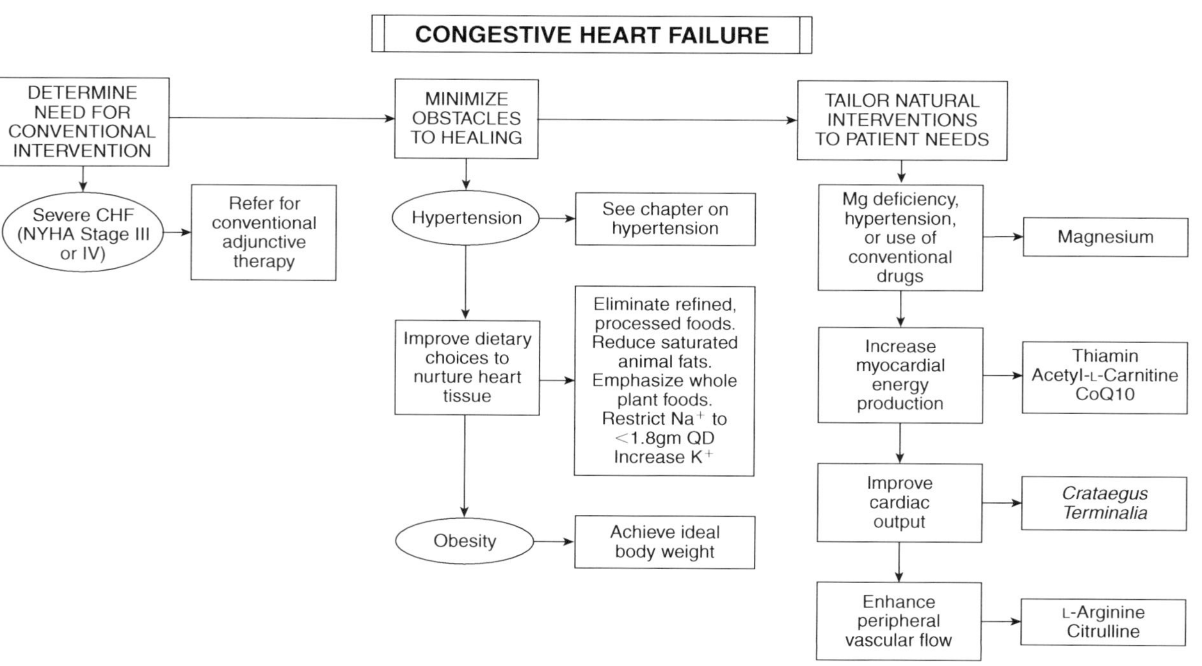
CONGESTIVE HEART FAILURE
DETERMINE NEED FOR CONVENTIONAL INTERVENTION
Severe CHF (NYHA Stage III or IV)
Refer for conventional adjunctive therapy
MINIMIZE OBSTACLES TO HEALING
Hypertension
See chapter on hypertension
Improve dietary choices to nurture heart tissue
Eliminate refined, processed foods. Reduce saturated animal fats. Emphasize whole plant foods. Restrict Na+ to <1.8gm QD Increase K+
Obesity
Achieve ideal body weight
TAILOR NATURAL INTERVENTIONS TO PATIENT NEEDS
Mg deficiency, hypertension, or use of conventional drugs
Magnesium
Increase myocardial energy production
Thiamin Acetyl-L-Carnitine CoQ10
Improve cardiac output
Crataegus Terminalia
Enhance peripheral vascular flow
L-Arginine Citrulline

- **Consequences of reduced cardiac output (CO):** reduced renal blood flow and glomerular filtration, causing sodium (Na) and fluid retention. Activation of renin-angiotensin-aldosterone (RAA) system increases peripheral vascular resistance, ventricular afterload, and levels of circulating vasopressin, a vasoconstrictor and antidiuretic.
- **Compensatory mechanisms for reduced CO:** tachycardia, increased sympathetic nervous system activation, ventricular dilation, and hypertrophy. These are a mixed blessing; increased sympathetic activity increases CO by increasing HR and force of contraction but it also increases vascular resistance.
- **Signs and symptoms of CHF:** depend on which ventricle has failed; left, pulmonary congestion and edema; right, systemic venous congestion and peripheral edema. Weakness, fatigue, and shortness of breath (SOB) are common to both, as is biventricular failure.

DIAGNOSTIC CONSIDERATIONS

CHF is most effectively treated by natural measures in early stages. Early diagnosis and prevention by addressing causative factors are imperative. First symptoms are SOB and chronic nonproductive cough. Conduct extensive cardiovascular evaluation—complete physical examination looking for characteristic signs (e.g., peripheral signs of heart failure, enlarged and sustained left ventricular impulse, diminished first heart sound, gallop rhythm), electrocardiogram, and echocardiogram.

THERAPEUTIC CONSIDERATIONS

During initial stages of CHF, natural measures for underlying causes (e.g., hypertension) or improving myocardial metabolic function (*Textbook,* "Angina") are often quite effective. At later stages, conventional treatments—diuretics, angiotensin-converting enzyme (ACE) inhibitors, and/or digitalis glycosides—are indicated in most cases. Measures described here are used as adjuncts in more severe cases. Expect excellent clinical results in New York Heart Association (NYHA) classes I and II with natural measures described later.

Stages of Congestive Heart Failure as Defined by the New York Heart Association

Stage	Symptoms
Stage I	Patient is symptom-free at rest and with treatment.
Stage II	Patient experiences impaired heart function with moderate physical effort. Shortness of breath with exertion is common. There are no symptoms at rest.
Stage III	Even minor physical exertion results in shortness of breath and fatigue. There are no symptoms at rest.
Stage IV	Symptoms such as shortness of breath and signs such as lower extremity edema are present when the patient is at rest

Nutritional Supplements

Improve myocardial energy production because CHF is always characterized by energy depletion, often from nutrient or coenzyme deficiency (e.g., magnesium [Mg], vitamin B_1, coenzyme Q10 [CoQ10], carnitine). Dietary recommendations for hypertension are appropriate for most CHF patients, especially if CHF is caused by hypertension. Recommend diet low in Na^+ and high in potassium (K^+); restrict Na^+ intake to less than 1.8 g q.d. Intake of several nutrients is deficient in CHF patients: Mg, calcium (Ca), zinc (Zn), copper (Cu), manganese (Mn), vitamins B_1 and B_2, folic acid. A high-potency multiple vitamin-mineral formula is critical, especially in diuretic therapy.

- **Mg:** critical nutrient for producing adenosine triphosphate (ATP). Low white blood cell Mg is common in CHF patients. Mg levels correlate directly with survival rates. Mg deficiency is linked to cardiac arrhythmias, reduced cardiovascular prognosis, worsened ischemia, and increased mortality rate in acute MI. Deficiency is probably caused by inadequate intake; increased wasting by overactivation of RAA system, common in patients with heart failure; and diuretics such as furosemide. Mg supplementation prevents Mg depletion caused by conventional drug therapy for CHF: digitalis, diuretics, and vasodilators (e.g., beta-blockers, Ca channel blockers). Mg supplements produce positive effects in CHF patients taking conventional drugs, even if serum Mg is normal. Mg supplementation is not indicated in renal failure because of predisposition to hypermagnesemia—a risk factor for death. ACE inhibitors have Mg-sparing effect in patients on furosemide. Dose: 200 to 300 mg q.d. to t.i.d. (citrate). Monitor serum Mg to prevent hypermagnesemia in patients with renal impairment and those on digoxin. Mg reduces frequency and complexity of ventricular arrhythmias in digoxin-treated patients with CHF even without digoxin toxicity, but too much Mg may interfere with digoxin.

- **Thiamine:** vitamin B_1 deficiency has cardiovascular effects: "wet beri beri," Na^+ retention, peripheral vasodilation, and heart failure. Furosemide (Lasix) causes B_1 deficiency in animals and patients with CHF. Severe B_1 deficiency is uncommon (except in alcoholics), but many do not get recommended daily allowance (RDA) (1.5 mg), especially elderly in hospitals or nursing homes. Significant percentage of geriatric population is deficient in B vitamins critical to cardiovascular and brain function. Daily doses of 80 to 240 mg of B_1 improve clinical picture; 13% to 22% increase of left ventricular ejection fraction (LVEF). Increased ejection fraction is linked to greater survival rate in CHF. The benefit, lack of risk, and low cost of 200 to 250 mg B_1 q.d. warrant its use in CHF, especially if the patient is taking furosemide.
- **L-Carnitine:** essential for transport of fatty acids into myocardial mitochondria for ATP production. The normal heart stores more carnitine and CoQ10 than it needs, but heart ischemia quickly decreases both. Carnitine supplements improve cardiac function in CHF patients. The longer carnitine is used, the more dramatic the improvement. A dosage of 500 mg t.i.d. for 6 months increases maximal exercise time by 16% to 25% and ventricular ejection fraction by 12% to 13%.
- **CoQ10:** Most studies used CoQ10 as adjunct to conventional drugs. The largest study included 2664 patients in NYHA classes II and III in open study in Italy. The daily dose was 50 to 150 mg orally for 90 days (majority of patients, 78%, took 100 mg q.d.). Proportions of patients with improved clinical signs and symptoms: cyanosis, 78.1%; edema, 78.6%; pulmonary edema, 77.8%; hepatomegaly, 49.3%; venous congestion, 71.81%; SOB, 52.7%; heart palpitations, 75.4%; sweating, 79.8%; subjective arrhythmia, 63.4%; insomnia, 66.2%; vertigo, 73.1%; nocturia, 53.6%. Improvement of at least three symptoms occurred in 54% of patients, with significantly improved quality of life with CoQ10. Mild side effects were not common—only 1.5%. CoQ10 may not achieve therapeutic benefit in more severe stages of CHF or if blood levels of CoQ10 do not reach suggested threshold of 2.5 mcg/mL.

- **L-Arginine:** amino acid of value in CHF. CHF patients are less able to achieve peripheral vasodilation during exercise. Endothelial cells make natural vasodilator nitric oxide from L-arginine. Dose of 5.6 to 12.6 g q.d. oral L-arginine increases peripheral blood flow by 29%. The 6-minute walk distance increases by 8% and arterial compliance increases by 19%. L-Arginine improves endothelial cell function and renal function (improved glomerular filtration rate, natriuresis, and plasma endothelin level) in patients with CHF.

Botanical Medicines

- ***Crataegus oxyacantha* (hawthorn):** quite useful in early stages as sole agent and later stages in combination with digitalis cardioglycosides. *Crataegus* extract standardized to 15 mg procyanidin oligomers per 80-mg capsule b.i.d. for 8 weeks was better than placebo in improving heart function. It mildly reduces systolic and diastolic blood pressure (BP) with no adverse reactions at recommended dosage. *Crataegus* given to patients with CHF (NYHA class II) at 600 mg standardized *Crataegus* extract q.d. for 56 days was better than placebo at increasing patient working capacity on bicycle ergometer (25 versus 5 W). The *Crataegus* group also had a drop in systolic BP from 171 to 164 mm Hg and HR from 115 to 110 beats per minute, with no change in BP or HR in the placebo group. In patients with NYHA class III CHF, *Crataegus* may not be sufficient to produce clinical effects. In such patients, hawthorn offers no significant improvement in 6-minute walk distance or in measures of quality of life, functional capacity, neurohormones, oxidative stress, or inflammation. However, it does effect a modest improvement in LVEF.
- ***Terminalia arjuna:*** traditional Ayurvedic botanical for cardiac failure. CHF patients (class IV NYHA) received bark extract (500 mg every 8 hours) for 2 weeks or placebo. The extract group had statistically significant improvement in end-systolic volume and LVEF (by echocardiogram). The uncontrolled phase of the study using combination of *T. arjuna* and conventional drugs for 2 years found nine patients showing remarkable improvement to NYHA class II and other three improving to class III.

THERAPEUTIC APPROACH

Diet and natural agents are effective in early stages (NYHA classes I and II); in later stages, adjunct drug therapy is necessary. Treatment is designed to address underlying pathophysiology and improve myocardial function through improved energy production.

- **Diet:** Achieve ideal body weight. Restrict Na^+ intake (<1.8 g q.d.). Increase whole organic plant foods. Reduce saturated fat. Follow other guidelines for lowering BP (see the chapter on hypertension).
- **Nutritional supplements:**
  — Mg: 200 to 400 mg t.i.d. (citrate)
  — Thiamin: 200 to 250 mg q.d.
  — L-Carnitine: 500 to 1000 mg t.i.d.
  — CoQ10: 100 to 300 mg q.d.
  — L-Arginine: 1000 to 2000 mg t.i.d.
- **Botanical medicines:**
  — *C. oxyacantha* (hawthorn extract) (1.8% vitexin-4′-rhamnoside or 10% procyanidin content): 200 to 300 mg t.i.d.
  — *T. arjuna* extract: 500 mg t.i.d.

Cystitis

DIAGNOSTIC SUMMARY

- Burning pain on urination
- Increased urinary frequency, nocturia
- Turbid, foul-smelling, or dark urine
- Lower abdominal pain
- Urinalysis showing significant pyuria and bacteriuria
- Pain in pelvis (suprapubic) or between vagina and anus in women or between scrotum and anus in men (perineal)
- Chronic pelvic pain (CPP)
- Persistent urgent need to urinate
- Pain during sexual intercourse

GENERAL CONSIDERATIONS

Bladder infections in women are common: 10% to 20% of all women have urinary tract discomfort at least once a year; 37.5% of women with no history of urinary tract infection (UTI) will have one within 10 years; 2% to 4% of healthy women have elevated bacteria in urine, indicating unrecognized UTI. A woman with history of recurrent UTI has an episode once a year. Recurrent bladder infections are significant problems; 55% eventually involve kidneys. Recurrent kidney infection causes progressive damage: scarring and, for some, kidney failure. UTIs are much less common in males, except infants, and indicate anatomic abnormality, prostate infection, or unprotected rectal intercourse.

Interstitial cystitis/painful bladder syndrome (IC/PBS) is a chronic bladder disorder characterized by CPP and irritative voiding symptoms. IC/PBS is not caused by infection; it is characterized by symptoms similar to cystitis; patients may report undiagnosed CPP. Symptoms of IC/PBS can overlap with endometriosis, recurrent UTI, CPP, overactive bladder (OAB) and vulvodynia.

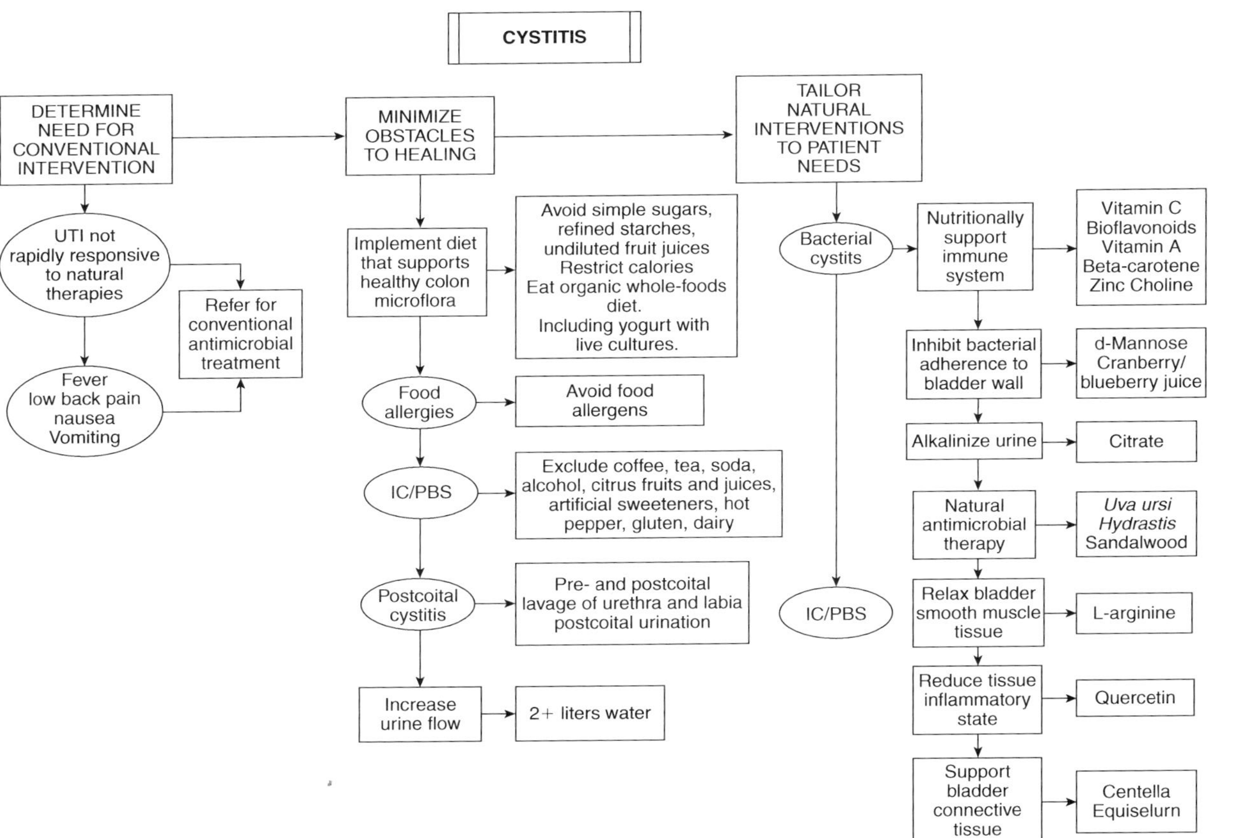
CYSTITIS
DETERMINE NEED FOR CONVENTIONAL INTERVENTION
UTI not rapidly responsive to natural therapies
Fever low back pain nausea Vomiting
Refer for conventional antimicrobial treatment
MINIMIZE OBSTACLES TO HEALING
Implement diet that supports healthy colon microflora
Avoid simple sugars, refined starches, undiluted fruit juices Restrict calories Eat organic whole-foods diet. Including yogurt with live cultures.
Food allergies
Avoid food allergens
IC/PBS
Exclude coffee, tea, soda, alcohol, citrus fruits and juices, artificial sweeteners, hot pepper, gluten, dairy
Postcoital cystitis
Pre- and postcoital lavage of urethra and labia postcoital urination
Increase urine flow
2+ liters water
TAILOR NATURAL INTERVENTIONS TO PATIENT NEEDS
Bacterial cystits
IC/PBS
Nutritionally support immune system
Vitamin C Bioflavonoids Vitamin A Beta-carotene Zinc Choline
Inhibit bacterial adherence to bladder wall
d-Mannose Cranberry/ blueberry juice
Alkalinize urine
Citrate
Natural antimicrobial therapy
Uva ursi Hydrastis Sandalwood
Relax bladder smooth muscle tissue
L-arginine
Reduce tissue inflammatory state
Quercetin
Support bladder connective tissue
Centella Equiselurn

DIAGNOSIS

Bladder infection diagnosis is imprecise; clinical symptoms and presence of significant amounts of bacteria in urine do not correlate well. Only 60% of women with UTI symptoms have abundant bacteria in urine; 20% have serious kidney involvement. Diagnosis is according to signs, symptoms, and urinary findings. Pelvic examination is indicated if history suggests vaginitis or cervicitis or if any diagnostic confusion exists. Microscopic examination of infected urine reveals high WBCs and bacteria. Urine culture determines quantity and type of bacteria. *Escherichia coli* (from the colon) are most common. Fever, chills, and low back pain suggest kidney involvement. Recurrent infections warrant intravenous urogram to rule out structural abnormality.

IC/PBS can also be difficult to diagnose because symptoms overlap with those of other disorders—endometriosis, UTI, chronic CPP, OAB, and vulvodynia. There is no definitive diagnostic test; IC/PBS remains a diagnosis of exclusion. Presence of additional symptoms caused by other pain generators can confuse diagnosis even further. Median time between development of IC/PBS symptoms and diagnosis is 5 years.

CPP is pain lasting 6 months or longer that is severe enough to affect daily functioning or requires medical care. The cause of CPP is often unknown and may be multifactorial. Gynecologic conditions that can cause CPP include endometriosis, adhesions, pelvic inflammatory disease (PID), cysts, and polyps. However, a retrospective cohort analysis of a large primary care database in the United Kingdom found that only 20.2% of all cases of CPP had a gynecologic cause. Gastrointestinal diagnoses represented 37.7% of cases, with irritable bowel syndrome (IBS) accounting for 29.1%. Cystitis accounted for 30.8% of diagnoses in this population of women with noncyclic pain lasting for 6 months or longer. Up to one half of the women in primary care practices who have CPP may have more than one diagnosis for their pain. It is common for a patient with CPP to have both endometriosis and IC/PBS.

Physical examination is a critical component of diagnosing IC/PBS. In IC/PBS patients, this can be emotionally distressing because of pain, so it is important that the physician proceed slowly and carefully. Because the bladder is a pain generator in IC/PBS, tenderness with single-digit examination of the trigonal area (bladder base or urethra) can help establish diagnosis of IC/PBS, as can pain in pelvic floor or levator ani. Patients with IC/PBS tend to have urethral or bladder tenderness, whereas those with vestibulodynia have vestibular tenderness. Tenderness on single-digit examination of vaginal fornices can help distinguish endometriosis from IC/PBS. Urinalysis rules out hematuria; urine culture identifies bladder infection. Cytology and computed tomography with double contrast when indicated (hematuria, history of smoking, 40 years of age and older) help rule out urinary tract malignancies. Patients with results suggesting a malignancy must be referred to a urologist. Optional diagnostic tests help diagnose IC/PBS. Glomerulations seen on cystoscopy with hydrodistention may aid diagnosis of IC/PBS. A negative cystoscopic evaluation never rules out IC/PBS; many patients with early IC/PBS will not have glomerulations. A potassium sensitivity test (PST) may indicate defective bladder lining. The PST involves intravesical instillation of a potassium solution, which triggers symptoms of pain and urgency in patients with abnormal permeability of the bladder lining. Intravesical instillation of anesthetic cocktail is a diagnostic tool as well as treatment. Known as anesthetic bladder challenge, this test helps localize pain to the bladder.

Collection of Urine Specimen for Culture

The optimal method is the voided midstream specimen. Clean the urethral meatus and vaginal vestibule before collecting. Spread the labia and cleanse the area with two gauze sponges moistened with cleansing solution and a dry gauze sponge. Wash by making single front-to-back motion with each of two moist sponges and then the dry sponge. While the labia are still held apart, a small amount of urine is allowed to pass into the toilet or bedpan. Then a midstream specimen is collected in a sterile container, and the container is immediately closed. Collection by catheterization is more invasive and carries a 1% to 2% chance of initiating UTI. Suprapubic aspiration is the most accurate method but also is the most invasive.

Examining Collected Urine

Routine methods include dipsticks, microscope, and culture. For the most accurate results, examine urine within 1 hour. If examination must be delayed, refrigerate at 5°C. Culturing requires that urine not be refrigerated for more than 8 hours.

- **Dipsticks:** reagent strips are dipped into urine and removed. Parts of the dipstick are impregnated with chemicals that react with specific substances in urine to produce various colors. Careful matching of dipstick color to color standard at appropriate time is essential. Dipsticks are invaluable for qualitative and rough quantitative analysis: pH, protein, glucose, ketones, bilirubin, hemoglobin, nitrite, and urobilinogen. Some dipsticks detect white blood cells (WBCs) and bacteria (including semiquantitative cultures). The leukocyte esterase test detects WBCs (80% to 90% sensitive). Many organisms reduce urine nitrate to nitrite (*Citrobacter* species, *E. coli, Klebsiella pneumoniae, Proteus* species, *Pseudomonas* species, *Serratia marcescens, Shigella, Staphylococcus* species [most]). Measuring nitrite (50% sensitive) is inexpensive and a rapid detector of bacteriuria; confirm by culture.

- **Microscopic examination:** Perform within first hour. Place a drop of fresh urine or a drop of resuspended sediment from centrifuged fresh urine on slide, cover with cover glass, and examine with high-dry objective under reduced illumination. More than 10 bacteria per field in unstained specimen suggests a bacterial count higher than 100,000/mL. Gram stain under oil immersion objective; WBCs indicate infection. Abundant protein and/or WBC casts indicate renal involvement, commonly pyelonephritis.
- **Urine culture:** Only quantitative cultures typically are used. Diluted urine is introduced to suitable medium and incubation. Colonies are counted and multiplied by dilution factor, giving bacterial count per milliliter. Bacteriuria is significant if this value exceeds 100,000/mL, but 1000 colonies/mL is clinically significant in the presence of UTI symptoms. Semiquantitative tests using dipsticks or glass slides coated with culture media commonly are used. Colonies are counted or appearance is compared 12 to 24 hours later. Recurrent or chronic infection warrants sensitivity studies. Roughly 95% of UTIs involve single bacterial species. Recurrence of UTI after the initial bacterial infection has resolved is common. Mixed species suggest contamination. *Staphylococcus epidermidis,* diphtheroids, and *Lactobacillus* are common in the distal urethra but rarely cause UTI. The most common organisms are *E. coli, Proteus mirabilis, K. pneumoniae, Enterococcus, Enterobacter aerogenes, Pseudomonas aeruginosa, Proteus* species, *S. marcescens, S. epidermidis,* and *Staphylococcus aureus.* Symptoms of recurrent UTI: urgency, frequency, nocturia, pelvic pain. Diagnosis is established by a positive urine culture.

Coexisting Conditions and Differential Diagnosis

- Although bacterial cystitis usually appears acutely and by itself, IC/PBS typically manifests with comorbidities—endometriosis, IBS, vulvodynia, and OAB. Detailed medical history and physical examination diagnose cause of CPP. Questionnaires (e.g., Pelvic Pain, Urgency, and Frequency [PUF] questionnaire; O'Leary-Sant [OLS] questionnaire) may elicit urinary symptoms. Tenderness of bladder base on pelvic examination is characteristic of IC/PBS and may help distinguish it from other causes of CPP. Optional tests—laparoscopy and diagnostic imaging—may help. PST or intravesical anesthetic challenge also helps.
- Endometriosis is characterized by presence of endometrial-like glands and stroma outside uterine cavity. Symptoms: pain in lower abdomen, dysmenorrhea, dyspareunia, dysuria, and frequency. Endometriosis and IC/PBS frequently coexist. In women with CPP and bladder tenderness on examination, more than 70% had both endometriosis and IC/PBS.
- OAB is characterized by urgency with or without urge incontinence and usually includes frequency and nocturia. Key symptom: urgency. OAB and IC/PBS can coexist. Urgency can be caused by detrusor overactivity, demonstrated through urodynamic testing. Urgency is a common symptom of both OAB and IC/PBS, but the cause differs. In OAB, urgency involves a strong desire to avoid leakage; but in IC/PBS, urgency entails strong need to void to relieve pain caused by bladder fullness.
- Vulvodynia is characterized by vulvar discomfort, often reported as burning pain. Pain can occur during intercourse, during vigorous activity, after intercourse, or even at rest. The cause of vulvodynia is unknown; diagnosis is one of exclusion. Symptoms of vulvodynia that overlap IC/PBS: pain and dyspareunia but not frequency or nocturia; this can help distinguish vulvodynia from IC/PBS. IC/PBS and vulvodynia can also coexist. The history and physical examination are important in diagnosing vulvodynia. A history of chronic pain at vestibule lasting more than 3 months can suggest vulvodynia. Infectious causes: viral, bacterial, or fungal organisms; rule out pathogens as causes of vulvar pain. Vulvar dermatoses may account for vulvar symptoms. Tenderness to pressure with a cotton swab at vestibule is a hallmark of vulvodynia; tenderness at bladder base is typical of IC/PBS.

THERAPEUTIC CONSIDERATIONS

Treatment

Primary goal is to enhance normal host defenses—to enhance urine flow by proper hydration, promote protective urine pH, prevent bacterial adherence to bladder endothelium, and enhance immune system. Use antimicrobial botanical medicines as needed.

Increase Urine Flow

Increase quantity of liquids consumed—purified water and herbal teas. Dilute fresh fruit and vegetable juices with twice the amount of water. Encourage intake of more than 2 L of liquid, with more than half being purified water. Avoid soft drinks, concentrated fruit drinks, coffee, and alcohol.

Chronic Interstitial Cystitis

- Chronic IC is an underdiagnosed persistent form of cystitis and a source of undiagnosed CPP not caused by infection. These patients have higher incidence of inflammatory bowel disease, lupus, IBS, and fibromyalgia. Focus on enhancing integrity of bladder interstitium and endothelium. "Leaky bladder urothelium" theory: lack of integrity in glycosaminoglycan layer of bladder epithelium, increasing permeability to potassium and causing inflammation and pain. Eliminate food allergens that can produce cystitis in some patients. *Centella asiatica* extracts improve integrity of connective tissue that composes interstitium and heal bladder ulcerations (*Textbook, "Centella asiatica* [Gotu Kola]").
- Educating patients with IC/PBS empowers them to control symptoms and to be active participants in therapy. Patients should avoid triggers that increase IC/PBS symptoms. Encourage reducing stress and using support groups to deal with IC/PBS. Although patients with IC/PBS are more likely to be food sensitive than patients with CP/CPPS (Chronic prostatitis/chronic pelvic pain syndrome), symptoms of patients with both IC/PBS and CP/CPPS are aggravated by similar comestibles (e.g., grapefruit juice, spicy foods, alcohol, and caffeinated coffee). Symptoms of both groups improve with certain comestibles (water and antacid containing calcium glycerophosphate). More than 90% of patients with IC experience increased symptoms when they consume coffee, tea, soda, alcohol, citrus fruits and juices, artificial sweeteners, and hot pepper.

- Food restrictions have not conclusively retarded progression of disease or improved its course. Usually food restriction should be weighed against decrease in quality of life. After 2 weeks, patients are asked to add one food item back into their diets every 3 days to identify any specific alimentary sensitivity.
- Medical treatments include antidepressants, anticholinergics to reduce urinary urgency, and antihistamines for decreasing mast cell activation and reducing inflammation.
- Mast cells can be critically important in IC. Histamine causes pain, swelling, and scarring and prevents bladder lining from healing.
- Pentosan polysulfate sodium (Elmiron) is a U.S. Food and Drug Administration (FDA)–approved oral heparinoid compound that is thought to replenish defective bladder lining. When taken orally, only 1% to 3% of active drug reaches the bladder. Treatment can be continued for 3 months and then extended as needed.
- Second-line therapies: immunosuppressive agents—prednisone. Cyclosporine relieves symptoms of severe IC/PBS. Symptoms generally recur after treatment is discontinued.
- Intravesical therapy can be used for flare management. Dimethyl sulfoxide (DMSO) is the only FDA-approved intravesical IC/PBS treatment. Intravesical instillation of anesthetic can bring immediate relief. Intravesical instillation of heparin and alkalinized lidocaine provides immediate and sustained relief of pain and urgency.
- Intravesical cocktails of combinations of heparin, lidocaine, sodium bicarbonate, gentamicin, and glucocorticoids are used to treat IC/PBS.
- Muscle relaxants for increased muscle spasticity of pelvic floor in CPP are beneficial. Cyclobenzaprine is related to tricyclic antidepressants. It is used at starting doses of 10 mg q.d., prescribed up to t.i.d. Tizanidine, a centrally acting $alpha_2$ agonist, treats spasticity in several conditions. Clonazepam treats neuropathic pain.

Alternative Treatments

Biofeedback allows the patient to learn to control musculature of the pelvic floor by visualizing activity of the muscle on a computer and using visual feedback to achieve conscious control over muscular contractions. Sessions of 30 to 60 minutes a week for 6 weeks dramatically reduced pain scores and muscle tenderness.

Herbs and Supplements

- Chinese herbs, *Cornus*, garden rhubarb, *Psoralea*, and *Rehmannia* decrease pain after 3 months.
- *C. asiatica: Centella* extracts improve integrity of connective tissue composing the interstitium and heal ulcerations of the bladder.
- Horsetail *(Equisetum arvense)* has astringent properties.
- *Aloe vera* ("burn plant"): heals and relieves pain of burns. A freeze-dried whole-leaf *A. vera* concentrate, 3 600-mg capsules b.i.d. for 3 months, may offer symptomatic relief.

L-Arginine

- Essential amino acid that increases production of nitric oxide (NO), dependent on enzyme nitric oxide synthetase (NOS). NO and NOS have antibacterial, smooth muscle relaxant, hormone-releasing, and immune-modulating (increasing T-cell counts) properties.
- NOS production is decreased in patients with IC and increased in patients with UTI compared with controls.
- L-Arginine (1.5 g/day) over 6 months increased urinary NOS and improved symptoms of frequency and nocturia. Other studies have revealed no benefit. Efficacy of L-arginine, NO, and NOS for IC remains controversial.

Quercetin

- Quercetin: naturally occurring flavonoid that inhibits histamine release from mast cells and has anti-inflammatory and antioxidant properties.
- Sources: onions, seeds, citrus fruits, olive oil, tea, and red wine.
- Quercetin given at 500 mg b.i.d. for 4 weeks has helped some patients experience decreases in OLS symptom and problem index scores and a decrease in global assessment of pain (Likert scale; range 0 to -10).

General Measures

- **Cranberry juice *(Vaccinium macrocarpon):*** effective in several clinical studies; 0.5 L q.d. cranberry juice is beneficial in 73% of male and female UTI subjects. Withdrawal of cranberry juice from people who benefited resulted in recurrence in 61%. To acidify urine, 1 L of cranberry juice or more must be consumed at one sitting; concentration of hippuric acid in urine from drinking cranberry juice is insufficient to inhibit bacteria.

Constituents in cranberry juice reduce ability of *E. coli* to adhere to bladder and urethral endothelium. Only cranberry and blueberry *(Vaccinium angustifolium)* contain this inhibitor; blueberry juice is a suitable alternative to cranberry juice in bladder infections. Avoid immunosuppressive effects of sweetened cranberry juice. Instead use fresh cranberry (sweetened with apple or grape juice) or blueberry juice. Cranberry extracts may be more cost-effective than juice; ensure that ample water is ingested if tablets are used. Recent studies of cranberry juice have cast some doubt on its ability to prevent recurrent UTIs. The theoretical concern that cranberry can induce kidney stone formation, because cranberry contains oxalate, may not be warranted. Urinary oxalate excretion does not increase after drinking cranberry juice; no cranberry studies have reported increased kidney stone incidence.

- **Acidify or alkalinize?** Acidifying urine is difficult. Popular methods (ascorbic acid, cranberry juice) have little effect on pH at commonly prescribed doses. Alkalinizing urine is more effective, especially in women without pathogenic bacteria in urine. The best method for alkalinizing is citrate salts (potassium citrate and sodium citrate) that are rapidly absorbed and metabolized without affecting gastric pH or producing laxative effect. They are excreted partly as carbonate, raising urine pH. Potassium citrate and/or sodium citrate are used to treat lower UTIs and are often used as a "holding exercise" until urine culture is completed. With a dosage of 4 g sodium citrate every 8 hours for 48 hours, 80% of 64 women had relief of symptoms, 12% had reduction of symptoms, and 91.8% rated treatment acceptable. Significant symptomatic relief experienced by 80% of another 159 women studied who were abacteriuric. Urine culture can be restricted to women who do not respond to alkalinization. Many herbs used to treat UTIs (*Hydrastis canadensis, Arctostaphylos uva-ursi*) contain antibacterial components that work most effectively in an alkaline environment. Enhance immune function (*Textbook,* "Immune Support").
- **Acupuncture:** Patients with IC/PBS can gain benefit from 10 to 20 sessions of acupuncture. Acupuncture for 6 to 8 weeks reduced pain of IC. In one study, 85% of patients treated with acupuncture were free of cystitis during a 6-month observational period. It is a reliable modality as primary or adjunctive treatment. Some practitioners effectively combine acupuncture with Chinese herbal tradition.

Nutritional Supplements

- **D-Mannose:** simple sugar that helps prevent pili of *E. coli* and other bacteria from adhering to bladder wall. D-Mannose is in cranberry juice but in lower concentrations than in specific supplements. No clinical trials are available, but clinical experience supports its use. Adult dose: 0.5 to 1 tsp t.i.d. mixed in a little water. It can be used in reduced doses for UTIs in children.

Botanical Medicines

- ***A. uva-ursi* (bearberry or upland cranberry):** Urinary antiseptic component is arbutin, composing 7% to 9% of leaves. Arbutin is hydrolyzed to hydroquinone in the body. Hydroquinone is most effective in alkaline urine. Crude plant extracts are more effective medicinally than isolated arbutin. Uva-ursi is especially active against *E. coli* and has diuretic properties. Prophylactic effect of standardized extract on recurrent cystitis continued over 1-year period of study without side effects. Regular use may prevent bladder infections. Uva-ursi increases susceptibility of bacteria to antibiotics such as β-lactams. Catechins, compound P, epicatechin gallate from green tea, and baicalin from *Scutellaria amoena* may have similar effects. **Avoid excessive doses of uva-ursi;** as little as 15 g ({½} oz) dried leaves can be toxic in susceptible individuals. Signs of toxicity include tinnitus, nausea and vomiting, sense of suffocation, shortness of breath, convulsions, delirium, collapse.
- ***Allium sativum* (garlic):** antimicrobial activity against many disease-causing organisms, including *E. coli, Proteus* species, *K. pneumoniae, Staphylococcus* species, *Streptococcus* species.
- ***H. canadensis* (goldenseal):** very effective antimicrobial agent against *E. coli, Proteus* species, *Klebsiella* species, *Staphylococcus* species *E. aerogenes* (requires large dose), and *Pseudomonas* species. Berberine constituent works better in an alkaline urine (*Textbook, "Hydrastis canadensis* [Goldenseal] and Other Berberine-Containing Botanicals").

THERAPEUTIC APPROACH

Most cases of cystitis are relatively benign but must be properly diagnosed, treated, and monitored. Patient must notify physician of any change in condition. If culture positive, follow up with another culture 7 to 14 days after treatment is started. Citrates can ameliorate symptoms. Pyelonephritis requires immediate antibiotic therapy and sometimes hospitalization. Patient must promptly inform physician of fever, low back pain, and nausea or vomiting. Occasional acute bladder infection is easily treated; chronic cystitis is a challenge. Find underlying cause: structural abnormalities, excessive sugar intake, food allergies, nutritional deficiencies, chronic vaginitis, local foci of infection (prostate, kidneys), current or childhood sexual abuse. Causative agents for cystitis have not changed, but bacterial multidrug resistance to antibiotics (trimethoprim-sulfamethoxazole, β-lactam drugs, fluoroquinolone) is an alarming trend. Natural therapeutics protect urinary tract, support immunity, and inhibit bactericidal attack as first-line therapy in nonpyelonephritic cases and as an adjunctive to efficacy of antibiotics, if needed.

- **General measures:** large amounts of fluids (2 L or more q.d.), including at least 0.5 L unsweetened cranberry or at least 0.25 L blueberry juice q.d. For recurrent postcoital cystitis, urinate after intercourse; wash labia and urethra with strong tea of *H. canadensis* (2 tsp/cup) before and after. If this is inadequate, use dilute solution of povidone-iodine.
- **Diet:** UTIs arise and ascend with stool bacteria. Diet alters stool bacterial composition; UTI risk can change with modification of diet. Avoid all simple sugars, refined carbohydrates, full-strength fruit juice (diluted is acceptable), and food allergens. Restrict calories. Eat unsweetened yogurt with live probiotics and liberal amounts of garlic and onions. Patients with IC/PBS should exclude coffee, tea, soda, alcohol, citrus fruits and juices, artificial sweeteners, and hot pepper. Suspect gluten and dairy products, based on clinical experience. An elimination and challenge diet may be worthwhile.

Bacteriologic Susceptibility to Nutrients and Botanical Medicines

Bacterial Species	Agent
Escherichia coli	*Allium sativum, Hydrastis canadensis, Arctostaphylos uva-ursi*
Klebsiella pneumoniae	*A. sativum, H. canadensis*
Proteus mirabilis	*A. sativum, H. canadensis*
Pseudomonas aeruginosa	*H. canadensis*
Staphylococcus saprophyticus	*A. sativum, H. canadensis*

- **Nutritional supplements for bacterial cystitis:**
  — D-Mannose powder: 0.75 tsp t.i.d.
  — Vitamin C: 500 mg every 2 hours

— Bioflavonoids: 1000 mg q.d.
— Vitamin A: 25,000 international units (IU) q.d. (<10,000 IU q.d. during pregnancy)
— Beta-carotene (mixed carotenoids): 200,000 IU q.d.
— Zinc: 30 mg elemental zinc q.d. (e.g., picolinate)
— Choline: 1000 mg q.d.

- **Nutritional supplements for nonbacterial IC/PBS**
  — L-Arginine: 1500 mg in divided doses
  — Quercetin: 500 mg b.i.d.
- **Botanical medicines for bacterial cystitis (t.i.d.):**
  — Uva-ursi: dried leaves or as a tea, 1.5 to 4.0 g (1 to 2 tsp); freeze-dried leaves, 500 to 1000 mg; tincture (1:5), 4 to 6 mL (1 to 1.5 tsp); fluid extract (1:1), 1.0 mL (0.25 to 0.5 tsp); powdered solid extract (10% arbutin), 250 to 500 mg
  — *H. canadensis:* dried root (or as tea), 1 to 2 g; freeze-dried root, 500 to 1000 mg; tincture (1:5), 4 to 6 mL (1 to 1.5 tsp); fluid extract (1:1), 2 to 4 mL (0.5 to 1.0 tsp); powdered solid extract (8% alkaloid), 250 to 500 mg
  — Sandalwood oil, 1 to 2 drops (natural, not artificial)
- **Botanical medicines for nonbacterial IC/PBS**
  — *C. asiatica:* Dried herb: as tea t.i.d. Powdered herb (capsules): 1000 to 4000 mg t.i.d.; tincture (1:2 w/v, 30% alcohol), 30 to 60 drops (1.5 to 3 mL; 5 mL in a tsp) t.i.d.; standardized extract, 50 to 250 mg b.i.d. to t.i.d. (40% asiaticoside, 29% to 30% asiatic acid, 29% to 30% madecassic acid, and 1% to 2% madecassoside)
  — *E. arvense:* standardized dose, 300 mg t.i.d. standardized to 10% to 15% silica; herbal infusion (tea), 2 to 3 tsp t.i.d. Hot water is poured onto herb, steeped for 5 to 10 minutes; tincture (1:5), 1 to 4 mL t.i.d.; external (compresses), 10 g of herb per 1 L water a day

Nitrates and Biologic Organisms

Organisms that Reduce Nitrates to Nitrites	Organisms that Do Not Reduce Nitrates to Nitrites
Citrobacter spp.	*Neisseria gonorrhoeae*
Escherichia coli	*Streptococcus faecalis*
Klebsiella pneumoniae	*Mycobacterium tuberculosis*
Proteus spp.	
Pseudomonas spp.	
Serratia marcescens	
Shigella	
Staphylococcus spp. (most)	

Dermatitis Herpetiformis

DIAGNOSTIC SUMMARY

- Pruritic, papulovesicular eruption, usually on extensor surfaces
- Most common in middle-aged white men, although may occur in individuals of any age
- Immunoglobulin A (IgA) deposits in dermal papillae; confirmed by immunofluorescence
- Asymptomatic celiac disease (gluten-sensitive enteropathy) in 75% to 90% of patients

GENERAL CONSIDERATIONS

- Dermatitis herpetiformis (DH), described as "celiac disease of the skin," is a cutaneous manifestation of gluten-sensitive enteropathy (celiac disease).
- Patients with DH have serum IgA antibodies against epidermal transglutaminase and tissue transglutaminase. The putative autoantigen of DH is epidermal transglutaminase. Most individuals with CD have celiac-associated antibodies and specific pairs of allelic variants in two human leukocyte antigen (HLA) genes, *HLA-DQA1* and *HLA-DQB1*. Only 3% of persons with one or both of these alleles develops CD, yet 30% of the general population has one of them. Therefore their presence is not diagnostic of CD, but their absence excludes CD diagnosis. Genetic testing is available for the assessment of CD.
- Jejunal biopsy in DH patients reveals villous atrophy characteristic of celiac disease, but gastrointestinal (GI) symptoms are rare. Absorption studies (*Textbook,* "Intestinal Permeability Assessment") are used to assess degree of enteropathy. Average age of onset of rash is 7.2 years, with a predilection for elbows, knees, and buttocks. Skin biopsy reveals granular IgA deposits. Skin lesions are itchy, grouped vesicles often located on extensor surfaces.
- Intense pruritus is predominate symptom; however, DH is a clinical chameleon and can cause excoriations, eczematous lesions, or minimal patterns of discrete erythema or digital purpura.

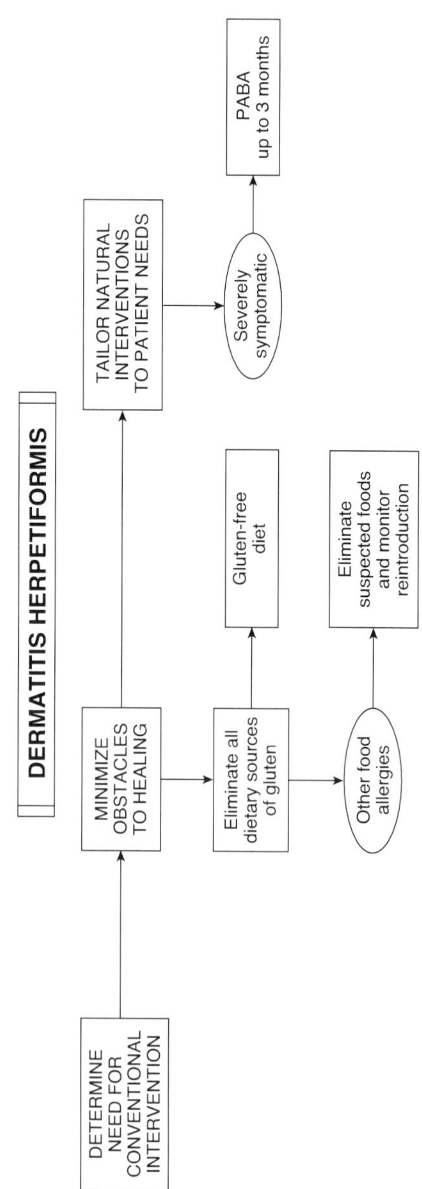
DERMATITIS HERPETIFORMIS
DETERMINE NEED FOR CONVENTIONAL INTERVENTION
MINIMIZE OBSTACLES TO HEALING
Eliminate all dietary sources of gluten
Gluten-free diet
Other food allergies
Eliminate suspected foods and monitor reintroduction
TAILOR NATURAL INTERVENTIONS TO PATIENT NEEDS
Severely symptomatic
PABA up to 3 months

THERAPEUTIC CONSIDERATIONS

- **Gluten:** most important factor in DH is to eliminate all sources of gluten. Frazer's criteria for diagnosing gluten-sensitive enteropathy (improvement on gluten-free diet and relapse after reintroduction) indicate rash and villous atrophy are largely gluten dependent. Gluten elimination improves virtually all patients, including disappearance of reticulin and gluten antibodies in DH. Gliadin polypeptide of gluten is key antigen; indirect immunofluorescence shows antibodies to gliadin in sera of 45% of DH patients. Titer and correlation increase with increasing disease severity. Approximately 81% of patients with severe jejunal abnormalities show antibodies to gliadin. Gluten connection is never mentioned in conventional medical textbooks. Gluten-free diet is superior to drugs such as dapsone, with its severe side effects. Beneficial effects of gluten-free diet: at least 65% of patients have complete resolution and the remainder substantially improve. DH enteropathy completely resolves; harsh medicines can be eliminated or substantially reduced; most patients experience improved sense of well-being. Those using gluten-free diet rather than drugs are protected against developing lipomas.
- **Food allergy:** 35% of patients are not adequately helped by gluten-free diet; only half of patients totally eliminate cutaneous IgA deposits and develop normal jejunal tissue. Other food allergies develop from increased leakage of macromolecules across damaged GI mucosa. Milk allergy is significant in some patients. According to enzyme-linked immunosorbent assay, 75% of DH patients have serum antibodies to gliadin, bovine milk, or ovalbumin. Thus other food sensitivities can also induce DH. Elemental diet, followed by careful food reintroduction, gives better results than gluten-free diet.
- **Para-aminobenzoic acid (PABA)** has been used successfully to control DH, even in those not controlling dietary gluten. It provides only symptom control and no repair of villous atrophy. It is not recommended as treatment of choice but as adjunct in unresponsive or severe cases.
- **Treatment of nutritional deficiencies:** investigate deficiencies of iron, zinc, calcium, fat-soluble vitamins, and folic acid. Consider and assess possibility of osteopenia and osteoporosis; treat according to findings.

THERAPEUTIC APPROACH

Eliminate all gluten and gliadin sources. Identify and eliminate other food allergens (*Textbook,* "Food Allergy Testing"). Use therapeutic regimen similar to atopic dermatitis. Patience is necessary because response may take several weeks to 6 months.

- **Diet:** normal, healthy, unprocessed diet free of all grains and allergenic foods
- **Supplements:**
  — Para-aminobenzoic acid: 5 g q.d. until remission (maximum of 3 months)

Diabetes Mellitus

DIAGNOSTIC SUMMARY

- Elevated blood glucose determination
  - — Fasting (overnight): venous plasma glucose level of 126 mg/dL or higher on at least two separate occasions
  - — After ingestion of 75 g glucose: venous plasma glucose level of 200 mg/dL or higher at 2 hours postingestion and at least one other sample during 2-hour test
  - — Random blood glucose level of 200 mg/dL or more plus presence of suggestive symptoms
- Classic symptoms: polyuria, polydipsia, polyphagia
- Presenting symptoms: fatigue, blurred vision, poor wound healing, periodontal disease, frequent infections

GENERAL CONSIDERATIONS

Diabetes mellitus (DM) is a chronic disorder of carbohydrate, fat, and protein metabolism characterized by fasting elevations of blood glucose and greatly increased risk of heart disease, stroke, kidney disease, retinopathy, and neuropathy. Two major categories of DM: types 1 and 2.

Classification

Two major categories:

- **Type 1 (T1DM):** most often in children and adolescents (juvenile-onset diabetes).
- **Type 2 (T2DM):** onset after age 40 years (adult-onset diabetes). Incidence of this type is rising in sedentary, obese children. Fifteen percent of adults diagnosed with type 2 actually have type 1.

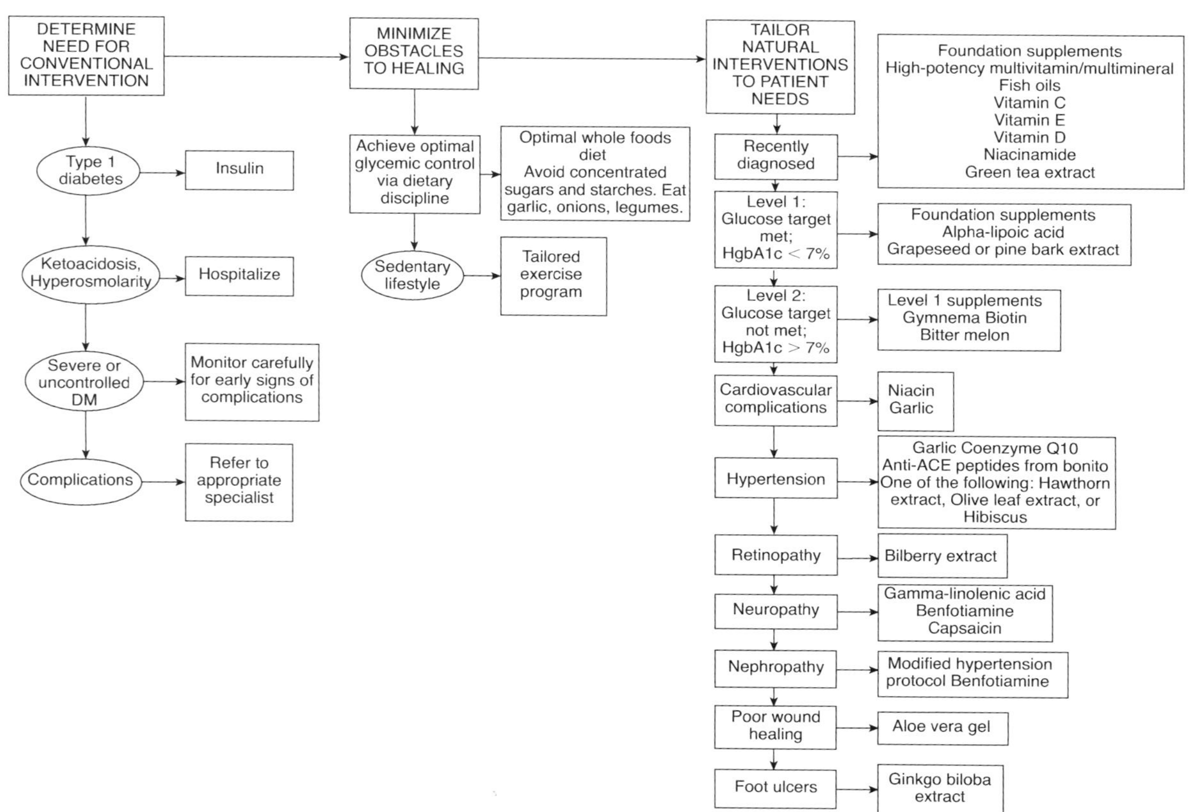
DIABETES MELLITUS TYPE 1
DETERMINE NEED FOR CONVENTIONAL INTERVENTION
Type 1 diabetes
Insulin
Ketoacidosis, Hyperosmolarity
Hospitalize
Severe or uncontrolled DM
Monitor carefully for early signs of complications
Complications
Refer to appropriate specialist
MINIMIZE OBSTACLES TO HEALING
Achieve optimal glycemic control via dietary discipline
Optimal whole foods diet Avoid concentrated sugars and starches. Eat garlic, onions, legumes.
Sedentary lifestyle
Tailored exercise program
TAILOR NATURAL INTERVENTIONS TO PATIENT NEEDS
Recently diagnosed
Foundation supplements High-potency multivitamin/multimineral Fish oils Vitamin C Vitamin E Vitamin D Niacinamide Green tea extract
Level 1: Glucose target met; HgbA1c < 7%
Foundation supplements Alpha-lipoic acid Grapeseed or pine bark extract
Level 2: Glucose target not met; HgbA1c > 7%
Level 1 supplements Gymnema Biotin Bitter melon
Cardiovascular complications
Niacin Garlic
Hypertension
Garlic Coenzyme Q10 Anti-ACE peptides from bonito One of the following: Hawthorn extract, Olive leaf extract, or Hibiscus
Retinopathy
Bilberry extract
Neuropathy
Gamma-linolenic acid Benfotiamine Capsaicin
Nephropathy
Modified hypertension protocol Benfotiamine
Poor wound healing
Aloe vera gel
Foot ulcers
Ginkgo biloba extract

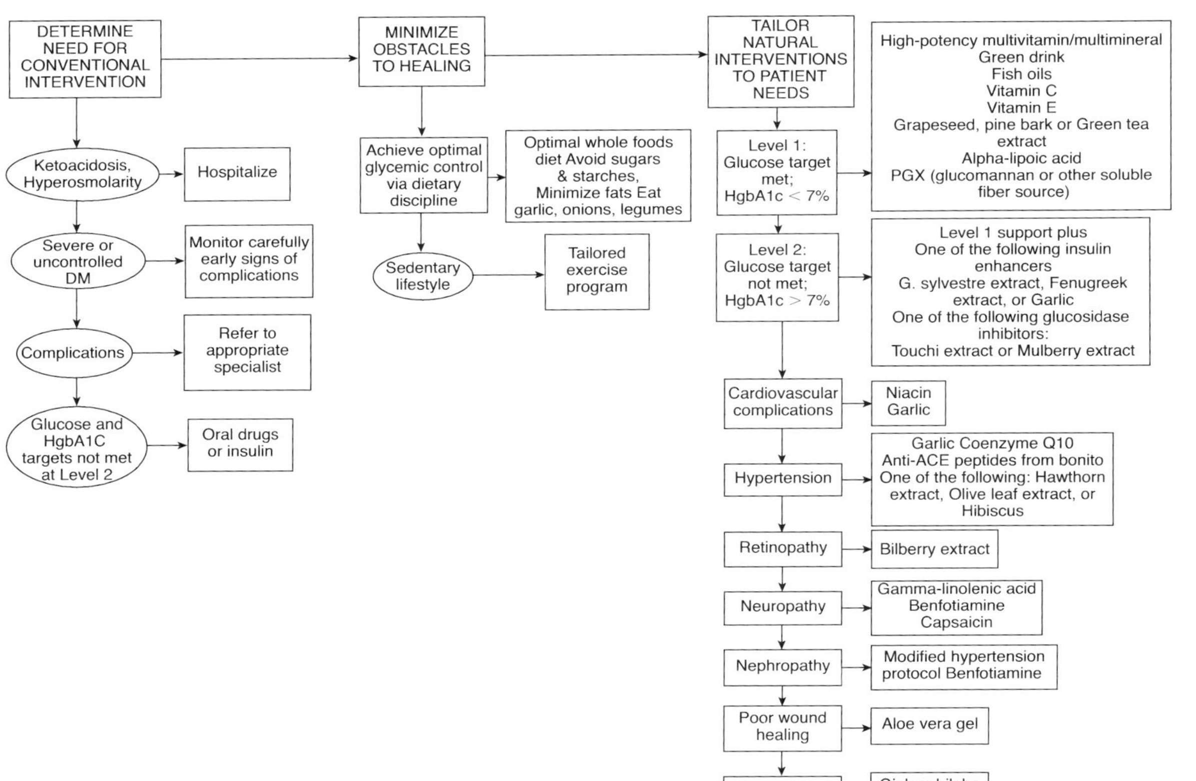
DIABETES MELLITUS TYPE 2
DETERMINE NEED FOR CONVENTIONAL INTERVENTION
Ketoacidosis, Hyperosmolarity
Hospitalize
Severe or uncontrolled DM
Monitor carefully early signs of complications
Complications
Refer to appropriate specialist
Glucose and HgbA1C targets not met at Level 2
Oral drugs or insulin
MINIMIZE OBSTACLES TO HEALING
Achieve optimal glycemic control via dietary discipline
Optimal whole foods diet Avoid sugars & starches, Minimize fats Eat garlic, onions, legumes
Sedentary lifestyle
Tailored exercise program
TAILOR NATURAL INTERVENTIONS TO PATIENT NEEDS
Level 1: Glucose target met; HgbA1c < 7%
High-potency multivitamin/multimineral
Green drink
Fish oils
Vitamin C
Vitamin E
Grapeseed, pine bark or Green tea extract
Alpha-lipoic acid
PGX (glucomannan or other soluble fiber source)
Level 2: Glucose target not met; HgbA1c > 7%
Level 1 support plus
One of the following insulin enhancers
G. sylvestre extract, Fenugreek extract, or Garlic
One of the following glucosidase inhibitors:
Touchi extract or Mulberry extract
Cardiovascular complications
Niacin
Garlic
Hypertension
Garlic Coenzyme Q10
Anti-ACE peptides from bonito
One of the following: Hawthorn extract, Olive leaf extract, or Hibiscus
Retinopathy
Bilberry extract
Neuropathy
Gamma-linolenic acid
Benfotiamine
Capsaicin
Nephropathy
Modified hypertension protocol Benfotiamine
Poor wound healing
Aloe vera gel
Foot ulcers
Ginkgo biloba extract

Differences between Type 1 and Type 2 Diabetes

Features	Type 1	Type 2
Age at onset	Usually younger than 40 years	Usually older than 40 years
Proportion of all diabetics	<10%	>90%
Family history	Uncommon	Common
Appearance of symptoms	Rapid	Slow
Obesity at onset	Uncommon	Common
Insulin levels	Decreased	Normal to high initially, decreased after several years
Insulin resistance	Occasional	Often
Treatment with insulin	Always	Usually not required

- **T1DM:** autoimmune disease caused by destruction of the beta cells of pancreas, which synthesize insulin. Positive antibodies against beta cells or insulin occur in 75% of patients with T1DM. Postulated triggers for autoimmunity: viral infection, food allergens, and chemical or free radical damage; combined with genes predisposing to T1DM. T1DM patients require lifelong exogenous insulin to control blood glucose. The T1DM patient must learn to manage glucose levels day by day, modifying insulin types and doses according to meals eaten, liver production of glucose, and results of regular blood glucose testing.
- **T2DM:** historical onset after age 40 in overweight persons; but today it is seen even in pediatric patients because of obesity epidemic affecting all age groups. Ninety percent of all diabetics have T2DM. Initially, insulin is elevated in T2DM, indicating loss of tissue sensitivity to insulin. Obesity is a major contributing factor to loss of insulin sensitivity. Ninety percent of persons with T2DM are obese. Achieving ideal body weight often restores normal blood glucose levels. Even if T2DM has progressed to insulin deficiency, weight loss can improve blood glucose control and reduce other health risks. T2DM characteristics: progressive worsening of glycemic control—starting with mild alterations in postprandial glucose homeostasis, followed by increasing fasting plasma glucose, lack of insulin production, and need for insulin therapy. Body load of persistent organic pollutants (POPs) that block insulin receptor sites is becoming a major causative factor.

- **Other types of diabetes:**
  - — Adult latent autoimmune diabetes ("DM type 1.5"): slower-onset autoimmune type of diabetes that occurs after age 35.
  - — Chronic pancreatitis and other insults to the pancreas.
  - — Gestational diabetes: affects 4% of all pregnant women who were not diabetic before pregnancy but developed diabetes during pregnancy. This occurs more frequently among African Americans, Hispanic/Latino Americans, and American Indians; obese women; and women with family history of diabetes. After pregnancy, 5% to 10% of women with gestational diabetes are found to have T2DM. Women who have had gestational diabetes have 20% to 50% chance of developing DM in subsequent 5 to 10 years.
  - — Genetic disorders; least common; examples are neonatal diabetes and mature-onset diabetes of youth—generally caused by faulty genes causing impaired insulin function.

Prediabetes and Metabolic Syndrome

Prediabetes (impaired glucose tolerance [IGT]) is characterized by fasting glucose between 100 and 125 mg/dL and/or postprandial glucose of 140 to 199 mg/dL. Many prediabetics will develop T2DM despite the fact that prediabetes is reversible and, in most cases, can be avoided through dietary and lifestyle changes. Contributing factors: refined starches and sugar, particularly high-fructose corn syrup; saturated fats; overeating as a result of increased portion sizes of food; increases in inflammatory markers; lack of exercise; industrial pollution; abdominal weight gain; hormonal imbalances; inadequate sleep; and nutritional deficiencies. It is the first step in insulin resistance. Prediabetes is accompanied by serious health risks—increased risk for cardiovascular disease. People with prediabetes often meet criteria for metabolic syndrome (MetS)—cluster of factors that together carry greater risk for cardiovascular disease and T2DM. They include the following:

- Greater waist-to-hip ratio
- Two of the following:
  - — Triglyceride level higher than 150 mg/dL
  - — High-density–lipoprotein cholesterol (HDL-C) level higher than 40 mg/dL for men and 50 mg/dL for women
  - — Blood pressure equal to or higher than 130/85 mm Hg

DIAGNOSIS

- **Classic symptoms of T1DM:** frequent urination, weight loss, impaired wound healing, infections, and excessive thirst and appetite. Patients may have diabetic ketoacidosis (DKA); they are usually lean in presentation.
- **T2DM symptoms:** milder and may go unnoticed for many years. Many people with T2DM do not know they have the disease. Abdominal obesity, fatigue, blurred vision, poor wound healing, periodontal disease, and frequent infections can be manifesting symptoms of T2DM.
- **Standard method for diagnosing diabetes:** measurement of blood glucose levels; initially after fasting for 10 hours but not more than 16. Normal reading: 70 to 99 mg/dL. Fasting blood glucose higher than 126 mg/dL (7 mmol/L) on two separate occasions indicates diagnosis of DM. Fasting glucose above 100 but below 126 mg/dL is classified as prediabetes.
- **Postprandial measurement:** usually made 1 to 2 hours after a meal. Random measurement is made at any time regardless of the time of the last meal. Reading above 200 mg/dL (11 mmol/L) indicates DM.

Criteria for Response to the Glucose Tolerance Test

Type	Criteria
Normal	No elevation >160 mg/dL (9 mmol/L); <150 mg/dL (8.3 mmol/L) at end of first hour, below 120 mg/dL (6.6 mmol/L) at end of second hour
Flat	No variation of more than ±20 mg/dL (1.1 mmol/L) from fasting value
Prediabetic	Blood glucose levels of 140 mg/dL (7.8 mmol/L) to 180 mg/dL (10 mmol/L) at end of second hour
Diabetic	>180 mg/dL (10 mmol/L) during first hour, 200 mg/dL (11.1 mmol/L) or higher at end of first hour, 150 mg/dL (8.3 mmol/L) or higher at end of second hour

- **Glycosylated hemoglobin (HbA_{1c}):** valuable test for evaluating long-term blood glucose levels. Proteins with attached glucose molecules (glycosylated peptides) are elevated severalfold in DM. Normal levels are 4.6% to 5.7% of hemoglobin. **HbA_{1c}** from 5.7% to 6.4% indicates prediabetes. **HbA_{1c}** of 6.5% or higher, particularly from a screening test, can diagnose DM and is revealing in patients with nondiagnostic fasting blood sugar levels. It is best coupled with fasting blood glucose and 2-hour postprandial glucose for a more accurate diagnosis. Because average lifespan of red blood cells (RBCs) is 120 days, **HbA$_{1c}$** represents time-averaged values for blood glucose over preceding 2 to 4 months. **HbA$_{1c}$** at 5% indicates that glucose median for previous 3 months was around 100 mg/dL. Each digit of elevation in percentage indicates an additional 35 mg/dL of glucose. Thus **HbA$_{1c}$** of 7% means that on average over preceding 3 months, blood glucose was 170 mg/dL. **HbA$_{1c}$** index is extremely valuable simple, useful method for assessing effectiveness of treatment and patient compliance; check it every 3 to 6 months.

CAUSES OF DIABETES

Risk Factors for Type 1 Diabetes Mellitus

In T1DM, insulin-producing cells of the pancreas are destroyed, in most cases, by the immune system; what triggers this destruction can vary. Genetic factors may predispose by impaired defense mechanisms, immune system sensitivity, and/or defects in tissue regeneration capacity. The entire set of T1DM genetic factors is termed *susceptibility genes;* but they are neither necessary nor sufficient for disease to develop. Genetic predisposition sets the stage for environmental or dietary factor to initiate destructive process. Less than 10% of those with increased genetic susceptibility for T1DM actually develop the disease.

- **Environmental and dietary risk factors:** abnormalities of gut immune development of antibodies by gut immune systems that ultimately attack beta cells. Possible underlying factor contributing to T1DM is poor protein digestion. Poorly digested dietary proteins can cross-react with antigens of pancreas beta cells. Two implicated dietary proteins: milk (bovine serum albumin and bovine insulin) and wheat (gluten). Bovine insulin activates T-cells in those predisposed to DM, leading to beta-cell destruction by direct attack from T-killer cells. Breastfeeding establishes proper intestinal immune function and reduces risk of T1DM. Breastfeeding confers reduced risk of food allergies and offers better protection against bacterial and viral intestinal infections. Patients with T1DM are more likely to have been breastfed for less than 3 months and to have been exposed to cow's milk or solid foods before 4 months of age. Early cow's milk exposure may increase risk by about 1.5 times. Ingestion at any age may increase risk of T1DM. Sensitivity to gluten—major protein component of wheat, rye, and barley—may play a role. Gluten sensitivity produces celiac disease, another autoimmune disorder. Celiac disease, like T1DM, is linked to abnormalities in intestinal immune function. Breastfeeding can be preventive; early introduction of cow's milk can be causative. Risk of developing T1DM is higher in children with celiac disease. The highest level of antibodies to cow's milk proteins is found in people with celiac disease.

- **Enteroviruses and type 1 diabetes:** T1DM can arise from gastrointestinal (GI) viral infection. Working theory: the immune system becomes slightly confused as to which proteins to attack—food-based dairy or gluten proteins or similar proteins on pancreatic beta cells or insulin. Viral infection increases stimulation of the immune system, prompting confused immune cells to damage the pancreas. Enteroviruses (polioviruses, coxsackieviruses, echoviruses) and rotavirus are common in children, can activate immune cells, and can infect beta cells, triggering a white blood cell attack. GI virus infections may increase intestinal permeability. Small intestinal leaky gut during and after rotavirus infections exposes gut immune cells to intact protein.
- **Vitamin D deficiency:** cod liver oil vitamin D may be protective. Supplementation during early childhood can prevent T1DM. Protective dose is 2000 international units (IU) daily. Children taking vitamin D from cod liver oil have an 80% reduced risk of T1DM; vitamin D–deficient children have a 300% increased risk. Vitamin D from cod liver oil during pregnancy reduces T1DM frequency. Lack of sun exposure during childhood may explain higher T1DM rates in Northern countries. Vitamin D can prevent autoimmune conditions, including those that attack beta cells, from developing, in a dose-dependent degree of protection. Vitamin D helps normalize immune system development and inhibit autoimmune reactions against beta cells.
- **Omega-3 fatty acid deficiency:** omega-3 fatty acids in cod liver and other fish oils are also protective. Compounds that generate free radicals (e.g., nitrosamines, alloxan) destroy beta cells. Fish oil can prevent chemically induced T1DM by improving cell membrane function, enhancing antioxidant status, and suppressing formation of inflammatory cytokines.

- **Nitrates:** the increase in nitrates in diet and water is linked to an increased rate for T1DM. Sources of nitrates include agricultural fertilizer runoff and cured and smoked meats. Nitrates are converted in the body into nitrosamines, which can cause DM. Infants and young children are particularly vulnerable. (*Note:* The U.S. Department of Agriculture [USDA] requires all manufacturers of processed meats to add vitamin C to their products to prevent the formation of nitrosamines.) Nitrates in water may be a key factor in the 3% annual growth in T1DM. High-quality water purifiers are recommended.

Early Treatment and Possible Reversal of Type 1 Diabetes Mellitus

Early intervention designed to reduce immune-mediated or oxidative damage may help to slow down or even reverse the disease process. In addition to elimination of the risk factors noted above, the following may be of benefit:

- **Niacinamide (nicotinamide):** may help prevent immune-mediated destruction of beta cells and reverse disorder. It must be given soon enough after onset of DM to restore beta cells or retard destruction. A dose of 3 g niacinamide daily may prolong non–insulin-requiring remission, lower insulin requirements, improve metabolic control, and increase beta-cell function as determined by C-peptide secretion. Timed-release niacinamide may not provide sufficient peak concentrations to block autoimmunity (e.g., cytokine production). Complete reversal in some patients makes its use worth the effort because no reasonable alternative is available. Dose is based on body weight: 25 to 50 mg niacinamide per kilogram (2.2 pounds) of body weight to maximal dose of 3 g q.d. in divided doses. No side effects were reported in T1DM clinical trials. It can harm the liver; monitor liver enzymes every 3 months.
- **Epicatechin:** bark from the Malabar kino tree *(Pterocarpus marsupium)* is used in India for DM. Epicatechin extract prevents beta-cell damage in rats. Epicatechin and crude extract of *P. marsupium* can regenerate beta-cell function in diabetic animals. Green tea *(Camellia sinensis)* extract has a higher epicatechin content and broader range of beneficial effects. Green tea polyphenols have antiviral activity against rotavirus and enterovirus, suspected of causing T1DM. Dose for children younger than 6 years is 50 to 150 mg; children 6 to 12 years, 100 to 200 mg; children older than 12 years and adults, 150 to 300 mg.

Decaffeinated green tea extracts with a polyphenol content of 80% are preferred.

Risk Factors for Type 2 Diabetes Mellitus

Risk Factors for Type 2 Diabetes Mellitus

- Family history of diabetes
- Obesity
- Increased waist/hip ratio
- Increasing age: beginning at age 45
- Race/ethnicity: African American, Hispanic American, Native American, Native Australian or New Zealander, Asian American, Pacific Islander
- Impaired fasting glucose or impaired glucose tolerance
- History of gestational diabetes: diabetes during pregnancy or delivery of baby weighing more than 9 lb
- Hypertension: blood pressure >140/90 mm Hg
- Triglycerides >250 mg/dL
- Low levels of adiponectin, elevated levels of fasting insulin
- Polycystic ovary syndrome (to be considered in any adult woman who is overweight with both acne and infertility)

- **Obesity (excess body fat):** 80% to 90% of type 2 diabetics are obese (body mass index above 30). Abdominal adipocytes, engorged with fat, secrete resistin, leptin, tumor necrosis factor, and free fatty acids that dampen the effect of insulin, impair glucose use in skeletal muscle, promote liver gluconeogenesis, and impair beta-cell insulin release by pancreatic beta cells. The increasing size of adipocytes reduces secretion of compounds (adiponectin) that improve insulin sensitivity, reduce inflammation, lower triglycerides, and inhibit atherosclerosis. Adipose is part of the endocrine system. Blood levels of adiponectin or adipohormone may predict T2DM. Increasing insulin resistance leads to compensatory increased insulin secretion to the point of beta-cell exhaustion or burnout.
- Family history: parent or sibling with T2DM
- Increased waist/hip ratio
- Increasing age beginning at age 45 years
- Race or ethnicity: African American, Hispanic, Native American/First Nation, Native Australian or New Zealander, Asian American, Pacific Islander
- Impaired fasting glucose (IFG) or IGT
- History of gestational diabetes or delivery of infant larger than 9 pounds
- Hypertension (blood pressure higher than 140/90 mm Hg)

- Triglyceride level higher than 250 mg/dL
- Low adiponectin, elevated fasting insulin
- Polycystic ovary syndrome (adult women: overweight, acne, infertile)

Under naturopathic care, the pancreas can recover and continue to secrete insulin for the rest of the patient's life. However, with conventional care, allowing the patient to eat a high-carbohydrate diet, diabetes is not well controlled, causing ultimately complete pancreatic failure to output insulin, thus requiring full use of basal and bolus insulin. This scenario is preventable with good diabetes care and if a patient's **HbA_{1c}** remains at 5.7 or less. (See box "Risk Factors for Type 2 Diabetes Mellitus.")

- **Genetics of type 2 diabetes and obesity:** even with the strongest genetic predisposition, DM can be avoided in most cases. When DM-prone ethnic groups follow the traditional diet and lifestyle of their original culture, DM incidence is extremely low. These groups are simply sensitive to the Western lifestyle.
- **Diet, exercise, lifestyle, and diabetes risk:** T2DM is a disease of diet and lifestyle: lack of exercise, failure to eat whole plant foods, high intake of harmful fat, and obesity. Lifestyle changes alone are associated with a 58% reduced risk of developing DM in people with IGT.
- **Glycemic index and glycemic load (GL):** glycemic index is the numeric value expressing a rise in blood glucose after a particular food has been eaten. The standard of 100 applies to the ingestion of glucose itself. The insulin response matches blood sugar elevation. Glycemic index reflects the quality of carbohydrates, not the quantity of sugar to be metabolized. Glycemic index is not related to portion size. GL is calculated by amount of carbohydrate in a serving multiplied by the food's glycemic index (compared with glucose), then divided by 100. The higher the GL, the greater the stress on insulin. GL has a stronger link in predicting DM than glycemic index. A high-GL diet increases risk for heart disease because of lower high-density lipoprotein (HDL) and higher triglyceride levels. Increased DM and heart risk start at daily GL of 161. GL should not exceed 150 daily.
- **Fiber and glycemic index or GL:** inadequate dietary fiber increases DM risk. Fibers most beneficial to glycemic control are water-soluble forms (hemicelluloses, mucilages, gums, and pectin, as in legumes, oat bran, nuts, seeds, psyllium seed husks, pears, apples, most vegetables). They slow down digestion and absorption, preventing rapid glycemic rises, increasing tissue

insulin sensitivity, and improving uptake of glucose by muscles and liver. Recommend at least 35 g of fiber daily from a variety of food sources, especially vegetables. Fiber supplements can also be used.

- **Wrong type of fats:** saturated fat and *trans* fats (hydrogenated vegetable oils, as in margarine, vegetable shortening) with relative insufficiency of monounsaturated and omega-3 fats. Cell membrane fluidity, affected by fatty acid composition, affects insulin binding to receptors. Monounsaturated fats (olive oil, nuts, nut oils) and omega-3 oils improve insulin action and protect against onset of T2DM. Eating nuts reduces risk of T2DM. Raw or lightly roasted and unsalted fresh nuts and seeds are preferred over commercially roasted and salted.
- **Low intake of antioxidants:** cumulative free radical damage ages cells and contributes to T2DM. Fruits and vegetables (even dark green salads) improve glycemic control and reduce risk. Vitamins C and E and carotenes lower risk. Antioxidant deficits and lipid peroxides increase risk.
- **Free radicals:** type 2 diabetics have higher levels of reactive oxygen species (ROSs) and reactive nitrogen species (RNSs), which exhaust antioxidant mechanisms and damage DNA, proteins, and membrane fatty acids. ROSs, RNSs, high blood glucose, and saturated fat activate inflammatory compounds (nuclear factor kappa B), increase insulin resistance, and impair insulin secretion.
- **POPs:** include polychlorinated dibenzo-*p*-dioxins (PCDDs), polychlorinated dibenzofurans (PCDFs), hexachlorobenzene (HCB), organophosphates, dichlorodiphenyldichloroethylene (DDE), and bisphenol A. These compounds are linked to development of T2DM. Body load of POPs is a strong predictor of T2DM and might be a more important risk factor than obesity. Unfortunately, direct measurement of POP levels is difficult and expensive. However, a good indirect measure is gamma-glutamyltransferase (GGTP). An elevated GGTP is a strong predictor of diabetes risk. Those with levels above 40 IU/L have a 20-fold increased risk. The apparent mechanisms of action are blocking of insulin receptor sites and impairment of insulin production.
- **Lifestyle versus drugs to prevent T2DM:** the benefits of drugs pale compared with the efficacy of diet and lifestyle changes.
- **Environmental toxicity:** reduce patients' exposure to environmental pollutants. Use organic foods and natural cleaning agents in the home and avoid chemical pesticides.

MONITORING THE DIABETIC PATIENT

- **Urine glucose monitoring:** kidneys conserve glucose until blood glucose reaches 200 to 250 mg/dL (10 mmol/L). A negative urine glucose means blood glucose since previous voiding has been below 200 to 250 mg/dL (10 mmol/L). Urine testing is crude; it gives no indication of blood glucose below 200 mg/dL. It is worthless for severe hypoglycemia or monitoring hyperglycemia.
- **Urine ketone testing:** when fat is the primary source of energy, ketones are produced. High ketone level spills over into urine. In the patient with T1DM or T2DM who underproduces innate insulin, ketonuria occurs with severe deficits in insulin availability or activity. This is associated primarily with T1DM, because the vast majority of patients with T2DM do not develop ketoacidosis. Examples: a patient with T1DM accidentally or purposefully fails to take insulin; or a diabetic is ill, is injured, or is given high doses of cortisone-related drugs. Loss of insulin effect impairs glucose uptake and use of glucose. The result is hyperglycemia, fat burning for energy, and toxemia from acidic ketones, with severe dehydration from water loss caused by glycosuria. This state is the deadly medical emergency termed *diabetic ketoacidosis,* necessitating intravenous (IV) insulin, IV fluids, and intensive care unit monitoring. Urine ketone testing is critical, especially in T1DM. Urine ketones (with hyperglycemia) may indicate impending or established ketoacidosis, requiring immediate intervention. Advise patients to test urine for ketones during acute illness; during severe stress, when blood glucose is consistently elevated (above 300 mg/dL [16.7 mmol/L]); regularly during pregnancy; or in the presence of symptoms of ketoacidosis (nausea, vomiting, abdominal pain).
- **Self-monitoring of blood glucose:** glycemic control is the most important factor in the long-term risk of serious complications in T1DM and T2DM. Self-monitoring of blood glucose allows the patient to modify treatment to maintain glycemic control, detect hypoglycemia, adjust care to daily circumstances (food intake, exercise, stress, illness), detect and treat severe hyperglycemia, increase therapeutic compliance, and improve motivation from immediate feedback.

Optimal Range for Self-Monitored Blood Glucose

- Fasting or before meals: 80 to 110 mg/dL (4.4 to 6.7 mmol/L)
- Two hours after eating (postprandial): <140 mg/dL (7.8 mmol/L)
- At bedtime: 100 to 140 mg/dL (5.6 to 7.8 mmol/L)
- Note that these are whole-blood values, which typically run 10 mg/dL (0.6 mmol/L) higher than serum values. To avoid confusing numbers, some home glucose-monitoring kits, even those using whole-blood samples, are now calibrating to serum levels. Check the glucose monitor's documentation to find out if it is set up to determine whole-blood or serum glucose levels.
- Slightly higher values may be acceptable in the elderly or in young children because of their higher risk of developing dangerous hypoglycemia.

Optimal Schedule for Self-Monitored Blood Glucose

1. Test on awakening and just before each meal. Ideal blood sugar before meals is <120 mg/dL (6.7 mmol/L).
2. Test 2 hours after each meal. Ideal blood sugar 2 hours after meals is <140 mg/dL (7.7 mmol/L).
3. Test at bedtime. Ideal blood sugar at bedtime is <140 mg/dL (7.7 mmol/L).

- **Type 1 diabetes and self-monitoring of blood glucose**: all type 1 diabetics must frequently monitor blood glucose to make ongoing adjustments to insulin injections, diet, and exercise. Until recently, type 1 diabetics often were prescribed combinations of short- and medium-acting or long-acting insulin one or two times per day. Diabetics are now trained to maintain ideal levels 24/7 by intensive insulin therapy (IIT) plus frequent glycemic monitoring. Using rapid-acting and short-duration insulins, IIT involves either frequent injections of insulins (Humalog [insulin lispro] or NovoLog [insulin aspart]) or an insulin pump (continuous electronic injection of very-short-acting insulins with extra boluses before meals) allows timing and size of doses to be adjusted to daily events. Despite multiple injections (before meals and at bedtime) and glycemic testing six or more times daily, IIT allows greater freedom, higher quality of life, and superior glycemic control.
- **Type 2 diabetes and self-monitoring of blood glucose:** every type 2 diabetic must own a monitor and be intimately familiar with its use. Even if glucose is well controlled by diet, lifestyle, and supplements, they should monitor regularly. T2DM patients with good glucose control according to regular laboratory testing, including A_{1c}, should designate a day every 1 to 3 weeks as intensive glycemic measuring day. Check before breakfast (fasting), just before meals, 2 hours after meals, and

before bed. Record measurements, diet, exercise, and supplements in a journal to increase awareness of the effects of factors on blood glucose. Type 2 diabetics with poor control should monitor intensively each day and seek professional help to regain control. Diabetics in advanced stages, with diminished insulin secretion, may need IIT. Blood test for C-peptide estimates insulin output. IIT requires self-monitoring of blood glucose as frequently as type 1 diabetics (before and 2 hours after each meal). Advanced type 2 diabetics with diminished insulin production have less than normal C-peptide. Common intervention trend: one injection of new, very-long-acting insulin (insulin glargine [Lantus]) for smooth, continual 24-hour release plus diet and medication. With this regimen, self-monitoring should be done before and 2 hours after each meal.

- **C-peptide determination:** assessing insulin secretion influences treatment, especially in a diabetic hoping to avoid or stop using insulin, and the type of pharmaceuticals and nutraceuticals likely to be effective. Pancreas manufactures proinsulin first. Enzymes snip off a piece of this proinsulin (C-peptide); both C-peptide and insulin are secreted. Injected insulin has no C-peptide, nor does the body produce antibodies against it, as it can against insulin. T1DM patients and those who have injected insulin even once are at high risk of having developed insulin antibodies. Measuring C-peptide helps both T1DM and T2DM patients, but T2DM patients more so. C-peptide can uncover how much insulin the pancreas is making, to determine how much of a T1DM pancreas is still active. It may even make it possible, with alternative care, to stabilize the patient's condition. In T2DM, high C-peptide confirms high insulin resistance. If C-peptide is low, it indicates that the pancreas is so damaged that insulin therapy is required.

Interpreting Levels of C-Peptide

C-Peptide results	Interpretation
Normal	Insulin production at normal level
Below normal	Newly diagnosed type 1 diabetic or chronic, long-term type 2 diabetic
Above normal	Newly diagnosed type 2 diabetic or a benign pancreatic tumor (insulinoma; rare)
Undetectable	Chronic type 1 diabetic or postsurgical removal of pancreas (rare)

- **Physician monitoring**: diabetics are rarely successful in controlling DM without professional guidance. Physician monitoring through laboratory testing of blood glucose has major impact on diabetic patient's long-term outcomes. A key determinant of glucose control is HbA_{1c}, reflecting average glucose levels over preceding 3 months. HbA_{1c} closely correlates with risk for diabetic complications. However, HbA_{1c} may not be entirely accurate because HbA_{1c} is an index that averages spikes and troughs in glucose levels. A patient with glucose levels that fluctuate wildly can have the same desirable HbA_{1c} under 6% as one whose glucose levels are steady and well controlled. HbA_{1c} below 5.5% is ideal and indicates glucose levels causing no tissue damage. Monitor HbA_{1c} every 3 to 4 months, depending on stability of condition. If HbA_{1c} level is not clearly known to result from good control or fluctuating highs and lows, the GlycoMark test measures blood levels of 1,5-anhydroglucitol (AG). 1,5-AG is found in nearly all foods. Ingested 1,5-AG is nearly 100% nonmetabolized and remains in a constant amount in blood and tissues. When blood glucose exceeds 180 mg/dL for any period of time, the kidneys attempts to reabsorb as much glucose back into the blood as possible. During glucosuria, the additional glucose in the kidneys blocks 1,5-AG reabsorption; 1,5-AG is excreted in urine at a higher rate than normal. Blood levels of 1,5-AG decrease immediately and continue to decrease until glucose values drop below 180 mg/dL. Competitive inhibition of 1,5-AG from glucose allows GlycoMark to reflect hyperglycemic episodes over 180 mg/dL. GlycoMark is more accurate than HbA_{1c} and offers clearer picture of glucose control and postprandial spikes. Early detection of problems through regular screening and monitoring is preventive. Table "Clinical Management of the Patient with Diabetes" provides a checklist for proper evaluation and monitoring.

Clinical Management of the Patient with Diabetes

	Quarterly	Annually
Review Management Plan		
Blood glucose self-monitoring results	X	X
Medication/insulin regimen	X	X
Nutritional plan	X	X
Exercise program	X	X
Psychosocial support	X	X
Physical Examination		

	Quarterly	Annually
Weight	X	X
Height (for child/adolescent)	X	X
Sexual maturation (for child/adolescent)	X	X
Skin, including insulin injection sites	X	X
Feet: pulses, capillary refill, color, sensation, nails, skin, ulcers	X	X
Neurologic: reflexes, proprioception, vibratory sensation, touch (distal temperature sensation, distal pinprick or pressure sensation, standardized monofilament)	-	X
Regular retinal examination	X	X
Dilated retinal examination	-	X
Electrocardiogram	-	X
Laboratory Tests		
Fasting or random plasma glucose (normal/ target range: 80–120 mg/dL before meals)	X	X
Glycosolated hemoglobin (A_{1c}) (target range: <7% in adults, 7.5 to 8.5, age dependent)	X	X
Urinalysis (glucose, ketones, microalbumin, protein, sediment)	X	X
Complete Cardiovascular Profile		
Test/Target	-	X
Cholesterol <200 mg/dL	-	X
Triglycerides <200 mg/dL	-	X
Low-density lipoprotein <130 mg/dL	-	X
High-density lipoprotein <35 mg/dL	-	X
Lipoprotein (a) <40 mg/dL	-	X
C-reactive protein <1.69 mg/L	-	X
Fibrinogen <400 mg/L	-	X
Homocysteine <16 μmole/L	-	X
Ferritin 60–200 mcg/L (if elevated, transferrin saturation; if elevated, genetic testing for hemochromatosis only once)	-	X
Lipid peroxides <normal	-	X
Serum creatinine (in adults; in children only if protein is present in urine)	X	X

COMPLICATIONS OF DIABETES

Risk of complications is a reflection of glucose control; good glucose control greatly reduces risk; monitoring and controlling hyperglycemia are critical to preventing complications.

Acute Complications

Acute complications of DM may represent a medical emergency or life-or-death situation. Any symptom even remotely suggestive of acute complications must be addressed immediately.

Major Complications of Diabetes

- Cardiovascular disease
- Hypertension
- Retinopathy
- Renal disease
- Neuropathy
- Amputations
- Periodontal disease
- Pain
- Depression
- Autoimmune disorders

- **Hypoglycemia:** in T1DM, occurs from taking too much insulin, missing a meal, or overexercising; with "brittle" type 1; or in any diabetic on insulin or sulfonylurea who neglects monitoring. Daytime hypoglycemic symptoms: sweating, nervousness, tremor, and hunger. Nighttime hypoglycemia may be asymptomatic or may cause night sweats, unpleasant dreams, or early morning headache. Earliest autonomic symptom of hypoglycemia is hunger when glucose is below 65 to 70 mg/dL. Other symptoms: irritability, anxiety, heart palpitations, pallor, and sweating. Neuroglycopenic symptoms, when the brain becomes starved of glucose: blurry vision, headache, fatigue, abnormal behavior, slurred speech, unconsciousness, and seizures. Treatment of hypoglycemia follows the 15 to 15 rule: ingest 15 g of starch or sugar source and recheck glucose in 15 minutes. If glucose is still below 80 mg/dL, ingest another 15 g of carbohydrate and recheck glucose in an hour. If glucose sinks below 55 mg/dL, the patient will need help from another person. When it is below 20 mg/dL, seizure is likely and glucagon should be injected. The patient should record any hypoglycemic events and report them to the physician.

- **DKA:** most commonly seen in patients with newly diagnosed T1DM when they have infections, when they have deliberately or accidentally omitted their insulin, and under other circumstances—trauma, myocardial infarction or stroke, surgery, dental abscess, and other physiologic stress. Lack of insulin leads to extremely high blood glucose and a buildup of acidic ketone molecules as fat stores are burned to provide energy. If progressive, ketoacidosis can lead to metabolic problems, coma, or death. Ketoacidosis is a medical emergency; prompt recognition is imperative. Instruct patients to check for ketones in urine or blood when glucose is above 250 mg/dL for more than a few hours, if they are feverish or have an infection, if they feel unwell, and regularly during pregnancy, because DKA is usually fatal to the fetus. Symptoms of DKA: fruity breath, disorientation, abdominal tenderness, polyuria and polydipsia, hyperventilation, and signs of dehydration. Treatment of DKA depends on severity of the situation and glucose level—it can require injecting insulin, eating, or referral to an emergency department.
- **Nonketogenic hyperosmolar hyperglycemia:** in T2DM with some insulin production or in T1DM on inadequate insulin for acute situation. It evolves over days with severe dehydration and electrolyte (sodium, potassium) disturbance. If patient is comatose, mortality rate is greater than 50%. Cause is profound dehydration from deficient fluid intake or precipitating events (pneumonia, burns, stroke, recent surgery, certain drugs [phenytoin, diazoxide, glucocorticoids, and diuretics]). Onset is insidious over period of days or weeks; symptoms include weakness, polyuria and thirst, and worsening signs of dehydration (weight loss, loss of skin elasticity, dry mucous membranes, tachycardia, hypotension). This condition is completely preventable by regular monitoring during illness or stress.
- **Hyperosmolar hyperglycemic state (HHS):** occurs mostly in older T2DM patients, usually in seventh decade of life. It develops gradually over days to weeks. There is no ketoacidosis in HHS, but it has a higher mortality because it occurs in patients with other serious problems—acute illness, recent surgery, congestive heart failure, renal dysfunction, or cardiovascular disease—or who are taking certain drugs, are victims of elder abuse or neglect, or are noncompliant with diabetic therapy. Diagnostic criteria: glucose level above 600 mg/dL, profound dehydration, other changes in pH, and some alteration in consciousness. Symptoms: drowsiness, coma, visual changes, sensory deficits, and even paralysis or

seizures. HHS is a medical emergency; transport patient to emergency department. Injecting insulin can cause severe complications; hospital care is best.

Long-Term Complications

More common than acute complications are long-term ones. Primary areas of the body affected most by diabetic complications: eyes, kidneys, nerves, and endothelial lining. These four areas do not require insulin to absorb glucose into their cells, as do the liver, muscle, and fat cells. When glucose is elevated in uncontrolled DM, unregulated glucose floods those cells and causes increased glycation and buildup of sorbitol.

Contributing factors include the following:

- **Poor glucose control:** glycemic control reduces risk of complications—retinopathy (up to 76%), nephropathy (up to 56%), neuropathy (up to 60%). Keep HbA_{1c} at 7.0% or less.
- **Glycosylation of proteins:** changing structure and function of proteins deactivates enzymes, inhibits regulatory molecule binding, and forms abnormal protein structures. Glucose binds to low-density lipoprotein (LDL), blocking its binding to liver receptors that signal cessation of cholesterol synthesis. Antioxidants, such as vitamins C and E, flavonoids, and alpha-lipoic acid, help reduce glycosylation.
- **Sorbitol accumulation:** sorbitol is a sugar molecule formed from glucose within cells. In nondiabetics, sorbitol is quickly converted into fructose to allow excretion from the cell. Intracellular sorbitol accumulation creates an osmotic effect that forces damaging leakage of amino acids, inositol, glutathione, niacin, vitamin C, magnesium (Mg), and potassium. These losses increase susceptibility to damage. Sorbitol buildup is a major cause of complications. Ascorbate and flavonoids (quercetin, grapeseed extract, and bilberry extract) help lower intracellular sorbitol.
- **Oxidative damage:** elevated free radicals and oxidative compounds destroy cellular compounds and increase inflammatory mediators (C-reactive protein).
- **Nutrient deficiency:** risk of complications is inversely proportional to micronutrient status. Symptoms of deficiency can mimic long-term complication of diabetes. (Vitamin B_{12} deficiency or dysmetabolism causes numbness, pins-and-needles sensation, or a burning feeling in the hands and/or feet—virtually identical to DM neuropathy.)

- **Homocysteine:** elevation is an independent risk factor for cardiocerebrovascular disease. In DM, homocysteine is linked to retinopathy.
- **Hypertension:** more than half of all diabetics have hypertension. A single layer of endothelial cells lining all blood vessels acts as the interface between blood components and blood vessels that regulates blood flow, coagulation, and formation of compounds controlling blood pressure. These cells are damaged by oxidized LDL and free radicals.

Specific Complications

- **Atherosclerosis:** major feature in many chronic complications. Diabetics have a fourfold to sixfold higher risk of dying prematurely of atherosclerosis than do nondiabetics; 55% of deaths in diabetics are caused by cardiovascular disease. The majority of those with T2DM have hypertension, and many of the diet and lifestyle habits of diabetics—eating poorly and not exercising—combined with nutrient deficiencies accelerate cardiovascular pathogenesis. Lesions in microvasculature reduce oxygen and nutrient supply to nerves, eyes, kidneys.
- **Diabetic retinopathy:** leading cause of blindness in the United States between ages 20 and 64 years. The retina is damaged by microhemorrhages, scarring, and glycosylation of proteins. Within 20 years of diagnosis, 80% of type 1 and 20% of type 2 diabetics have significant retinopathy. Diabetics are prone to cataracts.
- **Diabetic neuropathy:** loss of peripheral nerve function with tingling, numbness, loss of function, and burning pain (neuropathic pain). First comes a loss of sensation in the hands and feet ("stocking-glove" neuropathy). Elsewhere, DM affects autonomic nerves of the GI tract, causing diarrhea, constipation, and/or gastroparesis. Progression deeper to autonomic nerves disturbs stomach emptying and heart function; results in alternating diarrhea and constipation and inability to empty the bladder. Impotence is a common effect caused by damage to microvasculature of penis and neuropathy of autonomic nerves controlling penile blood flow. Sixty percent of diabetics eventually develop neuropathy. Main problem of peripheral neuropathy: lack of feeling in feet can result in development of unfelt sores or lesions that then ulcerate, leading to gangrene and amputation.

- **Diabetic nephropathy:** 40% of cases of severe nephropathosis and most common reason for hemodialysis and kidney transplant. It is a leading cause of death in DM. Monitor kidney function by laboratory tests: microalbuminuria, 24-hour urine protein, blood urea nitrogen (BUN), uric acid, creatinine, creatinine clearance, glomerular filtration rate). Angiotensin-converting enzyme (ACE) inhibitors or angiotensin II receptor blockers (ARBs) are part of standard care because they protect kidneys from diabetic damage.
- **Poor wound healing and foot ulcers:** poor wound healing and foot ulcers are common. Microvascular damage impairs circulation, causing functional deficiency of vitamin C and immune dysfunction that allows chronic foot infections. Fifty percent of lower limb amputations in the United States (70,000 yearly) are the result of DM foot ulcers.
- **Immune system dysfunction:** begins long before DM diagnosis. Recurrent vaginal or skin yeast infection is the clue. Serious infections or complications of simple infections are a risk, such as secondary pneumonia during influenza. Chronic, hidden infections induce cardiovascular disease. C-reactive protein, a biomarker of inflammation, is often elevated in diabetics.
- **Depression and cognitive difficulties:** common in diabetics. Depression may begin decades before onset of T2DM. Brain is sensitive to glycemic levels and may suffer from deprivation linked to insulin resistance. Depression is common in the overweight and obese because of insulin resistance and diminished self-esteem. Cognitive changes begin after severe hypoglycemic episodes stressful to the brain; repeated severe hypoglycemia can cause cognitive impairment. Glycemic awareness training with frequent monitoring and new insulins can optimize control. Uncontrolled DM is linked to a fourfold increased risk for Alzheimer's disease.

Contributors to Long-Term Complications of Diabetes

- **Poor glucose control:** good blood glucose control reduces development of complications.
- **Glycosylation of proteins:** the poorer the glucose control, the greater the binding of glucose to proteins, changing their structure and function. Examples include inactivation of enzymes, inhibition of regulatory molecule binding, and formation of abnormal protein structures. When glucose binds to low-density–lipoprotein cholesterol (LDL-C), glucose blocks

LDL from docking with liver receptors that signal cessation of cholesterol synthesis. Thus liver cell synthesis of cholesterol continues unabated, causing diabetics to have high cholesterol levels. High intakes of antioxidants—vitamins C and E, flavonoids, and alpha-lipoic acid—help to reduce glycosylation.

- **Intracellular accumulation of sorbitol:** sorbitol is a sugar molecule formed from glucose within cells. In nondiabetics, sorbitol is quickly broken down into fructose, which is excreted from cells; sorbitol cannot exit cells. If sorbitol levels rise within cells, sorbitol induces an osmotic effect. Cells then leak small molecules such as amino acids, inositol, glutathione, niacin, vitamin C, Mg, and potassium to maintain osmotic balance. Yet these compounds normally protect cells, so their loss increases susceptibility to damage. Accumulation of sorbitol is a major factor in most complications of DM within affected cells—eye lens, nerve cells, kidney cells, and blood vessel endothelium. Vitamin C and flavonoids (quercetin, grapeseed extract, and bilberry extract) help lower intracellular sorbitol. Sorbitol accumulation has nothing to do with eating foods that contain sorbitol.
- **Increased oxidative damage:** major factor in chronic complications of DM. Reactive oxidative compounds bind to and destroy cellular compounds and increase insulin resistance. They increase inflammation by increasing inflammatory mediators—C-reactive protein, interleukin-6, and tumor necrosis factor-alpha. High intake of antioxidants counteracts free radicals and prooxidants.
- **Nutrient deficiency:** deficiency of certain nutrients contributes to several chronic complications of DM. For example, insulin resistance or inadequate insulin results in vitamin C not being transported into cells. Supplements help diabetics control glucose; they also lower blood pressure and reduce diabetic complications. Risk of long-term complications is inversely proportional to micronutrient status. Symptoms of nutrient deficiency can mimic those of a DM complication. High-potency multivitamin-mineral is critical.
- **Elevated homocysteine:** constitutes independent risk factor for heart attack, stroke, peripheral vascular disease, and long-term complications, especially retinopathy.
- **Hypertension:** blood pressure control is essential in preventing renal disease, retinopathy, and stroke.
- **Endothelial cell dysfunction:** single layer of endothelial cells lines all blood vessels, serving as a metabolically active interface

between blood components and blood vessels. These cells help regulate blood flow by influencing coagulation, clot formation, blood pressure, and formation of regulatory compounds. Endothelial cells are susceptible to damage by oxidized LDL-C and other free radicals—hence the need for antioxidants.

THERAPEUTIC CONSIDERATIONS

- **Diet therapy:** strictly avoid foods with a high GL. Rigorous sugar and starch discipline is required for glycemic and A_{1c} control. Achieve and maintain ideal body weight. Initially, GL may need to be no more than 20 per meal; space these meals 3 hours apart. High-fiber, low-GL diets are beneficial in both adults and children and in both T1DM and T2DM. Similar results occur in adults with T1DM, including pregnant women with T1DM. Low–glycemic index or low-GL diet is the most scientifically proven dietary support for T1DM. Diet alone can be effective as the sole intervention to treat and reverse T2DM. Treating T2DM begins with diet. A low–glycemic index or low-GL diet has the most scientifically proven benefit on blood sugar and DM sequelae, including cardiovascular risk and hypertension. Key goal: increase total fiber intake from foods to at least 50 g daily, especially soluble type.
- **Psychological support:** help patient deal with the diagnosis, develop a sense of empowerment, and make lifestyle changes. Analyze emotional aspects of DM and manage any negativity or sense of being overwhelmed—common in diabetics and impairing adherence to DM therapy. Consider the book *Diabetes Burnout: What to Do When You Can't Take It Anymore,* by William Polonsky. Cognitive therapy is effective for adolescents with T1DM, improving mood and glycemic control.
- **Stress management:** higher stress is linked to higher blood glucose in T1DM and T2DM. Stress response increases adrenaline and cortisol, which elevate blood sugar and blunt insulin response. Implement stress management such as relaxation training.
- **Exercise:** exercise is essential to prevent and manage DM and pre-DM states of glucose intolerance and syndrome X. Insulin sensitivity and glycemic control improve because of increased lean muscle mass and metabolism. Cardiovascular health, HDL, anxiety, depression, sexual function, confidence, self-esteem, and weight management improve. Types of exercises for DM: aerobic (walking, jogging, dancing, cycling, swimming), strength training (light to moderate weights three times weekly), and stretching (daily).

Nutritional and Herbal Supplements

Objectives: achieve ideal glycemic control and metabolic targets; reduce risk of complications. (1) Establish optimal nutrient status, (2) reduce postprandial glucose elevations, (3) improve insulin function and sensitivity, and (4) prevent nutritional and oxidative stress. Treatment requires careful integration of diet, lifestyle, and natural medicines. All type 1 and many type 2 diabetics require conventional treatments depending on adequacy of pancreatic output (C-peptide) and response to diet and lifestyle measures. The most important factor determining need for drugs and insulin is glycemic control.

Establish optimal nutritional status: nutrient-dense diet plus high-potency multiple vitamin-mineral supplement to improve glycemic control, reduce complications, and boost immune function. Whenever a diabetic adds significant nutrient, fiber, or botanical medicines to the protocol, glucose monitoring is needed because oral or injectable medicines may have to be reduced. A physician should be involved in all decisions regarding natural supplementation. Special supplements include the following:

- **Chromium (Cr):** component of glucose tolerance factor that works closely with insulin, facilitating glucose uptake into cells. Cr deficiency is a factor in DM, hypoglycemia, and obesity. Supplementing Cr decreases fasting glucose, improves glucose tolerance, lowers insulin, decreases total cholesterol and triglycerides, and increases HDL. Reversing Cr deficiency lowers body weight and increases lean body mass. Its effects are from increased insulin sensitivity. Cr produces meaningful improvements in glycemic control only in people who are Cr deficient. Cr has no recommended daily allowance (RDA), but at least 200 mcg q.d. is necessary for optimal sugar regulation. Diabetics should take 200 to 400 mcg q.d. Cr is depleted by refining of carbohydrates and lack of exercise. Cr polynicotinate, Cr picolinate, and Cr-enriched yeast are preferred. Cr picolinate in combination with biotin at 600 mcg and 2 mg, respectively, may help T2DM patients improve blood sugar control: fasting glucose dropped 10 mg/dL and HbA_{1c} dropped 0.54%. Improvements in blood lipids and atherogenic index scores may also manifest.
- **Vitamin C:** insulin enhances transport of vitamin C into cells. Many diabetics have intracellular deficiency despite usually adequate intake. Diabetics need extra ascorbate. A major function of vitamin C is the manufacture of collagen, the main protein substance of connective tissue. Vitamin C is vital for wound

repair, healthy gums, prevention of excess bruising, immune function, manufacture of certain neurotransmitters and hormones, and absorption and use of other nutritional factors. Chronic latent vitamin C deficiency causes increased bleeding tendency (increased capillary permeability), poor wound healing, microvascular disease, elevated cholesterol, and depressed immune function. Ascorbate reduces generation of compounds linked to DM complications, reduces hypertension, and improves arterial stiffness and blood flow. Doses ranging from 100 to 2000 mg q.d. reduce accumulation of sorbitol in RBCs of diabetics, independent of glycemic control, by inhibiting aldose reductase, the enzyme that converts glucose to sorbitol. It also inhibits glycosylation of proteins. Encourage vitamin C–rich foods that also contain flavonoids and carotenes, which enhance effects of vitamin C. Dietary sources of vitamin C include broccoli, peppers, potatoes, Brussels sprouts, and citrus fruits.

- **Vitamin E:** antioxidant protecting cell membranes, especially nerve cells. Vitamin E improves insulin action, prevents free radical damage to LDL and vascular lining, improves the functioning of blood vessels and endothelium, increases intracellular Mg, decreases C-reactive protein (biomarker of inflammation), increases glutathione (intracellular antioxidant), improves nerve impulse conduction, improves blood flow to eyes in diabetic retinopathy, improves kidney function, and normalizes creatinine clearance in diabetics with mild elevations. Diabetics require lifelong supplementation. Dose: 400 to 800 IU daily. Vitamin E may help those with haptoglobin (Hp) 2-2 genotype, a subgroup that includes 20% to 30% of the general population. Hp, a major antioxidant protein, is a determinant of cardiovascular events in T2DM diabetics. *HP* gene is polymorphic with two common alleles, 1 and 2. Hp 2 allelic protein product provides inferior antioxidant protection compared with the Hp 1 product. Vitamin E (400 IU/day) lowered rates of myocardial infarction, stroke, and cardiovascular death over 18 months. *Note:* In some patients with T2DM who were given 500 mg of alpha-tocopherol or mixed tocopherols daily, systolic blood pressure increased (6 to 7 mm Hg). Thus some patients may have hypertensive reactions. Monitor patients to rule out this negative effect. Patients who are Hp 2-2 should be strongly encouraged to avoid all sources of wheat. They are especially susceptible to increased gut permeability because Hp 2 is a precursor to zonulin.

- **Niacin and niacinamide (nicotinamide):** niacin (vitamin B_3)-containing enzymes are important in energy production; metabolism of fat, cholesterol, and carbohydrate; and the synthesis of many body compounds (sex and adrenal hormones). Niacin is an essential component of glucose tolerance factor. Niacinamide supplements may prevent T1DM and help restore beta cells or at least slow their destruction. Niacinamide prolongs non–insulin-requiring remission, lowers insulin, improves metabolic control, and increases beta-cell function. Niacinamide can induce complete resolution in some newly diagnosed type 1 diabetics. The main difference between positive and negative studies in recent-onset IDDM is older age and higher baseline fasting C-peptide in positive studies. The mechanism of action involves inhibition of macrophage- and interleukin-1–mediated beta-cell damage, inhibition of nitric oxide production, and antioxidant activity. Niacinamide (500 mg t.i.d.) improves C-peptide release and glycemic control in type 2 diabetics unresponsive to oral antihyperglycemic drugs alone. The daily dose of niacinamide is 25 mg/kg. Children use 100 to 200 mg q.d. Niacin lowers cholesterol safely and extends life.
- **Inositol hexaniacinate:** useful in T1DM and T2DM to lower hyperlipidemia. It lowers cholesterol and improves blood flow in intermittent claudication and improves sugar regulation and is much better tolerated than niacin. High-dose niacin can disrupt glucose control in diabetics; closely monitor glucose and discontinue if diabetic control worsens.
- **Vitamin B_6:** supplements protect against diabetic neuropathy. Vitamin B_6 inhibits glycosylation of proteins. Diabetics tend to be deficient in B_6. Longstanding DM or signs of peripheral nerve abnormalities indicate need for B_6. At 100 mg q.d., it is a safe and effective treatment for gestational diabetes. Dose in general is up to 150 mg q.d.
- **Mg:** Mg deficiency is common in diabetics and lowest in those with severe retinopathy. Mg may prevent DM retinopathy and heart disease. Mg (at 400 to 500 mg q.d.) improves insulin response and action, glucose tolerance, and fluidity of RBC membranes. RDA is 350 mg q.d. for men and 300 mg q.d. for women. Diabetics may need twice this amount. Emphasize dietary sources: tofu, legumes, seeds, nuts, whole grains, green leafy vegetables. Add 300 to 500 mg of Mg q.d. as aspartate or citrate. Supplement at least 25 mg B_6 q.d. and vitamin E to ensure entry of Mg into cells.

- **Zinc (Zn):** cofactor in 200 enzyme systems and involved in all aspects of insulin metabolism. Marginal deficiency is common in the elderly and diabetics, increasing susceptibility to infections, poor wound healing, diminished sense of taste or smell, skin disorders, and onset of DM. Zn is protective against beta-cell destruction and has antiviral effects. Diabetics excrete Zn excessively in urine. Supplements improve insulin levels in T1DM and T2DM. Sources: whole grains, legumes, nuts, and seeds. Dose for diabetics is 30 mg q.d.
- **Manganese (Mn):** cofactor in many enzymes of glucose control, energy metabolism, thyroid hormone function, and antioxidant enzyme superoxide dismutase. Mn deficiency in laboratory animals results in DM and offspring with pancreatic abnormalities or no pancreas at all. Diabetics have only half the Mn of normal persons. Daily dose for diabetics is 3 to 5 mg.
- **Biotin:** functions in manufacture and use of carbohydrates, fats, and amino acids. Biotin deficiency impairs sugar metabolism. It is synthesized in intestines by gut bacteria; vegetarian diet alters intestinal flora to enhance synthesis and promote absorption of biotin. Supplements enhance insulin sensitivity and increase activity of glucokinase, the enzyme in the first step of use of glucose by the liver. Glucokinase is low in diabetics. Dose of 16 mg biotin q.d. significantly lowers fasting glucose and improves glucose control in T1DM; in T2DM, similar effects occur at 9 mg biotin q.d. Biotin also helps treat diabetic neuropathy. Insulin use must be adjusted.
- **Omega-3 fatty acids from fish:** help lower lipids and blood pressure. They are anti-inflammatory and promote insulin sensitivity. Omega-3s are lacking in diet of diabetics. Foods that contain these oils: oily fish; walnuts; grass-fed beef; wild game; omega-3 eggs; and ground flax, hemp, and chia seeds. Omega-3s protect against heart disease in DM. At doses of 3 to 18 g/day (18% eicosapentaenoic acid [EPA] and 12% docosahexaenoic acid [DHA]), fish oil has no adverse effect on glycemic control. Insist on pharmaceutical-grade products that are guaranteed not to be rancid or to contain mercury, solvents, polychlorinated biphenyl (PCBs), or other toxins. Take fish oil at or near beginning of meals to avoid fishy aftertaste or burping. Combined total EPA plus DHA omega-3 supplementation should be 1100 to 1600 mg q.d.
- **Fiber supplements:** enhance glycemic control, decrease insulin, and reduce calories absorbed from food. To reduce postprandial

glucose, lower cholesterol, and promote weight loss, choose water-soluble fibers: glucomannan (from konjac root), psyllium, guar gum, defatted fenugreek seed powder, seaweed fibers (alginate and carrageenan), ground flaxseed, and pectin. With water, they form a gelatinous, viscous mass, which slows absorption of glucose, reduces calorie absorption, and induces satiety. Glucomannan has greatest viscosity, which is enhanced when combined with alginate and xanthan gum. Viscosity of soluble fiber is directly related to physiologic effects and benefits: decreased postprandial glycemia, increased insulin sensitivity, diminished appetite, weight control, improved bowel movements, and decreased cholesterol. Glucomannan lowers postprandial glucose by 20% and insulin secretion by 40% and produces whole-body insulin sensitivity index improvement of 50%, which is unequaled by any drug or natural product. Glucomannan–alginate–xanthan gum blend improves all aspects of syndrome X. PGX is a novel natural polysaccharide matrix composed of three natural compounds (glucomannan, alginate, and xanthan gum) combined in a proprietary process that leads them to coalesce and form an entirely new matrix with a viscosity three to five times higher than that of glucomannan alone. PGX reduces glycemic index of any food or beverage by 15% to 70% and also reduces postprandial blood glucose.

- **Natural glucosidase inhibitors:** alpha-glucosidases that line intestines to break down carbohydrates into absorbable glucose. Inhibiting these enzymes can diminish postprandial glucose and insulin. The drugs acarbose (Precose) and miglitol (Glyset) inhibit alpha-glucosidase but have side effects: flatulence, diarrhea, and abdominal discomfort. Superior natural alternatives are touchi or mulberry extract.
- **Touchi:** ancient Asian fermented soy product concentrated for alpha-glucosidase inhibitors. In type 2 diabetics, 300 mg touchi extract before each meal for 6 months reduced fasting glucose by 10 mg/dL or more in 80% of patients and HbA_{1c} by 0.5% or more in 60% of patients. It also mildly lowered triglycerides and cholesterol. No side effects have been observed and no GI complaints were noted.
- **Mulberry plant *(Morus indica):*** food for silkworms that has an alpha-glucosidase inhibitor and other compounds that improve glycemic control. At a dose of 3 g/day versus 1 tablet of glyburide (5 mg/day) for 4 weeks, mulberry lowers

fasting glucose 27% in diabetics; no significant differences were observed in the blood glucose between before and after glyburide. Mulberry acts as an antioxidant, reducing lipid peroxidation in RBC membranes, and decreases membrane cholesterol of type 2 diabetics. Mulberry is superior to glyburide.

Improve Insulin Function and Sensitivity

Achieve ideal body weight: follow dietary and lifestyle recommendations, including high-potency vitamin-mineral supplement. As needed, add one or combination of the following:

- ***Gymnema sylvestre:*** plant native to tropical forests of India that is effective in T1DM and T2DM. It enhances production or activity of insulin and promotes regeneration of pancreas beta cells. In T1DM, leaf extract reduces insulin requirements and fasting glucose and improves glycemic control. It improves glycemic control in T2DM, reducing hypoglycemic drug needs. Applied to the tongue, gymnemic acid blocks sensation of sweetness. Subjects who had *Gymnema* applied to the tongue ate fewer calories at meals compared with control subjects. *Gymnema* decreases cravings for carbohydrates and enables patients with T2DM to follow a lower-carbohydrate diet. Capsules or tablets do not produce the same effect. Dose: 200 mg (standardized to 24% gymnemic acid) b.i.d. No side effects reported; diabetics on insulin must monitor blood glucose because insulin doses may have to be decreased.
- ***Momordica charantia* (bitter melon, balsam pear)**: charantin is hypoglycemic constituent composed of mixed steroids more potent than the drug tolbutamide. Insulin-like constituent polypeptide, polypeptide P, lowers blood glucose when injected subcutaneously as insulin is into type 1 diabetics, with fewer side effects than insulin. Fresh juice and extract of unripe fruit lower blood sugar in clinical trials. Dose: 2 oz fresh juice.
- ***Panax quinquefolius* and *Panax ginseng:*** American ginseng is the most evidence-based herbal therapy for T2DM. Whole powdered American ginseng root at 3 g before each meal reduces postprandial glucose in T2DM. *P. ginseng* at 200 mg elevates mood, improves psychophysiologic performance, and reduces fasting glucose and body weight. It also improves HbA_{1c}, serum amino terminal propeptide concentrations, and physical activity.

- **Fenugreek seeds** *(Trigonella foenum-graecum):* active principles are special soluble fiber, alkaloid trigonelline, and 4-hydroxyisoleucine. It is helpful in T1DM and T2DM. Defatted seed powder at 50 g b.i.d. in T1DM reduces fasting glucose and improves glucose tolerance, with 54% reduction in 24-hour urinary glucose excretion and significant reductions in LDL, very-low-density lipoprotein (VLDL), and triglycerides. In type 2 diabetics, 15 g powdered seed soaked in water significantly reduced postprandial glucose during meal tolerance test. Type 2 diabetics on 1 g/day fenugreek seed extract for 2 months had improved blood glucose (fasting glucose dropped from 148.3 to 119.9 mg/dL) but with decreased insulin output, indicating improved insulin sensitivity.
- ***Allium cepa* and *Allium sativum*:** onions and garlic have blood sugar–lowering action. The active principles are sulfur-containing compounds allyl propyl disulfide (APDS) and diallyl disulfide oxide (allicin), respectively. Flavonoids may play a role. APDS lowers glucose by competing with insulin (also a disulfide) for insulin-inactivating sites in the liver, thereby increasing free insulin. ADPS in doses of 125 mg/kg given to fasting human beings drops blood glucose and increases serum insulin. Allicin at doses of 100 mg/kg has similar effect. Graded doses of onion extracts (1 mL of extract = 1 g whole onion) at levels found in diet (1- to 7-oz onion) reduce glucose in dose-dependent manner. Effects are similar in raw and boiled onion extracts; they also lower cholesterol and blood pressure. Garlic improves glycemic control, lowers cholesterol and blood pressure, and inhibits increases in fibrinogen.

Preventing Nutritional and Oxidative Stress

Diabetics have elevated damaging, proinflammatory free radicals and oxidative compounds. Flood the body with antioxidants to counteract negative effects of free radicals and pro-oxidants. Use flavonoid-rich extracts and alpha-lipoic acid.

- **Flavonoids:** Quercetin promotes insulin secretion and inhibits glycosylation and sorbitol accumulation. Bilberry and hawthorn extracts help diabetic retinopathy and microvascular abnormalities. Flavonoids increase intracellular vitamin C, decrease leakiness and breakage of small blood vessels, prevent easy bruising, promote wound healing, and provide immune system support. Sources: citrus fruits, berries, onions, parsley, legumes, green tea, red wine. Tissue affinity of flavonoids allows targeting of specific tissues. Identify most appropriate flavonoids for specific patient needs.

Flavonoids for Diabetes and Diabetic Complications

Flavonoid-Rich Extract	Daily Dose	Indication
Bilberry extract (25% anthocyanidins)	160-320 mg	Best choice in diabetic retinopathy or cataracts.
Ginkgo biloba extract (24% *Ginkgo* flavon glycosides)	120-240 mg	Best choice for most people older than 50 years. Protects brain and vascular lining. Very important in improving blood flow to the extremities, neuropathy, and foot ulcers.
Grapeseed extract or pine bark extract (95% procyanidolic oligomers)	150-300 mg	Systemic antioxidant; best choice for most people younger than 50 years, especially if retinopathy, hypertension, easy bruising, and poor wound healing are present. Also specific for the lungs, varicose veins, and protection against cardiovascular disease.
Green tea extract (60%-70% total polyphenols)	150-300 mg	Best choice in the early stage of type 1 diabetes or a family history of cancer.
Hawthorn extract (10% procyanidins)	150-300 mg	Best choice in cardiovascular disease or hypertension.
Milk thistle extract (70% silymarin)	100-300 mg	Best choice if showing signs of impaired liver function.
Mixed citrus flavonoids	1000-2000 mg	Least expensive choice but may not provide same level of benefit. Acceptable if no complication is present.
Quercetin	150-300 mg	Good choice if allergies, symptoms of prostate enlargement or bladder irritation, or eczema is also present.

- **Alpha-lipoic acid:** vitamin-like substance termed "nature's perfect antioxidant." It is efficiently absorbed, easily crosses cell membranes, quenches both water- and fat-soluble free radicals within cells and in intracellular spaces, and extends biochemical life of other antioxidants. It is an approved drug in Germany for diabetic neuropathy. Dose: 300 to 600 mg q.d. It improves glucose metabolism, improves blood flow to peripheral nerves, stimulates regeneration of nerve fibers, and increases insulin sensitivity.

Recommendations for Specific Long-Term Complications

The most important method for reducing risk of complications is achieving optimal glycemic control.

- **Elevated cholesterol:** key natural products are soluble fiber, garlic, and niacin (see chapter on atherosclerosis). Niacin at higher doses (at least 3000 mg q.d.) can impair glucose tolerance, but lower doses (1000 to 2000 mg q.d.) have not adversely affected glucose regulation. Niacin addresses all of the most common blood lipid abnormalities in T2DM—elevated triglycerides, decreased HDL, and preponderance of smaller, denser LDL particles—better than lipid-lowering drugs. Side effects of niacin: skin flushing, gastric irritation, nausea, liver damage. Risk of liver damage is pertinent. Diabetic patients who are overweight often develop fatty livers—as damaging as livers injured by alcoholism and hepatitis C. Fatty liver may facilitate fibrosis and cirrhosis. Niacin supplementation with a fatty liver may add extra stress. In overweight diabetics, be cautious with high-dose niacin. To reduce flushing, use timed-release formulas at bedtime or inositol hexaniacinate. Some people respond only to regular niacin. Dosage for regular niacin or inositol hexaniacinate: start with 500 mg at bedtime for 1 week; increase to 1000 mg the next week and 1500 mg the following week. Stay at 1500 mg for 2 months before checking the response. Adjust dose up or down depending on response. Administer timed-release niacin at 1500 mg at bedtime from the beginning. Check cholesterol, A_1, and liver function every 3 months.
- **Retinopathy and cataracts:** two forms: simple (bursting of blood vessels, hemorrhage, swelling) and proliferative (newly formed vessels, scarring, hemorrhage, retinal detachment). Laser photocoagulation treats proliferative retinopathy but is not indicated in milder forms. Key factor in prevention: maintaining optimal glycemic control. Monitor HbA_{1c} frequently. Use flavonoid-rich extracts that have affinity for blood vessels of the eye and improve circulation to the retina (bilberry, pine bark, grapeseed).
- **Neuropathy:** alpha-lipoic acid and Mg are important.
  - Gamma-linolenic acid (GLA) improves and prevents neuropathy. GLA bypasses disturbances in fatty acid conversion. Sources: borage, evening primrose, black currant oils. GLA at

480 mg/day for 1 year improved 16 parameters, including conduction velocities, hot and cold thresholds, sensation, tendon reflexes, and muscle strength, with better results among patients with better glucose control.

— Benfotiamine is a fat-soluble form of thiamine or vitamin B_1 that is more effective in raising blood thiamine levels (up to 120% to 240% versus regular thiamine). In diabetics, benfotiamine decreased advanced glycosylated end-product formation, decreased aldose reductase pathway, and reduced oxidative cellular damage. However, results in treatment of diabetic neuropathy and nephropathy with benfotiamine alone are modest. In patients with T1DM, 600 mg of benfotiamine plus 300 mg of alpha-lipoic acid produced better results in reducing the effects of hyperglycemia than benfotiamine alone.

— Capsaicin from cayenne pepper *(Capsicum frutescens)* blocks small pain nerve fibers by depleting substance P. Topical capsaicin relieves pain of neuropathy in 80% of patients. Apply over-the-counter 0.075% capsaicin cream b.i.d. to affected area. (Cover hand with plastic wrap to avoid capsaicin contacting eyes or mucous membranes.) Allow a few days to take effect. It will continue to work only with regular application.

- **Nephropathy:** high-protein diets strain kidneys forced to excrete more waste—nitrogenous byproducts of protein metabolism (ammonia and urea). A low-protein diet is required only for progressed nephropathy, but it is wise to modulate protein intake. Dietary water-soluble fibers are fermented by colon bacteria into short-chain fatty acids that fuel colonic cells and increase waste removal capabilities of the colon, acting as a "third kidney" collecting and excreting nitrogenous wastes from the blood. Vitamin C (1250 mg) and vitamin E (680 IU) q.d. for 4 weeks reduce elevated urinary albumin by 20% in type 2 diabetics, indicating retardation of nephropathy progression. If a patient has serious kidney failure, low-protein, low-potassium standard diet becomes necessary; unfortunately, that does not promote good glucose control, which can then worsen kidney function. Main critical goal: prevent end-stage renal disease from developing in the first place. Normalize blood pressure with drugs (ACE inhibitors in low doses) if necessary.
- **Poor wound healing:** any nutrient deficiency can impair wound healing. Key nutrients: vitamin C and Zn. Use high-potency

multiple vitamin-mineral formulas. Topical: pure (100%) *Aloe vera* gel, which contains vitamins C and E and Zn. Apply it to affected areas (not open wounds) b.i.d. or t.i.d. AmeriGel, featuring oak extract *(Quercus rubra)*, contains tannins including quercitannic acid, catechin, ellagitannin, and proanthocyanidin, which are readily absorbed into damaged skin.

- **Foot ulcers:** causative factors: lack of blood supply, poor wound healing, and peripheral neuropathy. Strategies: proper foot care—receiving care of nails and calluses by podiatrist, undergoing regular physician examinations of feet, avoiding injury, avoiding tobacco, improving local circulation. Keep feet clean, dry, warm. Wearing well-fitted shoes. Support circulation with regular exercise; avoid sitting with legs crossed or positions that compromise circulation; massage feet lightly upward. *G. biloba* and grapeseed extract support circulation.

THERAPEUTIC APPROACH

Although the information here has focused on T2DM, it is equally appropriate for T1DM, with the exception that the type 1 diabetic will always require insulin.

- **Step 1:** Thorough diagnostic workup. Investigate DM complications, diet, environment, lifestyle issues, glucose intolerance. Stay alert to early signs and symptoms of acidosis and hyperosmolar nonketogenic coma, and have patient hospitalized at the first signs.
- **Step 2:** Develop individualized diet, exercise, supplement program. Normalize weight.
- **Step 3:** Monitor carefully, especially if on insulin—symptoms, home glucose monitoring, HbA_{1c}. Alter drug dosages via prescribing physician as therapies take effect. *Note:* Under no circumstances should a patient suddenly stop taking diabetic drugs, especially insulin. According to current information, a T1DM patient will never be able to stop taking insulin.
- **Diet:** optimal healthy food diet. Avoid simple, processed, and concentrated sugars and starches. Stress high-fiber foods. Minimize fats. Encourage legumes, onions, garlic.

Supplementation for Type 1 Diabetes

- Depends on degree of glucose control as evidenced by self-monitored blood glucose and HbA_{1c} levels.

Recently Diagnosed Type 1 Diabetes Mellitus

- **Foundation supplements**
  - — High-potency multivitamin-multimineral.
  - — Fish oils: 1000 mg each of EPA and DHA q.d.
  - — Vitamin C: 500 to 1500 mg q.d.
  - — Vitamin E (mixed tocopherols): 400 to 800 IU q.d.
  - — Vitamin D: 4000 to 8000 IU q.d.
  - — Niacinamide: 25 to 50 mg/kg q.d.
  - — Green tea extract: children 6 years or younger, 50 to 150 mg; children 6 to 12 years, 100 to 200 mg; children older than 12 years and adults, 150 to 300 mg. Ensure polyphenol content of 80% and decaffeinated.
- **Level 1:** achievement of targeted blood glucose, HbA_{1c} below 7%, no lipid abnormalities, no signs of complications
  - — High-potency multivitamin-multimineral.
  - — Fish oils: 600 mg each of EPA and DHA q.d.
  - — Vitamin C: 500 to 1500 mg q.d.
  - — Vitamin E (mixed tocopherols): 400 to 800 IU q.d.
  - — Alpha-lipoic acid: 400 to 600 mg q.d.
  - — Grapeseed, pine bark, or green tea extract (or other appropriate flavonoid-rich extract): 100 to 300 mg q.d.
- **Level 2:** failure to achieve targeted blood glucose levels, HbA_{1c} above 7%
  - — Level 1 supplements plus:
    - *G. sylvestre* extract (24% gymnemic acid): 200 mg b.i.d.
    - Biotin: 8 mg b.i.d.
    - Optional: bitter melon juice: 2 to 4 oz q.d.

Supplementation for Type 2 Diabetes

Depends on degree of glucose control as evident by self-monitored blood glucose and HbA_{1c}.

- **Level 1:** achievement of targeted blood glucose and HbA_{1c} levels less than 7%, no lipid abnormalities, no signs of complications
  - — High-potency multivitamin-multimineral
  - — Greens drink: one serving a day
  - — Fish oils: 600 mg each of EPA and DHA q.d.
  - — Vitamin C: 500 to 1500 mg q.d.
  - — Vitamin E: 400 to 800 IU q.d.
  - — Grapeseed, pine bark, or green tea extract (or other appropriate flavonoid-rich extract): 100 to 150 mg q.d.
  - — Alpha-lipoic acid: 400 to 600 mg q.d.

  - PGX (glucomannan, or other soluble fiber source at equivalent dosage to PGX): 2500 to 5000 mg before meals
- **Level 2:** failure to achieve targeted blood glucose levels, HbA_{1c} above 7%
  - Level 1 support plus:
    - One of the following insulin enhancers:
      - *G. sylvestre* extract (24% gymnemic acid): 200 mg b.i.d.
      - Fenugreek extract: 1 g q.d.
      - Garlic: minimum of 4000 mcg of allicin q.d.
    - One of the following glucosidase inhibitors:
      - Touchi extract: 300 mg t.i.d. with meals
      - Mulberry extract: equivalent to 1000 mg dried leaf t.i.d.

If self-monitored blood glucose levels do not improve after 4 weeks of following the recommendations for the current level, move to the next highest level. For example, if the patient starts out having an HbA_{1c} of 8.2% and fasting blood glucose of 130 mg/dL, he or she should start on level 2 support. After 4 weeks, if the average reading has not dropped to less than 110 mg/dL, a prescription medication (either an oral hypoglycemic drug or insulin) will be required.

Additional Supplements for the Prevention and Treatment of Diabetic Complications

For High Cholesterol and Other Cardiovascular Risk Factors

Total cholesterol greater than 200 mg/dL or LDL cholesterol greater than 135 mg (100 mg if history of heart attack); HDL cholesterol less than 45 mg/dL; lipoprotein(a) greater than 40 mg/dL; or triglycerides greater than 150 mg/dL

- Niacin (or inositol hexaniacinate): 1000 to 2000 mg at bedtime
- Garlic: minimum of 4000 mcg of allicin q.d.

For Hypertension

- Garlic: minimum of 4000 mcg of allicin q.d.
- Coenzyme Q10: 100 to 200 mg q.d.
- Anti-ACE peptides from bonito: 1500 mg/day
- Take one of the following:
  - Hawthorn extract (10% procyanidins or 1.8% vitexin with 4% rhamnoside): 100 to 250 mg t.i.d.
  - Olive leaf extract (17% to 23% oleuropein content): 500 mg b.i.d.
  - Hibiscus: three 240-mL servings a day or an extract providing 10 to 20 mg anthocyanidins a day

For Diabetic Retinopathy

- Bilberry extract 160 to 320 mg daily, or grapeseed extract 150 to 300 mg q.d.

For Diabetic Neuropathy

- GLA from borage, evening primrose, or black currant oil: 480 mg q.d.
- Benfotiamine: 600 mg q.d.
- Capsaicin (0.075%) cream: applied to affected area b.i.d.

For Diabetic Nephropathy

- Follow aforementioned recommendations for high blood pressure unless kidney function falls below 40% of normal. Be cautious in recommending Mg and potassium supplements.
- Benfotiamine: 600 mg q.d.

For Poor Wound Healing

- *Aloe vera* gel: applied to affected areas q.d.

For Diabetic Foot Ulcers

- *G. biloba* extract 120 to 240 mg/day, or grapeseed extract 150 to 300 mg q.d.

Endometriosis

DIAGNOSTIC SUMMARY

- **Triad of symptoms:** dysmenorrhea, dyspareunia, infertility
- **Physical examination:** reveals one or more of the following: tenderness of the pelvic area and/or cul-de-sac, enlarged or tender ovaries, a uterus that tips backward and lacks mobility, fixed pelvic structures, adhesions
- **Pelvic ultrasounds:** detection and consistency of endometriomas
- **Definitive diagnosis:** laparoscopy or laparotomy visualizing pelvic endometrial implants

GENERAL CONSIDERATIONS

- Endometriosis affects 10% to 15% of menstruating women aged 24 to 40 years.
- Main risk factor is heredity—a mother or sister with endometriosis. Other risk factors include shorter menstrual cycles; longer duration of flow; lack of exercise from an early age; high-fat diet; intrauterine device use; estrogen imbalance; natural red hair color; personal history of abuse; pelvic immune action with antibody to sperm; immune dysfunction; prenatal exposure to estrogens, xenoestrogens, endocrine disruptors (polychlorinated biphenyls [PCBs], weed killers, plastics, detergents, household cleaners, aluminum can liners), or dioxin; liver dysmetabolism of estrogens.
- Based on latest evidence, lack of proper immune surveillance in pelvic area causes endometriosis; impairment in other aspects of immune function are involved in progression of disease. Both types of immunity, cell-mediated and humoral, are implicated in endometriosis. Cytokines, macrophages, T lymphocytes, and tumor necrosis factors are elevated in peritoneal fluid in women with endometriosis, and level of elevation correlates with severity of disease. Growth factors, angiogenic factors, and lipid peroxidation in peritoneal fluid may stimulate endometrial cell growth. Targeting these proinflammatory compounds and blocking their action with antioxidants are aspects of treatment strategies.

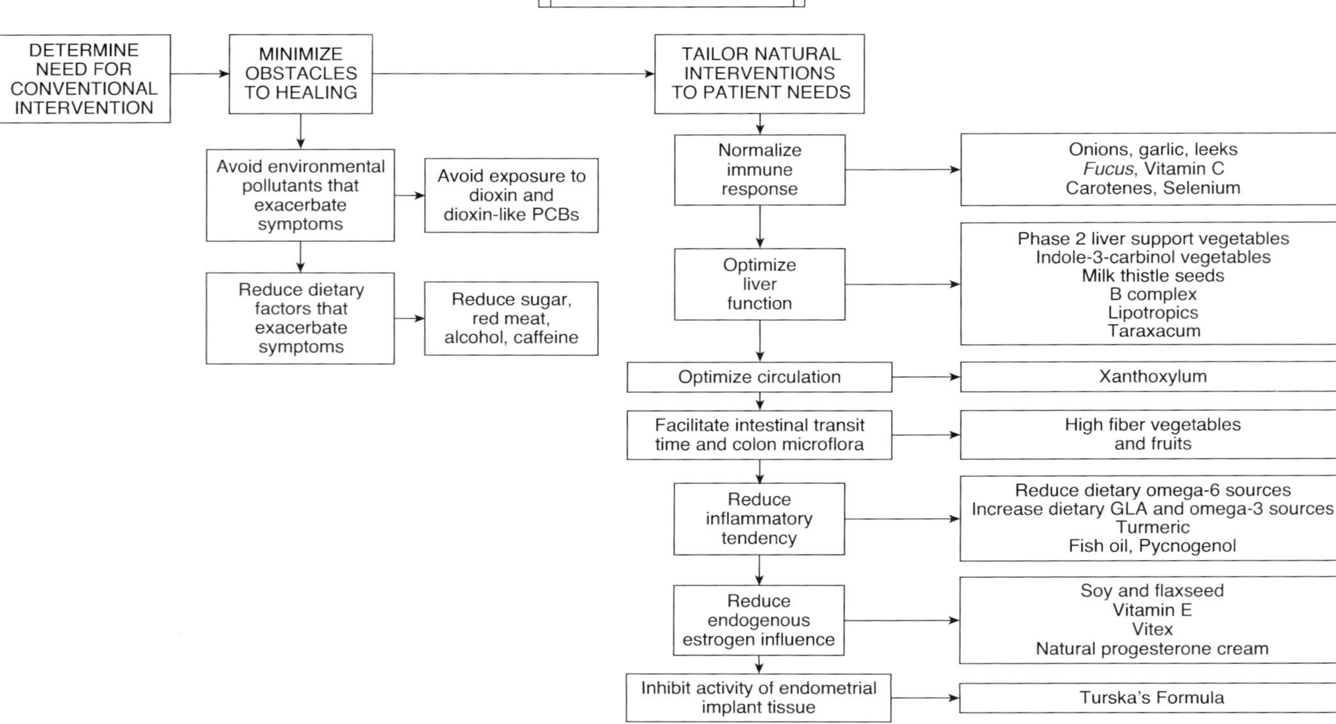
ENDOMETRIOSIS
DETERMINE NEED FOR CONVENTIONAL INTERVENTION
MINIMIZE OBSTACLES TO HEALING
Avoid environmental pollutants that exacerbate symptoms
Avoid exposure to dioxin and dioxin-like PCBs
Reduce dietary factors that exacerbate symptoms
Reduce sugar, red meat, alcohol, caffeine
TAILOR NATURAL INTERVENTIONS TO PATIENT NEEDS
Normalize immune response
Onions, garlic, leeks
Fucus, Vitamin C
Carotenes, Selenium
Optimize liver function
Phase 2 liver support vegetables
Indole-3-carbinol vegetables
Milk thistle seeds
B complex
Lipotropics
Taraxacum
Optimize circulation
Xanthoxylum
Facilitate intestinal transit time and colon microflora
High fiber vegetables and fruits
Reduce inflammatory tendency
Reduce dietary omega-6 sources
Increase dietary GLA and omega-3 sources
Turmeric
Fish oil, Pycnogenol
Reduce endogenous estrogen influence
Soy and flaxseed
Vitamin E
Vitex
Natural progesterone cream
Inhibit activity of endometrial implant tissue
Turska's Formula

- **Genetic influences:** abnormalities in detoxification enzymes, tumor suppressor genes, and other genetic factors occurring in multistep fashion may be involved in development and progression of disease.
- Endometriosis can cause infertility and miscarriage, producing excess free radicals involved in implantation. Endometriomas (ectopic endometrium on ovaries) are found in two thirds of endometriosis patients. Infertility may cause endometriosis from tubal scarring, adhesions, unruptured follicles.

DIAGNOSTIC CONSIDERATIONS

- **Symptoms begin at onset of menstruation or later,** worsening with time. Triad of symptoms: dysmenorrhea, dyspareunia, infertility. Features include acute pain before menses, lasting a day or two during menses or throughout the month; vomiting; diarrhea; fainting concurrent with pelvic or abdominal cramping and labor-like pains; chronic bearing-down pain; pressure on low back; pains radiating down legs; pain with urination or bowel movements; bleeding from nose, bladder, or bowels; fatigue. There is no correlation between pain intensity and extent of disease. Women with fixed ovaries and large endometriomas may report only mild discomfort, whereas those with smaller lesions may report severe chronic pain. These might be more influenced by circulating estrogens. Severity of symptoms is correlated with depth of lesions rather than number of lesions.
- **Curious feature:** pain and extent of disease correlate poorly. Symptom severity correlates with depth of lesions rather than number of lesions.
- **Physical examination:** one or more of the following: tenderness in pelvic area and/or cul-de-sac; enlarged or tender ovaries; uterus that tips backward and lacks mobility; fixed pelvic structure; adhesions. Other findings include endometrial tissue or surgical scar tissue in vagina or on cervix. Examination during the first or second day of menses: tender septum between rectum and vagina.
- **Pelvic ultrasound:** useful assessing pain and tumors but not definitive; detects mass on ovary; determines size, characteristics, consistency of endometriosis. Blood test CA 125 can be positive in endometriosis but cannot distinguish endometriosis, fibroids, malignancies, and even normal tissue.

- **Definitive diagnosis:** biopsy by laparoscopy or laparotomy of visualized tissue.
- **Estrogens stimulate growth of implants:** therapy manipulating endogenous hormones may be effective.

THERAPEUTIC CONSIDERATIONS

No single theory explains development of endometriosis in all cases. It probably stems from a combination of postulated mechanisms with variable influences from case to case. Therapeutic plans may vary, targeting one or more mechanisms.

Diet

- **Objectives:**
  - — Reduce inflammatory foods and increase anti-inflammatory foods
  - — Enhance detoxification mechanisms
  - — Increase dietary fiber to promote optimal transit time and proper gut flora
  - — Increase omega-3 fatty acids and reduce *trans* fats
- **Fatty acids:** *trans* fats appears to increase risk of endometriosis; long-chain omega-3 fats appear to be protective. Although there is no proven link between total fat intake and endometriosis risk, women with highest intake of long-chain omega-3s were 22% less likely to be diagnosed with endometriosis compared with women with lowest intake of omega-3s. Those women with highest intake of *trans* unsaturated fats were 48% more likely to be diagnosed with endometriosis.
- **High-fiber foods** optimize intestinal transit time and balance friendly gut microflora that displace undesirable strains that deconjugate estrogens, allowing them to recirculate. Lower-protein, high-fiber organic vegetarian diet: decreases plasma active unconjugated estrogens; reduce intake of proinflammatory arachidonic acid. Vegetable protein, soy, nut butters (almond), salmon are preferred. Emphasize phase II liver support vegetables: carrots, beets, artichokes, lemons, dandelion greens, watercress, burdock root, cabbage family vegetables. Indole-3-carbinol, in broccoli, Brussels sprouts, cabbage, cauliflower, favors less-active estrogen metabolites. Onions, garlic, and leeks contain immunity-enhancing organosulfur compounds and bioflavonoids (quercetin) that protect against oxidation, block inflammation, and inhibit tumor growth.

- **Phytoestrogens:** soy isoflavones and flaxseed lignans help alleviate endometriosis symptoms. Moderate intake of soy isoflavones may decrease need for premenopausal hysterectomy for endometriosis.
- **Seasonings:** turmeric (curcumin) protects against environmental carcinogens, decreases inflammation, increases bile secretion. Milk thistle seeds, soaked and ground, help liver function. Fresh flaxseeds increase anti-inflammatory fatty acids. *Fucus* (seaweed) stimulates T-cell production and absorbs toxins.
- **Decrease** sugar, caffeine, dairy, red meat, alcohol.

Nutritional Supplements

- **Vitamin C:** increases cellular immunity, decreases autoimmunity and fatigue, decreases capillary fragility and tumor growth.
- **Beta-carotene:** enhances immunity, increases T-cell levels, protects against early stages of tumor growth. Retinoids can moderate effects of interleukin-6, an inflammatory mediator implicated in endometriosis. One third of beta-carotene is converted to vitamin A (retinol). Immune function is from carotenoids rather than vitamin A. However, a significant portion of the population poorly converts beta-carotene to vitamin A, so supplemental vitamin A is still often needed to ensure proper immune function.
- **Vitamin E:** helps correct abnormal progesterone/estradiol ratios in patients with mammary dysplasia (increased growth of cells), which parallels abnormal growth of lesions in endometriosis. It inhibits the arachidonic lipid pathway, preventing release of inflammatory chemicals. Free radicals may contribute to inflammation and excessive growth of endometrial tissue; vitamin E and *N*-acetylcysteine, another antioxidant, can act to inhibit this proliferation.
- **Pine bark (pycnogenol):** special standardized extract from bark of French maritime pine. Constituents: polyphenols, phenolic acids, catechins, taxifolin, procyanidins. Pycnogenol selectively inhibits matrix metalloproteinases; it inhibits cyclooxygenases 1 and 2. Women surgically diagnosed with endometriosis, with confirmed regular menstruation and ovulation for 3 months postsurgery, started pycnogenol within 6 months of surgery at 30 mg b.i.d. for 48 weeks or gonadotropin-releasing hormone agonist leuprorelin acetate depot, 3.75 mg intramuscularly, every 4 weeks for 24 weeks. After 4 weeks on pycnogenol, patients slowly but steadily improved to a 33% reduction in symptoms. The leuprorelin group had greater response within treatment

period but relapsed 24 weeks after treatment. Pycnogenol patients maintained regular menses and normal estrogen levels during treatment. Leuprorelin patients had suppressed menstruation and drastically lowered estrogens during treatment. Some women taking pycnogenol became pregnant.

- **Essential fatty acids:** Gamma-linolenic acid (in borage, black currant, evening primrose oil) and alpha-linolenic acid (in flaxseed, canola, pumpkin, soy, walnuts) help decrease tissue inflammatory responses by increasing noninflammatory prostaglandins. The higher the ratio of omega-6 to omega-3 fatty acids, the longer the survival time and secretion of interleukin-8 in cells from women with or without endometriosis. The cells from women with endometriosis secrete higher levels of interleukin-8, and the levels are proportionately higher at higher ratios of omega-6 to omega-3.
- **B vitamins:** help the liver inactivate estrogen. Supplementation may cause the liver to become more efficient in processing estrogen.
- **Selenium:** aids synthesis of liver detoxification antioxidant enzymes and stimulates white blood cells and thymus function. Selenium deficiency impairs cell-mediated immunity, decreases T cells, and promotes inflammation.
- **Lipotropics:** enhance liver function and detoxification reactions. Choline, betaine, and methionine promote bile flow that facilitates excretion of estrogen metabolites.

Botanical Medicines

Use same herbs as for menstrual cramps: valerian, cramp bark, black cohosh.

- ***Vitex agnus-castus* (chaste tree):** treats hormone imbalances in women, acting on the pituitary to increase luteinizing hormone, which stimulates progesterone production. Uses: reducing estrogen excess linked to fibroids, premenstrual syndrome, perimenopause, symptoms of endometriosis.
- ***Taraxacum officinale* (dandelion root):** supports liver and gallbladder detoxification efforts to expel wastes and deactivate excess estrogens. Dandelion may have antitumor activity. Dandelion leaf contains vitamins A, C, and K; calcium; and lipotropic choline.
- ***Zanthoxylum americanum* (prickly ash):** treats capillary engorgement and sluggish circulation. It stimulates blood flow body-wide, enhancing oxygen and nutrient transport and removal of cellular wastes. It relieves pelvic congestion by enhancing pelvic circulation.

- *Leonurus* **(motherwort):** antispasmodic that gently soothes nerves. To alleviate uterine cramps and pain, it promotes relaxation during extreme bearing-down uterine or pelvic pain. It is a mild sedative for needed rest during menstrual cramps.
- **Turska's formula:** old naturopathic treatment for decreasing aberrant cancer cell growth, useful in endometriosis because of similarities to pelvic cell growth. Ingredients include monkshood *(Aconite napellus),* yellow jasmine *(Gelsemium sempervirens),* bryony *(Bryonia alba),* and poke root *(Phytolacca americana).* Monkshood and yellow jasmine alkaloids disrupt assembly of microtubules of undifferentiated mesenchymal cells and abnormal ectopic pelvic lesions. Bryony provides antitumor effects. Poke root glycoproteins stimulate lymphocyte transformation for immune enhancement and have anti-inflammatory properties. Tinctures of this formula are toxic if misused.

Other Considerations

- **Natural progesterone:** progesterone modifies the action of estradiol by decreasing retention of receptors and diminishing serum estradiol. Progesterone insufficiency causes estrogen excess imbalance. Progesterone sedates painful uterine contractions and relieves entire pelvic region. Natural progesterone is not used alone but as part of a comprehensive plan. For some women, cream preparations are applied—{¼} teaspoon t.i.d. for 3 weeks on and 1 week off (week off is week of menses). Others need it only the week before menses. And others require higher doses of natural oral micronized progesterone in a cyclic administration pattern.

THERAPEUTIC APPROACH

Diet

Increase high-fiber fruits and vegetables. Decrease omega-6 fatty acids (domesticated land animal products). Increase omega-3 fatty acids (wild fish, flax). Increase indole-3-carbinol (broccoli, Brussels sprouts, cabbage, cauliflower). Limit caffeine.

Supplements

- **Vitamin C:** 6 to 10 g q.d. in divided doses
- **Beta-carotene:** 50,000 to 150,000 international units (IU) q.d.
- **Vitamin E:** 400 to 800 IU q.d. (mixed tocopherols)

- **Fish oil:** 1000 mg EPA plus DHA q.d.
- **Vitamin B complex**: 50 to 100 mg q.d.
- **Selenium:** 200 to 400 mcg q.d.
- **Lipotropics:** 1000 mg choline and 1000 mg methionine or cysteine t.i.d.
- **Pycnogenol:** 60 to 150 mg q.d.

Botanical Medicines

- Chaste tree, dandelion root, prickly ash, and motherwort tincture (equal parts): {½} tsp to 1 tsp. t.i.d.
- Turska's formula (*Aconite* 1{½} drams plus *Bryonia* 1{½} drams plus *Gelsemium* 1{½} drams plus *Phytolacca* 3 drams plus {½} dram water): 5 drops q.i.d.
- Topical progesterone cream:
  - Option 1
    - Days 1 to 7, no cream
    - Days 8 to 28, {¼} to {½} tsp b.i.d.
  - Option 2
    - Days 1 to 14, no cream
    - Days 15 to 28, {¼} to {½} tsp b.i.d.
  - Option 3
    - Days 1 to 21, no cream
    - Days 22 to 28, {¼} to {½} tsp b.i.d.

Epilepsy

DIAGNOSTIC SUMMARY

- Recurrent seizures
- Characteristic electroencephalographic changes accompanying seizures
- Mental status abnormalities or focal neurologic symptoms may persist for hours postictally

GENERAL CONSIDERATIONS

Epilepsy is not a disease in itself, but a symptom of disease. Epilepsy describes a group of disorders characterized by sudden, recurrent, and episodic changes in neurologic function caused by abnormalities in electrical activity of the brain. An episode of neurologic dysfunction is called a *seizure.* Seizures are termed *convulsive* when accompanied by motor manifestations and *nonconvulsive* when accompanied by sensory, cognitive, or emotional events. Epilepsy can result from many abnormalities: neural injuries, structural brain lesions, systemic diseases. It is termed *idiopathic* when neither history of neural insult nor other apparent neural dysfunction is present. The common denominator is the epileptic attack or seizure.

- **Epidemiology:** prevalence of chronic, recurrent epilepsy is 10 in 1000. Ten percent of the population will have seizure at some point in life. Cumulative lifetime incidence is 3%. From 2% to 5% of the population will have a nonfebrile seizure at some point in life; an additional 2% to 5% of children have febrile convulsions during the first several years of life. Ten percent of these children, especially with prolonged febrile seizures, have epilepsy later in life. Sixty percent of newly diagnosed patients enter remission with conventional treatment.
- **Genetic factors:** prevalence of seizures in close relatives is three times that of the overall population.

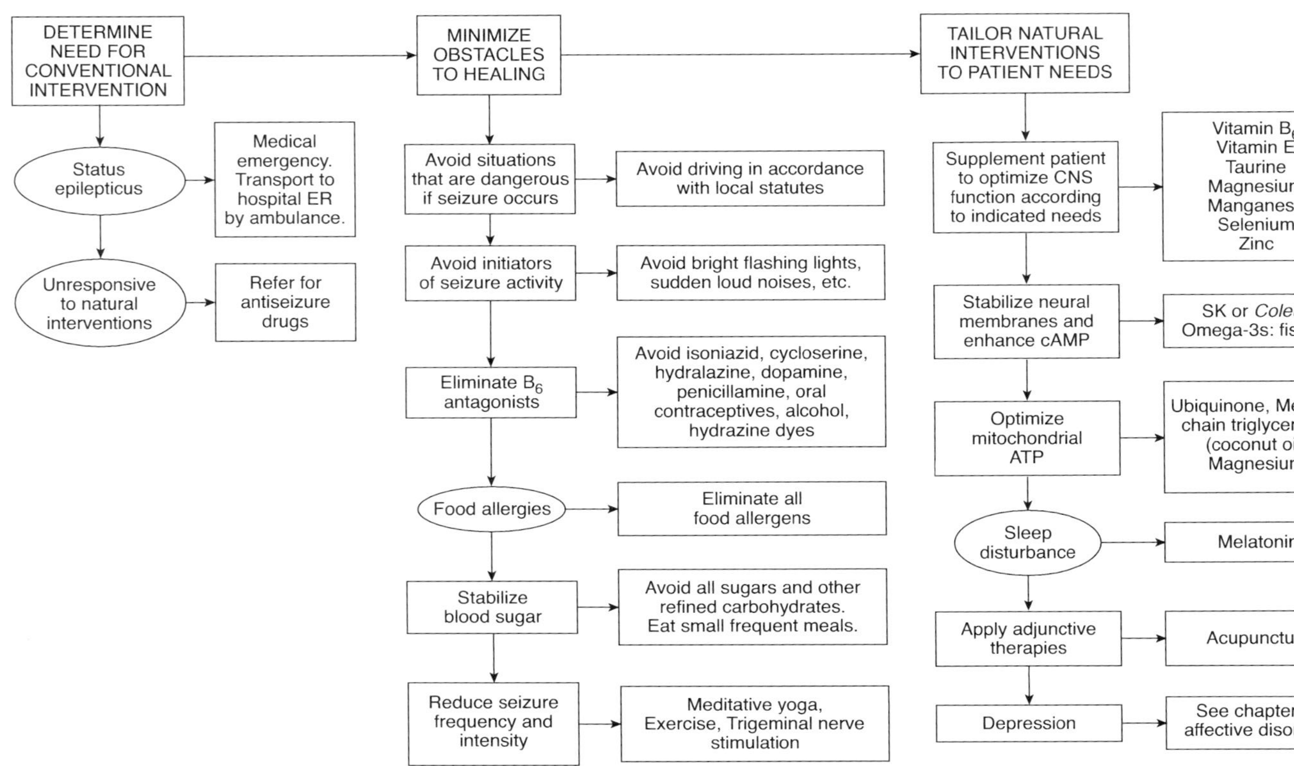
EPILEPSY
DETERMINE NEED FOR CONVENTIONAL INTERVENTION
Status epilepticus
Medical emergency. Transport to hospital ER by ambulance.
Unresponsive to natural interventions
Refer for antiseizure drugs
MINIMIZE OBSTACLES TO HEALING
Avoid situations that are dangerous if seizure occurs
Avoid driving in accordance with local statutes
Avoid initiators of seizure activity
Avoid bright flashing lights, sudden loud noises, etc.
Eliminate B6 antagonists
Avoid isoniazid, cycloserine, hydralazine, dopamine, penicillamine, oral contraceptives, alcohol, hydrazine dyes
Food allergies
Eliminate all food allergens
Stabilize blood sugar
Avoid all sugars and other refined carbohydrates. Eat small frequent meals.
Reduce seizure frequency and intensity
Meditative yoga, Exercise, Trigeminal nerve stimulation
TAILOR NATURAL INTERVENTIONS TO PATIENT NEEDS
Supplement patient to optimize CNS function according to indicated needs
Vitamin B6
Vitamin E
Taurine
Magnesium
Manganese
Selenium
Zinc
Stabilize neural membranes and enhance cAMP
SK or Coleus
Omega-3s: fish oil
Optimize mitochondrial ATP
Ubiquinone, Medium chain triglycerides (coconut oil)
Magnesium
Sleep disturbance
Melatonin
Apply adjunctive therapies
Acupuncture
Depression
See chapter on affective disorders

- **Etiology:** classified as symptomatic or idiopathic. Symptomatic means a probable cause can be identified. From 70% to 80% of cases are idiopathic.

Probable Causes Determined by Age of Onset

Age of Onset	Presumptive Causes
Birth to 2 yr	Birth injury, degenerative brain disease
2-19 yr	Congenital birth injury, febrile thrombosis, head trauma, infection (meningitis or encephalitis)
20-34 yr	Head trauma, brain neoplasm
35-54 yr	Brain neoplasm, head trauma, stroke
55 yr and older	Stroke, brain neoplasm

Common Causes of Seizures

- Brain damage before or at birth (congenital malformations, anemia, fetal infection)
- Head trauma injuring brain and gliosis
- Central nervous system infections (meningitis, encephalitis, brain abscess, neurosyphilis, rabies, tetanus, falciparum malaria, toxoplasmosis, cysticercosis of brain)
- Metabolic disorders (hypocalcemia, hypoglycemia, hypoparathyroidism, phenylketonuria, withdrawal from alcohol and drugs)
- Brain tumors and other space-occupying lesions
- Stroke and other vascular disorders
- Degenerative brain disease
- Genetic disease
- Toxic conditions
- Idiopathic

Classification

Classification is based on clinical and electroencephalographic criteria (International League Against Epilepsy).

Partial (Focal, Local) Seizures

- Simple partial seizures (consciousness not impaired)
  - — Motor signs
  - — Somatosensory or special sensory symptoms
  - — Autonomic symptoms or signs
  - — Psychic symptoms

- Complex partial (consciousness impaired)
  - Simple partial onset followed by impaired consciousness
  - Consciousness impaired at onset
- Partial seizures evolving to generalized seizures (tonic, clonic, or tonic-clonic)
  - Simple partial seizures evolving to generalized seizures
  - Complex partial seizures evolving to generalized seizures
  - Simple partial seizures evolving to partial seizures evolving to generalized seizures

Generalized Seizures (Convulsive or Nonconvulsive)

- Absence seizures
  - Typical (brief stare, eye flickering, no emotion)
  - Atypical (associated with movement)
- Myoclonic seizures
- Clonic seizures
- Tonic seizures
- Tonic-clonic seizures
- Atonic seizures
- Unclassified seizures

DIAGNOSIS

Differentiating between partial or focal seizures and generalized seizures is of great clinical significance. Partial seizures begin focally as a specific sensory, motor, or psychic aberration reflecting the affected part of the cerebrum. These seizures may remain localized. Generalized seizures affect consciousness and motor function. Partial seizures are indicative of focal brain disorders (e.g., tumors, gliosis). Generalized seizures rarely have a definable cause (perhaps metabolic disorders). Eyewitness account of the onset is valuable in classifying the seizure. Explore past trauma, infections, drugs, alcohol use, and family history. A complete neurologic examination is a preliminary screen for neoplasms. Epilepsy is not diagnosed from a solitary seizure; the recurrence rate after a single seizure is 27% over a 3-year period.

Diagnostic Workup

- Serum glucose and calcium
- Complete blood cell count
- Liver and kidney function tests
- Serologic test for syphilis

- Skull radiographs
- Electroencephalogram (EEG)
- Computed tomography (CT) scan
- Magnetic resonance imaging (MRI)

Cerebrospinal fluid examination is indicated if infection or meningeal neoplasm is suspected. MRI is the gold standard to investigate epilepsy; resolution is superior to computed tomographic scan. Electroencephalography during functional MRI maps normal and pathologic brain function.

PATHOPHYSIOLOGY

Hallmark of altered physiologic state of epilepsy is rhythmic, repetitive, synchronous discharge of many neurons in a localized brain area. Discharge pattern is recorded on EEG during attack. The cause of abnormal discharges is unknown. Synchronous depolarization of masses of neurons results from the combination of increased excitation and decreased inhibition. Gamma-aminobutyric acid (GABA) blockers are potent convulsants. Antiepileptic drugs (phenobarbital, benzodiazepines) enhance GABA. In some forms of chronic focal epilepsy, inhibitory terminals on neurons in areas around cortical gliotic lesions are diminished. Nerve cell membranes in epileptics are unstable; during seizures, stored intracellular calcium (Ca^{2+}) is released and moves toward inner cell membranes, binding to Ca^{2+}-receptive proteins, causing protein conformational changes. These changes trigger transmembranal Ca^{2+}, potassium (K^+), and sodium (Na^+) channels to remain open, potentiating excitation. Earliest symptoms (aura) generated by focal discharge are the best clue to localization and characterization of the responsible lesion.

THERAPEUTIC CONSIDERATIONS

Environmental Toxins

- **Heavy metals:** lead, mercury, cadmium, and aluminum induce seizures by disrupting neural function. Rule out heavy metal toxicity; hair mineral analysis is the most cost-effective screening method (*Textbook,* "Environmental Medicine" and "Metal Toxicity: Assessment of Exposure and Retention"). Urine analysis remains best method for quantifying stored heavy metals after administration of a chelating agent (e.g., calcium disodium ethylenediaminetetraacetic acid [EDTA], dimercaptosuccinic acid [DMSA], and/or

2,3-dimercapto-1-propanesulfonic acid [DMPS]). The protocol recommended is to collect first morning urine, which indicates current exposure; administer 500 mg of DMSA plus 300 mg of DMPS, and collect urine for 6 hours.

- **Neurotoxic chemicals:** many neuron-, axon-, and myelin-toxic chemicals are released into the ecosystem. Neurotoxins invade human tissues, instigating neurologic dysfunction. Minimize patient exposure and improve body's ability to eliminate neurotoxins. Explore possible exposure during detailed history taking (*Textbook,* "Environmental Medicine"). The most common source of neurotoxins is pesticides in conventionally grown foods. The 1000-fold variation in activity of liver detoxification enzymes helps explain individual susceptibility.

Dietary Considerations

- **Hypoglycemia:** important metabolic cause of seizures. Serum glucose is unusually low before a seizure. From 50% to 90% of epileptics have constant or periodic hypoglycemia. Seventy percent of epileptics have abnormal glucose tolerance test results. The correlation of glucose abnormalities and epilepsy is well documented, but the mechanism is unknown. Hypoglycemia may impair adenosine triphosphate (ATP) production in neurons, reducing efficacy of sodium (Na)–adenosine triphosphatase pump. Defective Na pump increases intracellular Na, depolarizing the cell membrane and lowering the firing threshold. Leptin is a factor that may help regulate occurrence of seizures. Injecting leptin reduces occurrence and severity of seizures. Low blood sugar results in low circulating leptin levels, leading to another possible mechanism of action. Single measurements of serum glucose are inadequate to determine glycemic status; extended glucose tolerance test is required.
- **Ketogenic diet (KD):** has a long history of use to reduce seizure activity. Components are large amounts of fat and minimal proteins and carbohydrates. Low carbohydrates inhibit fat metabolism, causing production of excess ketone bodies (acetone, acetoacetic acid, beta-hydroxybutyric acid), which are intermediary oxidation products. Beneficial effects are caused by metabolic acidosis, which corrects underlying tendency of epileptics toward spontaneous alkalosis. Acidification may normalize nerve conductivity, irritability, and membrane permeability. Another possible benefit of KD: augmenting ATP production by using ketone bodies in place of glucose. Many epileptics are

hypoglycemic, thus compromising mitochondrial ATP production. KD may provide an alternative route for balancing this deficit.

— Two types of KDs: classic ketogenic diet (CKD) and medium-chain triglyceride ketogenic diet (MCTKD). CKD limits carbohydrates and protein to less than 10% of calories combined. MCTKD diet uses medium-chain triglycerides to produce ketosis, allowing a larger intake of carbohydrates and protein. Forty percent of 27 children aged 1 to 16 years had a seizure reduction of more than 50%, with 25% becoming seizure free; 35% discontinued diet because of the difficulty following the rigorous guidelines. KD is effective in one third to one half of cases in children and partially effective in another third.

— Success rate of KD exceeds that of medications; KD is cheaper and has fewer side effects. Linear growth may be maintained or retarded, but body weight decreases in children on both diets because of inadequate energy intake. Protein intake is adequate. MCTKD resulted in a 0.7 decrease in ratio of total cholesterol to high-density–lipoprotein cholesterol at 4 months. Biochemical indexes, including albumin, were normal, but long-term studies are needed. MCTKD may be more nutritionally adequate. Long-term risks are associated with a high-fat diet, and it is unhealthy for a growing child.

— For children, recommend adequate calories and protein, a higher proportion of unsaturated to saturated fats; consider vitamin-mineral supplements. Do not allow children to eat very large meals, which predispose to seizures. Small, frequent meals may decrease hypoglycemia. Good long-term efficacy—on seizure frequency, EEG readings, and neurologic development—and tolerability of KD have been proven in pediatric drug-resistant epileptic patients.

— The Atkins diet also is ketogenic and is less restrictive on protein. The Atkins diet reduced intractable focal and multifocal epileptic seizures in a small pilot study.

Leptin

- Leptin is a protein hormone that helps regulate appetite and metabolism. Acting on receptors of hypothalamus, it inhibits hunger by counteracting effects of neuropeptide Y and anandamide, two powerful feeding stimulants.

- Leptins act on receptors that activate signaling proteins that reduce brain excitability and the frequency and intensity of seizures.
- Anticonvulsant action of leptin has been demonstrated in animal seizure models by either injecting leptin directly into the cortex or administering it intranasally. Theorized mechanism of action: leptin activates two signaling proteins—JAK2 (Janus kinase) and PI3K (phosphotidylinositol 3-kinase). These proteins block nerve impulses triggered by neurotransmitter glutamate, thus reducing severity and frequency of seizures. PI3K helps regulate glucose transporter type 4 (GLUT4), a cytoplasmic protein essential for sugar regulation. This may be another important mechanism of action of elevated leptins.
- Leptin's usefulness in chronic cases is yet to be determined. Leptin has a relatively short half-life (15 to 30 minutes), leading to dosage problems. However, creating a physiologic environment that improves blood leptin levels through dietary and supplemental intervention could prove therapeutic.
- KD diet increases levels of circulating leptins—perhaps another plausible mechanism of action of KD.
- Another anticonvulsant mechanism of leptin involves hypoglycemia. Low blood sugar is linked with increased seizure formation; hypoglycemic individuals also have low leptin levels. This may explain in part why hypoglycemia is associated with occurrence of seizures.
- **Food allergy:** little research has explored the correlation between food allergy and epilepsy. Epileptic patients may have allergic reactions in the brain similar to swelling, anoxia, and inflammatory chemical reactions of local allergic reactions. Suspect allergy in epileptics with multiple other symptoms of food allergy (*Textbook,* "Epilepsy" and "Food Allergy Testing"). Folic acid deficiency is a common side effect of most antiepileptic drugs. Link among celiac disease, epilepsy, and cerebral calcifications indicates that celiac disease be ruled out (even in the absence of gastrointestinal symptoms) in all patients with epilepsy and cerebral calcifications of unexplained origin, especially when epilepsy is characterized by occipital seizures and calcification is located bilaterally in posterior regions. Epileptic children have higher rates of eczema in mothers, rhinitis in siblings, allergic states in both of these groups, allergy to cow's milk, and asthma compared with control subjects.

Mitochondrial Adenosine Triphosphate

- Individuals with mitochondrial diseases compromising ATP production have increased seizure frequency. Mechanism: importance of respiratory chain ATP in controlling stability of cell membranes.
- Families with genetic mitochondrial disease (defect in reduced nicotinamide adenine dinucleotide [NADH] ubiquinone oxidoreductase step) show significant increase in seizures.
- Subjects with mitochondrial encephalopathies have epileptic seizures as a main symptom. Partial seizures, chiefly with elementary motor symptoms, and focal or multifocal EEG epileptiform activity characterize epileptic presentation in 71% of these patients.
- Theory: compromised ATP production plays a role in provoking seizures.
- Supplementing with ubiquinone improves symptoms produced by mitochondrial encephalopathies.
- Ubiquinone is beneficial in several neurologic disorders (e.g., Parkinson's disease, Huntington's chorea).
- Positive effects of KD may relate to mitochondrial functionality. Animals placed on KD had a 46% increase in density of mitochondria, source of ATP synthesis in neuronal tissues.

Nutritional Considerations

- **Pyridoxine:** two types of vitamin B_6–related seizures in newborns and infants younger than 18 months old—B_6 deficient and B_6 dependent—with similar neurologic symptoms, EEG abnormalities, and prognosis of mental retardation if untreated. B_6-dependent type is an autosomal recessive inherited error of metabolism with recurrent long-lasting seizures, with onset in infancy and up to age 3 years. Seizures resist anticonvulsants. It is fatal if diagnosis and pharmacologic administration of B_6 are delayed too long. Suspect B_6 dependency if convulsions in the first 18 months of life have the following clinical features:
  - — Seizures of unknown origin in previously normal infant without abnormal gestational or perinatal history
  - — History of severe convulsive disorders
  - — Long-lasting focal or unilateral seizures, often with partial preservation of consciousness
  - — Irritability, restlessness, crying, and vomiting preceding actual seizure

MRI with spectroscopy can assess parenchymal changes despite normal-appearing brain MRI in patients with B_6-dependent seizures. Atypical presentations of B_6-responsive seizures suggest empiric trial of parenteral B_6 for neonate or infant with long-lasting convulsions, especially with no clear-cut cause. Dose is 100 to 200 mg intravenously or 20 mg every 5 minutes to a total of 200 mg. If seizures stop, child has B_6-responsive seizures. Diagnosis of B_6 responsiveness is lost if B_6 is given together with, or after, anticonvulsant drugs. B_6 deficiency responds to dietary amounts, but B_6 dependency requires continuous high-dose supplementing at 25 to 50 mg q.d. The mechanism is not fully understood, but it is related to B_6 as a cofactor in synthesis of neurotransmitters dependent on amino acid decarboxylation. Absorbed B_6 is phosphorylated to pyridoxal-5-phosphate (P5P), a coenzyme in converting glutamic acid to GABA, an inhibitory neurotransmitter. Proposed mechanism: pyridoxal phosphate does not bind with usual affinity to glutamic acid decarboxylase, reducing GABA production; thus, higher levels of B_6 are required for activity of this enzyme. Uncontrollable infantile spasms or sequelae improve in 2 to 14 days with oral P5P (20 to 50 mg/kg). Adverse reactions include elevated transaminase levels, nausea, and vomiting. Administration of B_6 to epileptics must be strictly monitored and improvements noted; daily doses of 80 to 400 mg interfere with anticonvulsants.

- **Folic acid:** low serum and red blood cell folic acid occurs in 90% of patients using barbiturates or the anticonvulsants phenytoin or carbamazepine; these drugs interfere with intestinal uptake of folate by mucosa. Lamotrigine and zonisamide do not seem to cause this problem; valproate has mixed reports. Supplementing folic acid appears safe even up to 15 mg/day, protecting against birth defects for women of childbearing potential and elevated homocysteine, a cardiac risk factor for antiepileptic medicines. The activated folates would likely be more effective.
- **Thiamin:** deficiency may promote epileptic episodes in those with subclinical predisposition for seizures. Vitamin B_1 may play a significant role in nerve conduction. Vitamin B_1 deficiency may accompany low concentrations of GABA. In patients with late-onset epilepsy, thiamin deficiency may be a cause.
- **Taurine:** one of the most abundant amino acids in the brain, taurine is involved in hyperpolarizing neurons by changing ion permeability. It may mimic effects of GABA and glycine. Taurine's anticonvulsive mode of action is a membrane-stabilizing effect (normalizes flow of Na^+, K^+, and Ca^{2+} into and out of

the cell). Taurine acts as a GABA-like neurotransmitter and may increase GABA levels by enhancing action of glutamic acid decarboxylase. Epileptics have much lower taurine levels in platelets than do control subjects. Anticonvulsant effects have been demonstrated, but the rate of efficacy is far below the level warranting recommendation as standard treatment. No consensus exists on amenable seizure types, dosage, or whether taurine traverses the blood-brain barrier. Daily dose was 0.05 to 0.3 g/kg in one study and 750 mg in another—effective in some cases of intractable epilepsy, decreasing seizures by more than 30% in one third of subjects unresponsive to any other anticonvulsant. Partial epilepsy showed best results, with those achieving highest taurine concentrations showing the best response. Monitoring platelet or plasma taurine levels is useful.

- **Magnesium (Mg):** epileptics have much lower serum Mg compared with normal control subjects. Seizure severity correlates with level of hypomagnesemia. The mechanism is not fully understood. Mg may be lowered by antiepileptic drugs. Mg is beneficial in control of some seizures. Mg deficiency induces muscle tremors and convulsive seizures; dose is 450 mg q.d. If epilepsy is unresponsive to Mg, pyridoxal-5′-phosphate may also be needed to facilitate Mg transport into the cell.
- **Manganese (Mn):** low whole-blood and hair Mn levels are common in epileptics; those with lowest levels have the highest seizure activity. Mn is a critical cofactor for glucose use within neurons, adenylate cyclase activity, and neurotransmitter control. Optimal central nervous system function requires sufficient Mn. Supplements may help control seizure activity in some patients.
- **Zinc (Zn):** children with epilepsy have much lower serum Zn levels, especially in West or Lennox syndromes. Epileptics may have elevated copper (Cu)/Zn ratio. Seizures may be triggered when Zn levels fall, as in the absence of adequate taurine. The exact role of Zn or Cu/Zn ratio is unclear; it may involve storage or binding of GABA. Supplementation is warranted because anticonvulsants may cause Zn deficiency.
- **Choline, betaine (N,N,N,-trimethylglycine), dimethylglycine (DMG), and sarcosine:** produce anticonvulsant activity in human and animal studies. Choline is converted to betaine when acting as a methyl donor; betaine is converted to DMG when donating a methyl group to homocysteine to produce

methionine. Supplemental betaine is quite effective in alleviating seizures in human beings with homocystinuria. DMG blocks seizures induced in laboratory animals. DMG strikingly decreased seizure frequency in a patient with longstanding mental retardation at dose of 90 mg b.i.d. Glycine and betaine may act indirectly on glycine metabolism and glycine-mediated neuronal inhibition, enhance GABA activity, or simply have a nonspecific effect on biologic membranes.

- **Vitamin D:** anticonvulsant drugs are linked to disorders of mineral metabolism (hypocalcemia, rickets, osteomalacia). Studies of serum levels of vitamin D in epilepsy are conflicting. Supplemental vitamin D is recommended when the climate or lifestyle does not allow adequate exposure to sunlight (particularly important for people with dark skin pigmentation). Supplementing epileptics with 4000 to 16,000 international units (IU) vitamin D has significantly decreased the number of seizures. At high doses, serum levels of vitamin D and its active monohydroxy and dihydroxy forms need to be monitored.
- **Vitamin E and selenium (Se):** function synergistically. Vitamin E deficiency produces seizures; antiepileptic drugs decrease vitamin E and beta-carotene levels. Vitamin E and Se levels are low in epileptics. Phosphate diesters of vitamins E and C prevent epileptogenic focus formation or attenuate seizure activities in animal models. Vitamin E and Se supplements may improve control of seizures. Se is helpful in children with reduced glutathione peroxidase activity, intractable seizures, multiple infections, and resistance to anticonvulsants. Other antioxidants (green tea [−]-epigallocatechin and [−]-epigallocatechin-3-*O*-gallate; alpha-lipoic acid) scavenge radical oxygen species and may be prophylactic for epileptic discharges induced in animal models.
- **Essential fatty acids (EFAs):** long-chain polyunsaturated EFAs may alleviate or prevent cerebrovascular pathology and reinforce blood-brain barrier competency. Dose of 5 g q.d. 65% omega-3 fatty acid spread reduced frequency and strength of seizures. However, gamma-linolenic acid and linoleic acid (omega-6) as evening primrose oil (EPO) induced temporal lobe epilepsy in three hospitalized schizophrenics. Monitor closely when using EFAs for epilepsy. Omega-3 EFAs are best choice; use EPO (as well as borage and black currant oils) with caution.
- **Melatonin (5-methoxy-*N*-acetyltryptamine):** powerful antioxidant that treats abnormalities in sleep-wake cycle, jet lag, cancer, and Parkinson's disease. Epileptic children have a higher incidence of sleep problems; epilepsy is exacerbated by sleep

deprivation. Melatonin has antiepileptic activity. Mechanism may be antiexcitotoxic neuroprotection achieved by lowering lipid peroxidation and raising coenzyme Q10 within the central nervous system. In children aged 3 to 12 years seizure free on sodium valproate (10 mg/kg/day) for 6 months, fast-release 3-mg melatonin tablet 1 hour before bedtime improved attention, memory, language, anxiety, behavior, and other cognitive processes. Very high doses (up to 300 mg/day) are well tolerated in adults; slowly increasing dose beyond 3 mg gives better results.

Botanical Medicines

- **Chinese herbal medicine:** Chinese herbal combination Saiko-Keishi-To (SK) demonstrated dramatic therapeutic effects on some difficult cases unresponsive to anticonvulsants. SK is a combination of nine botanicals:
  - — *Bupleuri* radix: 5.0 g
  - — *Scutellaria* radix: 3.0 g
  - — *Pinelliae* tuber: 5.0 g
  - — *Paeoniae* radix: 6.0 g
  - — *Cinnamon* cortex: 2.0 g
  - — *Zizyphi* fructus: 4.0 g
  - — *Ginseng* radix: 30.0 g
  - — *Glycyrrhizae* radix: 1.5 g
  - — *Zingiber* rhizoma: 2.0 g

SK inhibits intracellular shift of Ca^{2+} toward cell membrane; inhibits binding of Ca^{2+} to Ca^{2+}-receptive membrane proteins and Ca^{2+}-calmodulin complex; inhibits conformational changes of Ca^{2+}-receptive membrane proteins; inhibits pathologic transmembrane current of Na^+, K^+, and Ca^{2+}. Attempts to isolate purified chemicals from component herbs failed to match crude drug's efficacy, revealing synergistic effect among herbal agents. SK also protects neurons from damage produced by various factors, including stress, as a result of antioxidant compounds within the formula. SK helps prevent abnormal expression of a seizure-related genes.

- ***Coleus forskohlii:*** cyclic nucleotides are involved in the pathophysiology of seizures—possible mechanism of action of several botanicals. Cyclic adenosine monophosphate (cAMP) depresses electrical activity in animal models. Cyclic guanosine monophosphate (cGMP) can produce seizure-like discharge in the same tissues. cAMP inhibits Ca^{2+} binding to intracellular proteins (calmodulin), decreasing extrusion of neurotransmitters into synapse. *Coleus* is an Ayurvedic herb that activates adenylate cyclase, increasing cAMP. The constituent forskolin, a diterpene, increases adenylate cyclase activity by 530%. Seven of the nine botanicals in SK (*Bupleuri* radix, cinnamon cortex, *Glycyrrhizae* radix, *Paeoniae* radix, *Ginseng* radix, *Scutellaria* radix, and *Zingiber* rhizoma) also increase cAMP by enhancing adenylate cyclase or inhibiting cAMP phosphodiesterase.

- ***Ginkgo biloba:*** antioxidant that improves memory and cerebral insufficiency. It may precipitate seizures in some people. *Gingko* flavonoids exert GABAergic activity as partial agonists at benzodiazepine receptors. Avoid *Ginkgo* in patients with seizure history.

Yoga and Meditation

Meditative types of yoga (Sahaja yoga) have the most benefits in reducing intensity and occurrence of seizures. Patients who practiced meditative yoga regularly had a 50% reduction in number of seizures at 1-year follow-up.

Trigeminal Nerve Stimulation

Intractable epilepsy, which affects more than 1 million Americans and is often resistant to drug treatment, may be ameliorated by trigeminal nerve stimulation (TNS). The trigeminal nerve, which extends into the brain from the face and forehead, plays a role in inhibition of seizures; stimulating this nerve can reduce their occurrence. TNS entails a stimulator the size of a cell phone that fits into a pocket. Its wires are connected to the forehead with adhesives. Electrical impulses are transmitted to the nerve. Patients have experienced 66% reduction of seizures in first 3 months, 56% after 6 months, 59% reduction after 12 months, and, in one subject, 90% reduction in seizures after 1 year. TNS is an alternative mode of neurostimulation that is not invasive (compared with vagus nerve stimulation, which requires surgery).

Exercise

Caution recommending exercise to epileptic patients is a result of fear of injury and possibility of seizure induction. Medical literature reveals no increase in frequency of seizures with exercise. Exercise may even reduce seizure frequency in drug-resistant patients. Exercise may reduce muscle spasms, improve sleep, and increase energy. In animals, exercise seems to modulate neuronal vulnerability to epileptic insults. Metabolic, electrophysiologic, and immunohistochemical evaluations have confirmed positive influence of exercise on epileptic patients. Consider integrating physical exercise to reduce intensity and frequency of seizures.

THERAPEUTIC APPROACH

Avoid situations that could be dangerous if seizures occur. Be aware of state laws regarding epilepsy and driving. Avoid known initiators of seizure activity (e.g., bright flashing lights, sudden loud sounds). Continue therapy at full doses until patient is seizure free for at least 2 years. Reduce dose gradually over several months. Epileptics not controlled with natural therapies require drug therapy. Eliminate pyridoxine antagonists (isoniazid, cycloserine, hydralazine, dopamine, penicillamine, oral contraceptives, alcohol, and hydrazine dyes [FD&C yellow No. 5]).

Note: Status epilepticus is a medical emergency causing serious neurologic damage or death if untreated. Immediate hospitalization is mandatory, preferably with emergency medical services transport to maintain airway, assist ventilation, and administer intravenous glucose and anticonvulsants.

Monitor for depression. Endogenous depression is more prevalent in epileptics than in the general population.

- **Diet:** eliminate all sugar and refined carbohydrates. Moderate protein intake. Identify and eliminate food allergens. Eat small, frequent meals. If ketotic effect is desired, strictly limit all carbohydrates and increase fat. Ensure adequate calories, protein, and omega-3 fatty acids. Use vitamin-mineral supplements with carefully supervised ketotic diets.
- **Lifestyle:** regular sleep patterns should be encouraged.
- **Nutritional supplements** (adult doses; reduce proportionately for children):
  - — Vitamin B_6: 50 mg t.i.d.
  - — Folic acid: 0.4 to 4 mg q.d.
  - — Vitamin E: 400 IU q.d. (mixed tocopherols)
  - — Taurine: 500 mg t.i.d.
  - — Mg: 300 mg t.i.d.
  - — Mn: 10 mg t.i.d.
  - — Se: 100 mcg q.d.
  - — Zn: 25 mg q.d.
  - — Ubiquinone: 100 mg q.d.
  - — Melatonin: 3 mg in children, increase up to 20 mg or more in adults
- **Botanical medicine:**
  - — SK: 300 mL before bedtime
- **Caution:**
  - — *G. biloba:* contraindicated at this time

Erythema Multiforme

DIAGNOSTIC SUMMARY

- Sudden onset of symmetric, erythematous, edematous, macular, papular, urticarial, bullous, or purpuric skin lesions
- Evolves into "target lesions" ("bull's eye" lesions with clear centers and concentric erythematous rings)
- Characteristic first site: dorsum of hand
- Characteristic distribution: extensor surfaces of extremities with relative sparing of head and trunk
- Rare oral manifestations: range from tender superficial erythematous and hyperkeratotic plaques to painful, deep, hemorrhagic bullae and erosions
- Tendency to recur in spring and fall

GENERAL CONSIDERATIONS

- The term *erythema multiforme* (EM) includes a wide range of expressions, from exclusive oral erosions (oral EM) to mucocutaneous lesions ranging from mild (EM minor) to severe multiple mucosal membranes (EM major, Stevens-Johnson syndrome [SJS]) or large area of total body surface (toxic epidermal necrolysis [TEN]). But the term *erythema multiforme* is not accepted worldwide; various clinical categories have overlapping features. EM minor, EM major, SJS, and TEN differ in severity and expression. All variants share two common features: cutaneous target lesions and satellite cell or more widespread necrosis of epithelium. Clinically, EM major is characterized by typical or raised atypical targets located on extremities and/or face. SJS is diagnosed when lesions are flat, atypical targets or purpuric maculae that are widespread or distributed on trunk.
- Suspected etiologic factors: herpes simplex or *Mycoplasma* are linked to 90% of cases of EM minor; SJS and TEN (80% of cases) arise from drugs—anticonvulsants, sulfonamides, nonsteroidal anti-inflammatories, and antibiotics. Vaccines (e.g., vaccinia, bacille Calmette-Guérin, polio), food allergy, and other infectious

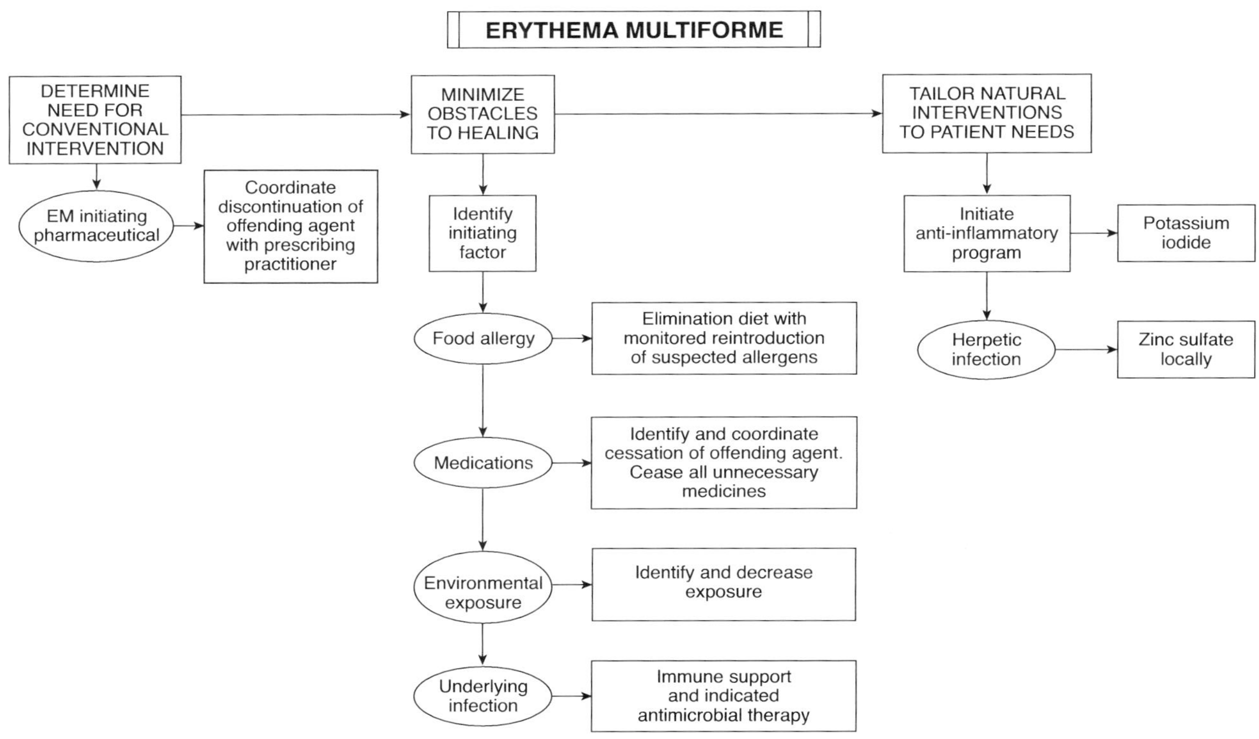
ERYTHEMA MULTIFORME
DETERMINE NEED FOR CONVENTIONAL INTERVENTION
EM initiating pharmaceutical
Coordinate discontinuation of offending agent with prescribing practitioner
MINIMIZE OBSTACLES TO HEALING
Identify initiating factor
Food allergy
Elimination diet with monitored reintroduction of suspected allergens
Medications
Identify and coordinate cessation of offending agent. Cease all unnecessary medicines
Environmental exposure
Identify and decrease exposure
Underlying infection
Immune support and indicated antimicrobial therapy
TAILOR NATURAL INTERVENTIONS TO PATIENT NEEDS
Initiate anti-inflammatory program
Potassium iodide
Herpetic infection
Zinc sulfate locally

organisms have all induced EM minor. Common factor: highly reactive, polymorphonuclear leukocyte oxygen intermediates trigger hypersensitivity and immune system–mediated tissue damage.
- Human leukocyte antigen (HLA) DQ3 correlates closely with recurrent EM and may be a marker to distinguish herpes-associated EM from other skin diseases. Biopsy can help predict disease progression from EM lesions to SJS or TEN.

THERAPEUTIC CONSIDERATIONS

- **Potassium iodide:** historically used to treat a variety of erythematous disorders, including EM, erythema nodosum, nodular vasculitis, acute febrile neutrophilic dermatosis, and subacute nodular migratory panniculitis. Potassium iodide has documented dramatic success. Mechanism: suppression of generation of oxygen intermediates (hydrogen peroxide, hydroxyl radical) by stimulated polymorphonuclear antibodies. Iodine therapy is occasionally associated with adverse skin reactions and gastrointestinal discomfort. Never use in pregnant women in last trimester because of suppression of fetal thyroid.
- **Zinc:** zinc sulfate (0.025% to 0.05%) is used locally at site of herpetic infection to prevent relapse of postherpetic EM.

THERAPEUTIC APPROACH

Carefully search to determine initiating factor; treat underlying infections; cease all unnecessary medicines; initiate anti-inflammatory program. In herpes-associated EM, antiviral treatment initiated after EM has erupted has no benefit. Symptomatic treatment—local skin care, analgesics, and soothing mouthwashes—is important. Liquid antiseptics help prevent superinfection. Liquid diet may be necessary. Intravenous fluid replacement with electrolytes and nutrients should be started as early as possible. Systemic corticosteroids are controversial, some believing that it may increase risk of complications.

- **Supplements:**
  - — Potassium iodide: 100 mg t.i.d. for 4 to 6 weeks. Discontinue if adverse reactions occur.
  - — Zinc sulfate: 0.025% to 0.05% solution applied locally to postherpetic lesions.

Fibrocystic Breast Disease

DIAGNOSTIC SUMMARY

- Very common: 20% to 40% of premenopausal women.
- Pain or premenstrual breast pain and tenderness common, although the condition is often asymptomatic.
- Cyclic and bilateral with multiple cysts of varying sizes giving breasts nodular consistency.

GENERAL CONSIDERATIONS

- **Benign breast discomfort:** conditions present in most women of reproductive age should never be labeled pathologic. Misconception: women with painful or lumpy breasts have increased breast cancer risk. Premenstrual pain and sensitivity are common; more prominent estrogen than progesterone effect at this time, when effect of progesterone is normally greater in luteal phase. This does not mean lower or higher levels of any particular hormone, but increased tissue sensitivity to estrogen with related fluid retention. This discomfort is tolerable in most women. Others need lifestyle changes or supplements. Oral contraceptives or hormone replacement therapy may cause breast discomfort: physiologic, cyclic pain and swelling.
- **Mastalgia:** breast pain of severity interfering with daily life and prompting medical attention. Cyclic mastalgia is this severe 15% of the time. Noncyclic mastalgia is rarer, caused by infection, old trauma, musculoskeletal conditions of chest wall.
- **Diffuse lumpiness:** cyclic or noncyclic and may or may not include pain. Normal breasts can have diffuse lumpiness—glands, fat, connective tissue. Prominent lumpiness and numerous lumps distinguish this from normal. Diffuse lumpiness is symmetric, distinguishing normal from suspicious lump.
- **Unilateral densities:** most are benign. If mass edge merges in one or more places with surrounding tissue, it is nondominant. Evaluate masses carefully to distinguish dominant mass or mass of concern. Fine-needle biopsy may be needed. Most show nonproliferative changes; 20% show proliferative changes without

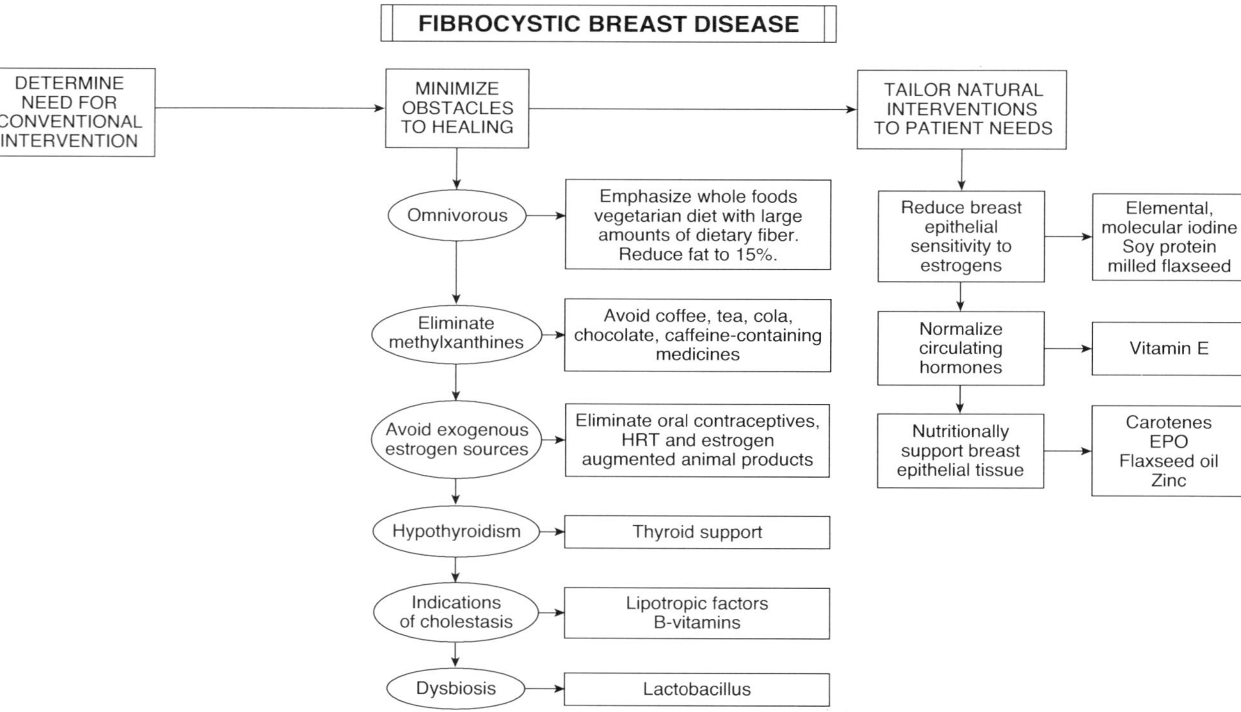
FIBROCYSTIC BREAST DISEASE
DETERMINE NEED FOR CONVENTIONAL INTERVENTION
MINIMIZE OBSTACLES TO HEALING
TAILOR NATURAL INTERVENTIONS TO PATIENT NEEDS
Omnivorous
Emphasize whole foods vegetarian diet with large amounts of dietary fiber. Reduce fat to 15%.
Eliminate methylxanthines
Avoid coffee, tea, cola, chocolate, caffeine-containing medicines
Avoid exogenous estrogen sources
Eliminate oral contraceptives, HRT and estrogen augmented animal products
Hypothyroidism
Thyroid support
Indications of cholestasis
Lipotropic factors B-vitamins
Dysbiosis
Lactobacillus
Reduce breast epithelial sensitivity to estrogens
Elemental, molecular iodine Soy protein milled flaxseed
Normalize circulating hormones
Vitamin E
Nutritionally support breast epithelial tissue
Carotenes EPO Flaxseed oil Zinc

atypical hyperplasia with no increased breast cancer risk. Approximately 5% show atypical hyperplasia with increased risk, especially if first-degree relative has or had breast cancer.

- **Dominant masses:** noncyclic, unilateral, distinct on all sides from surrounding tissue. They persist over time and require thorough assessment, except in the very young. They are either fibroadenomas or obvious cysts. Fibroadenomas are rubbery, smooth, benign, fibrous tumors that usually do not grow bigger. Cysts are softer and disappear by draining with needle aspiration. Fibroadenomas and cysts do not increase risk but must be distinguished from malignancy.

DIFFERENTIAL DIAGNOSIS

Fibrocystic breast disease (FBD) (cystic mastitis) cannot be definitively differentiated from breast cancer or breast fibroadenoma on clinical criteria alone. Pain, cyclic variations in size, high mobility, and multiplicity of nodules are indicative of FBD. Noninvasive procedures (mammography, ultrasonography) are helpful, but definitive procedures are needle aspiration, fine-needle biopsy, or excisional biopsy.

THERAPEUTIC CONSIDERATIONS

See *Textbook*, "Premenstrual Syndrome," for additional factors that can influence FBD.

Dietary Considerations

- **Methylxanthines:** caffeine, theophylline, and theobromine inhibit action of cyclic adenosine monophosphate (cAMP) and cyclic guanosine monophosphate (cGMP) phosphodiesterase and elevate their levels in breast tissue. Increased cyclic nucleotides excessively stimulate protein kinase, causing overproduction of cellular products (fibrous tissue, cyst fluid). Excess cyclic nucleotides in breast are one of the biochemical findings in breast cancer; caffeine promotes carcinogenesis in mammary gland of rats. Limiting dietary methylxanthines (coffee, tea, cola, chocolate, caffeinated medicines) improved 97.5% of 45 women who completely abstained and 75% of 28 who limited consumption. Women may have varying thresholds of response to methylxanthines. Stress plays a role; fibrocystic breasts are more responsive to epinephrine, which increases adenylate cyclase activity (cAMP).

- **Fiber:** an inverse association exists between dietary fiber and risk of benign, proliferative, epithelial breast disorders. Fiber may reduce risk of benign breast disease and cancer.
- **Soy:** in premenopausal women consuming soy protein daily for 1 year, their physicians reported subjective reduction in breast tenderness and FBD after use of breast-enhanced scintigraphy test imaging. Average and maximal count breast activity and variability of tissue activity declined.

Nutritional Supplements

- **Evening primrose oil (EPO):** some studies of EPO for cyclic and noncyclic breast pain have indicated a 45% response for cyclic mastalgia and a 27% response rate for noncyclic mastalgia. At 3 g of EPO per day for 3 months, pain and tenderness were significantly reduced in cyclic and noncyclic pain. Differences in sufficiency of dose and duration of dose of gamma-linolenic acid from EPO might be a reason for inconsistency in study results.
- **Vitamin E:** D-alpha-tocopherol can relieve premenstrual syndrome (PMS), including FBD and cyclic and noncyclic pain, in some patients. Results of early studies have not been duplicated. Mode of action is obscure—normalizes circulating hormones in PMS and FBD patients; 600 international units (IU) q.d. normalizes elevated follicle-stimulating hormone (FSH) and luteinizing hormone (LH) in FBD. Supplementing with a combination of beta-carotene, vitamin E, vitamin C, and garlic powder reduced severity of mastalgia, PMS, infrequent menses, and menstrual cramping. It also reduced symptoms of fibromatosis. Chewable tablets containing vitamin E (200 mg) given twice daily for 4 months reduced severity and duration of pain in 70% of women studied. Improvement was seen as early as 2 months, with no further improvement at 4 months. Although early research was done with alpha-tocopherol, mixed tocopherols may be more effective.
- **Vitamin A:** 150,000 IU q.d. for 3 months caused complete or partial remission of FBD in five of the nine patients who completed the study. Some developed mild side effects, causing two of the original 12 to withdraw for headache, and one patient had dose reduced. Beta-carotene may be a better source of retinol; it is much less toxic and triggers similar activity in ovarian and inflammatory disorders (*Textbook,* "Vitamin A" and "Vitamin Toxicities and Therapeutic Monitoring").
- **Thyroid and iodine:** iodine deficiency in rats induces mammary dysplasia histologically similar to human FBD. Hypothyroidism

and/or iodine deficiency are linked to higher incidence of breast cancer. Thyroid hormone replacement in hypothyroid (and some euthyroid) patients may give improvement. Thyroid supplement (0.1 mg Synthroid q.d.) decreases mastodynia, serum prolactin, and breast nodules in euthyroid patients; subclinical hypothyroidism and/or iodine deficiency may be causative factors in FBD. Iodine caseinate may be an effective treatment for FBD. The theory is that absence of iodine renders epithelium more sensitive to estrogen stimulation. Hypersensitivity produces excess secretions, distending ducts and producing cysts and later fibrosis. In animal models, iodides correct cystic spaces and partially correct excess cellular reproduction; elemental iodine corrects entire disease process. Elemental iodine is preferred form for breast metabolism. Oral iodine has acute and long-term anti-inflammatory and antifibrotic effects. Human studies: iodides effective in 70% of subjects but with high rate of side effects (altered thyroid function in 4%, iodinism in 3%, and acne in 15%). Elemental iodine gives same benefits but no significant side effects: short-term increased breast pain corresponding to softening of breast and disappearance of fibrous tissue plaques. Dose of molecular iodine is 70 to 90 mcg/kg body weight (iodine caseinate or liquid iodine).

Herbal Supplements

- ***Vitex agnus-castus* (chasteberry):** chaste tree berry is very important for PMS and premenstrual dysphoric disorder. In cyclic mastalgia as part of PMS, after 3 months of treatment, 81% of women rated *Vitex* as very good treatment for their mastalgia. After treatment daily with chaste tree for three consecutive menstrual cycles, cyclic mastalgia decreased significantly along with a smaller degree of improvement even 3 months after stopping the plant. Many women have rated its effectiveness as moderate to excellent; some report no effect.

Other Considerations

- **Liver function:** liver is primary site for estrogen clearance. Any factor (cholestasis, toxic liver syndrome, environmental pollution) compromising the liver can cause estrogen excess. Lipotropic factors and B vitamins are necessary for estrogen conjugation.
- **Colon function:** breast disease is linked to a Western diet and bowel function. Epithelial dysplasia in nipple aspirates of breast

fluid and frequency of bowel movements (BMs) are also linked. Women having fewer than three BMs per week have 4.5-fold greater risk of FBD compared with women having one or more BMs every day. Colon bacteria transform endogenous and exogenous sterols and fatty acids into toxic metabolites (polycyclic carcinogens and mutagens). Fecal microbes can synthesize estrogens and metabolize estrogen sulfate and glucuronate conjugates. The result is absorption of bacteria-derived and previously conjugated estrogens. Diet influences microflora, transit time, and concentration of absorbable metabolites. Vegetarian women excrete two to three times more conjugated estrogens than omnivores. Omnivorous women have 50% higher unconjugated estrogens. *Lactobacillus* supplements lower fecal beta-glucuronidase.

- **Fiber:** an inverse correlation exists between dietary fiber and risk of benign, proliferative, epithelial breast disorders. Increasing dietary fiber may reduce risk for benign disease and breast cancer.

THERAPEUTIC APPROACH

Some women have noncyclic FBD; others have cyclic premenstrual breast tenderness and lumpiness. Therapy given in the *Textbook,* "Premenstrual Syndrome," may be more appropriate for individual needs. Recommendations here include key factors in that chapter and this one.

- **Diet:** primarily vegetarian with large amounts of dietary fiber. Eliminate all methylxanthines until symptoms are alleviated, then reintroduce in small amounts. Reducing fat to 15% of total calories and increasing complex carbohydrates reduces premenstrual breast tenderness and swelling as well as actual breast swelling and nodularity in some women. Reducing fat intake decreases circulating estrogens. Avoid exogenous estrogens (oral contraceptives, hormone replacement therapy, estrogen-augmented animal products). Emphasize whole, unprocessed foods (whole grains, legumes, vegetables, fruits, nuts, and seeds). Drink at least 48 oz water daily.
- **Supplements:**
  - Lipotropic factors: 1000 mg choline and 1000 mg of either methionine and/or cysteine q.d. Alternatively, *S*-adenosylmethionine (SAM) can be used at a dose of 200 to 400 mg q.d.

— Vitamin E: 400 to 800 IU q.d. D-alpha tocopherol (mixed tocopherols?).
— Beta-carotene: 50,000-300,000 IU q.d.
— Iodine (aqueous iodine): 3 to 6 mg q.d. (prescription item).
— Zinc: 15 mg q.d.
— EPO: 1500 mg b.i.d.

- ***Vitex* (chasteberry):** chaste berry extract (standardized to contain 0.5% agnuside) in tablet or capsule form: 175 to 225 mg q.d. If using liquid extract: 2 to 4 mL (½–1 tsp) q.d.

Fibromyalgia Syndrome

DIAGNOSTIC SUMMARY

- Affects 2% to 13% of population; 80% to 90% of those affected are female.
- Chronic widespread pain involving axial pain; pain on left, right, upper, and lower parts of body.
- Abnormal tenderness at 11 or more of 18 specific anatomic tender point (TnP) sites.
- Associated symptoms include fatigue, stiffness, headache, sleep disturbance, irritable bowel, depression, cognitive dysfunction, anxiety, coldness, paresthesias, sicca (Sjögren's) symptoms, exercise intolerance, dysmenorrhea.

DIAGNOSIS

Most common symptoms of fibromyalgia syndrome (FMS): fatigue, stiffness, headache, sleep disturbance, irritable bowel, depression, cognitive dysfunction, anxiety, coldness, paresthesias, sicca (Sjögren's) symptoms, exercise intolerance, dysmenorrhea

Differential Diagnosis

- Two major criteria for FMS are chronic (>3 months) widespread pain and tenderness.
- Hypothyroidism and cellular resistance to thyroid hormone may manifest with symptoms of FMS. Thyroid testing and a trial of thyroid hormone therapy can determine whether FMS is related to these disorders.
- Main disorders for differentiation are arthritis, myopathy, polymyalgia rheumatica, diabetic polyneuropathy, ankylosing spondylitis, discopathy, cardiac or pleural pain, multiple muscle myofascial pain syndromes, and lupus erythematosus.
- Distinguish FMS (except for hypothyroidism or cellular resistance to thyroid hormone) by careful pathognomy. Symptoms and signs of most FMS patients are indistinguishable from the subclass of hypothyroid or thyroid hormone–resistant patients for whom pain is the predominant symptom.

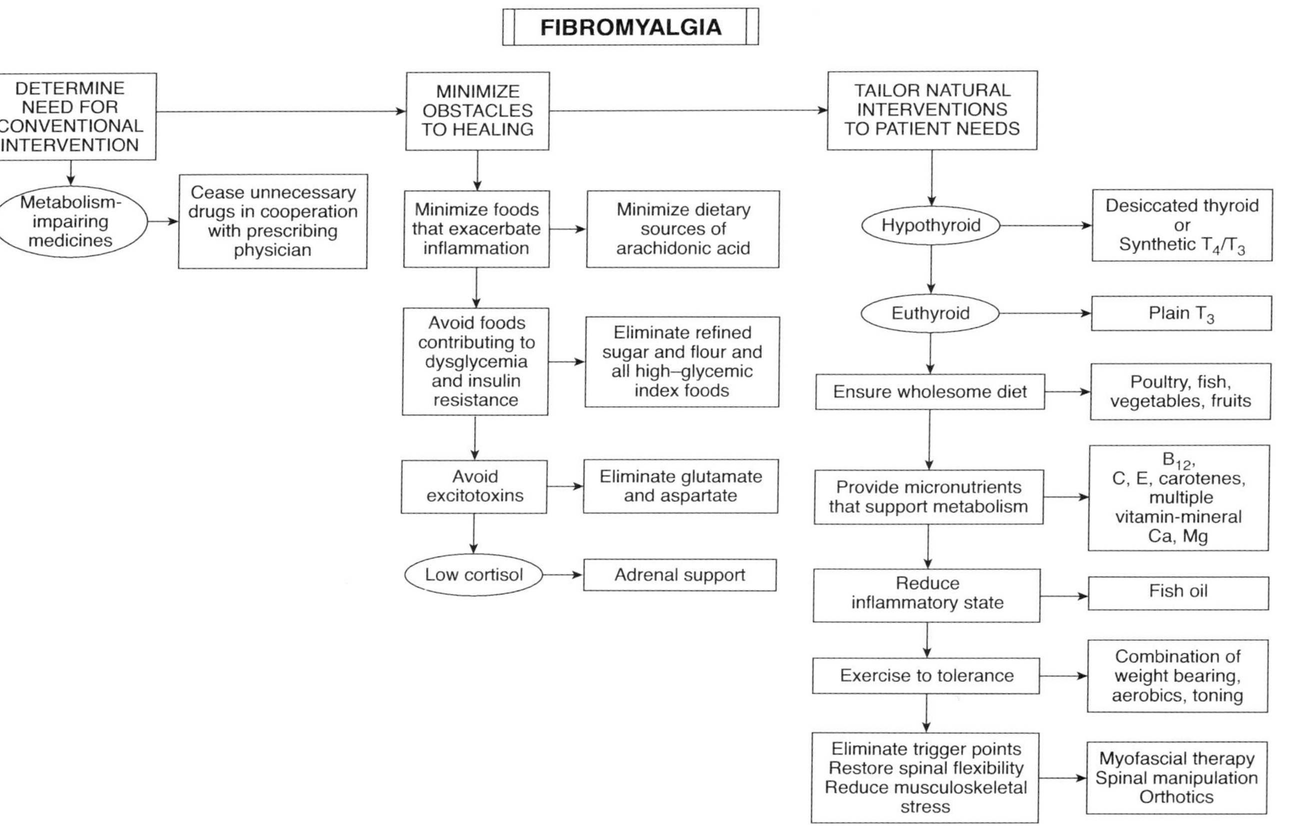
FIBROMYALGIA
DETERMINE NEED FOR CONVENTIONAL INTERVENTION
Metabolism-impairing medicines
Cease unnecessary drugs in cooperation with prescribing physician
MINIMIZE OBSTACLES TO HEALING
Minimize foods that exacerbate inflammation
Minimize dietary sources of arachidonic acid
Avoid foods contributing to dysglycemia and insulin resistance
Eliminate refined sugar and flour and all high–glycemic index foods
Avoid excitotoxins
Eliminate glutamate and aspartate
Low cortisol
Adrenal support
TAILOR NATURAL INTERVENTIONS TO PATIENT NEEDS
Hypothyroid
Desiccated thyroid or Synthetic T_4/T_3
Euthyroid
Plain T_3
Ensure wholesome diet
Poultry, fish, vegetables, fruits
Provide micronutrients that support metabolism
B_{12}, C, E, carotenes, multiple vitamin-mineral Ca, Mg
Reduce inflammatory state
Fish oil
Exercise to tolerance
Combination of weight bearing, aerobics, toning
Eliminate trigger points Restore spinal flexibility Reduce musculoskeletal stress
Myofascial therapy Spinal manipulation Orthotics

GENERAL CONSIDERATIONS

Current Focus of Conventional Research

- **Serotonin deficiency hypothesis:** core theoretical underpinning of rheumatology paradigm of FMS. Central nervous system (CNS) serotonin deficiency reduces efficiency of brainstem–spinal cord descending antinociceptive system, resulting in heightened pain perception in response to normal afferent input. This theory has been refuted. Central theoretical viewpoint has shifted from serotonin deficiency to augmented pain processing—hyperalgesic state plausibly explained by extraordinarily high levels of substance P in patients with FMS.
- **Hypometabolism hypothesis:** contributing factors are hypothyroidism and/or partial cellular resistance to thyroid hormone, pernicious diet, nutritional deficiencies, low physical fitness level, and metabolism-impeding drugs. Inadequate thyroid hormone regulation (ITHR) may be underlying mechanism of two main features of FMS: chronic widespread pain and abnormal tenderness. ITHR of metabolic processes in brainstem–spinal cord descending antinociceptive system can cause the following:
  — Spontaneous or ongoing pain
  — Tenderness (lowering pain threshold to mechanical stimuli)
  — Hyperalgesia (increased responsiveness to noxious stimuli)
  Following are two mechanisms of the syndrome:
- ITHR increases substance P, which is released from nociceptor neurons, is high in CSF of FMS patients, and facilitates summation of slow nociceptive signals, amplifying nociceptive signals in spinal cord. Thyroid hormone inhibits substance P synthesis and secretion in many CNS cells by repressing transcription of the gene for preprotachykinin A, a precursor of substance P, and its cognate substance P receptor. Thyroid hormone treatment lowers substance P level in the anterior pituitary, brain nuclei, and dorsal horns of the spinal cord. Excess thyroid hormone reduces substance P to subnormal levels.
- ITHR reduces synthesis and secretion of norepinephrine (NE) in the brainstem locus ceruleus cells, which are essential to the normal function of the descending antinociceptive system.

Antinociception pathways contain neurons that secrete serotonin or NE. Serotonin secretion is tonically augmented by NE secretion; normal serotonin secretion depends on NE secretion. Serotonin stimulates interneurons to secrete opiates that inhibit transmission by blocking release of the neurotransmitters glutamate and substance P from afferent neurons and block Calcium (Ca^{2+}) influx into and Potassium (K^+) efflux from afferent terminals (type C and A delta fibers), inhibiting nociceptive signals to spinothalamic neurons transmitting signals to the brain. Low NE from descending neurons may reduce serotonin selectively at dorsal horn interneurons, reducing opiates. Transmission of nociceptive signals heightens pain perception.

FMS patients have decreased NE (low dopamine and NE metabolites in cerebrospinal fluid [CSF]). The locus ceruleus has the brain's heaviest concentration of triiodothyronine (T_3). T_3 regulates two rate-limiting enzymes:

1. Tyrosine hydroxylase, which converts tyrosine to dihydroxyphenylalanine, which is converted to dopamine. Tyrosine hydroxylase activity in the locus ceruleus noradrenergic neurons is low in patients with hypothyroidism. Thyroid hormone therapy increases activity of tyrosine hydroxylase.
2. Dopamine beta-hydroxylase converts dopamine to NE. NE in the antinociceptive system and other tissues in thyroid disorders has not been studied extensively.

Other factors: most FMS patients are physically inactive because of pain; low motor drive from low dopamine contributes to inactivity. Low physical activity contributes to inefficiency of antinociceptive system.

ITHR can account for muscle and joint pain, paresthesias, cognitive dysfunction, depression, cold intolerance, exercise intolerance, weakness and fatigue, dry skin and mucous membranes, constipation, dysmenorrhea, menorrhagia, increased platelet $alpha_2$ adrenergic receptor density, reduced brain blood flow, reduced peripheral blood flow, sleep disturbance, deficient slow-wave sleep, hypotension, blunted sympathetic response to stress, stiffness and swelling, irritable bowel syndrome, excessive urination, high serum hyaluronic acid, low procollagen III, high ground substance proteoglycans, low pyridinoline and hydroxyproline, glycolysis abnormalities, low cell levels of high-energy phosphates, and low human growth hormone (HGH) and somatomedin C. Thyroid hormone's effect on the adrenergic system suggests that FMS is a condition of alpha adrenergic dominance.

Virtually identical presentations occur with FMS, hypothyroidism, and peripheral cellular resistance to thyroid hormone. Ninety percent of FMS patients have some form of thyroid disease or cellular resistance. The only clinical trials fully relieving FMS used oral thyroid hormone plus other metabolism-regulating therapies.

Other Metabolism-Regulating Therapies

Thyroid hormone is necessary but not sufficient for full recovery. Other therapies—wholesome diet, nutritional supplements, exercise to tolerance—provide some improvement but not full recovery. Additional intervention requires physical treatment.

- **Wholesome diet:** vegetarian diets; eliminate excitotoxins monosodium L-glutamate and aspartame; ingest *Chlorella pyrenoidosa;* uncooked vegan diet of berries, fruits, vegetables and roots, nuts, germinated seeds, sprouts; strict, low-salt, uncooked vegan diet rich in lactobacteria.
- **Nutritional supplements:** vitamins B_1, B_6, B_{12}, C, and E and beta-carotene have antinociceptive properties. "Myers' cocktail" (intravenous B vitamins, vitamin C, calcium [Ca], magnesium [Mg]); 5-hydroxy-L-tryptophan (5-HT); S-adenosyl-L-methionine (SAM); Mg; malic acid; combined *Aloe vera* extracts, plant saccharides, freeze-dried fruits and vegetables; *Dioscorea;* vitamin-mineral supplement; collagen hydrolysate; blend of ascorbigen and broccoli powder.
- **Exercise to tolerance:** results of exercise treatment for FMS are mixed. Cardiovascular exercise provides the most improvement, especially low-intensity endurance training. Endurance exercise reduces physical limitations of FMS. Low metabolic efficiency from ITHR renders some patients susceptible to FMS. Vigorous exercise exacerbates symptoms; high density of $alpha_2$ adrenergic receptors on FMS patients' platelets indicates receptor density in CNS. Binding catecholamines to high density of membrane receptors inhibits energy metabolism, worsening symptoms. During early phase of treatment, use mild exercise to minimize catecholamine secretion. Thyroid hormone therapy decreases density of $alpha_2$ adrenergic receptors and increases $alpha_2$ adrenergic receptors, enabling cells to respond appropriately to high catecholamines. Shifting from $alpha_2$ adrenergic receptor dominance explains the ability to engage in vigorous activity after thyroid hormone therapy.
- **Physical medicine:** necessary to eliminate FMS pain. Spinal manipulation, soft tissue manipulation, and trigger point therapy relieve pain. Lesions exacerbating FMS: myofascial trigger points and spinal joint fixations. Any nociception-generating neuromusculoskeletal lesion can exacerbate pain because of the impaired antinociceptive system. Neuromusculoskeletal lesions can disturb sleep, increasing symptoms in hypometabolic patients.

THERAPEUTIC CONSIDERATIONS

Laboratory Testing for Thyroid Status

Thyroid Function Tests

- Primary hypothyroidism (hormone deficiency from subnormal function of thyroid gland) is detected by two standard thyroid batteries:
  - Thyroxine (T_4), T_3 uptake, free T_4 index, thyroid-stimulating hormone (TSH)
  - Free T_3, free T_4, TSH

In untreated primary hypothyroidism, TSH is elevated; revised upper limit of serum TSH reference range is 2.5 μU/mL.

- Thyroid-releasing hormone (TRH) stimulation test distinguishes two conditions:
  - Euthyroidism (normal function of hypothalamic-pituitary-thyroid axis)
  - Central hypothyroidism (hormone deficiency caused by pituitary or hypothalamic dysfunction)

Basal blood TSH level is measured. TRH is then injected. Thirty minutes later, TSH is measured again. Subtract baseline TSH from 30-minute level to derive TSH response to injected TRH. Normal level is 8.5 to 20.0 μU/mL. Below 8.5 μU/mL suggests pituitary hypothyroidism; above 20.0 μU/mL suggests central hypothyroidism. (Exaggerated TSH response to TRH does not distinguish pituitary and hypothalamic hypothyroidism.) Diagnosis is tentative without evidence of other pituitary or hypothalamic hormone abnormalities (assays), pituitary or hypothalamic structural abnormalities (imaging), or mutations of TRH or TSH gene (nucleotide sequencing).

Thyroid Antibodies

The most common cause of primary hypothyroidism is autoimmune thyroiditis. Test is titer of thyroglobulin and thyroid microsomal (peroxidase) antibodies, which are important in FMS. Patients with elevated thyroid antibodies may also have thyroid function test results within reference ranges for years, but high thyroid microsomal antibodies occur in those with musculoskeletal symptoms. Prevalence of antibodies is higher in women than in men. In autoimmune thyroiditis, thyroid hormone levels too low to regulate the CNS antinociceptive system can escape detection by thyroid function tests, including TSH.

Thyroid Hormone Therapy Based on Initial Thyroid Status

- FMS with primary or central hypothyroidism: use preparation with both T_4 and T_3 in a T_4/T_3 ratio of 4:1. Dose: 2 to 4 grains (76 mcg T_4 and 18 mcg T_3 to 152 mcg T_4 and 36 mcg T_3). Hypothyroid and euthyroid FMS patients tend not to recover with conventional T_4 replacement. T_4/T_3 preparations and T_3 alone have been effective, in violation of conventional mandates for T_4 replacement:
  — Hormone therapy applied despite test results indicating euthyroid state.
  — Doses not titrated according to TSH levels but by clinical responses to particular doses.
- Effective doses suppressed TSH levels, but no symptoms of thyrotoxicosis arose and there was no evidence of thyrotoxicosis on electrocardiography, bone densitometry, or serum and urine biochemical tests.
- FMS with tests indicating euthyroidism: begin with plain T_3. Seventy-five percent of patients testing as euthyroid have partial peripheral cellular resistance to thyroid hormone according to four criteria:

1. Euthyroid (thyroid function tests including TRH stimulation) before beginning T_3
2. Recover from hypothyroid-like FMS symptoms and signs with supraphysiologic doses of T_3
3. Extremely high serum free T_3 after beginning T_3 therapy
4. No evidence of tissue thyrotoxicosis: serial electrocardiograms, serum and urine biochemical tests, bone densitometry

These patients benefit only from plain T_3 (not sustained-release T_3) in a single daily dose, responding only to supraphysiologic doses of T_3. T_3 dose is 75 to 125 mcg. For some patients, safe and effective dosages are far higher. Some FMS patients have both hypothyroidism and cellular resistance to thyroid hormone. Determine over time which form of hormone works best for an individual patient.

Dosage Adjustments

Titrate dosage changes according to tissue responses, not thyroid function test results, which have no value in finding the safest, most effective dose for any particular patient. Inference of the metabolic status of cells (other than thyrotrophs of anterior pituitary) from thyroid function tests is not justified. Levels of T_3 and T_4 in cells of different tissues cannot be accurately predicted from plasma TSH, T_3, or T_4. TSH levels correlate poorly with tissue metabolic status, such as speed of relaxation of the Achilles reflex. Symptoms and signs are more-accurate and more-reliable indicators of tissue metabolic status than are thyroid function tests. RMR measured with indirect calorimetry is most reliable measurement of metabolism, strongly regulated by thyroid hormone. TSH is not a useful tool for determining whether a patient's thyroid hormone dose is providing sufficient metabolism. Preferably, include indirect calorimetry. However, this instrument is not necessary for determining patients' safe and effective doses.

Rehabilitation Model: Data-Driven Clinical Decisions

Distinguish all factors impairing metabolism. Individualize treatment to correct, eliminate, or compensate for factors. A data-driven rehabilitation model requires baseline and repeated monitoring of clinical status by objective assessment methods.

Objective Assessment of Patient Status

Recovery gradually occurs over a 2- to 6-month period. Quantify patient's clinical status by objective measures weekly or biweekly. Post measurement scores as data points on line graphs after each evaluation, with baseline score before therapy as initial data point on each graph. Draw a line connecting data points to create a trend line to assess regimen efficacy. Typically, all measures change together in a direction of improvement, no improvement, or worsening. Patient subjective status usually closely corresponds to trend lines. False conclusions that no progress has occurred, despite minor setbacks, are quickly corrected by reviewing graphs objectively displaying real progress. Following are five objective assessments (in addition to physical examination at each evaluation):

- **Pain distribution body form:** the most sensitive indicator for changes in FMS status is pain distribution as percentage of body in pain. (Chronic widespread pain is one major criterion for assessing FMS.) Small changes in pain distribution are applied to drawings of body. Patient shades in location of aching, pain, soreness, or tenderness since last evaluation. Place a template over the patient's shaded form. The template divides the body into 36 areas, each with a percentage value. Total values of the shaded divisions. Place percentage number on a graph as a data point. Connect data points with a line to show trend of pain distribution over time.

- **Mean pressure and pain threshold of TnPs:** modified TnP examination measures pressure and pain threshold of TnPs with algometry (numeric values in kilograms per square centimeter), a more-precise quantification than the 1990 American College of Rheumatology method, enabling decisions that are more evidence based. Calculate mean of threshold values and post to a line graph.
- **FibroQuest Symptoms Survey:** 13 100-mm visual analog scales (VASs), one for each of 13 most common FMS symptoms also characteristic of hypothyroidism and peripheral cellular resistance to thyroid hormone. Patient estimates intensity of each symptom by marking appropriate point on scale (1 to 10). Total values for each marked symptom; divide total symptom intensity by number of symptoms marked at intake (baseline). Post mean score on a line graph.
- **Fibromyalgia Impact Questionnaire (FIQ):** measure of patient functional status. Post total score as a data point to a line graph. Assessment of functional ability is highly pertinent to care of FMS patients. For example, the average FMS patient has less ability in daily activities than the average community-dwelling woman in her 80s.
- **Zung Self-Rating Depression Scale:** depression is common in FMS. Use this scale in addition to VAS for depression. Post score on a line graph.

Physical examination: when FMS treatment includes thyroid hormone, use the five FMS measures plus physical tests that assess tissue responses to hormone: Achilles reflex (relaxation phase), pulse rate, basal body temperature. A combination of these is more reliable than thyroid function tests.

Integrated Metabolic Therapies Essential for All Fibromyalgia Syndrome Patients

Control or eliminate the following metabolism-impeding factors:

- **Thyroid hormone:** 90% of FMS patients have some form of thyroid disease.
- **Modify diet:** minimize arachidonic acid, which increases proinflammatory prostaglandin E_2 and leukotriene B_4, which contribute to chronic pain. Reduce refined carbohydrates. ITHR of glycolysis, citric acid cycle, and electron transport impedes production of adenosine triphosphate (ATP) and creatine phosphate. Dysglycemia and insulin resistance from refined carbohydrates worsen low production of high-energy phosphates from ITHR.

- **Wide array of nutritional supplements:** synergistic to thyroid hormone by optimal intracellular metabolism.
- **Exercise to tolerance:** sufficiently vigorous physical activity optimizes tissue metabolism and primes CNS descending nociceptive inhibitory system.

Additional Factors Needed for Some Patients

- **Adrenocortical hypofunction:** low cortisol can produce some symptoms similar to FMS (weakness, fatigue, inability to handle stress, exercise intolerance, hypotension, low nociception threshold). Low cortisol can create patient intolerant of dose of thyroid hormone high enough to be therapeutic. However, ITHR alone can cause adrenocortical hypofunction. If low cortisol stems from ITHR, thyroid hormone therapy may correct the deficiency. Low cortisol levels can also render patients intolerant of dose of thyroid hormone high enough to be fully therapeutic. The reason is that minimally effective dose of thyroid hormone can accelerate hepatic clearance of cortisol. This exacerbates symptoms of cortisol deficiency.
- **Neuromusculoskeletal lesion:** provide physical treatment for nociception-generating neuromusculoskeletal lesions (myofascial trigger points and spinal joint lesions) perpetuated by self-sustaining skeletal muscle contractures that may stem from low intramuscular, high-energy phosphate from ITHR.
- **Metabolism-impairing medicines:** some patients must cease some metabolism-impairing medicines and convert from maintenance to as-needed use of others.
  - — Beta-blockers: impair metabolism directly by reducing beta adrenergic receptor density on cell membranes and increasing $alpha_2$ adrenergic receptor density, exactly as hypothyroidism does. The isoform shift may impair CNS descending antinociceptive system, with pain and tenderness characteristic of FMS.
  - — Narcotics, tranquilizers, muscle relaxants are prescribed as FMS treatments but disincline patients from vigorous physical activity, increasing anergia and heightened pain perception.
  - — Some antidepressants (commonly prescribed for FMS) and decongestants can cause tachycardia when used concurrently with exogenous thyroid hormone. Wean patients off these drugs to increase hormone dose high enough to be therapeutic.

THERAPEUTIC APPROACH

Assess Fibromyalgia Syndrome Status

Determine FMS status before treatment is begun and at intervals throughout treatment. Reevaluate weekly to biweekly and before each increase in hormone dose. If patients have taken measurements at home (e.g., basal temperature), they should provide a record of these measurements. Conduct physical examination and review five FMS measures at each evaluation:

- Pain distribution as percentage of 36 body divisions containing pain, according to body drawing
- Mean TnP score in kilograms per square centimeter—algometry
- Symptom intensity estimate—VASs (FibroQuest Symptoms Survey)
- Functional status—FIQ
- Depression—Zung Self-Rating Depression Scale

Generate line graphs by using scores for each assessment instrument. Base changes in individualized regimen on trend of scores on line graphs combined with physical examination and clinician's and patient's subjective assessments. Continue process (2 to 6 months) until scores and line graphs normalize, patient no longer meets criteria for FMS, and patient is symptom free and fully functional.

Patient Safety

- Obtain electrocardiogram before metabolic rehabilitation and, if indicated, at intervals throughout treatment. Arrhythmias usually are not obstacles to metabolic treatment, but identify them before thyroid hormone intervention.
- Educate patients extensively on signs and symptoms of thyrotoxicosis and its management. As indicated by history, test for adrenocortical hypofunction. If cortisol production is diminished, treat with physiologic doses of cortisol at least temporarily before thyroid hormone therapy.

Thyroid Hormone Therapy

- **Hypothyroid:** begin with 1 grain (60 mg) of desiccated thyroid or synthetic T_4/T_3 preparation with a 4:1 ratio. Increase dose by 2-to-1 grain at 1-month intervals.
- **Euthyroid:** plain T_3 at start. Continue dose of 50 to 75 mcg. Increase dose at weekly to biweekly intervals by 6.25 to 12.5 mcg. Continue dose increases until patient is symptom free, no longer meets criteria for FMS, and is fully functional.

Serum and salivary thyroid hormone levels and TSH levels have no value in finding a safe and effective dose. Titrate according to tissue responses.

Wholesome Diet

Components: Lean meats (poultry and fish), fruits, vegetables; minimize whole grains and arachidonic acid, and additive excitotoxins (glutamate and aspartate). Use organic foods and filtered drinking water.

Nutritional Supplements

- **High-potency multiple vitamin-mineral**
- **Vitamin B_{12}:** 3000 to 5000 mcg q.d. of methylcobalamin (try for pain control)
- **Vitamin C:** 500 mg to 1 g t.i.d.
- **Vitamin E:** 800 to 1600 international units (IU) q.d. (mixed tocopherols)
- **Carotenoids (mixed):** 15 mg q.d.
- **Calcium:** 2000 mg elemental q.d. in divided doses
- **Mg (preferably as aspartate, citrate, malate, or glycinate):** 1000 mg q.d. in divided doses
- **Fish oils:** 1000 to 2000 mg combined EPA plus DHA q.d.
- **Exercise to tolerance:** choose form patient enjoys and gradually increase intensity as symptoms diminish. Use combinations: weight-bearing exercise to support bone health; aerobics to strengthen cardiovascular and pulmonary systems; toning to build lean muscle mass, improving metabolism. Warm water exercise is an ideal way to begin.
- **Physical medicine:** both trigger points and spinal lesions can be perpetuated by self-sustaining skeletal muscle contractures. Contractures may result from deficient intramuscular high-energy phosphate production caused by ITHR. Myofascial therapy to eliminate trigger points in muscles and spinal manipulation to regain flexibility of spine and other joints also can raise nociceptive threshold and increase mobility. If an examination indicates, prepare weight-bearing castings for flexible orthotics. For some patients, orthotics reduce musculoskeletal stress and consequent nociceptive input to CNS.

Abstention from Metabolism-Impairing Medicines

Cease beta-blockers, antidepressants, maintenance doses of narcotics, tranquilizers, and muscle-relaxing drugs.

Gallstones

DIAGNOSTIC SUMMARY

- May be asymptomatic or cause biliary colic with irregular pain-free intervals of days or months.
- Real-time ultrasonography provides definitive diagnosis.

GENERAL CONSIDERATIONS

Gallstones are a Western diet–induced disease affecting 20% of women and 8% of men older than 40 years. Twenty million Americans have gallstones. Each year 1 million more develop gallstones. More than 300,000 cholecystectomies are performed each year for gallstones. Gallstones are risk factor for gallbladder (GB) cancer. Bile components are bile salts, bilirubin, cholesterol, phospholipids, fatty acids, water, electrolytes, other organic and inorganic substances. Gallstones arise when solubilized bile components become supersaturated and precipitate.

- **Four categories:** (1) pure cholesterol; (2) pure pigment (calcium bilirubinate); (3) mixed, containing cholesterol and derivatives plus bile salts, pigments, and inorganic calcium salts; (4) mineral.
- **Pure stones** (cholesterol or calcium bilirubinate) are rare in the United States, where 80% are mixed and 20% are exclusively minerals (calcium salts, oxides of silicon and aluminum).

PATHOGENESIS

Three Steps of Pathogenesis

1. Bile supersaturation
2. Nucleation and initiation of stone formation
3. Enlargement of gallstone by accretion

Cholesterol and mixed stones require cholesterol supersaturation of bile within the GB. Bile solubility and supersaturation are based on relative molar concentrations of cholesterol, bile acids, phosphatidylcholine (lecithin), and water. Free cholesterol is water-insoluble—it must be in lecithin–bile salt micelle. Increased cholesterol secretion or decreased bile acid or lecithin secretion

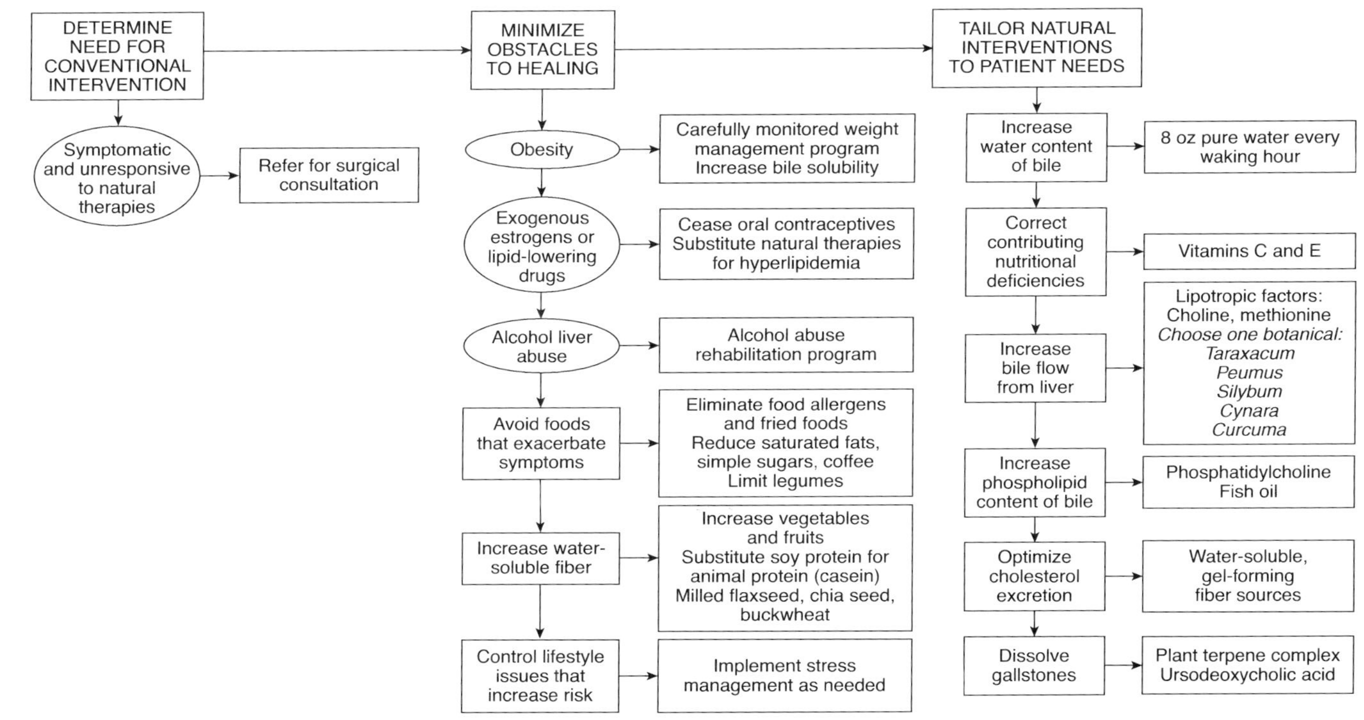
GALLSTONES
DETERMINE NEED FOR CONVENTIONAL INTERVENTION
Symptomatic and unresponsive to natural therapies
Refer for surgical consultation
MINIMIZE OBSTACLES TO HEALING
Obesity
Carefully monitored weight management program
Increase bile solubility
Exogenous estrogens or lipid-lowering drugs
Cease oral contraceptives
Substitute natural therapies for hyperlipidemia
Alcohol liver abuse
Alcohol abuse rehabilitation program
Avoid foods that exacerbate symptoms
Eliminate food allergens and fried foods
Reduce saturated fats, simple sugars, coffee
Limit legumes
Increase water-soluble fiber
Increase vegetables and fruits
Substitute soy protein for animal protein (casein)
Milled flaxseed, chia seed, buckwheat
Control lifestyle issues that increase risk
Implement stress management as needed
TAILOR NATURAL INTERVENTIONS TO PATIENT NEEDS
Increase water content of bile
8 oz pure water every waking hour
Correct contributing nutritional deficiencies
Vitamins C and E
Increase bile flow from liver
Lipotropic factors:
Choline, methionine
Choose one botanical:
Taraxacum
Peumus
Silybum
Cynara
Curcuma
Increase phospholipid content of bile
Phosphatidylcholine
Fish oil
Optimize cholesterol excretion
Water-soluble, gel-forming fiber sources
Dissolve gallstones
Plant terpene complex
Ursodeoxycholic acid

induces supersaturation. Stone formation is initiated by biliary stasis, infection, or mucin. Radius increases at 2.6 mm/yr, eventually reaching size of a few millimeters to more than a centimeter. Stone is symptomatic 8 years after formation begins. Cholelithiasis occurs in 95% of patients with cholecystitis.

Risk Factors for Cholesterol and Mixed Stones

Considerations are diet, gender, race, obesity, high caloric intake, estrogens, gastrointestinal diseases (Crohn's disease, cystic fibrosis), drugs, and age.

- **Gender:** frequency is two to four times greater in women than in men. Women are predisposed because of either increased cholesterol synthesis or suppression of bile acids by estrogens. Pregnancy, oral contraceptives, or other causes of elevated estrogen increase incidence.
- **Genetic and ethnic:** gallstones are most common in Native American women older than 30 years (70% have gallstones). Only 10% of black women older than 30 years have gallstones. Differences reflect extent of cholesterol saturation of bile. Dietary factors outweigh genetic factors.
- **Obesity:** increased activity of 3-hydroxy-3-methylglutaryl-coenzyme A (HMG-CoA) reductase and secretion of cholesterol in bile from increased cholesterol synthesis. Obesity is linked to much increased incidence because of biliary cholesterol saturation. During active weight reduction, biliary cholesterol saturation initially increases. Secretion of biliary lipids is reduced during weight loss, but secretion of bile acids decreases more than cholesterol. When weight is stabilized, bile acid output returns to normal and cholesterol output remains low. Net effect is a significant reduction in cholesterol saturation. Prolonged dietary fat reduction can promote biliary stasis, causing cholesterol saturation. Ten or more grams of fat daily are needed for proper GB emptying.
- **Gastrointestinal tract diseases:** Crohn's disease and cystic fibrosis involve malabsorption of bile acids from the terminal ileum that disturbs enterohepatic circulation by reducing bile acid pool and rate of bile secretion.
- **Drugs:** tamoxifen increases gallstones. Over 5 years, incidence of stones in tamoxifen-treated patients was 37.4% versus 2.0% in those not taking drug. Other problematic agents are oral contraceptives, other estrogens, cephalosporin ceftriaxone, octreotide, HMG-CoA reductase inhibitors, and possibly other lipid-lowering drugs.

- **Age:** average gallstone patient is 40 to 50 years old. Incidence increases with age because of inactivity of cholesterol 7-alpha-hydroxylase with increased biliary cholesterol hypersecretion, cholesterol saturation, and accelerated stone formation.
- **Risk factors for pigmented gallstones:** they are more common in Asia because of liver and GB parasites (liver fluke *Clonorchis sinensis*). Bacteria and protozoa cause stasis or act as nucleating agents. In the United States, pigmented stones are caused by chronic hemolysis or alcohol liver cirrhosis.

THERAPEUTIC CONSIDERATIONS

Gallstones are easier to prevent than reverse. Primary treatment is to reduce controllable risk factors. Therapeutic intervention is to avoid aggravating foods and increase solubility of cholesterol in bile. If symptoms persist or worsen, cholecystectomy is indicated. Eliminate foods producing symptoms. Increase dietary fiber. Eliminate food allergens. Reduce refined carbohydrates and animal protein. Gallstones increase risk for GB cancer. Vegetables and fruits protect against GB cancer; red meat (beef, mutton) increase risk of GB carcinogenesis. Use nutritional lipotropic compounds and herbal choleretics to increase solubility of bile. Biliary cholesterol concentration and serum cholesterol do not correlate, but increased serum triglycerides are linked to bile saturation.

Asymptomatic gallstones: natural history of silent or asymptomatic gallstones suggests elective cholecystectomy is not warranted. Cumulative chance for developing symptoms is 10% at 5 years, 15% at 10 years, and 18% at 15 years. If controllable risk factors are eliminated or reduced, the patient remains asymptomatic.

Diet

- **Dietary fiber:** diet high in refined carbohydrates and fat and low in fiber reduces liver synthesis of bile acids and lowers bile acids in the GB. Fiber reduces absorption of deoxycholic acid, produced from bile acids by gut bacteria, which lessens solubility of cholesterol in bile. Fiber decreases formation of deoxycholic acid and binds deoxycholic acid for fecal excretion. Prefer water-soluble fibers: vegetables, fruits, pectin, oat bran, and guar gum. Diets rich in legumes with water-soluble fiber (Native Americans) are linked to increased risk for cholesterol gallstones. Legumes increase biliary cholesterol saturation because of saponin content. A Dutch study showed just the opposite, because legume intake provided significant protection against gallstones. Until this issue is clarified, restrict legume intake in patients with existing gallstones.

- **Vegetarian diet:** protective against gallstones because of fiber content. Animal proteins (casein from dairy) increase formation of gallstones; vegetable proteins (soy) are preventive against gallstones.
- **Food allergies:** food allergies may cause GB pain. One study demonstrated 100% of patients to be symptom free while on elimination diet (beef, rye, soybeans, rice, cherries, peaches, apricots, beets, spinach). Foods inducing symptoms, in decreasing order of occurrence, are egg, pork, onion, fowl, milk, coffee, citrus, corn, beans, nuts. Ingestion of allergy-causing substances may cause swelling of bile ducts, impairing bile flow from GB.
- **Buckwheat:** decreases gallstone formation and reduces concentration of cholesterol in GB, plasma, and liver of animals compared with casein. Buckwheat is far more protective than soy. Buckwheat can enhance bile acid synthesis and fecal excretion of steroids. It may treat both hypercholesterolemia and gallstones and reduce colon cancer cell proliferation. Higher levels of arginine and glycine may help in buckwheat's protective function.
- **Sugars:** increase risk of biliary tract cancer based on relationship among sugars, blood lipids, and gallstone formation. Sugar increases cholesterol saturation of bile. Gallstones are linked to monosaccharides and disaccharides, independent of other energy sources.
- **Caloric restriction:** total calorie and carbohydrate intake and serum triglycerides are higher in gallstone patients than in control subjects. Refined carbohydrate intake is higher in female gallstone patients; fat intake is higher in male gallstone patients. Caloric intake of more than 2500 kcal/day and diets rich in carbohydrates and saturated fats increased gallstone risk. Alcohol intake at 20 to 40 g/day was protective. Caloric restriction must be instituted carefully because rapid weight loss and fasting increase risk of gallstones. Those who develop gallstones have higher baseline triglycerides and total cholesterol and greater rate of weight loss than those who did not.
- **Coffee:** can promote symptoms of gallstones but may also inhibit their formation. Avoid coffee until stones are resolved; coffee (regular and decaffeinated) induces GB contractions by cholecystokinin secretion. In women, 4 cups of caffeinated coffee daily induce 28% lower risk of developing symptoms of gallstones.

Drinking coffee regularly before or during early stone formation may inhibit development or clear small stones by enhanced GB contractions from multiple daily coffee doses. Large existing stones may exacerbate symptoms if contractions are induced by coffee.

Nutritional Factors

- **Lecithin (phosphatidylcholine):** main cholesterol solubilizer in bile. Low lecithin in bile may be a causative factor. A pure bile salt micelle requires 50 molecules to enclose a single molecule of cholesterol; a mixed bile salt–phospholipid micelle requires only seven molecules. Taking only 100 mg lecithin t.i.d. increases lecithin in bile, and larger doses (up to 10 g) provide greater increases. Increased lecithin content of bile usually increases solubility of cholesterol. No significant effects on gallstone dissolution are obtained by using lecithin alone.
- **Nutrient deficiencies:** deficiencies of either vitamin E or vitamin C caused gallstones in animal studies.
- **Olive oil:** olive oil "liver flush" is undesirable for patients with gallstones; consuming large quantities of any oil induces contraction of GB, increasing risk of stone blocking bile duct and causing a surgical emergency. Oleic acid increases development of gallstones in laboratory animals by increasing cholesterol in the GB.
- **Fish oils:** in animal studies, fish oil increased biliary phospholipid secretion and reduced cholesterol concentration in the GB and rate of gallstone formation. Omega-3 eicosapentaenoic acid (EPA) and docosahexaenoic acid (DHA) inhibit gallstone formation and decrease biliary calcium and total protein. Omega-3 fatty acids enhance stability of biliary phospholipid-cholesterol vesicles.
- **Lipotropic factors and botanical choleretics:** lipotropic factors are substances that hasten removal or decrease deposition of fat in the liver by interaction with fat metabolism. Lipotropic agents—choline, methionine, betaine, folic acid, and vitamin B_{12}—are used with herbal cholagogues and choleretics. Cholagogues stimulate GB contraction, whereas choleretics increase bile secretion by liver. Herbal choleretics have favorable effect on solubility of bile. Choleretics appropriate to gallstones are *Taraxacum officinale* (dandelion root), silymarin from *Silybum marianum* (milk thistle), *Cynara scolymus* (artichoke), *Curcuma longa* (turmeric), and *Peumus boldus* (alkaloid boldine helps treat gallstones).

Chemical Dissolution of Gallstones

Use complex of plant terpenes alone or, preferably, in combination with oral bile acids. Decreasing GB cholesterol and/or increasing bile acids or lecithin should result in dissolution of stone. Chemical dissolution is especially indicated for gallstones in the elderly who cannot withstand stress of surgery and in others for whom surgery is contraindicated.

- **Bile acids:** use of bile acids (ursodeoxycholic acid and tauroursodeoxycholic acid) is effective in dissolving small, uncalcified cholesterol gallstones. About 15% of all patients with cholesterol gallstones meet these criteria. Treatment with bile acids will lead to complete dissolution in 90% of cases after 6 months of therapy. Thereafter, it is imperative to follow gallstone prevention guidelines to reduce risk for recurrence. Bile acid preparations are available by prescription only; they are safe and effective nonsurgical alternative. Typical dose: 12 mg per kg body weight daily.
- **Terpenes:** natural terpene combination (menthol, menthone, pinene, borneol, cineol, camphene) is an effective alternative to surgery. It is safe even when consumed up to 4 years.
- **Combined therapy:** terpenes are effective alone, but best results come from combining plant terpenes and bile acids. Lower doses of bile acids can be used, reducing risk of side effects and cost of bile acid therapy. Menthol is a major component of formula; peppermint oil, especially enteric coated, may offer similar results.

Lifestyle

- **Sunbathing:** almost all cholesterol gallstones contain a central, pigmented nucleus with radial or lamellar pigmented bands, alternating with layers of crystalline cholesterol. Activation of the pigmentary system by ultraviolet light may increase concentrations of indole metabolites in bile, triggering their polymerization. Positive attitude toward sunbathing is linked to twice the risk of cholelithiasis compared with those with negative attitude. The association is almost entirely restricted to those who always burn after long sunbathing.
- **Social stress:** chronic social stress can increase bile retention, increase GB hypertrophy, and inhibit GB emptying. Chronic stress may be predictor of GB dysfunction and eventual gallstone formation.

THERAPEUTIC APPROACH

Healthy diet rich in dietary fiber, with controlled caloric intake and limited saturated fats, gives adequate prevention. After development of stones, implement measures to avoid GB attacks and increase bile solubility. Limit incidence of symptoms; intolerant or allergic foods and fatty foods must be avoided. Increase solubility of bile; follow dietary guidelines plus nutritional and herbal supplementation described here.

- **Diet:** increase vegetables, fruits, and dietary fiber, especially gel-forming or mucilaginous fibers (ground flaxseed, oat bran, guar gum, pectin). Increase intake of buckwheat. Reduce saturated fats, cholesterol, sugar, animal proteins. Avoid all fried foods. Allergy elimination diet reduces GB attacks (*Textbook,* "Food Reactions").
- **Water:** 8 fl oz of water every waking hour to optimize water content of bile.
- **Nutritional supplements:**
  - — Vitamin C: 1 to 3 g q.d.
  - — Vitamin E: 200 to 400 international units (IU) q.d. (mixed tocopherols)
  - — Phosphatidylcholine: 500 mg q.d.
  - — Choline: 1 g q.d.
  - — L-Methionine: 1 g q.d.
  - — Fiber supplement (guar gum, pectin, psyllium, or oat bran): minimum of 5 g q.d.
- **Botanical medicines:**
  - — Choose one of the following:
    - – *T. officinale* (t.i.d.): dried dandelion root, 4 g; fluid extract (1:1), 4 to 8 mL; solid extract (4:1), 250 to 500 mg
    - – *P. boldus* (t.i.d.): dried leaves (or by infusion), 250 to 500 mg; tincture (1:10), 2 to 4 mL; fluid extract (1:1), 0.5 to 1.0 mL
    - – *S. marianum* (milk thistle): sufficient dose according to form to yield 70 to 210 mg of silymarin t.i.d.
    - – *C. scolymus* (artichoke): extract (15% cynarin), 500 mg t.i.d.
    - – *C. longa* (turmeric): curcumin, 300 mg t.i.d.
  - — **Gallstone-dissolving formula:** menthol, 30 mg; menthone, 5 mg; pinene, 15 mg; borneol, 5 mg; camphene, 5 mg; cineol, 2 mg; citral, 5 mg; phosphatidylcholine, 50 mg; medium-chain triglycerides, 125 mg; chenodeoxycholic acid, 750 mg. Dose: t.i.d. if used in combination with meals. Note: peppermint oil in enteric-coated capsule can substitute at dose of 1 or 2 capsules (0.2 mL/capsule) t.i.d. between meals.

Glaucoma: Acute (Angle-Closure) and Chronic (Open-Angle)

DIAGNOSTIC SUMMARY

Acute Glaucoma

- Increased intraocular pressure (IOP), usually unilateral
- Severe throbbing pain in eye with markedly blurred vision
- Pupil moderately dilated and fixed
- Absence of pupillary light response
- Nausea and vomiting common

Chronic Glaucoma

- Persistent elevation of IOP is associated with pathologic cupping of optic discs
- Asymptomatic in early stages
- Gradual loss of peripheral vision resulting in tunnel vision
- Insidious onset in older individuals

Normotensive Glaucoma

- Normal IOP with no pathologic cupping of optic discs
- Asymptomatic in early stages
- Gradual loss of peripheral vision resulting in tunnel vision
- Insidious onset in older patients, more common in women than men
- Low blood pressure a common underlying feature

GENERAL CONSIDERATIONS

Glaucoma is increased IOP from imbalance between production and outflow of aqueous humor. Obstruction to outflow is the main factor in closed-angle glaucoma. Acute glaucoma occurs only with closure of preexisting narrow anterior chamber angle. In chronic open-angle glaucoma, anterior chamber appears normal.

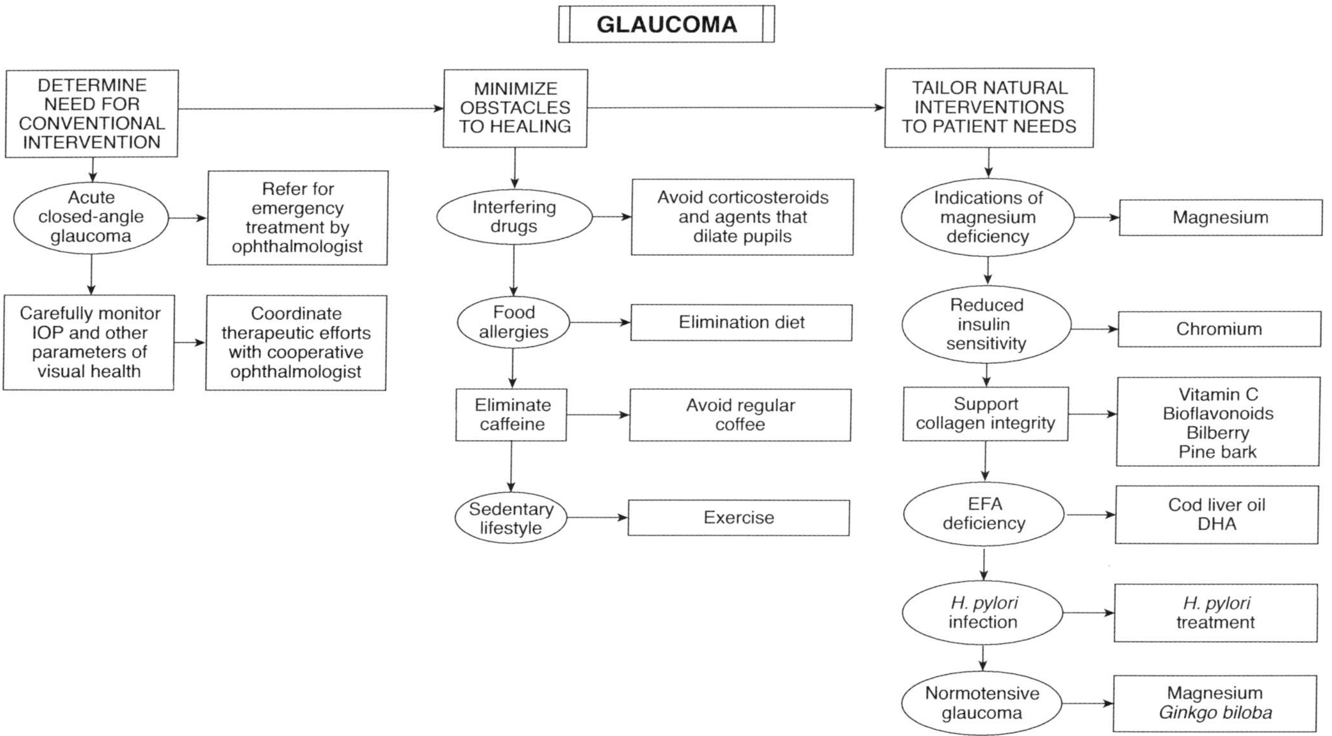
GLAUCOMA
DETERMINE NEED FOR CONVENTIONAL INTERVENTION
Acute closed-angle glaucoma
Refer for emergency treatment by ophthalmologist
Carefully monitor IOP and other parameters of visual health
Coordinate therapeutic efforts with cooperative ophthalmologist
MINIMIZE OBSTACLES TO HEALING
Interfering drugs
Avoid corticosteroids and agents that dilate pupils
Food allergies
Elimination diet
Eliminate caffeine
Avoid regular coffee
Sedentary lifestyle
Exercise
TAILOR NATURAL INTERVENTIONS TO PATIENT NEEDS
Indications of magnesium deficiency
Magnesium
Reduced insulin sensitivity
Chromium
Support collagen integrity
Vitamin C
Bioflavonoids
Bilberry
Pine bark
EFA deficiency
Cod liver oil
DHA
H. pylori infection
H. pylori treatment
Normotensive glaucoma
Magnesium
Ginkgo biloba

- **Three million cases in the United States:** 25% undetected; 90% are chronic open-angle type (no consistent anatomic basis for condition). Content and composition of collagen and glaucomatous eye are strongly correlated.
- **Collagen:** most abundant protein in the body, including eye. It provides tissue strength and integrity of cornea, sclera, lamina cribrosa, trabecular meshwork, and vitreous. Inborn errors of collagen metabolism (osteogenesis imperfecta, Ehlers-Danlos syndrome, Marfan's syndrome) have ocular complications: glaucoma, myopia, retinal detachment, ectopia lentis, and blue sclera. Morphologic changes in lamina cribrosa (scleral area pierced by optic nerve and blood vessels), trabecular meshwork (connective tissue network the aqueous humor must traverse to reach canal of Schlemm), and papillary blood vessels are found in glaucomatous eyes. Changes may elevate IOP or lead to progressive loss of peripheral vision.
- **Collagen structure changes:** may explain similar peripheral vision loss in patients with normal and elevated IOP, cupping of optic disc even at low IOP, and no apparent anatomic reason for decreased aqueous outflow.
- **Normotensive glaucoma (NTG; low-tension glaucoma):** develops in people with normal IOP. It accounts for 25% to 30% of all U.S. cases of glaucoma, is more common in women than men, and affects adults with average age of 60 years. The following are suggested causes:
  — Reduced blood flow
  — Early nerve cell death
  — Nerve irritation
  — Excess glutamate production
  — Autoimmune disease
  — Low blood pressure

DIAGNOSIS

There may be slight cupping of optic disc and narrowing of visual fields. Tonometry is the key to confirming diagnosis. Early recognition is critical; delayed surgical intervention increases risk of blindness.

THERAPEUTIC CONSIDERATIONS

- Treatment and prevention depend on reducing IOP and improving collagen metabolism in optic disc and trabecular meshwork.

- Optic disc is composed of lamina cribrosa, optic nerve fibers, and blood vessels. The lamina cribrosa is a meshlike network rich in collagen traversed by optic nerves and blood vessels. Collagen changes in lamina cribrosa, papillary vessels, and trabecular meshwork precede pressure changes. Intervention must prevent breakdown of ground substance and collagen.
- Corticosteroid use should be discouraged in glaucoma because of inhibition of biosynthesis of collagen and glycosaminoglycans (GAGs), causing glaucoma to develop.

Nutrition

- **Vitamin C:** achieving collagen integrity requires optimal tissue ascorbic acid (AA); AA lowers IOP in clinical studies. Daily dose of 0.5 g/kg body weight (single or divided doses) reduces IOP by 16 mm Hg. Near-normal tension was achieved in some patients unresponsive to acetazolamide (a carbonic anhydrase inhibitor) and 2% pilocarpine (a miotic agent). Hypotonic action of AA on eye is long lasting if supplement continued; intravenous administration gives greater initial reduction in IOP. Patient monitoring is necessary to determine required individual dose (2 to 35 g q.d.). Abdominal discomfort with high doses is common but resolves after 3 to 4 days. Proposed mechanisms: increased blood osmolarity, diminished production of aqueous fluid by ciliary epithelium, and improved aqueous fluid outflow; AA role in collagen formation may be key.
- **Flavonoids:** anthocyanosides (blue-red pigments in berries) elicit AA-sparing effect, improve capillary integrity, and stabilize collagen matrix by preventing free radical damage, inhibiting enzymatic cleavage of collagen matrix, and cross-linking with collagen fibers directly to form more stable collagen matrix. *Vaccinium myrtillus* (European bilberry) is rich in these compounds and is used in Europe to reduce myopia, improve nocturnal vision, and reverse diabetic retinopathy. Mirtogenol is a combination of bilberry anthocyanoside extract (160 mg Mirtoselect) and pine bark extract (80 mg pycnogenol). After 3 months of treatment, mean IOP decreased from baseline of 25.2 to 22 mm Hg. No further improvement was found after 6 months. No side effects were observed. Ocular blood flow (central retinal, ophthalmic, and posterior ciliary arteries) improved in systolic and diastolic components as measured by ultrasound. Rutin lowers IOP when used as an adjunct in patients unresponsive to miotics alone. In NTG, *Ginkgo biloba* extract (GBE) may be

helpful. In healthy human volunteers, GBE (120 mg daily) increased end-diastolic velocity in the ophthalmic artery (23% change). GBE did not alter arterial blood pressure, heart rate, or IOP. In patients with NTG, 40 mg GBE t.i.d. for 4 weeks improved visual field index scores, showing that GBE improves preexisting visual field damage in some patients with NTG.

- **Allergy:** chronic glaucoma has been successfully treated by antiallergy measures. Immediate rise in IOP of up to 20 mm (plus other allergic symptoms) occurred in patients challenged with appropriate allergen. Allergic responses (altered vascular permeability and vasospasm) may cause congestion and edema characteristic of glaucoma.
- **Magnesium (Mg):** channel blocking drugs benefit some glaucoma patients. Mg is "nature's physiologic calcium channel blocker." Mg administered at 121.5 mg b.i.d. for 1 month improved visual fields and peripheral circulation in patients with glaucoma. In patients with NTG, 300 mg of oral Mg (citrate) improved visual field measurements (e.g., mean deviation improved from −3.7 at baseline to −2.5, and pattern standard deviation improved from 3.6 baseline to 2.8). There was no change in ocular blood flow; exact mechanism of effect is not known.
- **Chromium (Cr):** primary open-angle glaucoma is strongly linked to deficiency of red blood cells, Cr, and AA and elevated red blood cell vanadium (Cr's principal antagonist). AA and Cr potentiate insulin receptors that help sustain strong ciliary muscle eye-focusing activity. AA or Cr deficiency is linked with elevated IOP, which stretches normal eye, reducing capacity for focusing power.
- **Fish oil:** cod liver oil reduces IOP dramatically in laboratory animals in a dose-dependent fashion. Preliminary human trials with docosahexaenoic acid (DHA) have been encouraging
- **Caffeine:** consumption of regular coffee (180 mg caffeine in 200 mL of coffee) by NTG or ocular hypertensive patients elevates IOP. This elevation may be clinically significant.

Other Recommendations

- **Exercise:** induces immediate and prolonged reduction in IOP. Within 5 minutes of starting exercise, IOP increases, then gradually decreases to lowest level 60 minutes after completion of exercise. Reduction: walking, 7.2%; jogging and running, 12.7%; more than decrease in IOP in normal eyes. Duration of IOP reduction: 84 minutes in glaucoma and 63 minutes in normal eyes. Mechanism is independent of systemic blood pressure and sympathetic stimulation but may be influenced by increased serum osmolarity. Moderate to heavy exercise is effective in sedentary subjects but less effective in physically fit subjects. Physically fit persons tend to have lower IOP, but if one stops exercising, effect wears off in 3 weeks. Still, many can benefit from exercise.

- ***Helicobacter pylori:*** infection is linked to open-angle glaucoma. Eradication of *H. pylori* can decrease IOP. See chapter on gastric ulcer for a discussion of *H. pylori* treatment.

Differential Diagnosis of the Inflamed Eye

	Acute Conjunctivitis	Acute Iritis	Acute Glaucoma	Corneal Trauma or Infection
Incidence	Very common	Common	Uncommon	Common
Discharge	Moderate to copious	None	None	Watery or purulent
Vision	No effect	Slightly blurred	Markedly blurred	Usually blurred
Pain	None	Moderate	Severe	Moderate to severe
Conjunctival injection	Diffuse, mostly fornices	Circumcorneal	Diffuse	Diffuse
Cornea	Clear	Usually clear	Steamy	Clarity may change
Pupillary size	Normal	Small	Dilated and fixed	Normal
Pupillary light response	Normal	Poor	None	Normal
Intraocular pressure	Normal	Normal	Elevated	Normal
Anterior chamber		Normal depth	Very shallow	Normal depth
Iris	Normal	Dull, swollen	Congested and bulging	Normal unless infected
Smear	Causative organisms	No organisms	No organisms	Causative organisms if there is infection

Modified from Distelhorst JS, Hughes GM. Open-angle glaucoma. *Am Fam Physician* 2003; 1937–1944.

THERAPEUTIC APPROACH

Acute closed-angle glaucoma is an ocular emergency; refer immediately to ophthalmologist. Unless treated within 12 to 48 hours, patient will be permanently blinded within 2 to 5 days. An asymptomatic eye with narrow anterior chamber angle may convert spontaneously to angle-closure glaucoma. The process can be precipitated by anything dilating pupil (atropine, epinephrine-like drugs). Signs and symptoms: extreme pain, blurring of vision, conjunctivitis, fixed and dilated pupil. Agents that dilate pupils must be strictly avoided if glaucoma is suspected.

- **Supplements:**
  - Vitamin C: 0.1 to 0.5 g/kg q.d. in divided doses
  - Bioflavonoids (mixed): 1000 mg q.d.
  - Mg: 300 mg elemental Mg q.d.
  - Cr: 100 mcg q.d.
- **Botanical medicines:**
  - To prevent and treat chronic open-angle glaucoma: either bilberry extract or proanthocyanoside extract, alone or in combination, as follows:
    - *V. myrtillus* extract (25% anthocyanidins): 160 to 240 mg q.d.
    - Pine bark extract (pycnogenol) or grapeseed extract (95% proanthocyanidin content): 150 to 300 mg q.d.
  - For NTG:
    - GBE: 120 to 320 mg q.d.

Gout

DIAGNOSTIC SUMMARY

- Acute onset, frequently nocturnal, of typically monarticular joint pain involving metatarsophalangeal joint of big toe in approximately 50% of cases
- Elevated serum uric acid level
- Asymptomatic periods between acute attacks
- Identification of urate crystals in joint fluid
- Aggregated deposits of monosodium urate monohydrate (tophi) chiefly in and around the joints of extremities but also in subcutaneous tissue, bone, cartilage, and other tissues
- Uric acid kidney stones
- Familial disease with 95% affected being male

GENERAL CONSIDERATIONS

Gout is a common arthritis condition caused by increased uric acid (final breakdown product of purine metabolism) in biologic fluid. Uric acid crystals (monosodium urate) deposit in joints, tendons, kidneys, and other tissues, causing inflammation and damage.

- Characterized biochemically by increased serum uric acid, leukotrienes, and neutrophil accumulation. It may debilitate from tophaceous deposits around joints and tendons. Renal involvement may cause kidney failure by parenchymal disease or urinary tract obstruction.
- Associated with affluence ("rich man's disease"). Meats (organ meats) are high in purines. Alcohol inhibits uric acid excretion by kidneys. Gout is primarily a disease of adult men (95% of cases are in men older than 30 years). Incidence rate is three adults in 1000; 10% to 20% of adults have hyperuricemia.
- Gout is a strong predictor of metabolic syndrome and increased risk for type 2 diabetes

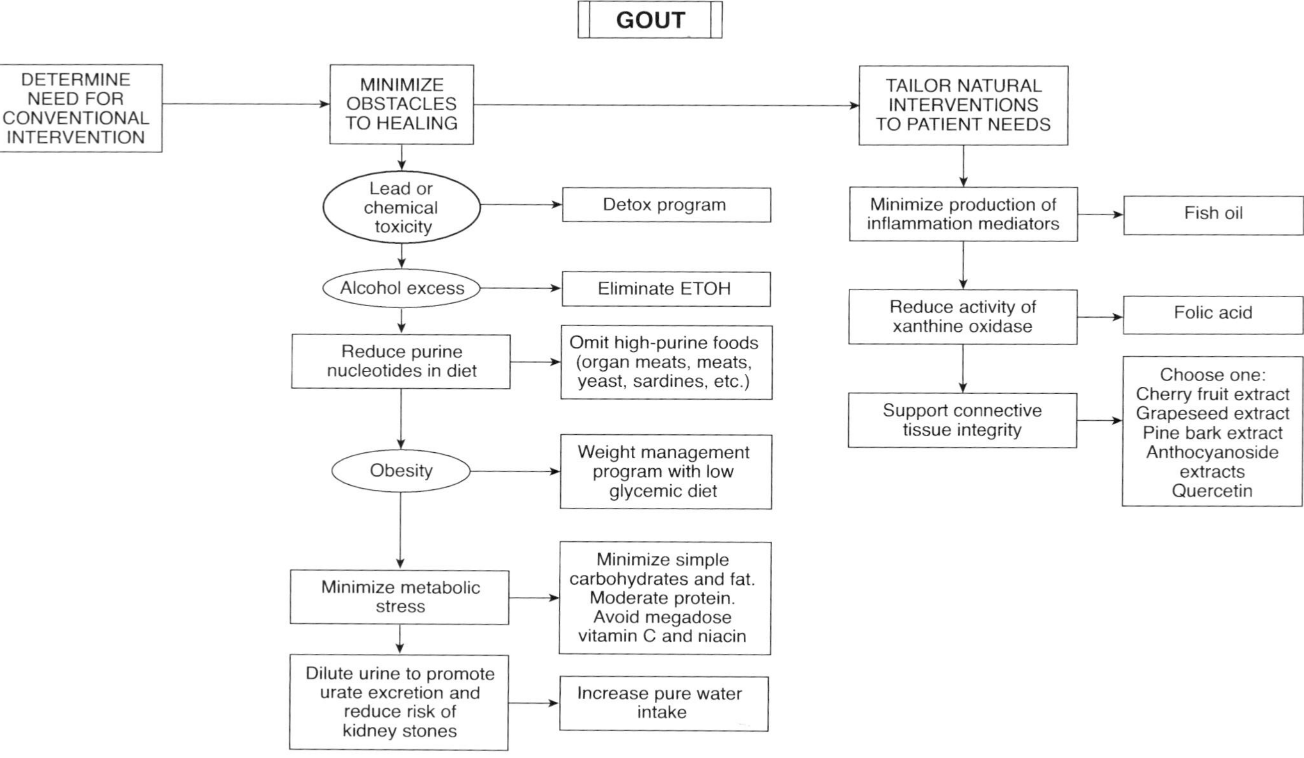
GOUT
DETERMINE NEED FOR CONVENTIONAL INTERVENTION
MINIMIZE OBSTACLES TO HEALING
Lead or chemical toxicity
Detox program
Alcohol excess
Eliminate ETOH
Reduce purine nucleotides in diet
Omit high-purine foods (organ meats, meats, yeast, sardines, etc.)
Obesity
Weight management program with low glycemic diet
Minimize metabolic stress
Minimize simple carbohydrates and fat. Moderate protein. Avoid megadose vitamin C and niacin
Dilute urine to promote urate excretion and reduce risk of kidney stones
Increase pure water intake
TAILOR NATURAL INTERVENTIONS TO PATIENT NEEDS
Minimize production of inflammation mediators
Fish oil
Reduce activity of xanthine oxidase
Folic acid
Support connective tissue integrity
Choose one: Cherry fruit extract Grapeseed extract Pine bark extract Anthocyanoside extracts Quercetin

Causes of Gout

- Two major categories:

1. **Primary gout:** 90% of all cases; usually idiopathic, but several known genetic defects cause elevated uric acid levels.
2. **Secondary gout:** 10% of cases; elevated uric acid is attributable to some other disorder (e.g., excessive breakdown of cells or renal disease). Diuretics for hypertension and low-dose aspirin are causes because they decrease uric acid excretion.

- Hyperuricemia of primary idiopathic gout has three causes:

1. **Increased synthesis of uric acid** (majority of cases)
2. **Reduced ability to excrete uric acid** (30% of cases)
3. **Overproduction of uric acid and underexcretion of uric acid** (minority of cases)

- Exact metabolic defect unknown in most cases, but the disease is controllable.
- From 200 to 600 mg uric acid are excreted daily in urine of adult male, two thirds of the amount produced. The remainder is excreted in bile and other gastrointestinal secretions. Dietary component of uric acid is 10% to 20%; in hyperuricemia, 1 mg/100 mL added to serum, enough to precipitate into tissues if individual is near saturation threshold.
- Almost all plasma urate is filtered at glomerulus; only a small amount bound to protein is not filtered. Renal excretion is peculiar; 80% of filtered uric acid is reabsorbed in proximal tubule of nephron. Distal tubule secretes most uric acid in urine. Distal to this site, postsecondary reabsorption occurs. Uric acid is highly insoluble. At a pH of 7.4 and at body temperature, serum is saturated at 6.4 to 7.0 mg/100 mL. An unknown factor in serum inhibits urate precipitation. The chance of acute attack is 90% when level is above 9 mg/100 mL. Lower temperatures decrease saturation point; urate deposits form in areas where temperature is lower than mean body temperature (e.g., pinna of ear). Uric acid is insoluble at pH below 6.0 and can precipitate as urine is concentrated in collecting ducts and passes to renal pelvis.

Signs and Symptoms

First attack includes intense pain, usually involving only one joint; first joint of big toe affected in 50% of first attacks and involved in 90% of cases. If attack progresses, fever and chills appear. First attacks usually occur at night, preceded by specific event (dietary excess, alcohol consumption, trauma, certain drugs, or surgery).

Subsequent attacks are common, usually within 1 year; but 7% never have a second attack. Chronic gout is extremely rare; dietary therapy and drugs lower urate levels. When it does occur, chronic gout is a result of poor compliance or inadequate response to treatment, or it may arise in patients with high flare frequency, tophi, and inability to maintain serum urate levels below 6 mg/dL. Some kidney dysfunction occurs in 90% of patients with gout, who have a higher risk of kidney stones.

THERAPEUTIC CONSIDERATIONS

- **Colchicine:** conventional acute treatment; an anti-inflammatory drug originally isolated from the plant *Colchicum autumnale* (autumn crocus, meadow saffron). Colchicine has no effect on uric acid levels; it stops inflammation by inhibiting neutrophil migration into areas of inflammation. Approximately 75% of patients improve within the first 12 hours of taking colchicine, but 80% of patients are unable to tolerate the optimal dose because of gastrointestinal side effects preceding or coinciding with improvement. Colchicine may cause bone marrow depression, hair loss, liver damage, depression, seizures, respiratory depression, and even death. Other anti-inflammatory agents also are used (indomethacin, phenylbutazone, naproxen, fenoprofen).
- **Post–acute episode measures to reduce risk of recurrence:** drugs to normalize urate levels, controlled weight loss in obese patients, avoidance of known precipitating factors (alcohol excess or diet rich in purines), low-dose colchicine to prevent attacks.
- **Dietary factors exacerbating gout:** alcohol, especially beer and hard liquor; high-purine foods (organ meats, meat, yeast, poultry), fats, refined carbohydrates, caloric excess. Gout patients typically are obese, hypertensive, prone to diabetes, and at greater risk for cardiovascular disease. Obesity is the most important dietary factor. Thiazide and loop diuretics are also linked to higher risk of incident gout and higher rate of gout flares.
- **Naturopathic approach:** similar to conventional approach—dietary and herbal measures instead of drugs to maintain normal urate levels, weight management to reduce obesity, control of known precipitating factors, nutritional substances to prevent acute attacks.
- **Lead (Pb) toxicity:** a secondary type of gout (saturnine gout) results from Pb toxicity. The source is leaded crystal (port wine elutes Pb when stored in crystal decanters). Pb level increases

with storage time, becoming toxic after several months. Even a few minutes in crystal glass produces measurable increases of Pb in wine. Mechanism of action is a decrease in renal urate excretion.

- **Persistent organic pollutants:** emerging research is showing that exposure to some persistent organic pollutants—currently shown in the fluorinated hydrocarbons—increases serum uric acid in proportion to total body load.

Dietary Guidelines

Eliminate alcohol; achieve ideal body weight; begin diet low in purines, high in complex carbohydrates, low in fat and protein, abundant in fluids, especially purified water.

- **Alcohol:** increases urate production by accelerating purine nucleotide degradation, which reduces urate excretion by increasing lactate (from alcohol oxidation) and impairing kidney function. Net effect is increased serum uric acid. Alcohol intake often initiates acute attack. Abstinence is the only change needed to prevent attacks in some patients.
- **Weight reduction:** obesity is linked to increased rate of gout. Weight reduction in obese persons reduces serum urate. Use low-glycemic, high-fiber, low-fat diet to improve insulin sensitivity and manage elevated cholesterol and triglycerides common in obesity.
- **Low-purine alkaline-ash diet:** reduces metabolic stress. Omit high-purine foods (organ meats, meats, shellfish, yeast [brewer's and baker's], herring, sardines, mackerel, anchovies). Curtail foods with moderate protein (dried legumes, spinach, asparagus, fish, poultry, mushrooms). Alkaline-ash diet is recommended because a more alkaline pH increases uric acid solubility. Alkaline-ash diet increases uric acid excretion from 302 mg/day at pH 5.9 to 413 mg/day at pH 6.5.
- **Carbohydrates, fats, and protein:** refined carbohydrates increase urate production; saturated fats increase urate retention. Enhance insulin sensitivity. Avoid excess protein (>0.8 g/kg body weight); high protein intake may accelerate urate synthesis in normal and gouty patients. Adequate protein (0.8 g/kg body weight) is necessary; amino acids decrease resorption of urate in renal tubules, increasing urate excretion and reducing serum urate.
- **Fluid intake:** liberal fluid (purified water) intake keeps urine dilute to promote urate excretion and reduce risk of kidney stones.

Nutritional Supplements

- **Eicosapentaenoic acid (EPA):** quite useful for gout; limits production of proinflammatory leukotrienes, mediators of inflammation and tissue damage in gout.
- **Folic acid:** inhibits xanthine oxidase, the enzyme that produces uric acid. A derivative of folic acid is an even greater inhibitor of xanthine oxidase than allopurinol. Folic acid at pharmacologic doses may be effective treatment. Positive results have been reported, but data are incomplete and uncontrolled.
- **Quercetin:** bioflavonoid that may offer significant protection by inhibiting xanthine oxidase in similar fashion to allopurinol, leukotriene synthesis and release, neutrophil accumulation, and enzyme release. Take with bromelain between meals.
- **Vitamin C:** megadoses of vitamin C are contraindicated in gout; vitamin C may increase urate in a small number of individuals.
- **Niacin:** high-dose niacin (>50 mg q.d.) is contraindicated in gout; niacin competes with urate for excretion.

Botanical Medicines

- **Cherries:** Consuming 0.25 kg fresh or canned cherries daily is effective in lowering uric acid and preventing gout attacks. Cherries decrease plasma urate within 5 hours by 30 μmol/L, correlating with increased urine urate excretion. Plasma C-reactive protein and nitric oxide decline slightly after 3 hours. Cherries, hawthorn berries, blueberries, and other dark red-blue berries are rich sources of anthocyanidins and proanthocyanidins. These flavonoids give fruits deep red-blue color and prevent collagen destruction. Effects of anthocyanidins and other flavonoids are to cross-link collagen fibers, reinforcing natural cross-linking of collagen matrix of connective tissue; prevent free radical damage by potent antioxidant and free radical scavenging action; inhibit cleavage of collagen by enzymes secreted by leukocytes during inflammation; prevent synthesis and release of compounds promoting inflammation (histamine, serine proteases, prostaglandins, leukotrienes).

THERAPEUTIC APPROACH

- **Basic approach:**
  - — Dietary and herbal measures that maintain normal uric acid levels
  - — Controlled weight loss for obesity

- — Avoidance of known precipitating factors (alcohol abuse, high-purine diet)
- — Nutritional substances to prevent acute attacks
- — Herbal and nutritional substances to inhibit inflammation

- **Diet:** Eliminate alcohol; maintain low-purine diet; increase complex carbohydrates; decrease simple carbohydrates; lower fat intake; optimize protein (0.8 g/kg body weight); drink liberal quantities of fluid (purified water); monitor dietary compliance with urinary 24-hour uric acid level (maintain below 0.8 g/day); eat liberal amounts (250 to 500 g q.d.) cherries, blueberries, other anthocyanoside-rich red-blue berries (or extracts).
- **Nutritional supplements:**
  - — Fish oils: 3000 mg combined EPA plus docosahexaenoic acid (DHA) q.d.
  - — Folic acid: 10 to 40 mg q.d.

Botanical Medicines

Choose one of the following:

- **Dark cherry fruit extract** (10:1): 500 to 1000 mg t.i.d.
- **Grapeseed extract** (>95% procyanidolic oligomers): 100 to 300 mg q.d.
- **Pine bark extract** (>90% procyanidolic oligomers): 100 to 300 mg q.d.
- **Anthocyanoside extracts** (e.g., *Vaccinium myrtillus*): equivalent to 80 mg anthocyanoside content q.d.
- **Quercetin**: 200 to 400 mg t.i.d. between meals

Causes of Hyperuricemia

Metabolic Causes

- Increased production of purine (primary)
- Idiopathic
- Specific enzyme defects (e.g., Lesch-Nyhan syndrome, glycogen storage disease)
- Decreased enzyme activity (e.g., hypoxanthine-guanine phosphoribosyltransferase is decreased in 1% to 2% of adults with gout)
- Increased enzyme activity (e.g., phosphoribosylpyrophosphate synthetase)
- Increased production of purine (secondary)
- Increased turnover of purines
- Myeloproliferative disorders

- Lymphoproliferative disorders
- Carcinoma and sarcoma (disseminated)
- Chronic hemolytic anemia
- Cytotoxic drugs
- Psoriasis
- Increased de novo synthesis (e.g., glucose-6-phosphatase deficiency)
- Increased catabolism of purines
- Fructose ingestion or infusion
- Exercise

Renal Causes

- Decreased renal clearance of uric acid (primary)
- Intrinsic kidney disease
- Decreased renal clearance of uric acid (secondary)
- Functional impairment of tubular secretion
- Drug induced (e.g., thiazides, probenecid, salicylates, ethambutol, pyrazinamide)
- Hyperlacticemia (e.g., lactic acidosis, alcoholism, toxemia of pregnancy, chronic beryllium disease)
- Hyperketoacidemia (e.g., diabetic ketoacidosis, fasting, starvation)
- Diabetes insipidus
- Bartter syndrome
- Chronic Pb intoxication
- Glucose-6-phosphatase deficiency

Hair Loss in Women

DIAGNOSTIC SUMMARY

- Increased hair loss not diagnosed as alopecia

GENERAL CONSIDERATIONS

Do not underestimate emotional impact of hair loss for some patients.

Physiology of the Hair Cycle

There are 100,000 to 350,000 hair follicles on the human scalp that go through cyclic phases of growth and rest:

- **Growth (anagen) phase:** active genetic expression of protein synthesis.
- **Resting (telogen) stage.**
- **Migratory phase:** hair bulb migrates outward and is sloughed. Stage is set for new hair to fill remaining papilla after old hair is lost.

Age, pathology, and nutritional and hormonal factors influence duration of hair cycle. Hair loss is a normal part of aging. Hair growth slows by age 40 years. Speed of replacing old hairs declines. The issue is more apparent in men because of the effects of androgens.

Hair-Pull Test

This helps determine relative formation of new hair. Take a few strands between thumb and forefinger and pull on them gently. Anagen hairs remain rooted in place; hairs in telogen come out easily. Knowing how many hairs were pulled and the number that came out, the provider can determine the percentage of hair follicles in telogen state. If 20 hairs were pulled and 2 came out, frequency of telogen hair follicles is 10%. A 10% telogen frequency is excellent; up to 25% is typical; over 35% is problematic. If after the pull test there are still hairs in balding areas, the test result is positive.

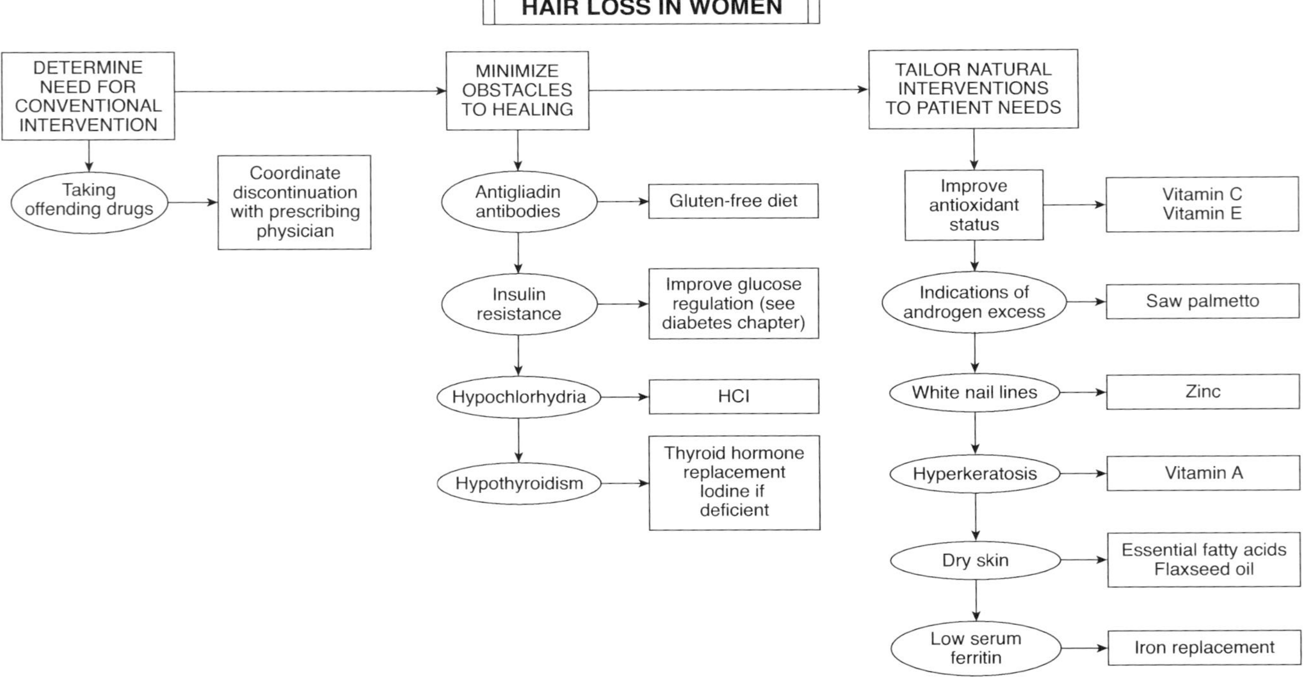

HAIR LOSS IN WOMEN
DETERMINE NEED FOR CONVENTIONAL INTERVENTION
Taking offending drugs
Coordinate discontinuation with prescribing physician
MINIMIZE OBSTACLES TO HEALING
Antigliadin antibodies
Gluten-free diet
Insulin resistance
Improve glucose regulation (see diabetes chapter)
Hypochlorhydria
HCl
Hypothyroidism
Thyroid hormone replacement Iodine if deficient
TAILOR NATURAL INTERVENTIONS TO PATIENT NEEDS
Improve antioxidant status
Vitamin C Vitamin E
Indications of androgen excess
Saw palmetto
White nail lines
Zinc
Hyperkeratosis
Vitamin A
Dry skin
Essential fatty acids Flaxseed oil
Low serum ferritin
Iron replacement

Differential Diagnosis

- Two types of hair loss: focal and diffuse.
- **Diffuse:** most often caused by telogen effluvium—umbrella term for nonscarring alopecia with diffuse hair shedding, often with acute onset, caused by metabolic or hormonal stress or by medicines. Recovery occurs when precipitating factors are resolved. Women can also experience male or female pattern hair loss (androgenic alopecia). Focal hair loss is often secondary to underlying disorder that may cause nonscarring or scarring alopecia. Nonscarring focal alopecia is usually caused by tinea capitis or alopecia areata, although patchy hair loss may also be caused by traction alopecia or trichotillomania. Scarring alopecia is rare, with numerous causes (e.g., discoid lupus erythematosus).

Differential Diagnosis of Hair Loss

Type of Hair Loss	Distinguishing Characteristics
DIFFUSE	
Female pattern hair loss	Manifests with hair thinning; frontal hairline intact; negative pull test
Male pattern hair loss	Manifests with hair thinning; M pattern; negative pull test
Diffuse alopecia areata	Distribution more patchy; positive pull test
Alopecia totalis or universalis	Total hair loss on the scalp and/or body
Telogen effluvium	30%–50% hair loss 3 months after precipitating event; positive pull test
Anagen effluvium	Sudden hair loss of up to 90% 2 weeks after chemotherapy
FOCAL	
Nonscarring alopecia areata	Normal scalp with surrounding exclamation point hairs
Tinea capitis	Scaly scalp with fungus visible on potassium hydroxide examination
Traction alopecia	Patchy; related to hair practices; may have some scarring
Trichotillomania	Patchy; possibly some scarring and associated psychological disturbance
Scarring (cicatricial) alopecia	Scarring and atrophy of scalp (e.g., discoid lupus erythematosus)

From Mounsey AL, Reed SW. Diagnosing and treating hair loss. *Am Fam Physician.* 2009;80(4):356-362.

THERAPEUTIC CONSIDERATIONS

Causes of Hair Loss in Women

- Androgenic female pattern hair loss
- Side effect of drug
- Nutritional deficiencies
- Hypothyroidism
- Antigliadin antibodies

Androgenic Female Pattern Hair Loss

Female pattern hair loss (diffuse androgen-dependent alopecia) is more diffuse than male pattern, affecting 30% of women before age 50 years. Factors include genetics, androgen excess, insulin resistance, polycystic ovarian syndrome, low antioxidant status (i.e., reduced glutathione).

- **Recommendations:**
  - — Improve blood glucose regulation through dietary, lifestyle, and supplementary measures (see chapter on diabetes mellitus)
  - — Increase antioxidant intake
  - — Saw palmetto extract
  - — Hormone replacement therapy

Reactive oxygen species (and testosterone) contribute to male pattern baldness and are found at higher levels in hair follicles of men (and presumably women) with this condition as a result of lower glutathione. Vitamins C and E help preserve glutathione.

- **Recommendations:**
  - — **Vitamin C:** 1000 to 1500 mg q.d. in divided doses
  - — **Vitamin E:** 400 international units (IU) q.d. (mixed tocopherols)

Saw palmetto extract, useful in benign prostatic hypertrophy, inhibits formation of dihydrotestosterone (DHT) by enzyme 5-alpha-reductase, also increased in male and female pattern baldness (the same mechanism as finasteride [Propecia] used in female pattern hair loss). Saw palmetto extract also inhibits transport of DHT to nuclear receptors.

- Dose: 320 mg q.d. of extract standardized to 85% to 95% fatty acids and sterols

Side Effect of Drugs

Hair loss concurrent with taking one of the drugs listed in the accompanying table does not indicate that the drug is the sole cause of hair loss. For chemotherapy agents (e.g., fluorouracil), the link is obvious. When medically appropriate, natural alternatives to suspected culprits should be used.

Classes of Drugs that Can Cause Hair Loss

Class	Examples
Antibiotics	Gentamicin, chloramphenicol
Anticoagulants	Warfarin, heparin
Antidepressants	Fluoxetine, desipramine, lithium
Antiepileptic drugs	Valproic acid, phenytoin
Cardiovascular drugs	Angiotensin-converting enzyme inhibitors, beta-blockers
Chemotherapy drugs	Doxorubicin, vincristine, etoposide
Endocrine drugs	Bromocriptine, clomiphene, danazol
Gout medications	Colchicine, allopurinol
Lipid-lowering drugs	Gemfibrozil, fenofibrate
Nonsteroidal anti-inflammatory drugs	Ibuprofen, indomethacin, naproxen
Ulcer medications	Cimetidine, ranitidine

Van Neste DJ, Rushton H. Hair problems in women. *Clin Dermatol.* 1997;15: 113-125.

Nutritional Deficiency

Zinc, vitamin A, essential fatty acids (EFAs), and iron should be considered first.

- **Zinc:** examine nails for white lines indicating poor wound healing of nail bed even with minor trauma—sign of zinc deficit.
- **Vitamin A:** examine backs of arms for hyperkeratosis—sign of vitamin A deficiency.
- **EFAs:** examine elbows and skin generally for dry skin of EFA deficiency.
- **Iron:** use serum ferritin test. If serum ferritin level is below 30 mcg/L, iron replacement is indicated. Low serum ferritin impairs hair growth and regeneration as the body seeks to conserve iron.

Women with noticeable generalized hair loss tend to have deficiencies in all these nutrients. Increase intake of these nutrients; supplement appropriately. Caveat: many may have hydrochlorhydria. Use hydrochloric acid supplements at meals. Use a high-potency vitamin-mineral supplement containing ferrous iron and 1 tbsp of flaxseed oil daily. If serum ferritin is below 30 mcg/L, supplement with additional iron: 30 mg iron bound to succinate, fumarate, or other chelate b.i.d. between meals. If abdominal discomfort ensues, recommend 30 mg with meals t.i.d. After 2 months, retest serum ferritin. Improved serum ferritin often correlates with improved hair health and reduced hair loss.

Hypothyroidism

Hair loss is a cardinal sign of hypothyroidism. Use blood thyroid hormone tests as criteria. From 1% to 4% of adults have moderate to severe hypothyroidism; another 10% to 12% have mild hypothyroidism. Prevalence among American women is 20%.

Antigliadin Antibodies

Gluten and its polypeptide derivative, gliadin, are found in wheat, barley, and rye grains. Antibodies to gliadin can cross-react and attack hair follicles, leading to alopecia areata—an autoimmune disease characterized by areas of virtually complete hair loss.

Celiac disease (nontropical sprue, gluten-sensitive enteropathy, or celiac sprue) entails malabsorption and abnormal small intestine structure that reverts to normal on removal of dietary gluten. Many people with gluten intolerance do not have overt gastrointestinal symptoms; instead, gluten intolerance may appear insidiously as hair loss. Instead of antigliadin antibody test, in patients with general hair loss or alopecia areata, test for human anti–tissue transglutaminase antibodies for greater sensitivity compared with antigliadin antibodies (see chapter on celiac disease). This test is especially indicated with gastrointestinal symptoms suggestive of celiac disease.

Key Diagnostic Features of Celiac Disease

- Bulky, pale, frothy, foul-smelling, greasy stools with increased fecal fat
- Weight loss and signs of multiple vitamin and mineral deficiencies
- Increased levels of serum gliadin antibodies
- Diagnosis confirmed by jejunal biopsy

Hepatitis, Viral

GENERAL CONSIDERATIONS

Defining Terms

Hepatitis refers to inflammation of the liver. Hepatitis lasting less than 6 months is termed *acute hepatitis;* that lasting longer than 6 months is called *chronic hepatitis.* In people with acute hepatitis who do not progress to chronic disease, all symptoms, signs, and blood abnormalities normalize without permanent or long-term sequelae. People who progress from acute to chronic hepatitis are at risk of progressing to cirrhosis and its complications—portal hypertension and hepatocellular carcinoma (HCC). Many inflammatory causes: autoimmunity, obesity, alcoholic liver disease, and some pharmaceuticals and herbs. Only hepatitis caused by a virus *(viral hepatitis)* is potentially infectious to others. This chapter focuses on viral hepatitis types A, B, and C.

Viral Hepatitis

- **Hepatitis A:** Picornaviridae family virus transmitted via fecal-oral (enteric) route by person-to-person contact; previously termed *infectious hepatitis;* most common cause of acute viral hepatitis in the United Statues. Although hepatitis A virus (HAV) does not lead to chronic disease, it accounts for 100 deaths annually in the United States.
- **Hepatitis B:** Hepadnaviridae family virus transmitted via parenteral route through blood or blood products, sexual contact, or from mother-child transmission during pregnancy and childbirth; previously termed *serum hepatitis;* can lead to chronic infection with hepatitis B virus (HBV), defined through blood work positive for hepatitis B surface antigen (HBsAg) and positive for hepatitis B core antibody (HBcAb). Chronic HBV is most common cause of cirrhosis and liver cancer.
- **Hepatitis C:** Flaviviridae family virus transmitted via percutaneous route of blood-to-blood contact; intravenous (IV) drug users; recipients of blood or blood-product transfusion before 1992; persons born to mothers infected. Those at risk for exposure to

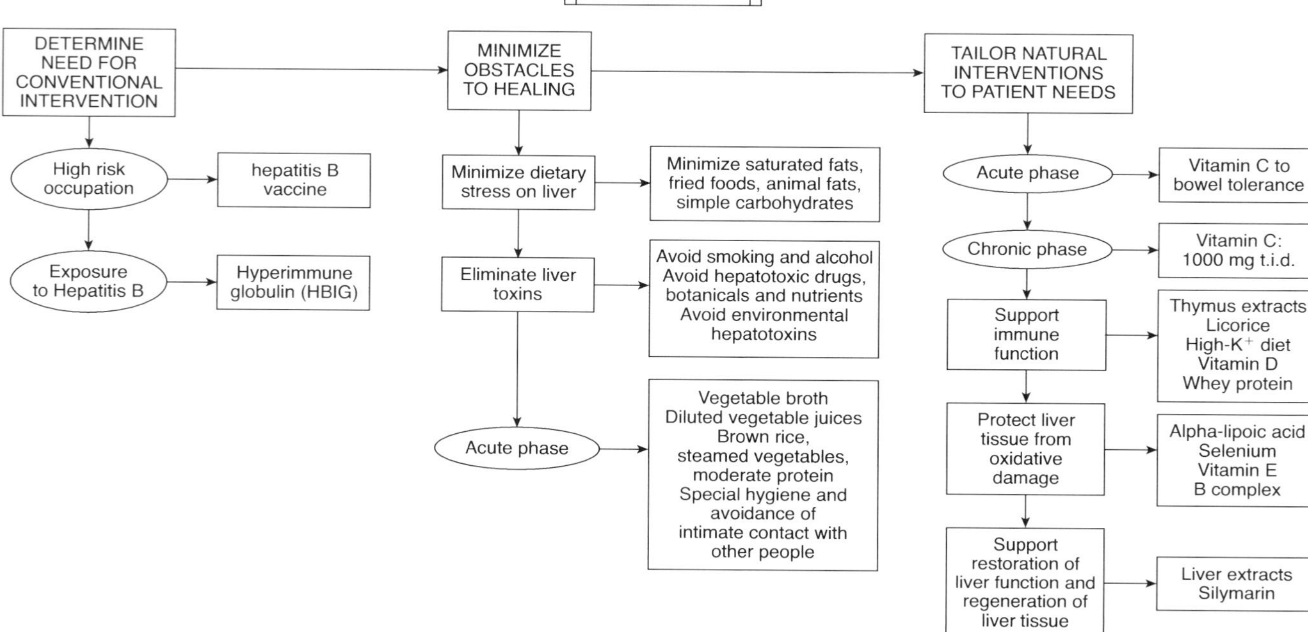
HEPATITIS
DETERMINE NEED FOR CONVENTIONAL INTERVENTION
High risk occupation
hepatitis B vaccine
Exposure to Hepatitis B
Hyperimmune globulin (HBIG)
MINIMIZE OBSTACLES TO HEALING
Minimize dietary stress on liver
Minimize saturated fats, fried foods, animal fats, simple carbohydrates
Eliminate liver toxins
Avoid smoking and alcohol
Avoid hepatotoxic drugs, botanicals and nutrients
Avoid environmental hepatotoxins
Acute phase
Vegetable broth
Diluted vegetable juices
Brown rice, steamed vegetables, moderate protein
Special hygiene and avoidance of intimate contact with other people
TAILOR NATURAL INTERVENTIONS TO PATIENT NEEDS
Acute phase
Vitamin C to bowel tolerance
Chronic phase
Vitamin C: 1000 mg t.i.d.
Support immune function
Thymus extracts
Licorice
High-K+ diet
Vitamin D
Whey protein
Protect liver tissue from oxidative damage
Alpha-lipoic acid
Selenium
Vitamin E
B complex
Support restoration of liver function and regeneration of liver tissue
Liver extracts
Silymarin

infected blood (health care or public safety workers) are at increased risk of infection. Unlike HBV, sexual contact is an inefficient means of hepatitis C virus (HCV) transmission. Before its identification in 1989, it was termed *non-A, non-B hepatitis.*

Symptoms and Signs

- **Acute viral hepatitis:** may be asymptomatic, or extremely debilitating with jaundice, flulike symptoms, anorexia, abdominal pain, nausea, diarrhea, vomiting, and fatigue. Typically, the more severely ill and jaundiced during acute phase, the better the chances of not progressing to chronic hepatitis.
- **Chronic viral hepatitis:** Probability of developing chronic disease is 1% to 5% in HBV-infected adults and 90% to 95% in HBV-infected infants. Hepatitis A never leads to chronic disease. Hepatitis C progresses to chronicity in 55% to 85% of infected persons, with females and children less likely to progress than male adults. Symptoms of chronic hepatitis vary from nonexistent to relentless fatigue and signs and symptoms of decompensated cirrhosis—ascites, variceal bleeding, and hepatic encephalopathy (HE).

DIAGNOSTIC CONSIDERATIONS

- Diagnosis made via combination of thorough history and physical examination; laboratory tests—serial liver function tests (aspartate aminotransferase [AST] and alanine aminotransferase [ALT], referred to as *transaminases*); hepatitis-specific serologies; imaging studies.
- These tests typically do not correlate with extent of liver damage; liver biopsy can determine grade (degree of inflammation) and stage (degree of fibrosis) of disease and need for therapy.

Prevention

- All people with chronic liver disease or hepatitis from any cause should receive immunizations for hepatitis A and B if not already exposed to these viruses.
- It is considered safe to administer the hepatitis B vaccine to pregnant women if needed. Infants born to HBsAg-positive mothers should receive both hepatitis B vaccination and hepatitis B immune globulin (HBIG) within 12 hours of birth.
- See "Individuals Needing Hepatitis B Vaccination" box for list of those at increased risk for hepatitis B, therefore needing hepatitis B vaccination.

- There is currently no vaccine to prevent HCV, because of complex HCV mutant strains—quasispecies—that can exist in a person infected with hepatitis C.
- HAV can be killed by boiling infected foods for more than 3 minutes and by disinfecting surfaces with bleach. Avoid eating raw or partially cooked mollusks (clams, oysters, mussels, scallops). In regions of the world with poor hygiene, eat well-cooked foods and drink only bottled water. Sanitize diaper-changing tables. Meticulous hand washing after excreting waste products, before eating, and before preparing food for others.
- Avoid unprotected sex. Employ barriers—condom, dental dam, female condom, finger cot—to decrease risk of transmission. Although risk of sexual transmission of HCV is rare, protected sex is recommended for anal sex and for those having multiple sex partners, patients with frequent prostate infections, those with open cuts or sores on genitalia, and those who are menstruating. People with HBV or HCV should avoid sharing anything that may contain even tiniest amount of their blood—toothbrushes, razors, nail clippers.
- People using injection drugs must never share needles with others or inject themselves with a used needle. Seek out needle-exchange programs. Alternatively, limit needle use to autodestruct syringes that self-destruct after one use. Engage in drug rehabilitation.
- Tattoos and body piercing: deal only with establishments that are clean and that adhere to meticulous sterilization practices.

Individuals Needing Hepatitis B Vaccination

- All newborns with hepatitis B surface antigen (HBsAg)–positive mothers
- At-risk children age 11 or 12 who did not receive the vaccine at birth
- People of any age who have more than one sex partner within a 6-month period
- People with a sexually transmitted disease
- Immigrants from geographic areas in which hepatitis B virus (HBV) is endemic—Asia, sub-Saharan Africa, Middle East, Amazon basin
- Children born in the United States to a person from an HBV-endemic area
- Adopted children from HBV-endemic areas
- Men who have sex with men
- Intravenous drug users and their sex partners
- People with blood-clotting factor disorders
- Those who have intimate or household contact with a person who is an HBV carrier (HBsAg positive).
- People who work in health care
- Public safety workers who may come into contact with blood
- People receiving hemodialysis
- People who live or work in an institution for the developmentally disabled
- Prison inmates
- Alaskan Natives and Pacific Islanders

THERAPEUTIC CONSIDERATIONS

Conventional Therapies

- **Goals of treatment of chronic hepatitis:** achieve sustained viral suppression or total elimination; slow or prevent progression to cirrhosis, hepatic decompensation, and HCC; prevent transmission to others.
- Chronic hepatitis B is not curable. Conventional treatment options: nucleoside or nucleotide analogues (NAs) or pegylated interferon (PI).
- **Interferons** (IFNs) are proteins, made naturally by the body, with antiviral, antiproliferative, and immunomodulatory properties. IFN and PI reduce HBV replication and induce disease remission. Efficacy of IFN is limited to a narrow population of HBV patients. Numerous side effects, difficult subcutaneous administration, cost, and high relapse rate hamper its use for chronic HBV.
- **NAs:** effective for suppressing HBV replication, inducing remission, and improving long-term outcomes. However, treatment period is not predefined and is determined by specific parameters that may differ from one patient to another. Treatment may be indefinite. Long-term use of NAs can be complicated by selection of antiviral-resistant mutations.
- Hepatitis C is curable in many patients; sustained virologic response (SVR) ranges from 20% to 90%. Length and success of HCV treatment are dependent on a variety of factors (see "Factors Affecting Hepatitis C Sustained Virologic Response" box).
  - **PI** given subcutaneously once a week, with oral **ribavirin (RBV)** daily for 24 to 48 weeks, has been standard of care (SOC) for chronic hepatitis C genotypes 2 and 3, and was SOC for genotype 1 (G1), the most common and most difficult to cure genotype.
  - **Protease inhibitors**—telaprevir (Incivek) or boceprevir (Victrelis)—have been elevated to SOC; SVR rates jumped from 42% to 86% for many G1 patients. From 44% to 60% of treatment-naive G1 patients are now capable of being cured in just 24 to 28 weeks. However, numerous adverse events (AEs), complex regimens, exorbitant costs, and potential for drug-resistance may decrease therapeutic usefulness.
  - **Nucleotide inhibitor of HCV NS5B RNA polymerase:** sofosbuvir (Sovaldi) is the latest exorbitantly expensive HCV antiviral to be added to others in combination, with very promising initial response rates.

— Natural and integrative therapies can positively affect progression of HCV, with or without SOC treatment for chronic hepatitis C.

Factors Affecting Hepatitis C Sustained Virologic Response

Host Factors
- Ethnicity
- Body mass index (BMI)
- Age
- Insulin resistance or diabetes mellitus (DM)
- Gender
- Alcohol use
- Nutritional factors

Viral Factors
- Genotype
- Viral load
- Interleukin-28B polymorphism

Disease Factors
- Degree of fibrosis
- Hepatitis C virus (HCV) and human immunodeficiency virus (HIV) coinfection

Adherence Factors
- Patient education
- Response-guided therapy
- Management of adverse events
- Alternative ribavirin (RBV) formulations
- Support team—medical and personal

Lifestyle Recommendations

Sleep

Sleep deprivation impairs immune function—reduced natural killer cell activity, suppressed interleukin-2 production, and increased proinflammatory cytokines. Survival is inversely associated with sleep disturbance among patients with cirrhosis. Tailored behavioral interventions might help to improve quality of life and outcomes. Sleep problems affect 60% to 65% of HCV patients. IFN-α treatment increases waking after sleep onset, decreases sleep efficiency, and reduces stage 3 and/or 4 sleep. Impairments in sleep quality exist independent of antiviral therapy and before advanced stages of liver disease. Sleep deprivation attenuates antibody response to hepatitis A immunization. Encourage proper sleep habits and duration of 8 hours.

Exercise

Benefits: changes the way HCV patients perceive their bodies and its capacities; improves self-confidence. Because fatigue is common and bothersome symptom of chronic hepatitis, exercise can boost energy and improve cardiovascular function. Exercise reduces total body fat, which tends to reduce fat content of the liver, inducing reduction in elevated liver enzymes. Encourage all patients with chronic hepatitis to exercise, combining weight training and aerobics as tolerated once they have been medically cleared.

Diet

- **Acute viral hepatitis:** Nutritional treatment for acute viral hepatitis should be symptom directed. Focus on replenishing fluids with vegetable broths, diluted vegetable juices (diluted with 50% water), and herbal teas to avoid dehydration if diarrhea is present. Eliminate alcohol.
- **Chronic viral hepatitis:** Nutritional treatments helps reduce obesity, alcohol consumption, and iron overload. Diet: low in saturated fats, sugar, white flour, fruit juice, honey, fried oils, sodium, and animal products. This diet may help patients with decompensated cirrhosis with ascites (fluid retention) and/or HE (brain fog). Focus on whole-plant foods (high-fiber diet) that increase elimination of bile acids, drugs, and toxic bile substances.

Fruit and Hepatitis C

- **Blueberries** inhibit replication of HCV and may protect against developing acute hepatitis. Antioxidant properties of flavonoid proanthocyanidin in blueberry leaves provide this benefit.
- **Grapefruit and other citrus fruits:** contain naringenin, a flavonoid that has anti-inflammatory, antioxidant, and lipid-lowering properties and may promote carbohydrate metabolism. Naringenin lowers very-low-density–lipoprotein cholesterol. HCV may "hitch a ride" on cholesterol. Naringenin can inhibit or reduce steatosis (deposition of fat in the liver) and can inhibit HCV viral replication. Special note: grapefruit contains furanocoumarins and flavonoids, which can inhibit cytochrome p450 drug metabolism pathway, leading to toxic levels of many medicines.

Caffeine and Hepatitis C

Hepatoprotective effects of caffeine: people consuming more than 2 cups of coffee a day are less likely to have elevated serum liver enzymes and less likely to have chronic liver disease compared with non–coffee drinkers. Higher coffee intake is linked to less hepatic steatosis, lower ratio of serum AST/ALT, and lower alpha-fetoprotein levels in patients with hepatitis C. Patients drinking more than 2 to 3 cups of coffee a day had lower disease progression rates and less fibrosis on histologic evaluation compared with HCV patients who drank less coffee. Similar results are not seen in patients ingesting other caffeine sources or decaffeinated coffee. Caffeine may reduce fatigue of HCV and/or chronic liver disease. Reasonable intake for HCV patients: 2 to 4 cups regular coffee daily.

Whey Protein

Whey may boost immune function, protect against free-radical damage, and increase cellular glutathione. At a dose of 24 g whey protein daily, it reduced serum ALT and increased plasma glutathione in people with HBV, but not those with HCV.

Nutrient Therapeutics

Vitamins C and E

- Patients with HCV who are treated with PI and RBV have higher SVR and are less likely to get RBV-associated anemia when supplemented with vitamins C and E_I.
- Vitamin C increases iron absorption; many patients with HCV already have elevated iron stores.
- Vitamin E levels are low in serum and liver tissue in people with hepatitis and in those who later develop liver cancer from chronic hepatitis. In adults with hepatitis C, vitamin E at 1200 international units (IU) per day for 8 weeks reduced liver damage.

Zinc and Hepatitis C

Zinc is essential to immunity and may protect the liver from chemical damage. Zinc may protect the body from viruses. Blood zinc levels inversely correlate with progression of chronic hepatitis C; zinc deficiency is often present in patients with both hepatitis C and HCC and/or cirrhosis. Oral zinc (150 mg/day) may slow HCV progression and reduce incidence of HCC. Zinc may improve response to IFN in patients with chronic hepatitis C. Daily doses of 100 mg of zinc may be immunosuppressive. Excessive zinc may lead to nausea, vomiting, and diarrhea, all possible side effects of HCV antiviral SOC therapy.

Vitamin D and Hepatitis C

Patients with chronic hepatitis C often have very low serum 25 hydroxy (OH) vitamin D. Such deficits are independently correlated with severity of inflammation and fibrosis, as well as with reduced incidence of SVR to SOC PI plus RBV. Supplementing vitamin D (1000 to 4000 IU/day) to achieve serum level above 32 ng/mL may improve SVR in some HCV patients treated with SOC antivirals. Immunomodulatory properties of vitamin D may act in synergy with this antiviral therapy. Tissue expression of cytochrome p450 25-hydroxylating liver enzyme CYP27A1 is parallel with vitamin D levels and inversely correlates with hepatic necroinflammatory activity. All patients with hepatitis C should add vitamin D to their antiviral regimens.

Selenium

Selenium is a trace element that is a cofactor for enzyme glutathione peroxidase, an oxidant mediator. Selenium deficiency is linked to immune dysfunction, cancer, and liver necrosis. Whole-blood and plasma selenium levels tend to be abnormally low in patients with chronic liver disorders—alcoholic and viral liver cirrhosis. Liver cancer cells are able to acquire a selective survival advantage prominent under conditions of selenium deficiency and oxidative stress. Oxidative stress is a feature in cirrhosis. Selenium deficiency correlates with development of HCC in patients with chronic hepatitis B; patients taking 200 mcg of selenium daily are less likely to develop HCC. Selenium is safe at daily doses below 1000 mcg.

S-Adenosylmethionine (SAM) and Hepatitis C

S-adenosylmethionine (SAM) is a methyl group donor. SAM enhances IFN's antiviral properties. At 400 mg daily, SAM has improved early viral kinetics and IFN signaling, leading to enhanced IFN responsiveness and higher percentage of patients achieving SVR.

Liver Extracts

Oral liver extracts have been used for many chronic liver diseases since 1896. These extracts promote hepatic regeneration and are quite effective in the treatment of chronic liver disease, including chronic active hepatitis. At 70 mg of liver extract t.i.d. for 3 months, patients had far lower liver enzyme (aminotransaminase) levels, suggesting an anti-inflammatory effect.

Thymus Extracts

Oral bovine thymus extracts in viral hepatitis induce broad-spectrum immune system enhancement presumably mediated by improved thymus gland activity. In acute and chronic hepatitis B, thymus extracts may be effective: they induced accelerated decreases of liver enzymes (transaminases), elimination of virus, and higher rate of seroconversion to anti-HBe, the antibodies produced against the hepatitis B envelope antigen (HBeAg). If HBeAg is detectable in a blood sample, this means that the virus is still active in the liver (and can be transmitted to others). If HBeAg is negative and anti-HBe is positive, this generally means that the virus is inactive.

Botanical Medicines

Glycyrrhiza glabra (Licorice Root)

- Glycyrrhizin component of licorice root provides benefits. Glycyrrhizin reduces serum ALT and AST. Glycyrrhizin inhibits

immune-mediated cytotoxicity against hepatocytes and antagonizes nuclear factor kappa B (NF-κB), a transcription factor that activates genes encoding inflammatory cytokines.
- Licorice's pharmacologic actions beneficial for acute and chronic hepatitis: antihepatotoxic, immune-modulating, antiviral, and choleretic effects.
- Licorice stimulates production of a natural supply of IFN. When used intravenously, licorice lowers liver enzymes and decreases risk of HCV-associated HCC.
- The IV product Stronger Neo-Minophagen C (SNMC) consists of 200 mg glycyrrhizin, 100 mg cysteine, and 2000 mg glycine in 100 mL physiologic saline. At dosage of 100 mL/day for 8 weeks, followed by treatments two to seven times weekly for up to 16 years, rates of cumulative HCC and cirrhosis were reduced dramatically. In HCV patients unresponsive to IFN, IV glycyrrhizin decreased risk of progression to HCC. However, results are not consistent. Although licorice may reduce ALT, long-term benefits for HCV-associated fibrosis are unclear.
- Main adverse effect of licorice: aldosterone-like effects; avoid it in patients with history of ascites, hypertension, or renal failure or who are currently using digitalis.

Silybum marianum (Milk Thistle)

- Active ingredient: located in seeds; consists of three flavolignans—silybin, silydianin, and silychristin, collectively termed *silymarin.* Silymarin is used in Europe to treat all types of liver disorders.
- Silymarin inhibits hepatic damage by the following actions:
  - — Acting as direct antioxidant and free radical scavenger
  - — Increasing intracellular glutathione and superoxide dismutase
  - — Inhibiting formation of leukotrienes
  - — Stimulating hepatocyte regeneration
- Silymarin is applicable for acute and chronic hepatitis of varying causes. Patients with acute viral hepatitis treated with silymarin show greater improvements in serum levels of bilirubin and liver enzymes compared with those treated with placebo.
- Oral silymarin does not have antiviral effect; it does not reduce ALT or improve ultrasound abnormalities related to hepatitis C.
- Silymarin phytosome: in humans, flavonoids have low bioavailability owing to first-pass metabolism. A newer form of

silymarin binds it to phosphatidylcholine—better absorbed and produces better clinical results. In patients with chronic hepatitis (viral, alcoholic, or chemically induced) who were treated with silymarin phytosome at either 120 mg b.i.d. or 120 mg t.i.d. for up to 120 days, liver function returned to normal faster with phytosome than with unbound silymarin and placebo.
- IV silybin is capable of greatest suppression of hepatitis C viral replication. HCV patient nonresponders to SOC treatment were able to achieve undetectable HCV RNA levels after IV silybin for 15 days. These results proved to be temporary; however, antiviral effect was permanent for one patient who received IV silybin for 2 weeks after liver transplantation. Silybin may be capable of preventing graft reinfection with HCV.

Phyllanthus amarus

P. amarus is a traditional Asian herb for liver disorders. Experimentally, 59% of patients with hepatitis B lost HBsAg when tested 15 to 20 days after treatment with *P. amarus* (200 mg dried, powdered, sterilized plant in capsules t.i.d.). These results have not been confirmed by other researchers, indicating that either the extract used was not effective or that *Phyllanthus* itself is not effective.

Berkson Combination Approach with Antioxidant and Botanical Therapy

Patients with advanced cirrhosis, portal hypertension, and esophageal varices secondary to chronic hepatitis C were effectively treated with low-cost combination protocol. Patients "recovered quickly," showed improved liver enzymes, and were able to resume normal daily activities. Patients progressed to health within 4 to 7 months. Berkson regimen is as follows:
- Alpha-lipoic acid (600 mg/day in two divided doses)
- Selenium (selenomethionine at 400 mcg/day in two divided doses)
- Silymarin (900 mg/day in three divided doses)
- B-complex vitamin
- Diet: high in fruits and vegetables; 4 oz or less of meat per meal; eight glasses of water daily
- Vitamin C: 1000 to 6000 mg daily
- Vitamin E: 400 IU/day
- Walk: 1 mile three times a week

Although this protocol is documented in only three cases, it makes reasonable sense from a naturopathic standpoint based on safety, cost, and efficacy of components. It is worth trying, especially in patients failing to respond to conventional therapies.

Acupuncture and Chinese Medicine Herbs

Chinese medicine diagnosis for hepatitis often includes consideration of damp heat in the liver and spleen channels. Acupuncture points and herbal formulas are often directed at clearing heat and damp to cool and drain these channels. Often efforts are made to nourish liver blood and tone the liver and spleen. Study: acupuncture once daily for 30 minutes for 4 to 6 weeks shortened recovery times, improved symptom, and lowered interleukin-8. Acupuncture has been helpful in reducing secondary and comorbid symptoms of depression and myalgia. Although acupuncture did not improve viral load, it may help other symptoms, improve immune balance, and lower comorbidity. Clean-needle technique minimizes risk of hepatitis from acupuncture.

Sho-Saiko-To or Xiao Chai Hu Tang

Sho-Saiko-To (named Xiao Chai Hu Tang in Chinese) is a botanical formulation containing seven herbs traditionally used to treat liver and GI disorders. In animal models, it prevents liver injury and promotes liver regeneration by inhibiting lipid peroxidation in hepatocytes and hepatic stellate cells. In humans, it prevents progression of cirrhosis to HCC and increases survival of those with chronic viral hepatitis by reducing progression to HCC. Contraindication with IFN therapy because of increased risk of pneumonitis; Sho-Saiko-To may cause acute hepatitis. Thus its use in patients with liver disease is not recommended.

Hepatotoxic Supplements

- **Niacin:** used for hyperlipidemia; contraindicated in compromised liver function. Side effects: flushing, headache, stomachache. Doses larger than 20 mg and/or sustained-release forms at 2 g/day or higher may contribute to liver toxicity. Used for mood and glycemic regulation, niacinamide seems not to induce abnormalities and is considered safer; avoid it in hepatitis when other options are available.
- **Vitamin A:** retinoid compound; 80% to 90% of total body stores of retinoids are in hepatic stellate cells. Excessive intake (acute

doses larger than 100,000 IU or chronic doses of 25,000 to 100,000 IU daily for a year) may cause hypervitaminosis A, leading to cirrhosis. Vitamin A's potential to cause liver toxicity is enhanced by alcohol, by excessive intake of other fat-soluble vitamins, and by a vitamin C deficiency.

- **Iron:** generates reactive oxygen species leading to point mutations, chromosomal damage, and inactivation of tumor suppressor genes (p53)—it is a direct hepatotoxin. Unless a patient is iron deficient, avoid iron supplements. Iron speeds progression and worsens course of alcoholic liver disease—alcohol and excess iron have an additive harmful effect on the liver.

Hepatotoxic Botanicals

- ***Symphytum officinale* (comfrey):** contains hepatotoxic pyrrolizidine alkaloids (PAs)—lasiocarpine and symphytine and related *N*-oxides. Comfrey is a topical vulnerary, but PAs may still be absorbed through skin. Avoid comfrey in patients with liver disease.
- ***Piper methysticum* (kava kava):** implicated in hepatic damage. Beware kava overdose or concomitant polypharmacy. Although considered safe at normal doses for people without liver disease, those with hepatic conditions should avoid kava kava.

THERAPEUTIC APPROACH

During contagious phase (2 to 3 weeks before symptoms appear to 3 weeks after), encourage patients to practice careful hygiene and avoid close contact with others. Once diagnosis has been made, avoid work in day care, restaurants, or similar employment venues. Chronic hepatitis requires a multifactorial integrative approach—lifestyle; dietary measures; combination of nutrients, botanicals, and conventional pharmaceuticals as needed on an individual basis.

Lifestyle

- Acute phase: bed rest; slow resumption of activities as health improves.
- Avoid strenuous exertion; recommend exercise commensurate with patents' health status. Avoid smoking and drinking alcohol. Encourage 8 hours of sleep.

Diet

- Whole foods, high-fiber diet
- Low saturated fats and fried oils; minimal simple sugar, white flour, and fruit juices.
- Drink vegetable broths, diluted vegetable juices (diluted with 50% water), herbal teas to prevent dehydration in the presence of diarrhea.
- Flavonoid-rich blueberry, coffee, and grapefruit (provided there are no interactions with medication) may be beneficial for chronic hepatitis.

Nutritional Supplements

- **Vitamin C:** to bowel tolerance (10 to 50 g q.d.) in acute cases; 1000 mg t.i.d. in chronic cases. Caution in cases of iron overload when taken with iron sources.
- **Vitamin D**: 1000 to 4000 IU q.d.
- **Vitamin E:** 1200 IU q.d. (mixed tocopherols).
- **Selenium:** 200 mcg q.d.
- **Whey protein:** for hepatitis B at 24 g q.d.
- **Liver extracts:** 70 mg t.i.d.
- **Thymus extracts**: equivalent to 120 mg pure polypeptides with molecular weights below 10,000 daltons or roughly 750 mg of crude polypeptide fraction q.d.

Botanical Medicines

- ***G. glabra*** **(licorice):** powdered root, 1 to 2 g three times daily; fluid extract (1:1), 2 to 4 mL (1 to 2 g) three times daily; solid (dry powdered) extract (5% glycyrrhetinic acid content), 250 to 500 mg t.i.d.
  - IV administration may be the most effective form. Note: chronic licorice therapy may require increased intake of potassium-rich foods.
- ***S. marianum*** **(milk thistle):** standard dose of milk thistle (70 to 210 mg t.i.d.) is based on silymarin content. Prefer standardized extracts. Best results are achieved at higher doses (i.e., 150 to 300 mg t.i.d.). Dose for silybin bound to phosphatidylcholine (phytosome) is 120 mg b.i.d. to t.i.d. between meals.
  - IV silibinin may be most effective form.

Berkson Combination Antioxidant Approach

See earlier section on this antioxidant botanical protocol.

Herpes Simplex

DIAGNOSTIC SUMMARY

- Acute recurrent viral infection of skin or mucous membranes characterized by grouped small vesicles on erythematous base, frequently occurring about the mouth (herpes gingivostomatitis), lips (herpes labialis), genitals (herpes genitalis), and conjunctiva and cornea (herpes keratoconjunctivitis).
- Incubation period 2 to 12 days, averaging 6 to 7 days.
- Vesicle scraping stained with Giemsa stain gives positive Tzanck's test result (type-specific glycoprotein testing for both herpes simplex virus [HSV] types 1 and 2).
- Regional lymph nodes may be tender and swollen.
- Outbreak may follow minor infections, trauma, hormonal fluctuations, stress (emotional, dietary, environmental), and sun exposure.
- Viral shedding, leading to possible transmission, during primary infection, recurrences, and (asymptomatically) between recurrences.

GENERAL CONSIDERATIONS

More than 70 viruses compose Herpesviridae. Of these, four are linked to human disease: herpes simplex virus (HSV), varicella-zoster virus (VZV), Epstein-Barr virus (EBV), and cytomegalovirus (CMV). Serology distinguishes two types of HSV: HSV-1 and HSV-2. HSV-1 is frequently acquired in early childhood. Recurrent HSV is present in more than one third of the world's population. Although 80% of seropositive persons do not have clinically apparent recurrences, they still shed virus asymptomatically. Recurrent HSV infections are present in 20% to 40% of the U.S. population. From 30% to 100% of adults have been infected with one or both HSV types. The greatest incidence is among lower socioeconomic groups; HSV-1 has replaced HSV-2 as the primary cause of genital lesions. People who are exposed to HSV and have asymptomatic primary infections may experience initial clinical

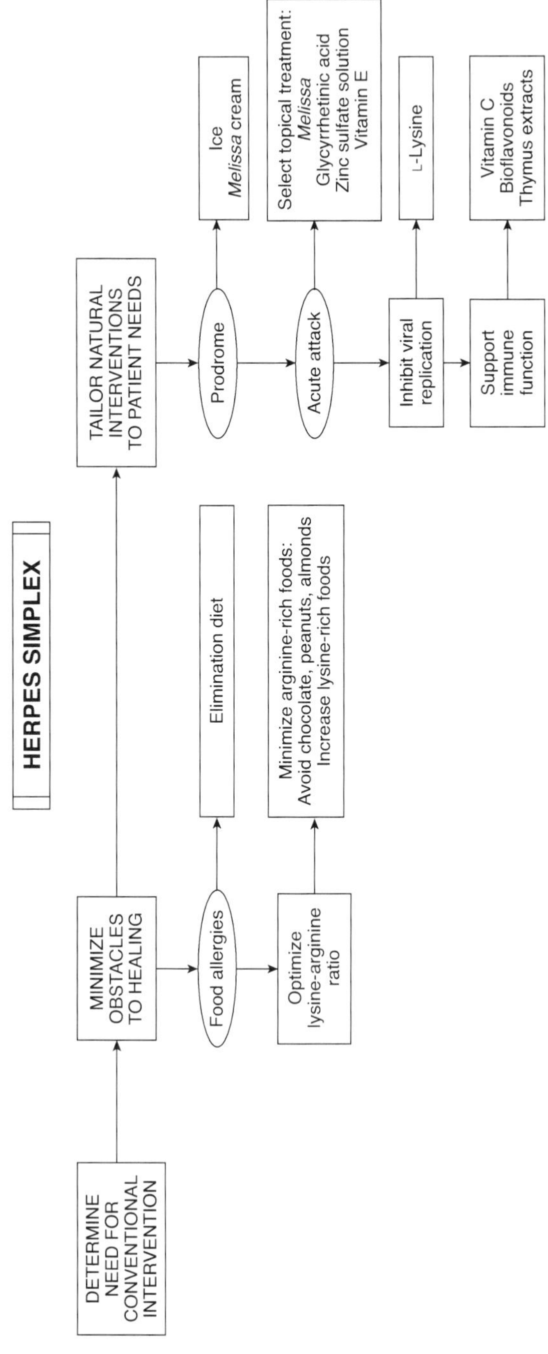
HERPES SIMPLEX
DETERMINE NEED FOR CONVENTIONAL INTERVENTION
MINIMIZE OBSTACLES TO HEALING
Food allergies
Elimination diet
Optimize lysine-arginine ratio
Minimize arginine-rich foods: Avoid chocolate, peanuts, almonds Increase lysine-rich foods
TAILOR NATURAL INTERVENTIONS TO PATIENT NEEDS
Prodrome
Ice Melissa cream
Acute attack
Select topical treatment: Melissa Glycyrrhetinic acid Zinc sulfate solution Vitamin E
Inhibit viral replication
L-Lysine
Support immune function
Vitamin C Bioflavonoids Thymus extracts

episode of genital herpes months to years after becoming infected. Herpes outbreaks on hands and fingers (herpes whitlow) is increasing, probably owing to digital-genital contact. Cigarette smoking is a risk: nicotine byproduct concentrates secretions and suppresses T-cell function.

- **Recurrence rate:** genital HSV-1 lesions have a recurrence rate of 14%; HSV-2 recurrence rate is 60%. Men are more susceptible to recurrences. After primary infection resolves, HSV is a dormant inhabitant in sensory and/or autonomic ganglia. Recurrences develop at or near site of primary infection, precipitated by sunburn, sexual activity, menses, stress, food allergy, drugs, certain foods. Risk of infection after sexual contact with partner with active lesions is 75%.
- **Immunologic aspects:** host defense is paramount in protecting against HSV infection. Persistent genital infections are seen in immunosuppressed individuals. Cell-mediated immunity is the major factor determining outcome of herpes exposure: resistance, latent infection, or clinical disease. HSV-neutralizing antibody found in saliva is decreased during active recurrence and is in immunoglobulin G (IgG) form, which is significant because IgA is the major immunoglobulin in saliva.

Diagnosis

Gold standard is isolation of HSV from tissue scrapings. Cytopathic effects are seen in 2 to 7 days. Direct staining of skin scrapings is a more-rapid test for mucocutaneous lesions. Type-specific serologic tests diagnose unrecognized infections or confirm suspected cases.

THERAPEUTIC CONSIDERATIONS

Prevent recurrent herpes to decrease number and severity of outbreaks, reduce asymptomatic viral shedding, and prevent transmission to partner and/or fetus. Three or more people may benefit when one person takes preventive measures. Education regarding transmission and asymptomatic viral shedding is imperative. Enhancing host immune status is the key to controlling herpes infection. A key natural measure to strengthen cell-mediated immunity is bovine thymus extracts. Thymus extracts reduce number and severity of recurrent infections in immune-suppressed persons and increase lymphoproliferative response to HSV, natural killer cell activity, and interferon production.

- **Zinc:** oral zinc (50 mg q.d.) is effective in clinical studies. Zn is an inhibitor of HSV replication in vitro; its effect in vivo is to enhance cell-mediated immunity. Topical 0.01% to 0.025% zinc sulfate solution ameliorates symptoms and inhibits recurrence.
- **Vitamin C:** oral and topical application of vitamin C increases rate of healing of herpes ulcers. Ascorbic acid–containing pharmaceutical (Ascoxal) applied with soaked cotton wool pad t.i.d. for 2 minutes reduces number of days with scabs, number of cases of worsening of symptoms, and frequency of culturing HSV from lesions. In herpes labialis, oral ascorbate-bioflavonoid complex (1000 mg water-soluble bioflavonoids and 1000 mg vitamin C in equal increments five times daily at first onset and continued 3 days) reduces outbreak of vesiculation and prevents disruption of vesicular membranes. This therapy is most beneficial when initiated at the beginning of disease. Optimal remission of symptoms occurs in 3 to 7 days with 600-mg dose of water-soluble bioflavonoid–ascorbic acid complex. Vitamin C administered intravenously benefits patients with HSV infection, including those with acquired immunodeficiency syndrome (AIDS).
- **Lysine and arginine:** lysine has antiviral activity in vitro from antagonism of arginine metabolism. HSV replication requires synthesis of arginine-rich proteins. Arginine may be an operon coordinate inducer. Preponderance of lysine over arginine may act as either allosteric enzyme inhibitor or operon coordinate repressor. Lysine at 1 g t.i.d. with dietary restriction of nuts, chocolate, and gelatin for 6 months was rated much better than placebo. Lysine and arginine are dibasic amino acids that compete with each other for intestinal transport. Rats fed lysine-rich diet show 60% decrease in brain arginine, although no change in serum levels. HSV resides in ganglia during latency. Supplemental lysine and arginine avoidance is warranted but not curative; this intervention only inhibits recurrences. In some patients, withdrawal from lysine is followed by relapse within 1 to 4 weeks.

Topical Preparations

- Melissa officinalis **(lemon balm):** concentrated extract (70:1) contains several components that work together to prevent virus from infecting human cells. It dramatically reduces recurrence; many patients never again have a recurrence. It rapidly interrupts infection and reduces healing time from 10 to 5 days.

Melissa either stops recurrences of cold sores or tremendously reduces frequency of recurrences (outbreak-free period longer than 3.5 months). Apply it fairly thickly (1 to 2 mm) to lesions q.i.d. during active recurrence. Extremely safe and suitable for long-term use.

- Glycyrrhiza glabra **(licorice root):** Preparations containing glycyrrhetinic acid (triterpenoid) inhibit growth and cytopathic effects of herpes simplex, vaccinia, Newcastle's disease, and vesicular stomatitis viruses. Topical glycyrrhetinic acid is quite helpful in reducing healing time and pain of cold sores and genital herpes. Extracts of other species of Lamiaceae (mint) family have in vitro efficacy against adsorption, but not replication, of HSV-1 and HSV-2 (e.g., *Mentha piperita, Prunella vulgaris, Rosmarinus officialis, Salvia officinalis,* and *Thymus vulgaris*).
- **Resveratrol (3,5,4′-trihydroxystilbene):** natural component of grapes that has anti-HSV activity in vitro. Topical application of resveratrol cream (12.5% to 25%) effectively blocks HSV replication and stops lesion eruption if applied early and frequently. No human studies have been reported. In vitro studies reveal that resveratrol suppresses HSV-induced activation of nuclear factor kappa B (NF-κB) within the nucleus and impairs expression of essential immediate-early, early, and late HSV genes and synthesis of viral DNA.
- **Vitamin E:** topical vitamin E has decreased pain and healing time in oral herpes. Lesions responded best when contents of a vitamin E capsule were applied every 4 hours.

THERAPEUTIC APPROACH

- **Goals:** shorten current attack and prevent recurrences. Support the immune system; control food allergens and optimize nutrients necessary for cell-mediated immunity. Inhibit HSV replication by manipulating dietary lysine/arginine ratio. No cure is known, but strengthening the immune system is quite effective in reducing frequency, duration, and severity of recurrences.
- **Diet:** develop diet that avoids food allergens and arginine-rich foods and promotes lysine-rich foods (*Textbook,* "The Optimal Health Food Pyramid"). Foods with worst arginine/lysine ratio are chocolate, peanuts, and almonds.
- **Supplements:**
  — Vitamin C: 2000 mg q.d.
  — Bioflavonoids: 1000 mg q.d.

- Zinc: 25 mg (elemental zinc as picolinate) q.d.
- L-Lysine: 1000 mg t.i.d.
- Thymus extract: equivalent to 120 mg pure polypeptides with molecular weights <10,000 daltons or roughly 500 mg crude polypeptide fraction q.d.

• **Topical treatment:**
- Sunscreen
- Ice: 10 minutes on, 5 minutes off during prodrome
- Zinc sulfate solution: apply 0.025% solution t.i.d.
- *Melissa* cream: apply b.i.d.
- Glycyrrhetinic acid: apply b.i.d.
- Vitamin E: apply every 4 hours

HIV/AIDS: Naturopathic Medical Principles and Practice

DIAGNOSTIC SUMMARY

- A diagnosis of human immunodeficiency virus (HIV)–positive infection is most commonly made after a positive test for HIV antibodies by enzyme-linked immunosorbent assay (ELISA); it is confirmed via Western blot analysis.
- An acute onset (acute antiretroviral syndrome) resembles common influenza. Most persons experience this syndrome 2 to 6 weeks after initial infection; it often goes undiagnosed as HIV owing to its similarity to influenza. Signs and symptoms can include fever, lymphadenopathy, skin rash, pharyngitis, myalgia, arthralgia, headache, diarrhea, and oral ulcerations. Laboratory findings might include leukopenia, thrombocytopenia, and elevated transaminases.
- An insidious onset may manifest as an acquired immunodeficiency syndrome (AIDS)–associated opportunistic infection (OI) or as unexplained progressive fatigue, weight loss, fever, diarrhea, or generalized lymphadenopathy.
- AIDS is diagnosed after positive serology and either a CD4+ T-cell count at or below $200/mm^3$ or the presence of a designated AIDS-indicator condition (from the Centers for Disease Control and Prevention [CDC] guidelines of 2008). Primary infection is also characterized by a high level of virus production, high concentrations of viral particles and RNA in plasma, and a rapid and steep decline in CD4+ T-helper cells. Peak viral titers can reach 10^7 virions per milliliter during this phase. Viral production can range up to 10 billion copies/day. After the initial viremia, high levels of viral p24 antigen appear.
- The lower the CD4+ count and the higher the viral load, the higher the risk of contracting OIs, neoplasms, or neurologic abnormalities and the higher the mortality rate.

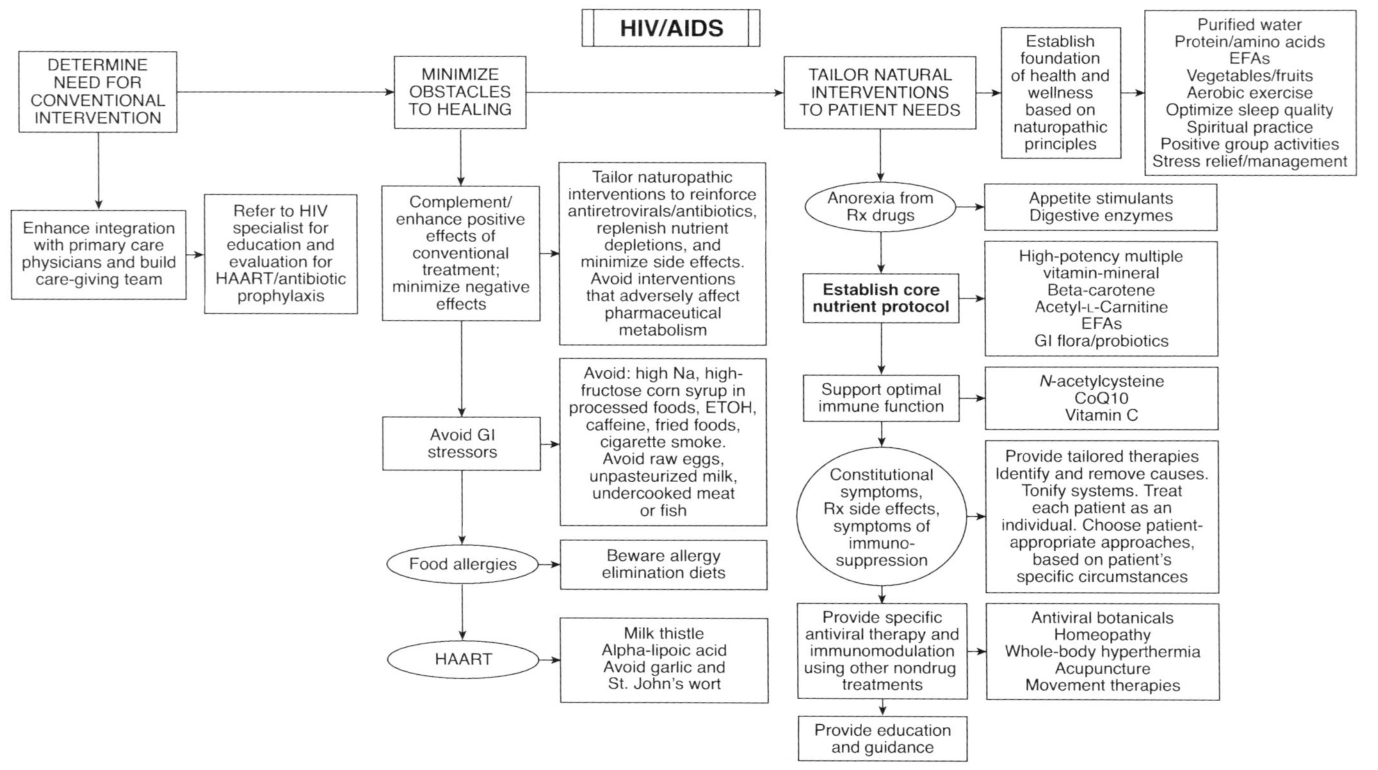
HIV/AIDS
DETERMINE NEED FOR CONVENTIONAL INTERVENTION
Enhance integration with primary care physicians and build care-giving team
Refer to HIV specialist for education and evaluation for HAART/antibiotic prophylaxis
MINIMIZE OBSTACLES TO HEALING
Complement/enhance positive effects of conventional treatment; minimize negative effects
Tailor naturopathic interventions to reinforce antiretrovirals/antibiotics, replenish nutrient depletions, and minimize side effects. Avoid interventions that adversely affect pharmaceutical metabolism
Avoid GI stressors
Avoid: high Na, high-fructose corn syrup in processed foods, ETOH, caffeine, fried foods, cigarette smoke. Avoid raw eggs, unpasteurized milk, undercooked meat or fish
Food allergies
Beware allergy elimination diets
HAART
Milk thistle
Alpha-lipoic acid
Avoid garlic and St. John's wort
TAILOR NATURAL INTERVENTIONS TO PATIENT NEEDS
Establish foundation of health and wellness based on naturopathic principles
Purified water
Protein/amino acids
EFAs
Vegetables/fruits
Aerobic exercise
Optimize sleep quality
Spiritual practice
Positive group activities
Stress relief/management
Anorexia from Rx drugs
Appetite stimulants
Digestive enzymes
Establish core nutrient protocol
High-potency multiple vitamin-mineral
Beta-carotene
Acetyl-L-Carnitine
EFAs
GI flora/probiotics
Support optimal immune function
N-acetylcysteine
CoQ10
Vitamin C
Constitutional symptoms, Rx side effects, symptoms of immuno-suppression
Provide tailored therapies
Identify and remove causes.
Tonify systems. Treat each patient as an individual. Choose patient-appropriate approaches, based on patient's specific circumstances
Provide specific antiviral therapy and immunomodulation using other nondrug treatments
Antiviral botanicals
Homeopathy
Whole-body hyperthermia
Acupuncture
Movement therapies
Provide education and guidance

- Groups at high risk for contracting HIV include injection drug users, homosexual and bisexual men, hemophiliacs and others receiving transfused blood or other blood products (highest risk to recipients before May 1985, when regular screening of the blood supply began), regular sex partners of people in the aforementioned groups, heterosexual people with more than one sex partner in the past 12 months, and those who have had unprotected sex during the past 6 months.

GENERAL CONSIDERATIONS

Clinical Progression to AIDS

- Within 2 to 3 weeks of initial infection, acute retroviral syndrome occurs. Recovery and seroconversion follow in 2 to 3 weeks. After recovery from acute syndrome, HIV plasma concentrations decline to viral set point and equilibrium is established between production and destruction of CD4+ cells. Level of viral replication after acute infection and seroconversion coupled with CD4+ count is predictive of long-term prognosis. Lower replication with higher CD4+ count indicates longer asymptomatic course. Conversely, higher replication with lower CD4+ counts indicates shorter asymptomatic course. Gradual decline in T-cell numbers begins with concurrent gradual increase in viral numbers over 5 to 15 years. Eventually T-cell decline impairs immune function; risk of OIs increases, ultimately ending in death.

Centers for Disease Control and Prevention Defining Guidelines

- See the box that lists the CDC 2008 revised surveillance case definition of AIDS for adults and adolescents (13 years of age or older). It creates stages of HIV infection based on CD4+ cell counts and percentages and/or clinical symptoms. Primary criterion: positive serology (i.e., positive for antibodies to HIV via ELISA and Western blot and/or positive HIV antigen detection via polymerase chain reaction [PCR] or other specific HIV antigen test). Given a positive serology, a diagnosis of stage 3 HIV or AIDS is given when CD4+ counts fall below $200/mm^3$ ($<14\%$), any of the noted AIDS-defining conditions occurs, or both.

Centers for Disease Control and Prevention (CDC) Surveillance Case Definition for HIV Infection among Adults and Adolescents Older than 13 Years*

- Stage 1: CD4+ T-lymphocyte count of >500/μl or >29%; no clinical evidence required and no AIDS-defining condition present
- Stage 2: CD4+ T-lymphocyte count of 200 to 299/μL or 14% to 28%; no clinical evidence required and no AIDS-defining condition present
- Stage 3 (AIDS): CD4+ T-lymphocyte count <200 /μL or <14% or documentation of an AIDS-defining condition
- Stage unknown: no information of CD4+ T-lymphocyte count or percentage; no information on presence of AIDS-defining conditions

The specific AIDS indicator conditions include the following:

- Candidiasis of esophagus, bronchi, trachea, or lungs
- Cervical cancer, invasive
- Coccidioidomycosis, disseminated or extrapulmonary
- Cryptococcosis, extrapulmonary
- Cryptosporidiosis, chronic intestinal (>1 month's duration)
- Cytomegalovirus disease (other than liver, spleen, or lymph nodes), onset at age >1 month
- Cytomegalovirus retinitis (with loss of vision)
- Encephalopathy, HIV-related
- Herpes simplex with chronic ulcers (>1 month's duration) or bronchitis, pneumonitis, or esophagitis (onset at age >1 month)
- Histoplasmosis, disseminated or extrapulmonary
- Isosporiasis, chronic intestinal (>1 month's duration)
- Kaposi's sarcoma
- Lymphoid interstitial pneumonia or pulmonary lymphoid hyperplasia complex
- Lymphoma—Burkitt's, immunoblastic, primary (brain or central nervous system)
- *Mycobacterium avium* complex (MAC) or *Mycobacterium kansasii,* disseminated or extrapulmonary
- *Mycobacterium tuberculosis* of any site, pulmonary, disseminated, or extrapulmonary
- *Pneumocystis jiroveci* pneumonia
- Pneumonia, recurrent
- Progressive multifocal leukoencephalopathy
- *Salmonella* septicemia, recurrent
- Toxoplasmosis of brain, onset at age older than 1 month
- Wasting syndrome caused by HIV—involuntary weight loss of greater than 10% of baseline plus chronic diarrhea (more than two loose stools per day for more than 30 days) or chronic weakness and documented enigmatic fever for longer than 30 days

From Schneider E, Whitmore S, Glynn KM, et al. Revised surveillance case definitions for HIV infection among adults, adolescents, and children aged <18 months and for HIV infection and AIDS among children aged 18 months to <13 years—United States, 2008. *MMWR Recomm Rep.* 2008; 57(RR-10);1-8.

- Patients are susceptible to complications (infectious and noninfectious) based on CD4+ counts. Higher viral load indicates greater risk for complications.
- When CD4+ cell count is above 500/mm^3, a patient could manifest acute retroviral syndrome, candidal vaginitis, persistent generalized lymphadenopathy (PGL), Guillain-Barré syndrome, myopathy, or aseptic meningitis.
- When CD4+ count is between 200 and 500/mm^3, possible complications include pneumococcal or other bacterial pneumonia, pulmonary tuberculosis, herpes zoster, oropharyngeal candidiasis or thrush, cryptosporidiosis (self-limited), Kaposi's sarcoma (KS), oral hairy leukoplakia, cervical and anal dysplasia or cancer, B-cell lymphoma, anemia, mononeuritis multiplex, idiopathic thrombocytopenic purpura, Hodgkin's lymphoma, or lymphocytic interstitial pneumonitis.
- When CD4+ count is below 200/mm^3, complications might include *P. jiroveci* pneumonia, disseminated histoplasmosis and coccidioidomycosis, miliary or extrapulmonary tuberculosis, progressive multifocal leukoencephalopathy (PML), wasting, peripheral neuropathy, HIV-associated dementia, cardiomyopathy, vacuolar myelopathy, progressive polyradiculopathy, or non-Hodgkin's lymphoma.
- When CD4+ count is below 100/mm^3, complications might include disseminated herpes simplex, toxoplasmosis, cryptococcosis, chronic cryptosporidiosis, microsporidiosis, or candidal esophagitis.
- When CD4+ count is below 50/mm^3, complications might include disseminated cytomegalovirus (CMV), disseminated MAC, or central nervous system lymphoma.

DIAGNOSIS AND WORKUP

Diagnostic Testing

- The accompanying box lists the most recent CDC guidelines for HIV testing. Standard serologic testing for presence of HIV begins with ELISA test using recombinant antigens to measure antibodies to HIV in blood. If the result of this test is positive, the test is repeated on the same blood sample. If it is positive a second time, a Western blot test (using electrophoresis to detect antibodies to specific HIV proteins) is used for confirmation. Together, these tests have a sensitivity and specificity approaching 100%.

Recommendations for HIV Testing of Adults, Adolescents, and Pregnant Women in Health Care Settings

Screening for HIV Infection

- Routine testing for all patients 13 to 64 years old
- Pregnant women
- All patients initiating treatment for tuberculosis
- All patients seeking treatment or evaluation at clinics treating sexually transmitted diseases
- All persons with signs or symptoms consistent with HIV or with an opportunistic infection (OI) consistent with HIV/AIDS

Repeat Screening

- Annual screening (minimally) for persons in high-risk groups (includes injection drug users and their sex partners, persons who exchange sex for money or drugs, sex partners of HIV-infected persons, men who have sex with men, and heterosexual persons who have had or whose sex partners have had more than one sex partner since their most recent HIV test).
- Patients and their prospective partners before initiating a new sexual relationship.
- Any person whose blood or body fluid is the source of an occupational exposure to a health care provider should be informed of the incident and tested at the time of the exposure.

Data from Branson BM, Handsfeld HH, Lampe MA, et al. Revised recommendations for HIV testing of adults, adolescents, and pregnant women in health-care settings. *MMWR Recomm Rep.* 2006;55(RR-14):1-17.

- Rapid HIV tests are currently approved by U.S. Food and Drug Administration (FDA). Options include OraQuick Advance, Uni-Gold Recombigen, Reveal G3, MultiSpot Rapid Test, Clearview Stat-Pak, Clearview Complete, and Vitros. Home Access Health Corporation produces a kit for specimens self-obtained at home and mailed in for analysis. Results are available in 1 to 5 days. These tests use whole blood, serum, plasma, or oral fluids and have sensitivity and specificity rates of 99% to 100%. If an ELISA result is negative and risk factors suggest likely infection, testing is repeated at 6-week, 3-month, and 6-month intervals.
- HIV testing remains voluntary. Discuss testing with each patient and obtain informed consent (either written or verbal) before testing. Patients have the right to opt out. Incorporate risk screening into routine primary care and risk reduction counseling offered. All states require that newly diagnosed cases of HIV/AIDS be reported to local health departments and that providers have case reporting forms available.

Medical History

- Detailed diet history, exercise patterns, complete review of systems. Additional historical details include those described in the accompanying box.

Historical Data Recommended for HIV-Positive Patients

- Dates of infection and subsequent diagnosis, as well as probable source of infection (intravenous drug use, sexual contact, transfusion). If date of infection is unknown, the naturopathic physician should determine whether there was any history of acute retroviral syndrome. In addition, past and current risk factors for HIV exposure should be determined. This information helps to estimate overall health and vital force and long-term prognosis.
- Vaccination history and adverse reactions to past vaccines.
- History of other sexually transmitted diseases. This information should include date and duration of infection as well as therapies (efficacy, adverse reactions, and duration of treatment). Particular infections to screen for include syphilis, gonorrhea, chlamydia, herpes simplex (all types), hepatitis (A, B, and C or E), and human papillomavirus (HPV) (skin, genital, or anal).
- Chronologic history of HIV-related problems including history of OIs or cofactor viruses or infections (mononucleosis, Epstein-Barr virus [EBV], molluscum contagiosum, CMV, or yeast infections—vaginal, gastrointestinal [GI], skin), skin rashes or other lesions, oral lesions or tongue coating, lymphadenopathy, fevers, night sweats, weight loss, diarrhea, anorexia, fatigue, malaise, shortness of breath, or cough.
- Specific for females, history of abnormal Pap smears and frequency of gynecologic examinations.
- HIV viral load and trend of CD4 count; good indicators of the patient's susceptibility to OIs, indication for and effectiveness of highly active antiretroviral therapy (HAART), as well as long-term prognosis.
- History of all past and present HAART as well as all other prophylactic antibiotic prescription medication with duration of treatment, response and side effects, intolerance, and allergies.
- Family history of chronic disease, with particular emphasis on cardiovascular disease (including lipid problems), diabetes, and cancer.
- History of psychoemotional trauma and issues (abuse history, anxiety, depression).
- Patients' spiritual lives and support systems, life goals, and meaning of HIV in their lives.
- Clear identification of complete medical care team as well as reasons for seeking naturopathic medical care.
- The initial physical examination must be both comprehensive and appropriately focused as directed by the history. In addition, all patients should have particularly thorough examinations of the mouth and throat, skin, and genitalia. If a full pelvic examination and Pap smear cannot be done on a new female patient at the initial evaluation, these should be scheduled for shortly thereafter.

Laboratory Assessment and Monitoring

- Complete blood count (CBC)
- Fasting serum chemistry panel (to monitor liver, kidney, pancreatic function; electrolytes; blood proteins; glucose; and lipids).
- Baseline serum albumin level serves as independent predictor of prognosis in HIV-positive women.
- Urinalysis, screening for sexually transmitted diseases (STDs) (syphilis, chlamydia, gonorrhea, herpes simplex), hepatitis (A, B, and C), toxoplasmosis, tuberculosis, varicella (if unknown history of chickenpox or shingles).
- Optional test: glucose-6-phosphate dehydrogenase (based on risk factors).
- Female patients: regular Pap smears with initial testing for HPV—increased cervical cancer rates in HIV-positive women.
- Anal Pap smear in male patients engaging in anal sex. Anal squamous cell cancer is linked to HPV infection; rates are elevated in HIV-positive men. There is no clear consensus on whether to make this test part of routine screening. Studies are ongoing.
- HIV-specific testing: viral load and T-cell counts as part of initial evaluation, then at 3- to 6-month intervals. Viral load test detects viral RNA in plasma or DNA in white blood cells (WBCs) and uses PCR branched-chain DNA (bDNA) or nucleic acid sequence–based amplification technology. The most sensitive test currently detects virus to 20 copies/mm^3 of plasma. Below any specific test's threshold, viral load is deemed undetectable—virus may be present below ability of given test to detect. These assays are not reflective of viral presence or concentration in body compartments beyond blood (tissues, cerebrospinal fluid, breast milk). Patients can still infect others even if virus is undetectable.
- T-cell counts: CD4+ helper cells and CD8+ suppressor cells are quantified (absolute numbers and relative percentages), along with CD4/CD8 ratio—used to stage HIV, predict susceptibility to OIs, monitor response to antiretroviral therapy. Factors that influence CD4+ cell counts: total WBCs, acute infection, certain medicines (corticosteroids, interferon), and others. There are also seasonal and diurnal variations in these counts.
- Resistance to antiretroviral medicines indicates resistance testing at time of diagnosis as baseline screening and before changing

therapy because of failure of current regimen. Two types of tests available: genotypic and phenotypic, each with pros and cons. This testing helps identify effective antiviral medicines to formulate most promising regimen.

THERAPEUTIC CONSIDERATIONS

Medical Management of HIV and AIDS

Conventional treatment of HIV/AIDS—treatment principles:

- Frequent monitoring—laboratory and physical examination
- Vaccinations—hepatitis A, hepatitis B, influenza, mumps-measles-rubella [MMR], pneumonia tetanus-diphtheria, varicella, HPV, travel-related vaccines
- Antiretroviral therapy (HAART) to inactivate or slow HIV replication and increase CD4+ cell counts
- Antibiotic prophylaxis for patients with abnormally low CD4 lymphocyte counts
- Antimicrobial treatment of opportunistic infections (OIs)
- Symptomatic care of HIV- or HAART-induced adverse drug reactions
- Radiation, chemotherapy, or both for HIV-related neoplasms
- Psychosocial support: counseling, clinical social work, and medication

Consult informed and current resources before making management decisions. AIDS websites:

U.S. Department of Health and Human Services (www.aidsinfo.nih.gov); and the Centers for Disease Control and Prevention (http://www.cdc.gov/hiv/).

Naturopathic Management of HIV and AIDS

Based on principles to optimize health, slow disease progression, improve quality of life, and improve immune function:

- Enhance integration with primary care physicians and build caregiving team.
- Complement and enhance positive effects of conventional treatment and minimize negative effects.
- Establish foundation of wellness based on naturopathic principles.
- Establish core nutrient protocol:
  - Replace nutrient deficiencies common with HIV.
  - Provide other nutrients to support immune function.

- Provide therapies to address constitutional symptoms, medication side effects, and symptoms of immunosuppression.
- Provide specific antiviral therapy and immunomodulation using other nondrug treatments.
- Educate and guide patients seeking alternatives to conventional treatment.

Resource for complementary practitioners: *AIDS and Complementary and Alternative Medicine, Current Science and Practice* by Standish LJ, Calabrese C, and Galantino ML, published by Churchill Livingstone in 2002.

Enhance Integration with Primary Care Physicians and Build a Caregiving Team

- Identify advantages of all available treatments and encourage positive relationships with all providers to create trusting relationships with patients who have a history of fear, discrimination, victimization, and abuse. Naturopathic medicine can empower HIV-positive patients.
- Ensure that each patient has a complete caregiving team beginning with conventional HIV specialists who will ensure access to HAART when appropriate and have great familiarity with multitude of signs, symptoms, adverse reactions, and other issues unique to HIV-positive population. HIV-positive patients who work with HIV specialists have better objective indexes of health, therapeutic compliance, and long-term survival.

Complement and Enhance Positive Effects of Conventional Treatment and Minimize Negative Effects

- Minimize need for higher-force (drug, surgery, radiation) interventions.
- There are no complementary and alternative medicine (CAM) therapies known to be as effective as HAART in suppressing viral load or increasing CD4 T-lymphocyte numbers. There are no realistic alternatives to HAART.
- Current standard of care: initiate HAART when CD4 count drops below 350/μL in asymptomatic patients, those with AIDS-defining illness (regardless of CD4 count), pregnant women, patients with HIV-associated nephropathy, or hepatitis B coinfection (when treatment of hepatitis is indicated). Consider HAART when CD4 counts are above 350/μL in discordant relationships (one partner is HIV positive and the other HIV negative), rapid CD4 decline, advanced age, or high viral load (>100,000 copies/mL).

- Most current recommendations: "Guidelines for the Use of Antiretroviral Agents in HIV-1–infected Adults and Adolescents," on AIDS website (https://aidsinfo.nih.gov/contentfiles/lvguidelines/AdultAndAdolescentGL.pdf).
- Factors in HIV holistic care: complications, from immune suppression, from pre-HIV health issues; social, psychoemotional, and spiritual challenges.
- Ensure that patient is safe from adverse drug-nutrient interactions. Understand mechanisms of HAART and those of common nutrients used by HIV-positive patients.

Five main classes of HAART are currently used in various combinations:

- Nucleoside or nucleotide reverse transcriptase inhibitors (NRTIs, or "nukes")
- Non-nucleoside reverse transcriptase inhibitors (NNRTIs, or "non-nukes")
- Protease inhibitors (PIs)
- Entry inhibitors (including fusion inhibitors and CCR5 inhibitors)
- Integrase inhibitors

Fixed-dose formulations combine multiple drugs and classes to simplify administration and decrease pill burden.

Because of increasing viral resistance, new antivirals are fast-tracked through FDA approval process. Full range of adverse side effects of new drugs is unknown.

Establish a Foundation of Health and Wellness on the Basis of Naturopathic Principles

- Large quantities of medicines, nutritional supplements, or both put biochemical stress on the body. Establish dietary habits that ensure optimal GI health and nutritional intake.
- **Optimize hydration:** high intake of filtered or safe water to decrease oxidative stress and reduce toxic load.
- **Optimize protein intake:** 100 to 150 g daily, particularly with malabsorption or diarrhea. Supplement protein to prevent weight loss. Whey protein and amino acids (L-glutamine, L-arginine) reverse or prevent HIV-induced wasting.
- **Essential fatty acids (EFAs):** deficient in HIV-positive patients. EFAs increase body cell mass (BCM) and decrease risk of progression to AIDS.
- **Antioxidants:** HIV-positive patients ingesting fruit juices or fruit-vegetable concentrate long term have higher micronutrient and antioxidant levels. Encourage eating colorful vegetables and fruits.

- **GI support:** digestive enzymes and appetite stimulants to combat adverse effects of HIV, HAART, and prophylactic antibiotics on GI system. Avoid GI stressors—high-sodium, high-fructose corn syrup in processed foods, alcohol (ETOH), caffeine, fried foods, and cigarette smoke. Raw eggs, unpasteurized milk, undercooked meat or fish, and potentially contaminated foods must be eliminated to prevent GI OIs and parasites.
- Beware allergen elimination; likelihood of nutrient deficiencies, maldigestion, and malabsorption caused by HIV itself and HAART. Recommend replacing food allergens one at a time to maintain caloric and nutrient intake.
- **Lifestyle factors:** aerobic exercise benefits immunodeficiency patients by alleviating stress and elevating mood. HIV-positive patients see increases in CD4, CD8, and natural killer (NK) cells immediately after aerobic exercise, and long-term exercise has demonstrated increases in immune parameters. Tai chi improves overall perception of health and several measures of physical function. Yoga increases self-confidence and speeds return to athletic activities after medical interventions.
- **Sleep:** encourage patients to create optimal sleeping environment and to sleep 8 to 10 hours nightly to repair and rebuild tissues and increase circulating NK cells and lymphocytes.
- **Group activities:** improve prognoses and decrease stress and anxiety. Long-term AIDS survival is linked to a positive attitude, health-promoting behaviors, spiritual activities, and HIV-positive community activities. Structured, brief group intervention for grief from loss of loved ones decreases plasma cortisol and improves several immune markers. Cognitive behavioral stress management improves quality of life, decreases herpes simplex 2 antibody titers, and improves HIV laboratory values.
- **Prayer, distance healing:** lead to fewer new AIDS-defining illnesses, less severity, fewer doctor visits, fewer hospitalizations, and improved mood. For those not on HAART, spiritual practice (prayer, meditation, affirmations, psychic healing, visualizations) reduces risk of death over a 1-year period. Laughter improves WBC values and decreases stress.

Establish a Core Nutrient Protocol

Replace Known Nutrient Deficiencies Caused by HIV

- Vitamin and mineral replenishment delays progression to AIDS and requirement to initiate antiretroviral therapy. Numerous deficiencies are identified with HIV disease progression. These deficiencies are likely the result of loss, poor absorption, or rapid use and consumption.

- The accompanying box summarizes nutrients deficient in HIV patients. Typical daily doses required, taken in divided doses, are noted in parentheses followed by rationale or benefits.

Nutrient Deficiencies in HIV Patients

- Vitamin A (15,000-30,000 international units [IU] taken with food) slows progression to AIDS and decreases mortality, improves growth in infants, decreases stunting associated with chronic diarrhea, and prevents gastrointestinal (GI) deterioration in mothers and infants. May increase the risk of HIV transmission by breastfeeding but has no effect on mortality by 24 months. Deficiencies can be caused by decreased dietary intake, poor GI absorption, high urinary loss, impaired hepatic protein synthesis, and increased needs as a result of chronic infection.
- Beta-carotene (60-120 mg/150,000 IU taken with food) replenishment—increased CD41 count, CD4/CD8 ratios, total lymphocyte count, and decreased mortality. Deficiency found in all HIV-positive patients is likely caused by poor digestion, decreased free radical elimination, and high lipid peroxidation.
- Folate (400 mcg) normalizes cell differentiation. Deficiency is most likely caused by malabsorption; AZT (azidothymidin)-induced deficiency may increase risk of bone marrow toxicity.
- Vitamin B_1 (50 mg) replenishment is associated with increased survival in HIV-positive patients and decreased progression to AIDS.
- Vitamin B_6 (50 mg) is essential in cellular and humoral immune responses. Vitamin B_6 repletion both alone and in conjunction with coenzyme Q10 (CoQ10) increases circulating immunoglobulin G (IgG), CD4+ cells, and CD4/CD8 ratios.
- Vitamin B_{12} (1000 mcg hydroxocobalamin, methylcobalamin, or cyanocobalamin best taken via intramuscular injections three times a week—alternate form is daily 1000 mcg sublingual) is important in several parameters of immune function, proper cell differentiation, and nerve function and in decreasing homocysteine levels. Vitamin B_{12} repletion can improve lymphocyte counts, CD4/CD8 ratios, and NK cell activity. Supplementation has also been found to reverse AIDS dementia complex when associated with low levels. Deficiency has been associated with increased risk of progression to AIDS and with HIV disease in general.
- Vitamin D (5000 IU) deficiency commonly found in urban HIV-infected men with suppressed viral load and CD4 count above 200; tobacco use was correlated with severe deficiency. Undetectable levels of vitamin D in HIV-positive patients correlated with more-advanced HIV infection, lower CD4 count, higher levels of tumor necrosis factor-alpha (TNF-α). Lower bone mineral density was found HIV patients using tenofovir/emtricitabine combination.
- Vitamin E (800 IU daily—mixed tocopherols taken with food) is indicated to decrease lipid peroxidation, protect against AZT-induced oxidative damage to cardiac mitochondria, normalize immune function, and slow progression to AIDS. Deficiency is found in most HIV-positive patients, with wasting, and in progression to AIDS.

- Copper (2 mg) can inhibit HIV protease and viral replication. Deficiencies of copper are associated with AZT therapy and AIDS.
- Magnesium (300 mg) deficiency is found in AIDS patients.
- Selenium (400 mcg) to suppress the progression of HIV-1, reduce viral burden, and provide indirect improvement of CD4 count. Decreases HIV-associated mortality, decreases anxiety in HIV-positive recreational drug users, and decreases hospitalizations and costs of caring for HIV-positive patients. Severity of deficiency in patients progressing to AIDS may be caused by decreased calorie and protein intake, malabsorption, and various infections.
- Zinc (15 mg—optimal intake levels have not been determined) has been found to decrease frequency of opportunistic infections (OIs). Deficiency is noted in all HIV-positive patients progressing to AIDS.
- Acetyl-L-carnitine (2-6 g best taken away from other proteins to optimize absorption) is essential for proper energy supply as well as critical metabolic functions. Deficiency is common in HIV-positive patients and increases the risk for alterations in fatty-acid oxidation. Repletion has also been linked with a reduction in serum triglycerides, decreased risk of wasting, increase in CD4 cells, reduced apoptosis, increased levels of serum insulin-like growth factor, reduction in mitochondrial neurotoxicity, and treatment of peripheral neuropathy. It has also been demonstrated as an effective treatment for nucleoside or nucleotide reverse transcriptase inhibitor (NRTI)–induced lactic acidosis.
- Dehydroepiandrosterone (DHEA) (15-50 mg taken with food) repletion helps to increase CD4 count, stimulate immune function, and improve quality of life.
- Testosterone (intramuscular injection weekly) is indicated if serum levels are low, to decrease loss of lean body and muscle mass.
- Glutathione (GSH; increased through selenium and *N*-acetylcysteine (NAC) or whey protein powder) has been found to decrease disease progression and mortality. Deficiencies are found in both symptom-free HIV-positive and AIDS patients.

Many of these nutrients can be replenished through the use of a highly nutritious diet and a good multivitamin. A few multivitamins have been specifically developed to replace the deficiencies of HIV-positive patients and include high doses of carotenoids, B vitamins, antioxidants, and sometimes digestive enzymes. Taking one multivitamin designed specifically for HIV reduces pill burden and enhances compliance. Conversely, it is generally more cost-effective to use a basic multivitamin and supplement individually with additional nutrients.

- Nutrient deficiencies (high doses of beta-carotene, vitamin D, acetyl-L-carnitine, dehydroepiandrosterone [DHEA], testosterone, reduced glutathione [GSH], and catalase) not commonly included in a multivitamin-multimineral supplement must be replaced through specific dietary regimens or through additional supplements. Use natural forms of beta-carotene; synthetic forms can increase risk of lung cancer in smokers. Consider acetyl-L-carnitine as a high priority, despite high cost, because of number of benefits.

Provide Other Nutrients to Support Optimal Immune Function

- The accompanying box summarizes nutrients that replace or reduce other nutrient deficiencies or benefit HIV patients, daily divided doses, and desirable effects. All these nutrients have value, but they increase overall cost and pill burden. Give priority to the most essential (EFAs and DHEA) and lower-cost (vitamin C) nutrients or to address specific symptoms as described in the next section.

Nutrients that Have Been Found to Replace or Reduce Other Nutrient Deficiencies or Have Beneficial Actions in HIV Patients

- *Silybum marianum* (milk thistle; 300 mg standardized extract away from highly active antiretroviral therapy [HAART]) is indicated for all patients on HAART to improve liver function, decrease liver damage, and increase the antioxidant activity of blood cells.
- *N*-acetylcysteine (NAC; 2-8 g best taken away from other nutrients but may need to be taken with food to decrease gastrointestinal distress) is indicated to prevent loss of sulfur-containing amino acids, increase GSH, decrease tumor necrosis factor-alpha (TNF-α) activity, and increase CD4 cell count.
- Coenzyme Q10 (CoQ10; 100-300 mg) optimized mitochondrial function and replaced deficiency. Repletion with CoQ10 increased circulating IgG, CD4+ cells, and CD4/CD8 ratios.
- Vitamin C (2-6 g) when combined with vitamin E significantly lowered oxidative stress and has demonstrated a trend toward lowered viral load.
- Alpha-lipoic acid (600 mg) protected the liver, inhibited viral replication, increased intracellular GSH, increased CD4/CD8 ratios, and potentially decreases peripheral neuropathic pain by its antioxidant effect on nervous tissue.
- L-Arginine (7.4 g taken away from food) improved lean body mass and increased natural killer cell activity. Must be used with caution because large amounts of arginine can aggravate herpesvirus outbreaks. Prophylactic L-lysine may prevent or reduce this effect.
- Essential fatty acids (EFAs) (5 g taken with food; best from fish oil) improved lean body mass, increased NK cell activity, and was beneficial as adjuvant therapy in patients with tuberculosis.
- L-Methionine (1000 mg taken away from other proteins) slowed decline of CD4 cells.

Provide Therapies to Address Constitutional Symptoms, Medication Side Effects, and Symptoms of Immunosuppression

Candida albicans and Oral Thrush.

Overgrowth of fungus may occur from low CD4+ count or secondary to prophylactic antibiotics. Thrush causes pain and makes eating difficult, reducing caloric intake. Intestinal infestation can compromise nutrient absorption. Esophageal cases must be dealt with swiftly via antifungal drugs. Instruct patients to avoid foods that promote yeast growth—simple sugars, baked goods, and starchy vegetables. Consider the following options:

- **Probiotics:** fermented foods and supplements with 8 billion or more colony-forming units (CFUs), best taken with food. Beneficial species: *Lactobacillus acidophilus* or *bifidus;* Lactobacillus rhamnosus; *Saccharomyces boulardii* (best for antibiotic-induced colitis and can help displace pathogenic flora).
- **Garlic** (1 to 2 g before meals): potent antifungal that spares nonpathogenic flora; patients on HAART should not take supplemental garlic.
- **Oregano oil** (300 mg away from food): potent antifungal.
- **Nystatin** and **fluconazole:** prescription antifungals.

Cardiovascular Disease.

Adverse effects on serum lipids and glucose from HAART promote cardiovascular disease, particularly in patients already at high risk (predisposing factors—positive family history). Encourage all patients on HAART to institute preventive diet, healthy lifestyle, and exercise per recommendations to promote cardiovascular health. Exercise increases functional aerobic capacity, eliminates functional aerobic impairment, and improves exercise performance (improved peak oxygen consumption, oxygen pulse, tidal volume, ventilation, and leg power). Avoid garlic owing to its adverse interaction with HAART. Consider the following specific nutrients:

- **Acetyl-L-carnitine** (2 to 6 g away from proteins to optimize absorption) repletion is linked with reduction in serum triglycerides.
- **Coenzyme Q10** (CoQ10) (100 to 300 mg) may enhance cardiovascular function.
- **Arginine** (7.4 g away from food) decreases atherosclerosis.
- **EFAs** (5 g with food) may lower lipids.

Diarrhea.

Diarrhea is common and diminishes quality of life. Specific cause guides choice of treatment. Causes: HIV-associated enteropathy, HAART side effects, antibiotic side effects, GI infections, and food allergies or intolerances. Osmotic-type diarrhea can occur from ingesting too many indigestible gelcaps. First treatment priority: remove cause, if possible. Rule out gluten intolerance, lactose intolerance, irritable bowel syndrome, food allergies and sensitivities. Consider stool cultures and testing for ova and parasites. Cease all nutrient supplementation temporarily to screen for osmotic cause; reintroduce one at a time to determine offending agent. Steps for prevention: avoid unfiltered tap water, unpasteurized milk or dairy products, ice made from unfiltered tap water, raw fruits and vegetables unless they can be peeled personally or washed with appropriate antimicrobial agents, raw or rare meat and fish, meat or shellfish that is not hot when served, and food from street vendors. Prevent dehydration by replacing electrolytes—broths, soups, fruit and vegetable juices, or high-nutrient drinks. Prevent malnutrition; ensure adequate micronutrients and macronutrients—multivitamin-mineral supplement, adequate protein (requirements may increase to 100 to 150 g/day). Consider initially simplifying the diet (*BRAT* diet: *b*ananas, *r*ice, *a*pplesauce, *t*oast) or using 1 tbsp tomato juice combined with 1 tbsp sauerkraut juice (Dr. John Bastyr). Carob powder is an astringent that helps symptomatically. Begin with 1 tsp in applesauce and increase up to 6 tsp/day as needed. Consider these additional supplements:

- Healthy flora earlier in care of candidal infection.
- L-Glutamine (9 to 40 g away from other proteins): amino acid fuel for small intestinal enterocytes. Powder form is most efficient and cost-effective. Start with 3 g t.i.d. Increase up to 40 g daily if needed. High dose can lead to psychoses; monitor patients closely.
- Diphenoxylate and atropine (Lomotil), loperamide (Imodium), and psyllium husk (Metamucil) are common pharmaceutical interventions.

Herpes Simplex Virus, Herpes Zoster, Shingles.

Herpes-type virus conditions are treated similarly. Herpes zoster lesions manifest as skin dermatomal patterns. They can occur secondary to stress, hormonal fluctuations, or poor immune response. First and foremost, identify and remove causes of stress (dietary, emotional, sunlight exposure); support immune function. Second, address symptoms (pain). Consider the following:

- **Diet:** eliminate foods high in L-arginine (promotes herpes replication)—chocolate, nuts, peanuts; increase foods high in L-lysine (antagonizes L-arginine)—whole grains, dairy, fish, lima beans, soy.
- **L-Lysine:** 1000 mg t.i.d., away from food, during outbreak; 500 mg t.i.d., away from food, prophylactically.
- **Olive leaf extract:** 2000 mg—effective antiviral.

- **Monolaurin:** antiviral, taken at 300 to 600 mg t.i.d.; effective against encapsulated DNA viruses.
- ***Melissa officinalis:*** antiviral botanical; ointment concentrate used topically.
- ***Glycyrrhiza glabra:*** antiviral oral and topical botanical.
- **Herbal tincture** (as parts): *Hydrastis* (1), *Taraxacum officinale* (the root) (2), *Lomatium* (2), *Passiflora* (1), *Astragalus* (1), *Gelsemium* (15 drops/oz); dose—60 drops every 2 hours during prodrome, q.i.d. during an outbreak, b.i.d. for prevention.
- **Acyclovir and valacyclovir:** pharmaceutical antivirals.

Kaposi's Sarcoma.

KS is an HIV-associated neoplasm of vascular origin that occurs when CD4+ counts fall below 500/mm^3. KS is rare outside of HIV-positive population. Etiology relative to AIDS is poorly understood. Contributing factors: human herpesvirus (HHV) type 8, compromised immunity, and hormones (KS is rare in women; androgen therapy increases proliferation). It is most common in iron-rich geographic areas; 90% of U.S. AIDS-related cases occur in homosexual men; it is rare in heterosexual men, women, and intravenous drug users. KS begins as macules or elevated papules and can progress to large plaques or nodules. Color ranges from pink to purple or brownish-black. Lesions may be round or oval and do not blanch under applied pressure. Lesions appear first on skin of upper body or mucosal surfaces. Aggressive form becomes widely disseminated and manifests anywhere on skin, mucous membranes, lymph nodes, or viscera (GI tract from mouth to anus, lungs, liver, spleen, pancreas). KS tumors secrete increased angiogenic growth factors, tumor necrosis factor-alpha (TNF-α), interleukin-6 (IL-6), basic fibroblast growth factor, platelet-derived growth factor, and oncostatin M. Level of immunosuppression determines clinical course of KS in AIDS. Currently there are no known cures; local and systemic approaches are aimed at palliation. Treatment: chemotherapeutic agents—doxorubicin, standard HAART. Surgical excision removes a lesion, but lesion often recurs at affected site. Other therapies: radiation, cryotherapy with liquid nitrogen, and electrical stimulation with direct current. Consider the following:

- Topical and systemic retinoids.
- Topical vitamin D (1,25-dihydroxyvitamin D_3).
- Iron stimulates growth of KS cells in vitro; iron chelators reduce growth. Limit iron intake; ensure that serum iron and ferritin levels are normal.

- Cytokine inhibitors and antiangiogenesis compounds might reduce proliferation of these vascular tumors.
- No known cure and difficult palliation means naturopaths can and must be creative. Given KS link to HHV type 8, consider antiherpetic therapies if patients are herpes simplex virus positive. Topical medicinal peat has induced remission of skin KS lesions in several patients. GSH (NAC as precursor) may also help.

Lipodystrophy.

Lipodystrophy (LD) is redistribution of fat tissue from extremities to the trunk, often with a cushingoid buffalo hump over upper thoracic area of the back or with truncal obesity. Self-image issues are common and problematic. LD arises form altered lipid metabolism secondary to HAART or chronic HIV infection (longer than 15 years). Adrenal abnormalities may contribute. Elevated serum cortisol induces insulin elevation, driving blood glucose into adipose cells. LD increases with lack of exercise. Increase exercise; ensure that blood glucose is regulated. Consider the following:

- L-glutamine (10 g in divided doses away from food).
- Acetyl-L-carnitine (2 to 6 g away from food) to optimize mitochondrial function.
- Uridine (36 g t.i.d. for 10 consecutive days monthly) to normalize subcutaneous fat.
- Testosterone (10 g of testosterone gel daily) in HIV-positive men with abdominal obesity and low testosterone; decreased whole-body, total, and abdominal fat mass; and increased lean body mass.
- Nandrolone decanoate (150 mg intramuscularly [IM] every 2 weeks) may increase lean body mass more effectively than testosterone.
- Tesamorelin, a growth hormone–releasing factor analogue (2 mg per subcutaneous injection), decreases visceral fat tissue and triglycerides without aggravating glucose.
- Dimethyl sulfoxide (DMSO) and bromelain (5% bromelain compounded in DMSO gel applied b.i.d. or t.i.d.). Topically reduces cushingoid fat deposits.
- Conventional treatment: surgical removal of truncal fat deposits. Despite invasiveness, patients tend to be happy afterward because of positive self-image.
- Buccal injections of polylactic acid (PLA; New-Fill) can be safe and reduce cosmetic signs and depressive symptoms of LD and wasting.

Macrocytic Anemia.

Macrocytic anemia (MA) can be secondary to malabsorption of nutrients or a side effect of HAART. Consider the following treatments:

- Vitamin B_{12} (hydroxocobalamin, methylcobalamin, cyanocobalamin 1000 mcg/mL given IM three times a week) for proper cell division and differentiation. If an intramuscular injection is unavailable, sublingual tablets at 1000 mcg q.d. bypass intestinal absorption issues.
- Folic acid (400 mcg q.d. (multivitamin-multimineral supplements) and vitamin B complex (3 mL IM weekly) are indicated for proper cell division and differentiation.

Neuropathy.

Neuropathy manifests in the periphery—feet. It can progress proximally as it increases in severity. It emerges from long-term HIV infection or as toxic effect of HAART on mitochondria in neurons. Diabetes mellitus type 2 can also be a factor, as can overdoses of vitamin B_6 (>200 mg/day). Consider the following:

- Acetyl-L-carnitine (2 to 6 g away from other proteins to optimize absorption) decreases risk for altered fatty-acid metabolism and decreases pain.
- EFAs (5 g/day with food) are anti-inflammatory agents and components of healthy cell membranes.
- Vitamin B_{12} (1000 mcg/mL IM three times weekly) for proper cell division and differentiation.
- Vitamin B complex (1 mL IM three times weekly) for proper cell division and differentiation.
- CoQ10 (100 to 300 mg) to optimize mitochondrial function.
- Alpha-lipoic acid (600 mg/day) may decrease pain.

Psychological Conditions.

Depression, anxiety, posttraumatic stress disorder, sexual dysfunction, and substance abuse are common in HIV-positive individuals, with physiologic effects. Suicidal ideation and attempts can be an issue. As quality of life declines, burdens of treatment increase, and friends die, will to live can wane. Be observant for suicidal thinking or loss of hope. Immediately engage experienced professionals to assist. Exercise extreme caution owing to issues of polypharmacy and drug-nutrient interactions. Interactions among many nutrients and numerous HIV drugs and even among drugs are likely. Before instituting treatment, rule out potential interactions.

Example: St. John's wort, commonly used herbal antidepressant, induces cytochrome p450 detoxification enzyme 3A4 in the liver and reduces serum levels of HAART medicines. It may reduce efficacy of those drugs and lead to increased resistance. Avoid St. John's wort in any patient undergoing HAART. Helpful modalities: counseling, lifestyle modification, homeopathy, meditation, mindfulness mantra practice. These modalities can help stabilize CD4+ T-lymphocyte counts independent of antiretrovirals, reduce anger, and increase spiritual faith and connectedness. Therapies to consider include the following:

- Multivitamin supplementation (B complex, C, and E) can reduce risk of elevated depressive symptoms and improve quality of life.
- Androgens (DHEA 50 mg or testosterone 300 mg IM weekly) can improve mood, quality of life, and overall survivability and also decrease fatigue.
- Amino acids (if levels are low by specialty laboratory analysis): prescribed in combinations tailored to replenish deficiencies.
- Zinc (25 mg/day) normalizes levels and improves efficacy of antidepressants.
- EFAs (5 g/day with food) are adjunctive treatment in depressive disorders.
- *S*-adenosylmethionine (SAM; 1600 mg/day) is as effective as imipramine (150 mg) in treating major depression and is better tolerated.

Wasting.

See definition from *The AIDS Reader* in box "AIDS Wasting Syndrome Criteria." BCM is measured via bioimpedance assay. BCM is a better predictor of survival than CD4 counts. Key issues to be addressed with patients: perceived weight loss, changes in appetite, diarrhea, energy level, and difficulty performing daily tasks.

AIDS Wasting Syndrome Criteria

AIDS wasting syndrome must meet one of the following criteria:

- Unintentional weight loss of >10% over 12 mo
- Unintentional weight loss of >7.5% over 6 mo
- BCM loss of <5% over 6 mo
  - Men: BCM <35% of TBW and BMI <27 kg/m^2
  - Women: BCM <23% of TBW and BMI <27 kg/m^2
- BMI <20 kg/m^2

BCM, body cell mass; BMI, body mass index; TBW, total body weight.

The etiology of wasting is as follows:

- Decreased food intake—anorexia (loss of appetite) or nausea secondary to medication, systemic illness, or GI pathosis; finances; dependence on others; poor food choices.
- Malabsorption or chronic diarrhea—decreased nutrient absorption resulting from GI infections, medication side effects, enzyme deficiencies, and malignancies.
- Alterations of metabolism—resting energy expenditure (REE) is higher in HIV/AIDS patients than in controls; REE does not downregulate if anorexia or malabsorption is present.
- Cytokine abnormalities—TNF, IL-1 may induce anorexia and affect lipid, protein, and carbohydrate use.
- Endocrine abnormalities—thyroid abnormalities, adrenal insufficiency (cortisol, DHEA), hypogonadism (testosterone), growth hormone deficiency.
- Alcohol abuse—progression to AIDS is quicker in HIV-positive patients who abuse alcohol; ETOH can stimulate HIV production, suppress immune defenses (lower CD4 counts), and deplete tissue antioxidants.

Identify and remove causes of wasting, if feasible; then identify and remove foods to which patient is allergic or intolerant (gluten and dairy in particular). Ensure optimal nutritional intake via dietary counseling. Help patients access social service assistance if necessary. Patients are likely to need superdoses of nutrients. Increase protein intake to 100 to 150 g/day. Encourage engagement with life, daily exercise, and so on. Consider the following therapies:

- EFAs (5 g/day with food)
- Acetyl-L-carnitine (2 to 6 g/day) to optimize fatty acid metabolism
- L-Glutamine (10 to 40 g), essential amino acid for enterocytes
- DHEA (50 mg) to promote lean body mass
- Melatonin (20 mg at bedtime) to decrease cachexia and TNF
- Marijuana (smoked q.i.d.) or oral dronabinol (5 to 10 mg q.i.d.) to increase daily caloric intake and body weight
- Progesterone (800 mg) to decrease cachexia
- Testosterone in hypogonadal men to increase lean body mass and muscle strength
- Anabolic steroids (nandrolone decanoate, oxandrolone, oxymetholone) to increase lean body mass
- Thalidomide, a cytokine modulator, to increase BCM and extracellular fluid

Provide Specific Antiviral Therapy and Immunomodulation Using Other Nondrug Treatments

Botanical, homeopathic, and physical medicine therapies are not substitutes for HAART. They are additional nondrug solutions that resonate with the unique needs of individual HIV-positive patients.

Botanical Medicines.

Botanicals that have demonstrated efficacy in treating HIV include the following:

- *G. glabra* (licorice; 1500 mg) inhibited HIV fusion and viral transcription. It should not be used in patients with a history of hypertension or with renal or cardiac problems.
- *Curcuma longa* (turmeric; 1200 mg) inhibited HIV integrase and proteases and viral transcription and decreased nuclear factor kappa B (NF-κB).
- *Olea* species (olive leaf extract; 2 to 6 g) increased NK-cell function and was effective against HIV and herpesviruses.
- *Phyllanthus amarus* (1200 mg) demonstrated in vitro and ex vivo HIV-1 inhibition of reverse transcriptase, receptors, and proteases and is also effective against HBV.
- *Lentinus edodes* (shitake mushrooms; 1 to 5 mg IV twice weekly) inhibited reverse transcriptase, increased CD4 counts, and decreased p24 (surface marker).
- *Andrographis paniculata* (1500 mg) inhibited fusion, viral replication, and HIV-1 cell-to-cell transmission. It also stimulated objective measures of immune function, increased the effectiveness of azidothymidin (AZT), protected against liver damage, and decreased diarrhea. Toxicity questions remain; further study is necessary.
- *Silybum marianum* (milk thistle; 300 mg extract) improved liver function and antioxidant activity of blood cells.
- *Hyssopus officinalis* (hyssop; 1 to 4 mL tincture) exhibited anti-HIV activity and inhibited integration of proviral genome into host genome.
- *Prunella vulgaris* (self-heal; 10 mg/mL IV) inhibited HIV replication and binding and prevented cell-to-cell infection.
- *Rosmarinus officinalis* (rosemary; use liberally in food) decreased HIV replication and protease activity.
- *Momordica charantia* (bitter melon; 6 oz fresh juice) normalized CD4+/CD8+ ratios and inactivated viral DNA.
- *Spirulina platensis* (blue-green algae; use liberally in food) reduced fusion and viral production.

- *Scutellaria baicalensis* (skullcap; 6 to 15 g whole root) inhibited HIV-1 reverse transcriptase.
- *Podophyllum* resin (25% solution as a single topical application) resulted in resolution of hairy leukoplakia.
- *Melaleuca leucadendron* (tea tree oil solution) was effective for fluconazole-refractory oropharyngeal candidiasis in patients with AIDS.
- *Hypericum perforatum* (St. John's wort; 900 mg) inhibited protein kinase C and viral uncoating, fusion, and assembly. Do not use in patients taking NNRTIs or PIs.
- *Allium sativa* (garlic; 4 g fresh garlic) selectively killed HIV-1–infected cells in vitro. It should not be used in patients taking NNRTIs or PIs.

Homeopathy.

Constitutional homeopathic remedies (30C to 1M doses) have caused some patients to became ELISA negative after 3 to 16 months. These medicines have increased CD41 T-cell counts after 6 months. Homeopathy can help with symptom care. Homeopathic remedies have also been able to reduce hypersensitivity to certain drugs. Homeopathic growth hormone has improved CD4 cells, CD8 cells, erythrocyte sedimentation rate (ESR), weight gain, and viral load; reduced occurrences of OIs; and increased platelet counts. Consider constitutional homeopathy an essential aspect of care of all HIV-positive patients, especially considering the amazing potential, minimal side effects, and overall affordability.

Physical Medicine and Acupuncture.

Physical medicine is another low-cost therapy that can play a pivotal role.

- Whole-body hyperthermia (twice weekly at 108°F for 20 minutes) may elevate CD4 count, but use extreme caution in heat-intolerant patients.
- Ozone (rectal and aural insufflation) may inactivate HIV-1.
- Acupuncture and moxibustion (three times weekly) can decrease diarrhea and illicit drug (cocaine and heroin) cravings.
- Electroacupuncture (by continually stimulating acupuncture or conductance skin points associated with nervous and immune systems) ameliorates complications of HIV-related peripheral neuropathy, raises CD4+ counts, and raises other lymphocyte counts.
- Massage therapy increases NK cells, CD3 and CD4 cell counts, and CD4/CD8 ratios; improves quality of life; and decreases health care costs.

Studies have demonstrated increased growth and development and overall behavior in HIV-exposed newborns and improved immune preservation in HIV-positive children in the absence of antiretroviral therapy.

- Therapeutic touch reduces anxiety in children.
- Cranioelectrical stimulation (microcurrent 0.1 mA at 100 Hz to alligator clips attached to earlobes 20 minutes b.i.d.) can decrease anxiety, insomnia, and depression.

Movement therapies include the following:

- Aerobic exercise to alleviate stress and enhance mood. HIV-positive patients derive improvements in CD8 and NK cells.
- Tai chi has improved overall perception of health and all functional measures in HIV-positive persons compared with controls.
- Yoga has improved self-confidence and sparked a return to athletic activities.

Provide Education and Guidance to Patients Seeking Alternatives to Conventional Treatment

There are currently no known therapies as effective as HAART in suppressing viral load or increasing CD4 cells. Avoid temptations to allow patients to believe otherwise. Ensure that the patient has access to a conventional HIV specialist to provide clear education on conventional Western medical approaches to HIV and help diagnose and treat OIs should they arise. Initiate a foundation of care—healthy diet and lifestyle, nutritional support, and additional therapies as described. Ensure that the patient is scheduled for frequent follow-ups with health care providers to regularly screen for and monitor potential or existing OIs. If a sole practitioner is treating a patient who refuses to undergo conventional medical or pharmaceutical intervention, specific use of the following therapies should be considered to decrease viral load and increase CD4 cell count:

- *C. longa* (turmeric; 1200 mg) to inhibit HIV integrase, proteases, and viral transcription.
- *Olea* species (olive leaf extract; 2 to 6 g) to increase NK-cell function and oppose HIV and herpesviruses.
- *P. amarus* (1200 mg), which inhibits HIV-1, reverse transcriptase, receptors, and proteases in vitro and ex vivo.
- *L. edodes* (shitake mushrooms; 1 to 5 mg IV twice a week) can increase CD4 and decrease p24 (a surface marker).
- Ozone (rectal and aural insufflations) may inactivate HIV-1.

For patients seeking advice on the discontinuation or interruption of HAART (a structured treatment interruption [STI] or "drug holiday"), ensure that patients clearly communicate this desire to their primary care physicians and HIV specialists. Treatment interruptions may be indicated in the following situations:

- Severe or life-threatening toxicity, unexpected inability to take oral medicines, or antiretroviral medication nonavailability (a short-term interruption).
- Patient has to be relieved of inconvenience, toxicity, and cost of antiretroviral therapy.
- Response to salvage therapy (treatment regimens used when other HAART regimens have failed) can be improved by allowing reemergence of wild-type virus (predominant virus type in a given individual as unaffected by HAART therapy).

Potential problems with treatment interruptions include viral rebound, immune decompensation, and clinical progression of HIV. There is no consensus on the safety of discontinuations. Current view of U.S. Department of Health and Human Services: do not interrupt HAART except in case of clinical trials or acute problem.

THERAPEUTIC SUMMARY

Diet

- Natural, whole-foods diet; high caloric intake.
- Low in sugar, white flour, fruit juice, honey, processed foods; low in natural and synthetically saturated fats; low in oxidized or *trans* fatty acids.
- High in protein, fiber, filtered water.
- Abstain from alcohol, nicotine, caffeine.
- Digestive stimulation, if appropriate.
- Avoid broad-spectrum allergy-elimination diets.

Lifestyle

- Aerobic or mind-body exercise (e.g., tai chi, yoga)
- Sleep: 8 to 10 hours nightly
- Prayer, spiritual activities, activities that support HIV-positive community, guided stress relief, relaxation training

Nutritional Supplements

Potential interactions with HAART must always be investigated in considering any nutrient or botanical.

- High-potency hypoallergenic multivitamin-mineral, preferably designed specifically to replace known nutrient deficiencies of HIV
- Beta-carotene: 150,000 international units (IU) q.d. as food

- Vitamin D: 5000 IU q.d. with food
- DHEA: 15 to 50 mg q.d. with food
- Acetyl-L-carnitine: 2 to 6 g q.d. in divided doses away from other proteins
- EFAs: 5 g q.d. with food
- Probiotics: 8 to 12 billion CFUs q.d. with meals
- Botanical medicines: *S. marianum* (milk thistle extract; 300 mg/day) for all patients on HAART
- Homeopathic medicines:
  - — Constitutional intake and remedy provided for each patient
  - — Acute remedies as indicated
- Physical medicine and acupuncture:
  - — Whole-body hyperthermia—use extreme caution in patients with heat intolerance or peripheral neuropathies.
  - — Movement therapies—as indicated.
  - — Acupuncture and electroacupuncture—as indicated.

Hypertension

DIAGNOSTIC SUMMARY

- Prehypertension: 120 to 139/80 to 89 mm Hg
- Stage 1 hypertension: 140 to 159/90 to 99 mm Hg
- Stage 2 hypertension: 160 and higher/100 and higher mm Hg

GENERAL CONSIDERATIONS

Hypertension is a major risk factor for myocardial infarction (MI) or stroke and is the most significant risk factor for stroke. More than 60 million Americans have hypertension, including 54.3% of all Americans aged 65 to 74 years and 71.8% of all black Americans in the same age group. In addition, 37% of U.S. adults have a blood pressure (BP) of 120 to 139/80 to 89 mm Hg, classified as prehypertension, linked to not only greater risk of developing hypertension and cardiovascular disease, but also diabetes and cognitive impairment.

- Normal diastolic (<80 mm Hg) but elevated systolic (>140 mm Hg) pressure (increased pulse pressure) suggests decreased compliance of aorta (arteriosclerosis) and is associated with twofold increase in cardiovascular death rates. Other causes of increased pulse pressure are increased stroke volume from aortic regurgitation, thyrotoxicosis, and fever.
- Classification of hypertension by cause: more than 90% of cases are classified as essential hypertension—no discernible cause. Essential hypertension groups are based on level of renin (enzyme secreted by kidney juxtaglomerular cells, linked to aldosterone in negative feedback loop). Renin helps generate vasoconstricting peptide angiotensin II. Renin secretion is influenced by fluid volume and sodium (Na) intake.
- Low-renin essential hypertension involves low renin activity. Aldosterone production is not being suppressed, leading to mild hyperaldosteronism with Na retention, increased fluid volume, and increased BP. This also occurs with normal-renin hypertension; low-renin hypertension may be at the end of the

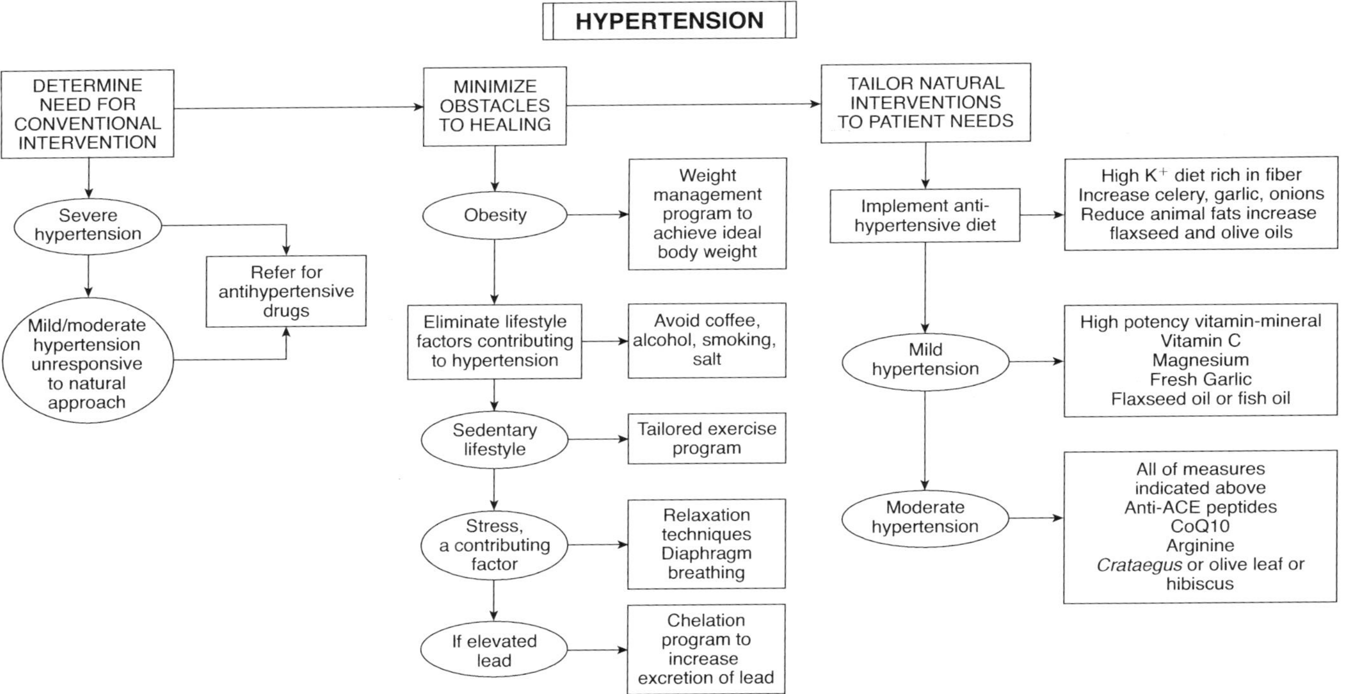
HYPERTENSION
DETERMINE NEED FOR CONVENTIONAL INTERVENTION
Severe hypertension
Mild/moderate hypertension unresponsive to natural approach
Refer for antihypertensive drugs
MINIMIZE OBSTACLES TO HEALING
Obesity
Weight management program to achieve ideal body weight
Eliminate lifestyle factors contributing to hypertension
Avoid coffee, alcohol, smoking, salt
Sedentary lifestyle
Tailored exercise program
Stress, a contributing factor
Relaxation techniques Diaphragm breathing
If elevated lead
Chelation program to increase excretion of lead
TAILOR NATURAL INTERVENTIONS TO PATIENT NEEDS
Implement anti-hypertensive diet
High K+ diet rich in fiber
Increase celery, garlic, onions
Reduce animal fats increase flaxseed and olive oils
Mild hypertension
High potency vitamin-mineral
Vitamin C
Magnesium
Fresh Garlic
Flaxseed oil or fish oil
Moderate hypertension
All of measures indicated above
Anti-ACE peptides
CoQ10
Arginine
Crataegus or olive leaf or hibiscus

continuum with essential hypertension. Patients with low renin levels have increased sensitivity to angiotensin II.

- Normal-renin essential hypertensives typically are insulin resistant with abdominal obesity. Hyperinsulinemia and insulin resistance are present even in lean hypertensives without non–insulin-dependent diabetes mellitus, suggesting a strong relation between insulin sensitivity and BP. Because insulin modifies ion transport across cell membranes, insulin insensitivity decreases cytosolic magnesium (Mg) and increases cytosolic calcium (Ca) in vascular smooth muscle, increasing vascular reactivity. Normal-renin essential hypertensives typically do not respond to Na restriction.
- High-renin essential hypertensives comprise 15% of essential hypertension patients. Renin elevation (and high BP) may arise from increased adrenergic system activity.
- Categories based on renin can identify therapeutic interventions, but renin levels do not remain constant in a given patient. In low-renin essential hypertension caused by insulin resistance secondary to obesity, weight loss regains insulin sensitivity but BP may not normalize. The patient would then have normal- or high-renin essential hypertension.
- **White coat hypertension:** persistent elevation of BP only at clinic or physician's office. Prevalence may be 20% to 45% of diagnosed hypertensives; is more frequent in women, older patients, and persons with mild hypertension. This should not be confused with "white coat effect"—the difference in BP between office and daytime ambulatory BP that occurs in patients with white coat hypertension and other causes. Treat white coat hypertension as if it were essential hypertension; it mirrors real-life reactions to stress. It is not an innocent phenomenon because it is linked to higher mortality and twice the risk of developing sustained hypertension as normotensives.
- **Ambulatory BP monitoring:** clinically useful for assessing suspected white coat hypertension and cardiovascular risk. If white coat hypertension is confirmed, drug treatment is not indicated; treat with lifestyle and dietary modification, weight reduction, exercise, smoking cessation, and correction of glucose and lipid abnormalities. Follow up with semiannual or annual ambulatory BP monitoring.
- **Etiology:** vascular, hormonal, renal, and neurologic factors function in complex interrelations to maintain normal BP. Disruption of any single facet creates a cascading effect on regulatory mechanisms. Genetic factors play a role, but dietary,

lifestyle, psychological, and environmental factors are underlying causes. Dietary factors: obesity; high Na/potassium (K) ratio; low-fiber, high-sugar diet; high saturated fat and low omega-3 fatty acid intake; low Ca, Mg, and vitamin C intake. Lifestyle factors: stress, lack of exercise, smoking. From 40% to 60% of hypertensives are Na sensitive. The heavy metals lead (Pb), mercury, cadmium, and arsenic target kidneys as end organs. Bone Pb studies indicate that exposure to heavy metals is linked to increased risk for hypertension. Pb has an acute effect on BP via recent or cumulative dose. Blood Pb is a strong and consistent predictor of both systolic and diastolic BP. Tibial Pb is also associated with hypertension status.

THERAPEUTIC CONSIDERATIONS

Eighty percent of patients with hypertension are in the borderline to moderate range; thus most cases can be brought under control by diet and lifestyle. Many nondrug therapies (diet, exercise, relaxation therapies) are superior to drugs in cases of borderline to mild hypertension. Patients on diuretics and/or beta-blockers have unnecessary side effects and an increased risk for heart disease. Calcium channel blockers and angiotensin-converting enzyme (ACE) inhibitors may be safer, with fewer side effects, but not without problems.

Current Pharmacotherapy

- **Most common:** diuretics used alone or in combination with calcium channel blockers and ACE inhibitors.
- **Step 1 drug:** used alone (thiazides, calcium channel blockers, ACE inhibitors); **step 2,** two drugs; **step 3,** three drugs; **step 4,** four drugs. Use single therapies before going on to combinations, unless compelling indications are present (e.g., diabetes or heart failure).
- **Other types of BP-lowering drugs (steps 3 or 4):** those acting on the central nervous system (clonidine, methyldopa, reserpine), vasodilators (nitroprusside sodium, hydralazine, prazosin, minoxidil, hydralazine), newer calcium channel blockers, and ACE inhibitors.

Lifestyle and Dietary Factors

See the chapter on atherosclerosis.

- **Lifestyle factors:** coffee, alcohol, lack of exercise, stress, smoking.

- **Dietary factors:** obesity; high Na/K ratio; low-fiber, high-sugar diet; high saturated fat and low essential fatty acids; low Ca, Mg, and vitamin C.
- **Stress:** causative factor of hypertension in many patients; key issue is response and processing of stress rather than stress itself. Relaxation techniques (deep breathing exercises, biofeedback, autogenics, transcendental meditation, yoga, progressive muscle relaxation, hypnosis) are useful in lowering BP. Effect is modest, but stress reduction is a necessary component in natural BP-lowering protocol. Diaphragmatic breathing significantly reduces stress and increases energy. Regular short exercise sessions of slow and regular diaphragmatic breathing lower BP in hypertensives. Shallow breathing induces Na retention. Slow breathing (six breaths per minute) improves oxygen saturation, exercise tolerance, and baroreflex sensitivity. Emphasize slow, deep diaphragmatic breathing. RESPeRATE is a medical device that interactively guides user toward slow, regular breathing by synchronizing voluntary respiration to musical tones. When used for 15 minutes daily, it can help reduce BP—systolic BP by 10.0 mm Hg and diastolic BP by 3.6 mm Hg. Greater BP reduction occurs in those who demonstrate greater compliance with the device.
- **Exercise:** physical activity (or fitness) and hypertension are inversely related. Regular exercise is effective treatment for high BP. Even mild to moderate aerobic exercise three times weekly of 20 minutes' duration has a hypotensive effect. BP reductions: 5 to 10 mm Hg for systolic and diastolic. Exercise can normalize borderline or mild hypertension.
- **Diet:** obesity is the major dietary cause of hypertension. Achieving ideal body weight is the most important therapeutic goal for most patients with any form of hypertension. From prehypertension all the way to chronic renal failure, weight loss can lead to complete elimination of the health issue, significant improvement, or at least a reduction in number of prescriptions needed. Attain ideal body weight. Increase proportion of whole organic plant foods in diet. Vegetarians have lower BP and lower incidence of hypertension and other cardiovascular diseases than do nonvegetarians. Dietary levels of Na do not differ between these two groups, but vegetarian diet contains more K, complex carbohydrates, essential fatty acids, fiber, Ca, Mg, and vitamin C and less saturated fat and refined carbohydrates. Increasing fruit and vegetable intake lowers BP, perhaps from the antioxidants.

Hypertensives have increased oxidative stress; antioxidants block angiotensin II–induced increases in BP and promote proper nitric oxide (NO) synthesis. Most useful foods for hypertensives are celery, garlic and onions, nuts and seeds or their oils (essential fatty acids), cold-water ocean fish (e.g., salmon, mackerel), green leafy vegetables (Ca and Mg), whole grains and legumes (fiber), foods rich in vitamin C (broccoli and citrus fruits), foods rich in active flavonoids (berries, cherries, grapes, small red kidney beans). Celery contains 3-n-butylphthalide, which lowers BP and cholesterol. Dose: four to six ribs of celery. Garlic and onions lower BP in hypertension. Garlic's BP reductions are 8 to 11 mm Hg for systolic and 5 to 8 mm Hg for diastolic.

DASH Diet (Dietary Approaches to Stop Hypertension)

The National Heart, Lung, and Blood Institute studied the efficacy of a system of dietary recommendations for hypertension—a diet rich in fruits and vegetables; low in dairy, saturated and total fat, and cholesterol; high in fiber, K, Ca, and Mg; and moderately high in protein. The DASH diet with lower Na lowered systolic BP by 7.1 mm Hg in nonhypertensives and by 11.5 mm Hg in hypertensives. Na intake less than 2400 mg q.d. can significantly and quickly lower BP. DASH components include those in the accompanying table.

- **K and Na**: A diet low in K and high in Na is linked to hypertension. Total K content of food plus Na/K ratio; a low-K, high-Na diet is linked to cancer and cardiovascular disease; a diet high in K and low in Na is protective against these diseases and therapeutic for hypertension. Dietary sodium chloride (NaCl; salt) is a major cause of raised BP; modest reduction in salt intake can lower BP. Salt intake directly correlates with cardiovascular risk. Ensure that patients get enough iodine from alternative sources. Excess NaCl intake, with diminished K, causes high BP in salt-sensitive persons. Na restriction alone is insufficient without high K intake. Typical Western diet: only 5% of Na is a natural constituent in food; 45% is added to prepared foods, 45% is added during cooking, and 5% is added as a condiment. Most Americans have K/Na ratio below 1:2. Studies indicate a K/Na ratio above 5:1 is necessary to maintain health. A natural diet rich in fruits and vegetables provides K/Na ratio above 100:1 (most fruits and vegetables have K/Na ratio of 50:1). Increasing dietary K can lower BP. K supplements alone can reduce BP in hypertensives at a dose of 2.5 to 5.0 g q.d. of K. Supplements are quite useful in persons older than 65 years.

The Food and Drug Administration restricts the amount of K in over-the-counter supplements to a mere 99 mg/dose because of problems with high-dose prescription K salts; yet salt substitutes (NoSalt, Nu-Salt) are potassium chloride, providing 530 mg K per {1/6} tsp. Supplement forms: salts (chloride, bicarbonate) bound to mineral chelates (e.g., aspartate, citrate) or food-based sources. High-dose salts in pills can cause nausea and vomiting, diarrhea, and ulcers. These effects are not seen when K is increased with diet only. Foods or food-based supplements are preferred. They are relatively safe except for patients with kidney disease; their inability to maintain K homeostasis may cause heart arrhythmias and other consequences of K toxicity. K supplements also are contraindicated when using some drugs (digitalis, K-sparing diuretics, and ACE inhibitor antihypertensive drugs).

Food Group	Daily Servings	Serving Sizes	Examples	Significance of Each Food Group to the DASH Diet Pattern
Grains and grain products	7-8	1 slice bread ½ cup dry cereal ½ cup cooked rice, pasta, or cereal	Whole-wheat bread, English muffin, pita bread, bagel, cereals, grits, oatmeal	Major sources of energy and fiber
Vegetables	4-5	1 cup raw leafy vegetable ½ cup cooked vegetable 6 oz vegetable juice	Tomatoes, potatoes, carrots, peas, squash, broccoli, turnip greens, collards, kale, spinach, artichokes, sweet potatoes, beans	Rich sources of potassium, magnesium, and fiber
Fruits	4-5	6 oz fruit juice 1 medium fruit ¼ cup dried fruit ½ cup fresh, frozen, or canned fruit	Apricots, bananas, dates, oranges, orange juice, grapefruit, grapefruit juice, mangoes, melons, peaches, pineapple, prunes, raisins, strawberries, tangerines	Important sources of potassium, magnesium, and fiber

Food Group	Daily Servings	Serving Sizes	Examples	Significance of Each Food Group to the DASH Diet Pattern
Low-fat or nonfat dairy foods	2-3	8 oz milk 1 cup yogurt 1.5 oz cheese	Skim or 1% milk, skim or low-fat buttermilk, nonfat or low-fat yogurt, part-skim mozzarella cheese, nonfat cheese	Major sources of calcium and protein
Meats, poultry, and fish	2 or fewer	3 oz cooked meats, poultry, or fish	Select only lean; trim away visible fats; broil, roast, or boil instead of frying; remove skin from poultry	Rich sources of protein and magnesium
Nuts, seeds, and legumes	4-5 per week	1.5 oz or ⅓ cup nuts ½ oz or 2 tbsp seeds ½ cup cooked legumes	Almonds, filberts, mixed nuts, peanuts, walnuts, sunflower seeds, kidney beans, lentils	Rich sources of energy, magnesium, potassium, protein, and fiber

- **Mg**: K interacts in many body systems with Mg. Low intracellular K may result from low Mg intake. Supplement Mg (400 to 1200 mg q.d. in divided doses) with K. This may lower BP. Mg lowers BP in a dose-dependent way; a drop of 4.3 mm Hg systolic and 2.3 mm Hg diastolic occurs for each 10-mmol/day increase in Mg dose. Mg lowers BP by activating cellular membrane Na^+-K^+ pump, which pumps Na out of and K into cells. High intake of Mg is linked to lower BP. Water high in minerals such as Mg is called *hard water.* Water hardness is inversely coordinated with high BP. Hypertensive patients who respond to Mg supplements are those taking diuretics, with high level of renin, with low red blood cell Mg, and/or with elevated intracellular Na or decreased intracellular K. Recommended daily intake for hypertensives is 6 to 10 mg/kg body weight. Mg bound to aspartate or Krebs cycle intermediates (malate, succinate, fumarate, citrate) is preferred. Mg supplements are well tolerated but sometimes cause looser stool (Mg sulfate [Epsom salts], hydroxide, or chloride). Use with great care in patients with kidney disease or severe heart disease (high-grade atrioventricular block).

- **Ca:** hypertension is linked to low intake of Ca, but the association is not as strong as for Mg and K. Ca supplements can lower BP in hypertension, but results are inconsistent. Ca supplements reduce BP in blacks and salt-sensitive patients but not patients with salt-resistant hypertension. Better results occur with Ca citrate compared with Ca carbonate. Elderly patients with mild to moderate hypertension respond to Ca.
- **Vitamin C:** The higher the intake of vitamin C, the lower the BP. A modest BP-lowering effect (drop of 5 mm Hg) occurs in people with mild hypertension. Daily dose of 500 mg produces the same benefit as higher doses (1000 or 2000 mg q.d.). It promotes excretion of Pb, which is linked to hypertension and increased cardiovascular mortality. Soft water supplies have increased Pb in drinking water because of the increased acidity of the water (soft water also is low in Ca and Mg, minerals protective against hypertension). Enhance efficacy by using ascorbate with other antioxidants. Combination 500 mg vitamin C, 600 mg alpha-tocopherol, 200 mg zinc sulfate, 30 mg beta-carotene q.d. has mildly reduced systolic BP.
- **Folic acid and vitamin B_6**: reduce plasma homocysteine, a contributor to atherosclerosis. B_6 alone lowers BP. B_6 oral dosage of 5 mg/kg body weight for 4 weeks reduced systolic and diastolic BP and serum norepinephrine. Mean systolic pressure dropped from 167 to 153 mm Hg and diastolic pressure dropped from 108 to 98 mm Hg.
- **Omega-3 oils:** increased intake can lower BP. Fish oil and flaxseed oil are quite effective. Dose of fish oils used: 3000 mg omega-3 eicosapentaenoic acid (EPA) and docosahexaenoic acid (DHA) q.d. Products with higher content of DHA are preferred. In one double-blind trial comparing 4 g q.d. of purified EPA, DHA, or olive oil (placebo), only DHA reduced 24-hour and daytime ambulatory BP. Fish oil laboratory certified as purified against pollutants and peroxides is preferred. Flaxseed oil may be a better cost-effective choice, requiring reduced intake of saturated fat and omega-6 fatty acids. One tablespoon daily of flaxseed oil reduces systolic and diastolic BP by up to 9 mm Hg. For every absolute 1% increase in body alpha-linolenic acid content, systolic, diastolic, and mean BPs decrease by 5 mm Hg.
- **L-Arginine:** amino acid precursor to NO that relaxes arteries, improving blood flow, renal plasma flow, and glomerular

filtration rate. Even in mild hypertension cases, endothelial NO production may be disordered, especially in the kidneys. By increasing NO, arginine improves blood flow, reduces blood clot formation, and improves blood fluidity. Arginine may be most beneficial in younger subjects with essential hypertension; aging hypertensives have disturbed NO-dependent renal mechanisms. In general, a dose of 4 g t.i.d. will produce only modest decreases (e.g., 5 mm Hg) in systolic BP with little meaningful change in diastolic BP. Intravenous infusion of arginine induces a significant increase in renal plasma flow, glomerular filtration rate, natriuresis, and kaliuresis without changes in filtration fraction in younger essential hypertensives but not in older subjects.

- **Anti-ACE peptides:** naturally occurring peptides in milk, chicken, and fish can inhibit ACE. Purified mixture of nine small peptides from muscle of the fish bonito (tuna family) do not produce the side effects of ACE inhibitor drugs and do not lower BP in normotensive people, even at dose 20 times greater than therapeutic dose for hypertensives. ACE converts angiotensin I to angiotensin II by cleaving off a small peptide. Drugs indiscriminately block this action. Anti-ACE peptides work as a decoy, causing ACE to react with the peptides instead of angiotensin. Anti-ACE peptides are transformed into even more potent inhibitors of ACE. Bonito anti-ACE peptides are prodrugs that exert an 800% greater activity. Bonito peptides and sardine dipeptide reduce systolic pressure by 10 or more mm Hg and diastolic by 7 mm Hg in borderline and mild hypertensives. Greater reductions occur in people with higher initial BP.
- **Coenzyme Q10 (CoQ10) (ubiquinone):** essential mitochondrial component synthesized within the body but deficient in 39% of hypertensive patients. Most studies exploring CoQ10 for high BP have been poorly designed or have used CoQ10 with drugs, making findings hard to interpret. In hypertensives, CoQ10 may lower systolic and diastolic BP with few side effects. Decreases in systolic BP range from 11 to 17 mm Hg; in diastolic BP from 8 to 10 mm Hg. Many patients were able to cease taking at least one antihypertensive drug. Average dose: 225 mg/day. The antihypertensive effect of CoQ10 is not seen until after 4 to 12 weeks of therapy. CoQ10 is not a typical BP-lowering drug; it corrects metabolic abnormality, favorably influencing BP.
- **Caffeine:** coffee and tea can produce short-lived immediate increases in BP. Regular coffee drinking slightly increases BP.

Coffee drinking ranging from 14 to 79 days at an average dose of 5 cups of coffee per day is linked to persistent increase in systolic and diastolic BP. Long-term avoidance of caffeine (coffee, tea, chocolate, cola drinks, some medications) is indicated because some patients respond quite favorably. Recent research suggests that caffeine is only a problem for those with low liver CYP1A2 activity.

Botanical Medicines

- ***Crataegus* species:** extracts of hawthorn berries and flowering tops lower BP and improve heart function. BP-lowering effect of hawthorn is quite mild and requires at least 2 to 4 weeks before effect is apparent.
- **Olive *(Olea europaea)*:** leaves of olive trees are antihypertensive and lower cholesterol. Active substances: oleuropein (a polyphenolic iridoid glycoside); oleacein and oleanolic acid act as natural calcium channel blockers. Hydroxytyrosol is a metabolite of oleuropein with antioxidant effects. Often olive extracts are standardized for hydroxytyrosol, a compound devoid of antihypertensive effect. Benolea (EFLA943), standardized to oleuropein (16% to 24%) and polyphenols, given at 1000 mg/day (500 mg b.i.d.), reduced systolic BP by 11.5 mm Hg and diastolic by 4.8 mm Hg.
- ***Allium sativum* (garlic) and *Allium cepa* (onion):** antihypertensive additions to diet along with garlic extracts. Meta-analysis conclusions: dried garlic powder standardized to contain 1.3% alliin at dose of 600 to 900 mg q.d. (corresponding to 7.8 to 11.7 mg of alliin or 1.8 to 2.7 g fresh garlic q.d.) can lower systolic BP by 11 mm Hg and diastolic BP by 5.0 mm Hg over a 1- to 3-month period.
- ***Hibiscus sabdariffa*:** Hibiscus tea and extracts from dried flowers (calyces) have demonstrated antihypertensive properties in clinical trials. Active components are anthocyanidin glycosides. Three 240-mL servings of brewed tea daily for 6 weeks lowered systolic BP by 7.2 mm Hg. Patients with higher systolic BP at baseline showed greater response to hibiscus. Among diabetic patients with hypertension who were not taking antihypertensive drugs, hibiscus lowers systolic BP by 22 mm Hg. It has very modest effect on diastolic BP. In one double-blind study, 193 patients with hypertension were given either hibiscus extract (250 mg of total anthocyanins daily) or 10 mg of lisinopril (control group). Results showed that the hibiscus extract decreased blood pressure from 146.48/97.77 to 129.89/85.96 mmHg, reaching an

absolute reduction of 17.14/11.97 mm Hg. Hibiscus shows therapeutic efficacy of 65.12% and tolerability and safety of 100%. Hibiscus has lowered plasma ACE activity from 44 to 30 U/L. Standardized extracts (9.6 mg of total anthocyanins) are as effective as captopril (50 mg/day).

- ***Viscum album* (mistletoe):** hypotensive action in animal studies. Mechanism of action is not fully understood. It inhibits excitability of vasomotor center in medulla oblongata. It possesses cholinomimetic activity. Hypotensive activity may depend on form in which mistletoe is administered and host tree from which it was collected. Aqueous extracts are more effective; the highest hypotensive activity is derived from macerate of leaves of mistletoe parasitizing on willow and gathered in January (*Textbook, "Viscum album* [European Mistletoe]").

THERAPEUTIC APPROACH

Borderline Hypertension

For borderline (120 to 160/90 to 94 mm Hg) or white coat hypertension or mild hypertension (140 to 160/90 to 104 mg):

- Reduce excess weight.
- Reduce salt (NaCl) intake substantially. Be sure to add other sources of iodine.
- Lead healthy lifestyle. Avoid alcohol, caffeine, smoking. Exercise and use stress-reduction techniques.
- Follow high-K diet rich in fiber consistent with either Mediterranean or DASH diet.
- Increase consumption of celery, garlic, and onions.
- Reduce or eliminate animal fats and increase olive oil.
- Check for Pb (oral dimercaptosuccinic acid [DMSA] challenge best for body load) and if elevated, put on an appropriate chelation protocol.
- Supplement diet with the following:
  — High-potency multiple vitamin-mineral formula
  — Vitamin C: 500 to 1000 mg t.i.d.
  — Mg: 800 to 1200 mg q.d. in divided doses
  — Fresh garlic: equivalent of 4000 mg q.d.
  — Omega-3 fatty acids: flaxseed oil: 1 tbsp q.d. or fish oils at 3 g total EPA and DHA content q.d.

If, after these recommendations have been followed for 3 months, BP has not normalized, consider recommendations for stage 1 hypertension given here.

Stage 1 Hypertension

For **stage 1 hypertension (140 to 159/90 to 99 mm Hg),** use all aforementioned measures with the addition of the following:

- CoQ10: 100 mg b.i.d. to t.i.d.
- Anti-ACE peptides from bonito: 1500 mg q.d.
- L-Arginine: 0.5 g/10 kg body weight in divided doses throughout the day
- Take one of the following:
  — Hawthorn extract (10% procyanidins or 1.8% vitexin-4′-rhamnoside): 100 to 250 mg t.i.d. *or*
  — Olive leaf extract (17% to 23% oleuropein content): 500 mg b.i.d.
  — Hibiscus: three 240-mL servings of tea or an extract providing 10 to 20 mg anthocyanidins daily

Follow these guidelines for 1 to 3 months. If BP has not dropped below 135/85, the patient may need antihypertensive medicines.

Stage 2 Hypertension

For **stage 2 hypertension (160+/100+ mm Hg),** drug intervention is required. All the measures delineated earlier should be employed. When satisfactory BP control is achieved, the patient can taper off drugs gradually.

Hyperthyroidism

DIAGNOSTIC SUMMARY

- Weakness, sweating, weight loss, nervousness, loose stools, heat intolerance, irritability, fatigue
- Tachycardia; warm, thin, moist skin; stare; tremor
- Diffuse, nonpainful goiter
- Increased thyroxine (T_4), free T_4, and free T_4 index
- Failure of thyroid suppression with triiodothyronine (T_3) administration
- In Graves' disease: goiter (often with bruit), ophthalmopathy

GENERAL CONSIDERATIONS

Hyperthyroidism (thyrotoxicosis) is a group of disorders characterized by increased free T_4 and/or T_3. The autoimmune disorder Graves' disease comprises 85% of all cases of hyperthyroidism. The disease is much more common in women than in men (8:1 ratio) and begins between ages 20 and 40 years. Diffuse, nonpainful goiter with hyperthyroidism is the most common presentation of Graves' disease. Less-common signs and symptoms are exophthalmos, pretibial myxedema and other skin changes, nail changes (acropachy), and paralysis in some groups. The common denominator is the antibodies against thyroid-stimulating hormone (TSH) receptors. Exophthalmos and skin changes can progress independently from thyroid dysfunction (euthyroid Graves' disease); predicting the course of disease in a given patient is difficult.

Disease Risk

Following are patterns of susceptibility in autoimmune disease (especially Graves' disease):

- **Gender:** female/male ratio is 7:1 to 10:1; the ratio in those with ophthalmic complications is 1:1.
- **Stress:** recent stress is a precipitating factor. The most common precipitating event is "actual or threatened separation from person on whom patient is emotionally dependent." The onset of

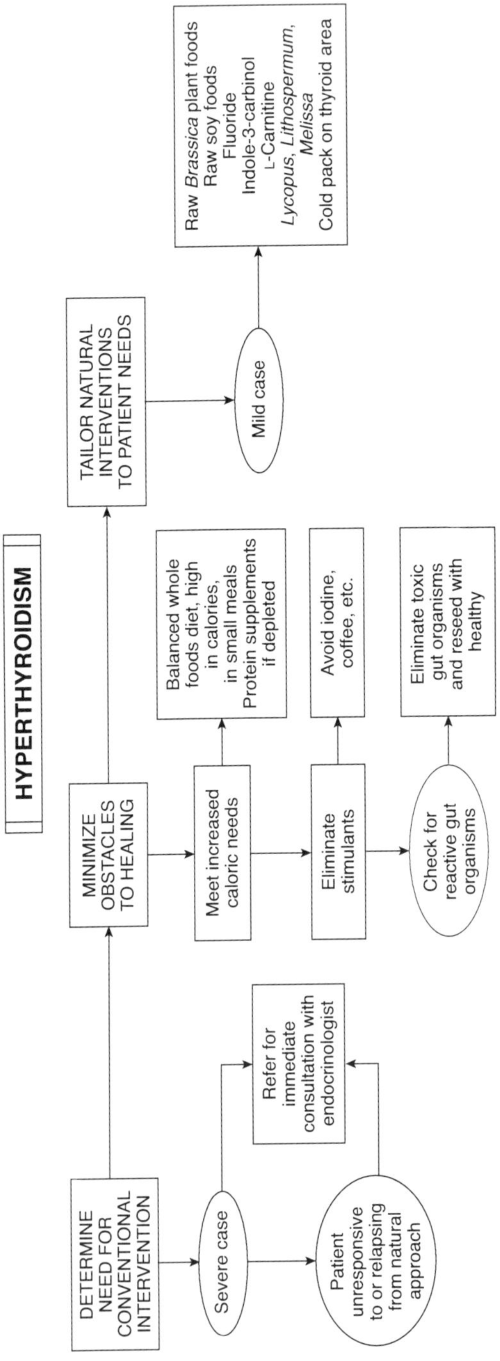
HYPERTHYROIDISM
DETERMINE NEED FOR CONVENTIONAL INTERVENTION
Severe case
Patient unresponsive to or relapsing from natural approach
Refer for immediate consultation with endocrinologist
MINIMIZE OBSTACLES TO HEALING
Meet increased caloric needs
Balanced whole foods diet, high in calories, in small meals Protein supplements if depleted
Eliminate stimulants
Avoid iodine, coffee, etc.
Check for reactive gut organisms
Eliminate toxic gut organisms and reseed with healthy
TAILOR NATURAL INTERVENTIONS TO PATIENT NEEDS
Mild case
Raw *Brassica* plant foods
Raw soy foods
Fluoride
Indole-3-carbinol
L-Carnitine
Lycopus, *Lithospermum*, *Melissa*
Cold pack on thyroid area

Graves' disease often follows emotional shock—divorce, death, or difficult separation.

- **Genetics:** Graves' disease is more prevalent in some human leukocyte antigen (HLA) haplotypes (HLA-B8 and HLA-DR3 in whites, HLA-Bw35 in Japanese, HLA-Bw46 in Chinese). HLA identical twins have a 50% chance of manifesting Graves' disease if one twin is affected; fraternal twins have a 9% chance. Some haplotypes are protective against Graves' disease. Genetic haplotype does not affect clinical course of disease or response to treatment.
- **Left-handedness:** a statistical trend exists for left-handed people to manifest Graves' disease and other autoimmune diseases. Seventy percent of male Graves' patients had some degree of left-handedness compared with 24% of control subjects. Some evidence exists for a higher rate of dyslexia in Graves' patients.
- **Smoking:** raises risk and severity of ophthalmopathy among patients with Graves' disease.
- **Iodine supplementation:** dietary iodine supplementation in iodine-sufficient areas can increase incidence of thyrotoxicosis (elevated T_4 and suppressed TSH with both nodular and diffuse goiters) in susceptible individuals. The rate of increase for women (8.03) was much greater than for men (1.34). When a population's intake of iodine suddenly increases, even to appropriate levels, many persons lapse into hyperthyroid states. This is more common among those who are elderly, have positive thyroid antibodies, or have marginal selenium status. Iodine from other sources in doses above 600 mcg can trigger Graves' disease and toxic multinodular goiter in susceptible individuals. Common iodine sources: potassium iodide, iodine/potassium iodide (Iodoral) supplement, medicines (e.g., amiodarone), and imaging contrast agents.
- **Mercury (Hg) and cadmium (Cd) exposure:** exposing animals to toxic levels of Cd or Hg induces immediate hyperthyroidism. Confirmatory anecdotal human clinical cases have been reported.
- **Infection:** TSH receptor antibodies in Graves' disease share a similar structure with antibodies against several pathogenic organisms in the gut. Cases of Graves' have started during or shortly after acute infection with *Yersinia enterocolitica* and *Borrelia burgdorferi* (Lyme disease).
- **Other factors** that may initiate Graves' disease: corticosteroids and local trauma to thyroid tissue.

- **Drugs:** in older patients with hyperthyroidism, consider toxic reaction to prescription drugs. Exposure to iodine-containing contrast agents during medical procedures is a common scenario. Some sources recommend TSH screening before administration of iodine-containing contrast agent. The most common causes of hyperthyroidism in the elderly are low iodine intake and higher use of amiodarone (an antihypertensive drug). Symptoms of hyperthyroidism vary in the elderly; apathy, tachycardia, and weight loss are more common. This response is more probable in those with subclinical hyperthyroidism (lack of symptoms, normal T_4, but low TSH).

DIAGNOSIS

Clinical Presentation

- **Graves' disease in young adult women:** nervousness, irritability, sweating, palpitations, insomnia, tremor, frequent stools, weight loss despite good appetite.
- **Physical examination:** smooth, diffuse, nontender goiter; tachycardia, especially after exercise; loud heart sounds (often systolic murmur); mild proptosis, lid retraction, lid lag, and tremor.
- **Other signs and symptoms:** muscle weakness and fatigue, anxiety, heat intolerance, pretibial myxedema.
- **Atypical cases (elderly):** in apathetic thyrotoxicosis, the aforementioned symptoms are absent. In the elderly, only symptom may be depression.
- Screening laboratory test for suppressed TSH.
- Increased thyroid hormone can manifest as worsening of already present cardiac symptoms (angina pectoris, congestive heart failure, and atrial fibrillation).
- **Characteristic skin changes:** moist, warm, and finely textured; perspiration increases in response to increased body temperature; pigment changes (vitiligo) and increased pigmentation of areas (skin creases, knuckles).
- Hair may thin or fall out in patches or altogether (alopecia).
- Nails may separate prematurely from nail bed (onycholysis).
- Localized, nonpitting edema along shins (myxedema) or elsewhere, such as extensor surfaces. It is often pruritic and red.
- **Other symptoms of Graves' disease:** glucose intolerance, osteoporosis, dyspnea, polyurea and polydipsia, myopathy, paralysis, parkinsonian or choreoathetoid affect.

- Although in severely hyperthyroid states symptoms are predictable, some symptoms can be paroxysmal, manifesting in both mild hyperthyroid and hypothyroid states (e.g., anxiety, palpitations, weight gain, fatigue, and insomnia). In managing patients for either hypothyroidism or hyperthyroidism, it is not safe to assume that they have too much or too little thyroid hormone based solely on symptoms.

Differential Diagnosis of Hyperthyroidism

- Graves' disease is the most common diagnosis of hyperthyroidism. The second most common is toxic nodular goiter. Others include toxic adenoma and multinodular goiter.
- Several types of thyroiditis cause hyperthyroidism: Hashimoto's thyroiditis (early stage), subacute thyroiditis, painless thyroiditis, and radiation thyroiditis.
- Hyperthyroidism from exogenous causes: iatrogenic hyperthyroidism, factitious hyperthyroidism (dieters taking T_4 for weight loss), and iodine-induced hyperthyroidism (Jod-Basedow disease).
- Toxic nodular goiters: toxic adenoma and multinodular goiter.
- Rare causes: thyroid carcinoma, ectopic hyperthyroidism, trophoblastic tumors (hydatidiform mole, choriocarcinoma, embryonic carcinoma of testis), excess TSH (pituitary adenoma, nonneoplastic pituitary secretion of TSH), and struma ovarii.

Laboratory Diagnosis

Definitive diagnosis includes the following:

- Serum T_3, T_4, thyroid resin uptake, and free T_4 usually are elevated.
- TSH assay is suppressed below 0.2.
- TSH receptor antibodies or thyroid-stimulating immunoglobulins (TSIs) are present in 80% of patients.
- If nodule or diffuse swelling can be palpated, use thyroid scan to rule out cancer and guide treatment.
- Serum antibodies can help rule out cancer in patients with lobular firm goiters. High antibody levels suggest chronic thyroiditis.
- A nodule in the absence of abnormal thyroid function tests always warrants ultrasound and possible biopsy. Iodine scans show diffuse heightened iodine uptake in Graves' disease and localized heightened iodine uptake ("hot" nodules) in toxic nodular goiter. "Cold" nodules on scans are regions of poor iodine uptake and are assumed to be cancerous until proved otherwise.

THERAPEUTIC CONSIDERATIONS

The chief objective of natural treatment of Graves' disease and hyperthyroidism is to establish normal thyroid status. Few treatments, short of antithyroid drugs (ATDs), radiation, or surgery, have a significant impact on immediate severity of symptoms. Nonetheless, adjunctive treatments and naturopathic lifestyle improvements can lower dose or duration of ATDs or raise likelihood of disease remission with conventional treatment.

- Reduce risk factors such as stress, smoking, excess iodine intake. Stress control is the single most important action. Avoid anything that will excite the patient and increase agitation. Counseling can prevent return to stress-generating life strategies. Increase rest—daily nap after lunch plus full night's sleep.

Comorbidities

Patients with autoimmune thyroid disease have elevated risk for celiac disease, osteoporosis, mitral valve prolapse, type 1 diabetes.

Treatment of Hyperthyroidism

- Conventional treatment focuses on radioactive iodine (RAI) ablation as first-line treatment. Advantages: high rate of response and obviating of need for ongoing suppression. Disadvantages: progression to hypothyroidism and elevated risk of nonlocalized cancers and parathyroid disease.
- Partial or total thyroidectomy is less common and considered when patient is very young or pregnant, iodine or ATDs are less preferred, enlarged gland causes anatomic impingement on adjacent structures, or cosmetic concerns are an issue. Disadvantages: laryngeal nerve damage, parathyroid abnormalities from localized trauma or inadvertent removal, and surgical complications.
- ATDs are mainstays of treatment for hyperthyroidism. A trial of an ATD for 18 to 24 months may obviate ongoing treatment afterward. Disadvantage: hepatic and hematologic toxicity that requires monitoring.
- ATDs enter thyroid via active transport mechanisms, accumulate inside thyroid tissue, and inhibit binding of iodine to tyrosine, disrupting hormone synthesis. This is first-line therapy in Europe and Japan, for Graves' and Plummer's diseases. Most cases resolve within 18 months, and patients remain euthyroid or hypothyroid for life.

- In the United States, RAI is first-line therapy; ATDs are used for initial management.
- Fluoride, as sodium fluoride, is a natural compound with antithyroid properties suitable as alternative to conventional ATD or in conjunction with ATDs for lower doses. Historically, sodium fluoride or fluorotyrosine were oral antithyroid agents before propylthiouracil (PTU) and methimazole. Common doses to manage adult hyperthyroidism: 200 to 450 mg/day in divided doses for PTU and 5 to 20 mg/day in divided doses for methimazole. Fluoride is Pregnancy Category C and causes gastrointestinal side effects at 3 mg/kg and toxicity at 5 mg/kg.
- It takes 4 to 6 weeks of ATD to see benefit owing to high amount of protein-bound iodine stored within thyroid tissue.
- Excess T_4 and T_3 are reabsorbed through enterohepatic recirculation. Cholestyramine can speed elimination of thyroid hormone by blocking enterohepatic recirculation. Dietary fibers—rice bran or milled flax—may have similar properties.

Diet

- **Balanced, whole-foods diet:** diet high in calories in the form of small, frequent meals to compensate for increased metabolism. Supplement protein if patient is nutritionally depleted. Avoid iodine supplements, caffeine, and other stimulants.
- **Dietary goitrogens:** substances that prevent use of iodine are isothiocyanates, which are similar in action and structure to PTU. Sources include turnips, cabbage, rutabagas, mustard, rapeseeds, cassava root, soybeans, peanuts, pine nuts, and millet. Goitrogens are transmitted from cow's milk to human beings. These foods are unreliable in treating hyperthyroidism.
  - Goitrogen content is quite low compared with doses of PTU used in hyperthyroidism (100 to 200 mg t.i.d. to q.i.d.).
  - Cooking inactivates goitrogens.
  - No solid evidence exists that natural goitrogens significantly interfere with thyroid function if dietary iodine is adequate.

Naturally occurring goitrogens may be used in mild cases instead of PTU and related drugs. Large amounts of these foods must be consumed raw, and iodine intake must be restricted. The highest levels of isothiocyanates are in raw soy milk (0.46 to 2.5 mg/dL). The *Brassica* genus (e.g., rutabagas, cabbage, and turnips) has the highest levels, but quantity varies according to climate and soil factors. A half head of raw cabbage daily is a typical prescription. Avoid iodine sources such as kelp, other seaweeds, and vegetables grown near the ocean; seafood; iodized salt; and iodine-containing nutritional supplements. Great care must be exercised in using this approach because results are inconsistent and delay in effective treatment can harm the patient. If the patient does not respond within a few weeks of treatment, conventional intervention is required.

Nutritional Supplements

- **Iodine:** dietary excess is common in developed nations. Sources include food additives (salt and iodine used to sterilize pipes in dairies) and medical products (povidone-iodine washes, iodine-containing drugs such as amiodarone, radiographic dyes). Effects of iodine in patients with hyperthyroidism include the following:
  - — Temporary symptom reduction by stopping hormone synthesis (Wolff-Chaikoff effect).
  - — Thyroid can remain suppressed or resume hormone synthesis at reduced, former, or increased rate (escape from Wolff-Chaikoff).
  - — Excess iodine can trigger hyperthyroidism (Jod-Basedow disease) in euthyroid person or trigger overactive thyroid to return to normal.
- The action of iodine is unpredictable. Keep iodine intake on the low end of normal therapeutic range: 150 to 250 mcg/day for adults.
- **Calcium (Ca):** Ca metabolism is altered in hyperthyroidism. Patients with Graves' disease are more susceptible to osteoporosis than normal individuals. Natural antithyroid treatments may be beneficial in early, mild cases or to lower dose of ATDs. Rarely are they adequate as monotherapies for significantly hyperthyroid patients.
- **L-Carnitine:** transports long-chain fatty acids into mitochondrial matrix. L-Carnitine is an antagonist of thyroid hormone effect in peripheral tissues by inhibiting its entry into cell nucleus. Carnitine's effect can even prevail over administered T_4. Because of its low toxicity, consider carnitine for Graves' disease–induced thyrotoxicosis during pregnancy, lactation, or other conditions in which ATDs are unwanted, such as liver disease and blood disorders.

Botanical Medicines

Medicinal Plants Traditionally Used in the Treatment of Hyperthyroidism

Medicinal Plant	Traditional Indications
Valeriana officinalis (valerian)	Nervine effect
Scutellaria lateriflora (skullcap, madweed)	Nervine effect
Cactus grandiflora (night-blooming cereus)	Heart tonic; use with elevated pulse
Iris versicolor (blue flag)	Traditional use for hyperthyroidism
Fucus spp. (kelp)	Use with caution; high iodine content can first improve symptoms then later cause aggravation
Lycopus spp. (e.g., bugleweed)	Blocks the thyroid-stimulating hormone (TSH) receptors and peripheral conversion of T_4 to T_3
Lithospermum officinale	Blocks the TSH receptors
Melissa officinalis (lemon balm)	Blocks the TSH receptors

Unfortunately, the plants in the accompanying table have not been adequately evaluated in clinical studies.

Lycopus Species, *Lithospermum officinale*, and *Melissa officinalis*

- Aqueous, freeze-dried extracts of *Lycopus* species, *L. officinale*, and *M. officinalis* have been studied in vivo and in vitro. Preliminary results support their use in Graves' disease; clinical research is needed.
- Inhibit effects of exogenous TSH on rat thyroid glands; block effects of TSH on TSH receptor sites on thyroid membranes; inhibit peripheral deiodination of T_4 to T_3; and block effects of antithyroid immunoglobulins on TSH receptors.
- Oxidation products of derivatives of 3,4-dihydroxycinnamic acid are responsible for most of the effects. Blocking effects of isolated compounds of TSH receptors are reversible. None of the compounds combined irreversibly or damaged or altered TSH receptors in situ.
- Alcohol extract of *Lycopus europaeus* given orally to rats caused long-lasting decrease in T_3 from reduced peripheral T_4 deiodination. TSH was reduced 24 hours later with a drop in luteinizing

hormone (LH) and testosterone. Water extracts are less potent; active constituents are unoxidized alcohol-soluble phenolic compounds.

- Dose recommendations from the British Herbal Pharmacopoeia for *Lycopus* species and *M. officinalis* (no mention is made of *L. officinale*) are given later.

THERAPEUTIC APPROACH

Acute Graves' disease is not easily treated by naturopathic methods. In severe cases no guarantee exists that natural treatments will adequately alleviate symptoms. Thyroid storm is a potentially fatal complication that must be treated aggressively with ATDs and/or iodine. In mild cases natural therapeutics can manage symptoms well, but monitor carefully to avoid sudden exacerbation. Relapse is quite possible. Treat mild cases symptomatically. Allow patient to return to euthyroid status if possible. If iodine is used, ablative treatment is needed; risk of escape (potential for more-intense symptoms) increases with time.

- **Allopathic treatment:** three equal treatments are possible. Decision making may be difficult for the patient while in thyrotoxic state; symptomatic relief is mandatory before a decision is made. ATDs can manage symptoms indefinitely pending return to euthyroid status. If drugs are not well tolerated, consider ablative therapies. Surgery has a higher rate of euthyroid results than does RAI but carries greater risk of serious complications. Render supportive natural treatment no matter the choice.
- **Diet:** whole-foods diet with increased calories, micronutrients, and protein to meet increased metabolic needs. In mild cases, use large amounts of raw *Brassica* foods and raw soy products and restrict iodine.
- **Supplements:**
  - — Fluoride: 3 to 10 mg q.d.
  - — Indole-3-carbinol: 200 to 600 mg q.d.
  - — L-Carnitine: 2 to 4 g q.d.
- **Botanical medicines:**
  - — *Lycopus* species, *L. officinale,* and/or *M. officinalis:* dried herb, 1 to 3 g or by infusion t.i.d; tincture (1:5), 2 to 6 mL t.i.d.; fluid extract (1:1), 1 to 3 mL t.i.d.
- **Hydrotherapy:** cold packs placed over thyroid t.i.d.

Hyperventilation Syndrome/ Breathing Pattern Disorders

DIAGNOSTIC SUMMARY

Hyperventilation Syndrome/Breathing Pattern Disorders Defined

- Hyperventilation is pattern of overbreathing in which depth and rate exceed metabolic needs at that time; usually seen at 30 breaths or more per minute.
- Breathlessness at rest or with only mild exercise.
- Physical, environmental, or psychological stimuli override automatic activity of respiratory centers, tuned to maintain arterial carbon dioxide ($Paco_2$) levels within narrow range.
- Although at any given time carbon dioxide (CO_2) production is set at a certain level, exaggerated breathing depth and rate of hyperventilation syndrome/breathing pattern disorders (HVS/ BPDs) eliminate CO_2 faster, causing arterial hypocapnia (low CO_2 in blood).
- Arterial hydrogen ion (pH) (acid-alkaline balance) rises into alkaline region, inducing respiratory alkalosis.
- HVS/BPDs causes multiple symptoms, some of which mimic serious disease. However, blood tests, electrocardiograms (ECGs), and physical examinations may reveal nothing abnormal. Up to 10% of patients in primary care experience HVS/BPDs. Symptoms can be severe and distressing.

Gender

More females than males have HVS/BPDs, from 2:1 to 7:1. Peak age is 15 to 55 years. Women may be more at risk because of hormonal influences. Progesterone stimulates respiratory rate; in luteal (postovulation, premenstrual) phase, CO_2 levels drop 25%. Stress can increase ventilation when CO_2 is already low. Progesterone (medroxyprogesterone) therapy can cause hyperventilation.

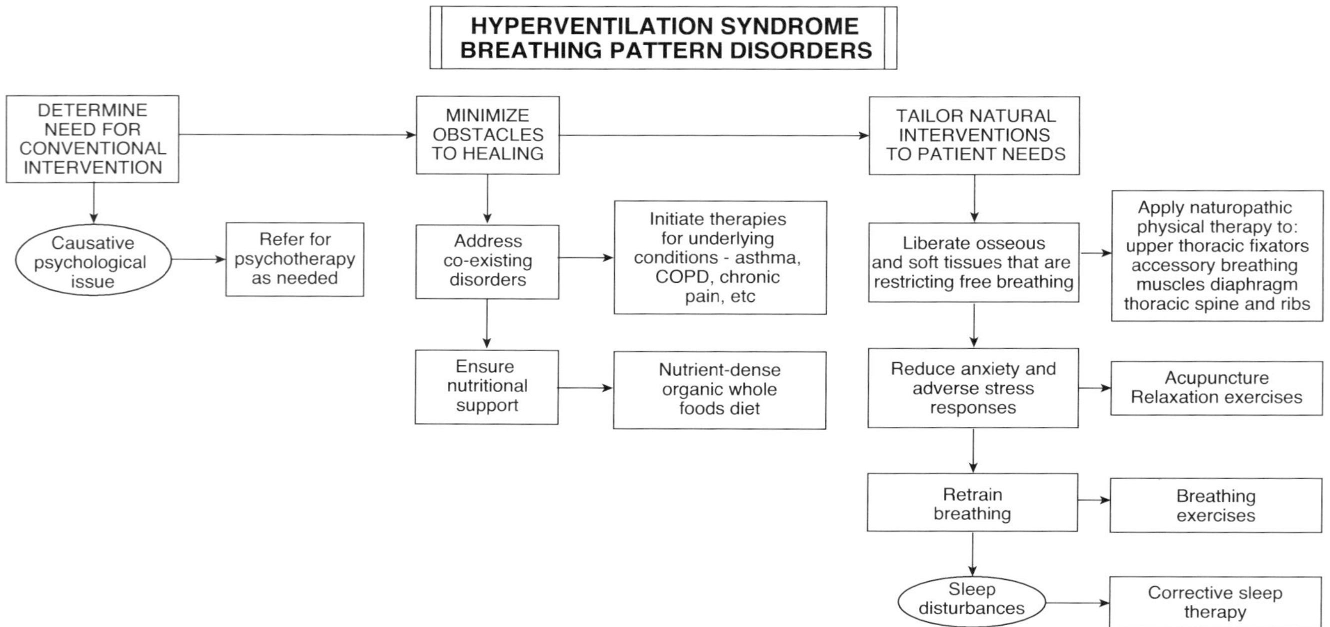
HYPERVENTILATION SYNDROME
BREATHING PATTERN DISORDERS
DETERMINE NEED FOR CONVENTIONAL INTERVENTION
Causative psychological issue
Refer for psychotherapy as needed
MINIMIZE OBSTACLES TO HEALING
Address co-existing disorders
Initiate therapies for underlying conditions - asthma, COPD, chronic pain, etc
Ensure nutritional support
Nutrient-dense organic whole foods diet
TAILOR NATURAL INTERVENTIONS TO PATIENT NEEDS
Liberate osseous and soft tissues that are restricting free breathing
Apply naturopathic physical therapy to: upper thoracic fixators accessory breathing muscles diaphragm thoracic spine and ribs
Reduce anxiety and adverse stress responses
Acupuncture
Relaxation exercises
Retrain breathing
Breathing exercises
Sleep disturbances
Corrective sleep therapy

Normal Breathing Pattern

- Breathing rate: 10 to 14 breaths per minute, moving 3 to 5 L of air per minute through chest airways.
- During active inhalation phase, air flows in through nose where it is warmed, filtered, and humidified before being drawn into lungs by downward movement of diaphragm and outward movement of abdominal wall and lower thoracic structures.
- Upper chest and accessory breathing muscles remain relaxed.
- Expiratory phase is effortless: abdominal wall and lower intercostals relax downward and diaphragm ascends to original domed position, aided by elastic recoil of lung.
- Relaxed pause at end of exhalation releases diaphragm briefly from negative and positive pressures exerted during breathing.
- Normally people are unaware of their breathing.
- Breathing rates and volumes increase or fluctuate in response to physical or emotional demands, but in normal subjects they return to relaxed low chest patterns after stimuli cease.

Patients with chronic fatigue, anxiety, or both who have a number of the following signs or symptoms might be candidates for respiratory treatment (see also "Diagnostic Considerations").

Benefits of Normal Respiratory Function

- Normal performance of brain, organs, tissues
- Normal speech and nonverbal expression (e.g., sighing)
- Fluid movement (lymph, blood)
- Spinal mobility through regular, mobilizing, thoracic cage movement
- Digestive function via rhythmic positive and negative pressure fluctuations, via normal diaphragmatic function

Impact of habitual HVS/BPDs can exacerbate wide range of disorders.

The Carbon Dioxide–Oxygen Balancing Act

Maintaining oxygen and CO_2 within normal limits is a complex task, even more so because supply of each gas fluctuates with each breath.

Respiratory Homeostasis

- Neural control system maintains constant arterial $Paco_2$. Volume of CO_2 expired continually balances volume produced by tissue metabolism.

- In rest and activity, when system is left to itself, it is so efficient that matching occurs virtually breath by breath, even when metabolic activity is continuously changing.

Pathophysiology

Physiologic and Pathophysiologic Causes of Altered Patterns of Breathing

Hyperventilation can be appropriate physiologic response to metabolic needs. Organic causes of HVS/BPDs that should be excluded and/or identified before breathing rehabilitation is initiated include the following:

- Respiratory: asthma, chronic obstructive respiratory disease, pneumonia, pulmonary embolus, pneumothorax, and pleural effusion.
- Cardiovascular: acute and chronic left-sided heart failure, right-sided heart failure, tachyarrhythmias
- Hematopoietic: anemia
- Renal: nephrotic syndrome, acute and chronic kidney failure
- Endocrine: Diabetes with ketoacidosis, pregnancy
- Metabolic: liver failure
- Pharmaceutic: aspirin, caffeine, amphetamine, nicotine, progesterone therapy

BPDs may emerge from established pathosis (e.g., asthma, cardiovascular disease, kidney failure, chronic pain). Even tumor infiltrates into brain respiratory centers and central chemoreceptors have caused hyperventilation. Fluctuating blood glucose levels may trigger HVS/BPD symptoms in patients with high-starch and high-sugar diets, which produce rapid rises followed by sharp falls to fasting levels or below. The following factors could lead to altered breathing patterns through pH shifts:

- Ketoacidosis promotes deeper, faster breathing because breathing centers respond to higher CO_2 content.
- Diarrhea results in loss of alkaline plasma bicarbonate ions (HCO_3^-), which if prolonged, leads to acidosis. This stimulates corrective overbreathing to remove CO_2 (as carbonic acid [H_2CO_3]) and normalizes the pH.
- Excessive vomiting causes loss of hydrochloric acid, shifting body toward alkalosis, slowing breathing to allow CO_2 to build up and restore pH. Hypoventilation results.
- Use of steroids and diuretics can lead to alkalosis.

Categorization of Causes

- Common etiologic features of HVS/BPD: biomechanical, biochemical, psychological, environmental, pathologic, and habitual categories.
- Structural, biomechanical causes: restricted thoracic spine, rib immobility; shortness of key primary and accessory respiratory muscles.
- Biochemical etiology: allergy or infection, which triggers narrowing of breathing passages and subsequent asthmatic-type responses; acidosis, as in kidney failure, directly alters breathing function to reduce acid via elimination of CO_2 through hyperventilation.
- Psychological distress: anxiety or depression.
- Environmental factors (e.g., altitude, humidity).

The Hydrogen Ion Factor

- pH (relative acidity): influences every organ; facilitates many metabolic exchanges; must be kept in careful balance; describes proportion of hydrogen ions available for combination.
- pH is on a log scale; a small change in pH means a big change in hydrogen ion concentration.
- Binding of positively charged hydrogen to negatively charged sites helps regulate enzymatic action, endocrine secretion, integrity of protein molecules, and cellular metabolism, including oxygen absorption and release.
- Physiologic normal pH in arterial blood is 7.4; acceptable range 7.35 to 7.45.

The Carbon Dioxide–Hydrogen Ion Connection

- Acidity of blood is determined mainly by CO_2.
- CO_2 is end product of aerobic metabolism, deriving from mitochondria.
- CO_2 in the atmosphere is at two hundredths of 1%, harmless to humans but adequate to sustain plant life.
- Transport of CO_2 occurs from tissues into blood and then to lungs for exhalation. The body converts CO_2 to H_2CO_3 in perpetual surplus.
- Lungs exhale 12,000 mEq of H_2CO_3 per day, compared with 100 mEq of fixed acids excreted by kidneys.
- Any increase in bodily activity produces CO_2, acidifying blood, unless more CO_2 is excreted and/or exhaled.

- Changes in breathing volume relative to CO_2 production regulate moment-to-moment pH of bloodstream (longer-term regulation of pH is shared with kidneys).
- Concentration of CO_2 in blood, not oxygen, regulates breathing drive.
- Higher CO_2 immediately stimulates more breathing.

The Bicarbonate Buffer

- HCO_3^- is derived from the union of CO_2 and H_2O in the blood to form H_2CO_3, which dissociates into hydrogen ions (H^+) and HCO_3^-.
- Bicarbonate reserve is adjustable as needed, up to a point, and is a major alkaline buffer system that opposes rises in acidity.
- Kidneys regulate the regulators by adjusting amount of bicarbonate returned to bloodstream. If kidneys detect excess acidity, they retain more bicarbonate to balance acid. This is not a fast process; it takes hours to days.
- In the short run, if bicarbonate buffering is not sufficient or if bicarbonate is depleted, the faster backup buffering system is hyperventilation. Excessive breathing exhales more CO_2 (acid), bringing pH closer to normal.

Oxygen Delivery and Smooth Muscle Constriction

- Blood carries oxygen mainly in hemoglobin, contained in red blood cells. In an appropriate environment, hemoglobin combines readily with oxygen (to form oxyhemoglobin).
- This process varies according to local pH and partial pressure of oxygen (Po_2), causing hemoglobin to absorb oxygen through alveoli and release oxygen through capillary walls, where oxygen diffuses into tissues.
- When pH is low (i.e., blood is more acidic), hemoglobin in that area is stimulated to release additional oxygen. This is true of metabolically active tissues in general but especially of muscles.
- An exercising muscle needs all the oxygen it can get, and this is assisted by its chemical nature. Exercising muscle is hypercarbic and hot, and it benefits from increased unloading of oxygen from capillaries. The effect of pH on oxyhemoglobin dissociation is called the *Bohr effect*.
- The lungs bind oxygen to hemoglobin; therefore lungs have a more-alkaline environment.
- The fact that shifting blood toward acidity promotes dissociation and release of oxygen from hemoglobin is key when considering hyperventilation, because resulting alkalinity causes

hemoglobin to retain more oxygen than usual. With increased alkalinity encouraging smooth muscle contraction and therefore diminished diameter of blood vessels, as well as the reluctance of hemoglobin to release oxygen, a relative oxygen deficit arises in tissues and brain, leading to symptoms—fatigue, aching, cramping, and cognitive problems.

Psychology and Hyperventilation Syndrome/Breathing Pattern Disorders

- "Cascade of symptoms": original cause (emotional or physical) leads to tension and anxiety that results in hyperventilation.

Influence of Emotion on Breathing

- Increased variability from breath to breath correlates with anxiety states. Low P_{CO_2} and increased frequency of sighing typify panic disorder even when individual is not panicking.
- These generalizations miss persons who do not have chronic HVS/BPD but experience disrupted breathing under particular conditions.
- These conditions provoke either amygdala alarm discharge or some specific, learned breathing response and occasional panic.
- Emotional events—loss, separation, grief, and anger—precipitate hyperventilation trend. Hypnosis might be helpful in discovering underlying cause of hyperventilation.
- Successful intervention must take all factors into account, focusing on priorities of survival. Human tendency to imagine, project, and recall stimulates breathing reflexes without apparent reason.

DIAGNOSTIC CONSIDERATIONS

Symptoms

Acute hyperventilation represents 1% of all cases of hyperventilation, well outnumbered by chronic hyperventilation. Symptoms and signs of HVS/BPD are variable; none are absolutely diagnostic. Indications of possible breathing pattern dysfunction are as follows:

- Feeling of constriction in the chest
- Shortness of breath
- Accelerated or deepened breathing
- Inability to breathe deeply
- Feeling tense (Nijmegen questionnaire avoids use of the word *anxiety*)
- Tightness around the mouth

- Stiffness in the fingers or arms
- Cold hands or feet
- Tingling fingers
- Bloated abdominal sensation
- Dizzy spells
- Blurred vision
- Feeling of confusion or losing touch with environment

Most Common Symptoms and Signs of Hyperventilation Syndrome/Breathing Pattern Disorders

System	Symptoms	Suggested causes
Cardiovascular	Chest pain and angina, palpitation and arrhythmias, tachycardia, lightheadedness and syncope, altered electrocardiographic features	Reduced coronary blood flow, altered excitability of sinoatrial and atrioventricular nodes of cardiac muscle, reduced cardiac output, peripheral vasodilatation
Gastrointestinal	Discomfort in lower chest and epigastric area, esophageal reflux and heartburn, bloating or distention, exacerbation of hiatal hernia symptoms, dry mouth, air swallowing and belching	Aerophagia, increased swallowing rate, mouth breathing
Neurologic	Headache; numbness and tingling (mainly involving extremities and perioral); positive Trousseau's and Chvostek's signs; dizziness, giddiness; ataxia and tremor; blurred and tunnel vision; anxiety and panic; phobias; irritability; depersonalization; detachment from reality; impaired concentration, cognition, performance; easy fatigue; insomnia; hallucinations	Cerebrovascular constriction (see notes on smooth muscle contraction later); vasoconstriction of vertebral or carotid arteries or both; reduced oxygen delivery, neuronal excitability resulting from alkalosis; hypocalcemia
Respiratory	Breathlessness; restricted sensation around thorax; sighing, yawning; obvious use of upper chest, accessory breathing muscles (e.g., scalenes) on inhalation; chest tenderness	Overuse of accessory breathing muscles and fatigue of primary respiratory muscles

System	Symptoms	Suggested causes
Muscular	Stiffness and aching, weakness in limbs, cramping, carpopedal spasm, tetany	Hyperexcitability of motor nerves, muscle fatigue, calcium/magnesium imbalance

Metabolic Disturbances and Hyperventilation Syndrome

- Two tests of nerve hyperexcitability produced by hypocapnia-induced hypocalcemia are Trousseau's and Chvostek's signs.
- Common chest pain of HVS/BPDs requires that heart disease be specifically excluded. Adrenaline-induced electrocardiographic changes can occur in hyperventilation, uncomplicated by coronary heart disease.
- In older patients, established coronary artery disease can be exacerbated by vasoconstriction arising from hypocapnia, which puts them at risk of coronary occlusion and myocardial damage.
- Hyperventilation can trigger spasms of normal caliber coronary arteries.
- Rapid breathing or mouth breathing instigates aerophagia from air gulping, causing bloating, burping, and extreme epigastric discomfort. Irritable bowel syndrome is a common symptom of chronic overbreathing. Fear and anxiety may induce abdominal cramps and diarrhea.
- Hyperventilation leading to hypocapnia causes cerebral arterioles to constrict, increasing vascular resistance and reducing cerebral blood flow. This is a natural response to changes in CO_2 to regulate oxygen delivery to the brain.

Acute Hyperventilation Progression

- The patient with acute hyperventilation appears distressed.
- The pattern of respiration is of deep, rapid breaths with use of accessory muscles visible in neck and upper chest.
- Wheezing may be heard as a result of bronchospasm triggered by hypocapnia.
- Stressful precipitating event is usually reported.
- Hypocapnia reduces blood flow to the brain (2% decrease in flow per 1-mm Hg reduction in arterial $Paco_2$), causing frightening central nervous system symptoms. Reduced oxygenation results from contraction of smooth muscle surrounding arteries and reluctance of hemoglobin to release oxygen in increasingly alkaline environment caused by excessive loss of CO_2.

- Poor concentration and memory lapses may occur with tunnel vision and onset in those susceptible to migraine headaches or tinnitus.
- Sympathetic dominance brings on tremors, sweating, clammy hands, palpitations, and autonomic instability of blood vessels causing labile blood pressures.
- Bilateral perioral and upper extremity paresthesia and numbness. Unilateral tingling is often confined to left side.
- Dizziness, weakness, visual disturbances, tremor, and confusion; sometimes fainting or seizures.
- Spinal reflexes become exaggerated owing to increased neuronal activity caused by loss of CO_2 ions from neurons.
- Tetany and cramping may occur in severe bouts.

Chronic Hyperventilation

- Diagnosis of chronic and intermittent hyperventilation is more difficult than acute hyperventilation.
- A careful history and systemic inquiry, checking all symptoms in other systems, highlights suspicious pattern. Examination must exclude organic diseases of brain and nervous system; heart disease, particularly angina and heart failure; respiratory disease; and gastrointestinal conditions, especially with suspicious symptoms in these systems.
- Inquire into precipitating causes of attacks.
- There may be no preceding stressful event. In chronic hyperventilators the respiratory center may have been reset to tolerate a lower-than-normal partial pressure of $Paco_2$. In such patients, a single sigh or one deep breath may reduce CO_2 enough to trigger symptoms.

Laboratory and Office Tests for Hyperventilation Syndrome/Breathing Pattern Disorders

- Preliminary tests to rule out respiratory and cardiac disease including peak expiratory flow rate, chest radiograph, ECG, and exercise ECG if chest pain is present.
- Palpation and observation can demonstrate paradoxical breathing pattern in which the abdomen retracts and the upper chest expands on inhalation (as opposed to normal abdominal protrusion and lower thorax expansion).
- Breath-holding time test does not require additional measurements or equipment. The time a hyperventilating patient can hold his or her breath is usually greatly reduced, often not beyond 10 to 12 seconds. Thirty seconds is dividing line between

hyperventilators and normal individuals for some clinicians. Breathless patients without hyperventilation may have equal difficulty in breath holding.

- A peak expiratory flow rate measurement, compared with age, sex, and height tables, provides a simple, quick exclusion of significant respiratory restriction.
- If a hyperventilation provocation test (HVPT) is performed (during which the patient is asked to voluntarily overbreathe to bring on symptoms), ECG should be monitored (see "Caution" later).
- Elevated erythrocyte carbonic anhydrase (ECA) might be a clinical marker for hyperventilation. Values of ECA are elevated (approximately 31 U/g hemoglobin) in patients who hyperventilate compared with controls (24.7 U/g hemoglobin). Other conditions might elevate ECA—glucose-6-phosphate dehydrogenase deficiency and different anemias (aplastic, iron deficiency, autoimmune hemolytic, β-thalassemia).
- Arterial blood gas measurement is invasive and painful (arterial puncture) but appropriate in emergency department, where diagnosis of acute hyperventilation is required. For patients in whom chronic hyperventilation is suspected, the pressure of end-tidal CO_2 ($PetCO_2$) can be measured noninvasively from a continuous sampling through nasal prongs or cannula with mouth occluded, or the tube can be situated in oral airway for those with nasal obstruction to monitor CO_2 deficits. The $PetCO_2$ is the level of CO_2 released at the end of expiration.
- Capnography: $PetCO_2$ can be evaluated after a 4-minute quiet breathing rest period, followed by exercise and recovery, or a HVPT can be conducted in the recovery period. Most patients with chronic hyperventilation have a $PetCO_2$ at or below 30 mm Hg and a markedly delayed recovery from hypocapnia after overbreathing, sometimes lasting 30 minutes after testing. By measuring $PetCO_2$ or transcutaneous CO_2 while a hyperventilation-provoking activity is performed, a potential link can be made between symptoms and CO_2 levels.
- The think test is initiated 3 to 4 minutes into recovery period. The patient is asked to recall a painful emotional experience during which symptoms developed. If $PetCO_2$ drops 10 mm Hg, the test supports hyperventilation. In some patients with hyperventilation. $Paco_2$ and $PetCO_2$ may be in normal range. In those asymptomatic at time of testing, this finding could be accepted. However, a normal level during experiencing of symptoms negates hypocapnia as cause of symptoms. It prompts search for alternative cause.

- Simple breath holding after expiration can predict percent of alveolar CO_2 and therefore the degree of hyperventilation to a high degree of accuracy. Optimal levels of alveolar Pco_2 correlate with postexpiratory breath-holding time of 40 to 60 seconds. Many asthmatics and hyperventilators are able to hold the breath out for less than 10 seconds.

Caution

Conduct HVPT before explanations of symptoms, to prevent suggestion and bias. Patients are warned only of a dry mouth. Ask the patient to concentrate on how he or she feels during 1- to 2-minute period while overbreathing at 30 to 40 breaths per minute. Rate is set by examiner's hand movements. Stress the importance of the test and the need to continue for as long as the patient can. Arterial blood gas measurement at the end of the test can establish depth of hypocapnia. Try as few as 12 deep breaths that the patient can recover from easily. Record subjective symptoms produced. In both breath-holding and voluntary overbreathing tests, strive to maintain trust and cooperation of patients.

The Nijmegen Questionnaire

- Gold standard for chronic HVS
- Noninvasive with high sensitivity (up to 91%) and specificity (up to 95%)
- Can be used to monitor progress of treatment by reevaluating symptoms
- Can help indicate whether initiating trigger causing HVS/BPDs resolved, suggesting that the patient had to deal with only "bad breathing" habit and musculoskeletal and motor pattern changes, or whether initiating triggers were ongoing or unresolved and might necessitate further cognitive help
- May be neither sensitive nor specific for chronic idiopathic hyperventilation without physiologic testing because many symptoms on the questionnaire are common to organic respiratory disease

BIOMECHANICAL (STRUCTURAL) CONSIDERATIONS

The Structure-Function Continuum

Prolonged changes in patterns of use, such as an inappropriate breathing pattern (hyperventilation), induce structural changes involving muscles and joints (e.g., rib) of respiration. These changes ultimately prevent normal function. Ultimately, the self-perpetuating cycle of functional change creating structural modification, leading to reinforced functional tendencies, can become complete, from whichever direction dysfunction derives. Examples are as follows:

- Structural adaptations can prevent normal breathing function.
- Abnormal breathing function ensures continued structural adaptational stresses.

Restoration of normal function demands restoration of adequate structural mobility. Maintenance of restored biomechanical flexibility requires that function (how the individual breathes) be normalized through reeducation and training.

Most useful approach: combination of restoration of structural integrity, combined with functional improvement. Address other underlying etiologic features—psychosocial, biochemical, or biomechanical factors.

The Muscles of Breathing

- Muscles of breathing function can be grouped as either inspiratory or expiratory. They are either primary in that capacity or provide accessory support.
- Expiration is primarily elastic response of lungs, pleura, and "torsion rod" elements of ribs; all muscles of expiration can be considered accessory because they are recruited only during increased demand. They include internal intercostals, abdominal muscles, transverse thoracis, and subcostales.
- With increased demand, iliocostalis lumborum, quadratus lumborum, serratus posterior inferior, and latissimus dorsi may support expiration, including during high demands of speech, coughing, sneezing, singing, and other special functions.

Neural Regulation of Breathing

Respiratory centers in the brainstem unconsciously influence and adjust alveolar ventilation to maintain arterial blood oxygen and CO_2 pressures at relatively constant levels, to sustain life under varying conditions and requirements.

Three main groups are as follows:

- Dorsal respiratory group: distal portion of medulla; receives input from peripheral chemoreceptors and other receptors via vagus and glossopharyngeal nerves. These impulses generate inspiratory movements and are responsible for basic rhythm of breathing.

- Pneumotaxic center: in superior part of the pons; transmits inhibitory signals to dorsal respiratory center, controlling filling phase of breathing.
- Ventral respiratory group: located in the medulla; causes either inspiration or expiration. It is inactive in quiet breathing but is important in stimulating abdominal expiratory muscles during levels of high respiratory demand.

The Hering-Breuer reflex prevents overinflation of lungs and is initiated by nerve receptors in walls of bronchi and bronchioles, sending messages to dorsal respiratory center via vagus nerve. The reflex switches off excessive inflation during inspiration and excessive deflation during exhalation.

The **autonomic nervous system** enables automatic unconscious maintenance of internal environment of the body in ideal efficiency and adjusts to the various demands of the external environment, be it sleep with repair and growth, quiet or extreme physical activity, or stress.

A **"third" nervous system** regulating airways—**nonadrenergic noncholinergic (NANC) system.** The NANC system contains inhibitory and stimulatory fibers; nitric oxide is the NANC neurotransmitter.

- NANC inhibitory nerves cause calcium ions to enter the neuron, mediating smooth muscle relaxation and bronchodilation.
- NANC stimulatory fibers—C fibers—are present in the lung supporting tissue, airways, and pulmonary blood vessels, involved in bronchoconstriction after exercise-induced asthma.

Chemical Control of Breathing

- Central role of respiration: maintain balanced concentrations of oxygen and CO_2 in the tissues. Increased CO_2 acts on central chemosensitive areas of respiratory centers, increasing inspiratory and expiratory signals to respiratory muscles.
- Oxygen acts on peripheral chemoreceptors located in carotid body (in bifurcation of common carotid arteries) via glossopharyngeal nerves and aortic body (on aortic arch), which sends appropriate messages via vagus nerves to dorsal respiratory center.

Voluntary Control of Breathing

- Automatic breathing can be overridden by higher cortical conscious input (directly via spinal neurons, which drive respiratory muscles) in response to fear, sudden surprise, and so on.

- Speaking, singing, playing wind instrument require voluntary control to interrupt normal rhythmicity of breathing.
- Cerebral cortex and thalamus also supply part of the drive for normal respiratory rhythm during wakefulness. (Cerebral influences on the medullary centers are withdrawn during sleep.)
- Habitual HVS/BPDs probably originate from some of these higher centers.

THERAPEUTIC CONSIDERATIONS AND THERAPEUTIC APPROACH

Treatment and Rehabilitation of Hyperventilation Syndrome/Breathing Pattern Disorders

- Different models of care in managing HVS/BPDs are available.
- Exclude all organic causes of breathing pattern changes.
- Attend to coexisting problems—asthma, chronic obstructive airway disease, chronic pain, and hormonal imbalances.
- Incorporate manual therapy approaches as essential element of rehabilitation.
- Bradley acronym: *BETTER* approach:
  - — Breathing retraining
  - — Esteem and self-image
  - — Total body relaxation
  - — Talk and breath control
  - — Exercise prescription
  - — Rest and sleep

Breathing retraining incorporates a number of elements:

- Awareness of faulty breathing patterns
- Relaxation of upper chest, shoulders, accessory muscles
- Abdominal and low chest breathing pattern retraining
- Awareness of normal breathing rates and rhythms both at rest and during activity

Elements of physical therapy protocol involving relaxation, exercise, talk and breath control, and sleep are all individualized and are not described here.

Osteopathic and Naturopathic Protocol for Care of Patients with Hyperventilation Syndrome/Breathing Pattern Disorders

- Initial (and continual or periodic) assessment of breathing function based on functional evidence and palpation determines what needs to be done to improve breathing function.

- Education and information are vital for creating motivation and awareness as to why homework is essential in normalizing BPDs.
- The patient must understand clearly that the practitioner or therapist can do no more than create an environment, a possibility, for restoration of more-normal function, but the breathing work itself is up to the patient.
- Treatment of muscles and joints alone, no matter how appropriate, can never restore normal breathing patterns without cooperative effort.
- Conversely, breathing retraining without the freeing of restricted structures is far more difficult to achieve.
- Psychotherapy and counseling are also unlikely to be successful unless retraining is introduced and structural factors are dealt with.
- Manual attention to the upper fixators and/or accessory breathing muscles (upper trapezius, levator scapulae, scalene, sternocleidomastoid, pectoral, and latissimus dorsi muscles) is usually required.
- The diaphragm area also requires direct attention as a rule (lower anterior intercostals, sternum, costal margin, beneath costal margin, abdominal attachments, quadratus lumborum, and psoas).
- Active trigger points in these muscles may need deactivating manually or via acupuncture.
- Acupuncture being administered for 30 minutes twice weekly for 4 weeks showed reduction in Nijmegen score from 31 to 24. The focus was on reducing anxiety, thereby reducing hyperventilation. The points used were colon 4, liver 3, and stomach 36 bilaterally.
- The thoracic spine and ribs may require mobilization (osteopathic or chiropractic adjustments).
- Osteopathic lymphatic pump methods may be required if there is evidence of stasis.
- Retraining: various breathing exercises should be introduced and individualized to the specific needs of the patient, commonly on the basis of pursed lip breathing and pranayama yoga methods.
- Relaxation methods, including autogenic training or progressive muscular relaxation or both, might usefully be introduced.
- Sleep pattern disturbances might require attention.
- Exercise of aerobic nature should be carefully introduced.

- Dietary advice and counseling should be introduced as appropriate.

Breathing Rehabilitation Exercises

"Breathing Rehabilitation Exercises" box describes three breathing rehabilitation exercises.

Chronic HVS/BPDs are commonly successfully treated; however, a time frame of 12 to 26 weeks may be required, with active patient participation throughout to break well-established habits. For anxious and phobic patients, employ breathing retraining, physical therapy, and relaxation.

Symptoms can resolve in 1 to 6 months, with some younger patients requiring only a few weeks. Therapy can be conducted in the following sequence:

- Brief, voluntary hyperventilation to reproduce reported complaints
- Reattribution of cause of symptoms to hyperventilation
- Explaining rationale of therapy involving reduction of hyperventilation by acquiring abdominal breathing pattern, with slowing down of expiration
- Breathing retraining for 2 to 3 months, working with physiotherapist

A canonical correlation analysis relating changes of various complaints to modifications of breathing variables showed that improvement of complaints was correlated mainly with slowing down of breathing frequency.

Breathing Rehabilitation Exercises

1. Pursed lip breathing—Essentially, blowing firmly and slowly through a narrow aperture such as pursed lips effectively tones the diaphragm via eccentric isotonic activity.
2. Antiarousal breathing.
3. Recitation of mantra or prayer.
   - The respiratory (and cardiovascular) effects of rosary prayer ("Ave Maria" in Latin) and recitation of a yoga mantra were assessed.
   - Results were similar, showing a slowing of respiration to approximately 6 counts per minute and synchronization of all cardiovascular rhythms (Traube-Hering-Mayer oscillations), representing blood pressure, heart rate, cardiac contractility, pulmonary blood flow, cerebral blood flow, and movement of cerebrospinal fluid.
   - This influence on autonomic activity, represented by the Traube-Hering-Mayer oscillations, is clearly health enhancing because it slows respiratory rate to the level considered optimal in breathing rehabilitation.

Hypoglycemia

DIAGNOSTIC SUMMARY

- Blood glucose level below 40-50 mg/dL
- Normal response curve during first 2 to 3 hours of glucose tolerance test (GTT) followed by decrease of 20 mg or more below fasting glucose level during final hours of test, with symptoms developing during decrease

GENERAL CONSIDERATIONS

Hypoglycemia is divided into two main categories:

- **Reactive hypoglycemia:** most common form. Symptoms of hypoglycemia occur 3 to 5 hours after a meal and may herald onset of early type 2 diabetes mellitus (T2DM). Gastric surgery may induce this condition, and anorexia nervosa may be a cause. It may also result from oral hypoglycemic drugs; these sulfa drugs (sulfonylureas) stimulate secretion of additional insulin by the pancreas and enhance tissue sensitivity to insulin. (See list of other hypoglycemic drugs later.) Some call this category "idiopathic postprandial syndrome" because symptoms exist and are related to rapid glucose drops, but absolute glucose levels are not reliable indicators of syndrome. Many asymptomatic control subjects have glucose levels below 50 mg/dL, and many symptomatic patients have normal postprandial glucose.
- **Fasting hypoglycemia:** rare; appears in severe disease states (pancreatic tumors, extensive liver damage, prolonged starvation, autoantibodies against insulin or its receptor, various cancers, excessive exogenous insulin in diabetics). Pregnant diabetic women taking insulin or oral glycemic drugs also can have asymptomatic hypoglycemia.

Hypoglycemia promotes untoward physiologic changes in the body. Insulin-induced hypoglycemia increases C-reactive protein, a cardiac risk factor. Glucose is the primary fuel for the brain; low levels affect brain first. Symptoms of hypoglycemia include headache, depression, anxiety, irritability, blurred vision, excessive

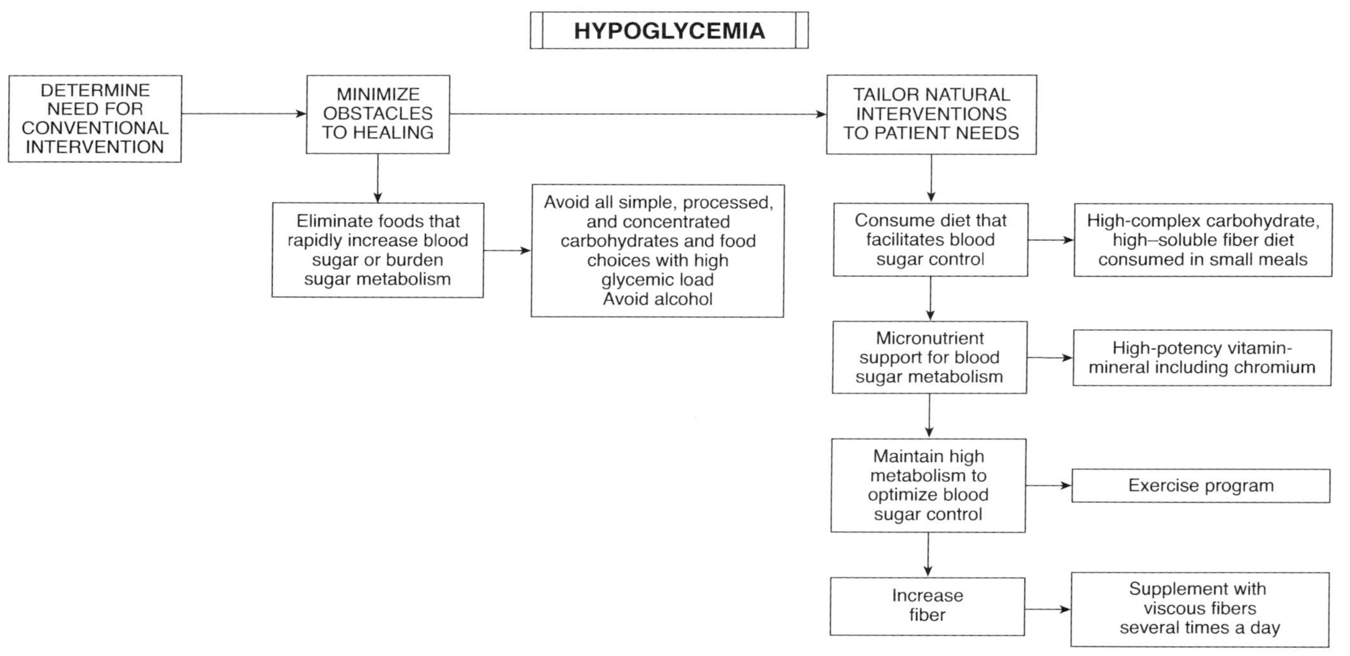
HYPOGLYCEMIA
DETERMINE NEED FOR CONVENTIONAL INTERVENTION
MINIMIZE OBSTACLES TO HEALING
TAILOR NATURAL INTERVENTIONS TO PATIENT NEEDS
Eliminate foods that rapidly increase blood sugar or burden sugar metabolism
Avoid all simple, processed, and concentrated carbohydrates and food choices with high glycemic load
Avoid alcohol
Consume diet that facilitates blood sugar control
High-complex carbohydrate, high–soluble fiber diet consumed in small meals
Micronutrient support for blood sugar metabolism
High-potency vitamin-mineral including chromium
Maintain high metabolism to optimize blood sugar control
Exercise program
Increase fiber
Supplement with viscous fibers several times a day

sweating, mental confusion, incoherent speech, bizarre behavior, convulsions.

Complex hormonal fluxes are largely the result of ingesting too many refined carbohydrates. Syndrome X is a cluster of abnormalities caused by a high intake of refined carbohydrates, leading to hypoglycemia, hyperinsulinemia, and glucose intolerance followed by diminished insulin sensitivity, further leading to hypertension, hypercholesterolemia, obesity, and T2DM. The U.S. government recommends that no more than 10% of total calories be derived from refined sugars. The average American consumes more than 100 pounds of sucrose and 40 pounds of corn syrup each year.

DIAGNOSTIC CONSIDERATIONS

Clinical hypoglycemia is identified by modified Whipple's criteria: (1) central nervous system symptoms of confusion, aberrant behavior, or coma; (2) simultaneous blood glucose level of 40 mg/dL or lower; and (3) relief of symptoms by administration of glucose. Standard methods of diagnosing hypoglycemia include measuring blood glucose; normal fasting level is 65 to 109 mg/dL. Fasting plasma blood glucose above 126 mg/dL on two separate occasions is diagnostic of diabetes mellitus (DM). Blood glucose below 50 mg/dL should arouse suspicion.

- **Glucose tolerance test (GTT):** used to diagnose reactive hypoglycemia and DM, but rarely required for DM. After patient has fasted for more than 12 hours, measure baseline blood glucose. Give patient glucose drink; the amount consumed is based on body weight (1.75 g/kg body weight). Measure blood sugar at 30 minutes, 1 hour, and then hourly for up to 6 hours. Levels above 200 mg/dL indicate DM. Levels below 50 mg/dL indicate reactive hypoglycemia (see table on page 456).
- **Glucose-insulin tolerance test (G-ITT):** blood sugar levels alone are often not enough to diagnose hypoglycemia; signs and symptoms of hypoglycemia occur in persons with glucose above 50 mg/dL. Wide overlap exists between symptomatic patients and asymptomatic control subjects. Symptoms linked to hypoglycemia arise from increases in insulin or epinephrine (adrenaline). Measure insulin or epinephrine during GTT because symptoms often correlate better with hormones than glucose. G-ITT has greater sensitivity in diagnosing hypoglycemia and DM than does GTT. Use standard 6-hour GTT coupled with measurements of insulin. Two thirds of patients with suspected

DM or hypoglycemia with normal GTT result demonstrate abnormal G-ITT result. However, G-ITT is costly.

- **24-Hour continuous glucose monitoring:** continuous glucose monitors (CGMs) are electronic diagnostic systems requiring insertion of a sensing catheter under abdominal skin. These miniaturized electronic devices measure glucose and send information every few minutes to a computer module worn on the belt for a week. The monitor provides 288 glucose readings per day, studied relative to food intake, appetite, food cravings, symptoms, medication, and exercise. Most people with obesity and insulin resistance have remarkably fluctuating glucose, or increased glycemic volatility. Rather than absolute glucose level determining hypoglycemic symptoms, feelings of hypoglycemia occur when glucose drops rapidly, even when it was above normal (70 to 100 mg/dL). Symptoms of hypoglycemia can range from mild to severe (e.g., food cravings, headache, depression, anxiety, irritability, blurred vision, excessive sweating, and mental confusion). Rather than having *hypoglycemia,* these patients may have *elevated glycemic volatility.* Such volatility may underlie most weight problems. Rapidly fluctuating blood sugar levels relate to some degree of insulin resistance and are worsened by immoderate consumption of high glycemic foods.
- **Hypoglycemic index:** helps diagnose borderline hypoglycemia. The value is determined by calculating the fall in blood glucose during a 90-minute period before the lowest point divided by the value of the lowest point. Hypoglycemic index above 0.8 indicates reactive hypoglycemia.
- **Hypoglycemia questionnaire:** most useful and cost-effective method of diagnosing hypoglycemia is to assess symptoms. When symptoms appear 3 to 4 hours after eating and disappear with ingestion of food, consider hypoglycemia (see questionnaire on page 457).

Health Impact of Hypoglycemia

- **Brain:** dependent on glucose as energy source. Hypoglycemia causes brain dysfunction. Hypoglycemia is involved in various psychological disorders. Depressed individuals show high percentage of abnormal GTT and G-ITT, but rarely is hypoglycemia considered and dietary therapy prescribed.
- **Aggressive and criminal behavior:** Reactive hypoglycemia is common in psychiatric patients and habitually violent and impulsive criminals. Abnormal and emotionally explosive behavior

often is seen during GTT. A sugar-restricted diet reduced antisocial behavior among male juvenile inmates. Behavior improved most in those charged with assault, robbery, rape, aggravated assault, auto theft, vandalism, child molestation, arson, and possession of a deadly weapon. Dietary changes did not seem to affect female prisoners. Men may react to hypoglycemia in a different manner from women; hypoglycemia is an innate internal signal for men to hunt for food. In noncriminal men, aggressiveness often coincides with hypoglycemia.

- **Premenstrual syndrome (PMS):** PMS-C is linked with increased appetite, craving for sweets, headache, fatigue, fainting spells, and heart palpitations. GTT on PMS-C patients 5 to 10 days before menses displays flattening of early part of curve and reactive hypoglycemia. GTT is normal during other parts of menstrual cycle. Flat, early part of GTT curve implies excessive insulin secretion in response to sugar consumption. Excessive secretion is hormonally regulated, but other factors are involved. Sodium chloride ingestion enhances insulin response to sugar, and decreased magnesium in pancreas increases insulin secretion (see the chapter on PMS).
- **Migraine headaches:** caused by excessive dilation of blood vessels in the head. Migraines are surprisingly common (15% to 20% of men and 25% to 30% of women). More than half of patients have a family history of migraine. Hypoglycemia is a common precipitating factor. Eliminating refined sugar from diets of migraine patients with confirmed hypoglycemia greatly improves the condition (see the chapter on migraine headaches).
- **Atherosclerosis, intermittent claudication, and angina:** reactive hypoglycemia or impaired glucose tolerance is a significant factor in atherosclerosis. High sugar intake elevates triglycerides and cholesterol. Abnormal GTT result and hyperinsulinism are common in patients with heart disease. High sugar intake and reactive hypoglycemia can cause angina and intermittent claudication.
- **Metabolic syndrome:** a set of cardiovascular risk factors (glucose or insulin disturbances, hyperlipidemia, hypertension, and android obesity). Other terms: *metabolic cardiovascular risk syndrome, Reaven's syndrome, insulin resistance syndrome,* and *atherothrombogenic syndrome.* The underlying metabolic denominator is hyperinsulinemia from elevated intake of refined carbohydrates. Development of T2DM is preceded by hyperinsulinemia and insulin insensitivity. In most cases these defects present

themselves decades before the development of DM. Hypoglycemia, hyperinsulinemia, metabolic syndrome, and T2DM are progressive stages of the same illness—maladaptation to the refined Western diet.

THERAPEUTIC CONSIDERATIONS

Dietary Factors

In whole, unprocessed foods, sugars are slowly absorbed because they are contained within cells and associated with fiber. A high–complex carbohydrate, high-fiber, low-sugar diet is recommended. Natural, simple sugars in fruits and vegetables have an advantage over sucrose and other refined sugars attributable to balance by a wide range of nutrients aiding the use of sugars. Sugars in whole, unprocessed foods are more slowly absorbed because of the integration within cells and fiber. Refining removes vitamins, trace minerals, and fiber. More than half of carbohydrates consumed in the United States are sugars added to processed foods.

- **A closer look at simple carbohydrates:** most diabetic and hypoglycemic persons can tolerate moderate amounts of fruits and fructose without a loss of blood sugar control. These foods produce less-sharp elevations in blood sugar compared with starch. Fructose decreases the amount of calories and fat consumed. Regular fruit consumption may help control sugar cravings and reduce obesity.
- **Glycemic index and glycemic load:** glycemic index expresses a rise in blood glucose after a particular food is eaten; serves as a guideline for dietary recommendations for people with DM or hypoglycemia. Glycemic index must not be the sole dietary guideline. High-fat foods (e.g., ice cream, sausage) have low glycemic indexes because fat impairs glucose tolerance and are poor food choices for hypoglycemic or diabetic patients. The standard value of 100 is based on the rise seen with ingestion of pure glucose. Glycemic index ranges from 20 for fructose and whole barley to 98 for a baked potato. Insulin response to carbohydrate-containing foods is similar to the rise in blood sugar. Avoid foods with high values and choose foods with lower values.
- **Glycemic load:** value of a food's glycemic index divided by 100, then multiplied by its available carbohydrate content. A glycemic load of 20 or more is high; 11 to 19 is intermediate; 10 or less

is low. This provides more-comprehensive assessment of impact of carbohydrate intake. Even though glycemic index for a food is fairly high, its glycemic load can be low, indicating that with reasonable serving sizes it does not adversely stress glycemic control. Foods containing natural soluble and insoluble fibers and minimally processed whole foods are better choices for glycemic influence and insulin response. Diets with high glycemic load are directly linked to DM; coronary heart disease; and colon, ovarian, and pancreatic cancer risk.

- **Fiber:** blood sugar disorders are related to inadequate dietary fiber. Increase intake of complex carbohydrate sources rich in fiber. Dietary fiber is composed of the plant cell walls plus indigestible residues from plant foods. Water-soluble forms are most beneficial to blood sugar control: hemicelluloses, mucilages, gums, and pectin. The majority of fiber in most plant cell walls is water soluble. Good sources of water-soluble fiber are legumes, oat bran, nuts, seeds, psyllium seed husks, pears, apples, and most vegetables. Daily intake of 50 g is recommended. Beneficial effects include the following:
  - Slow digestion and absorption of carbohydrates, preventing rapid rises in blood sugar
  - Increase human tissue cell sensitivity to insulin, preventing hyperinsulinism
  - Improve uptake of glucose by liver and other tissues, preventing sustained hyperglycemia (*Textbook,* "Role of Dietary Fiber in Health and Disease")
- **PolyGlycopleX (PGX):** although low glycemic diet helps reduce blood sugar, it does not reduce blood sugar volatility. Instead, use low glycemic diet along with a novel matrix of soluble fibers (PGX). PGX reduces postprandial hypoglycemia in a dose-dependent manner, independent of food form. PGX matrix has higher viscosity, gel-forming properties and better expansion with water than any other known fiber. This reduces glycemic impact of any food or meal. Dose: 1.5 to 5 g before meals.
- **Chromium (Cr):** key constituent of glucose tolerance factor. Cr deficiency may be a contributing factor to hypoglycemia, DM, and obesity. Marginal Cr deficiency is common in the United States and may be a cause of many cases of reactive hypoglycemia. Cr alleviates hypoglycemic symptoms, improves insulin binding, and increases number of insulin receptors.

Lifestyle Factors

- **Alcohol:** severely stresses blood sugar control and is a contributing factor to hypoglycemia. It induces reactive hypoglycemia by interfering with normal glucose use and increases secretion of insulin. Resultant drop in blood sugar produces craving for foods that quickly elevate blood sugar plus cravings for more alcohol. Increased sugar consumption aggravates reactive hypoglycemia. Hypoglycemia is a complication of short- and long-term alcohol abuse. Hypoglycemia aggravates mental and emotional problems of the withdrawing alcoholic: sweating, tremor, tachycardia, anxiety, hunger, dizziness, headache, visual disturbance, decreased mental function, confusion, and depression. Acute alcohol ingestion induces hypoglycemia. Long-term abuse leads to hyperglycemia and DM. The body becomes insensitive to chronic augmented insulin release caused by alcohol. Alcohol causes insulin resistance even in healthy persons. Alcohol intake is strongly correlated with DM; the higher the alcohol intake, the more likely a person will have DM.
- **Exercise:** an important part of hypoglycemia treatment and prevention. Regular exercise prevents T2DM and improves insulin sensitivity and glucose tolerance in patients with existing DM. Exercise increases tissue Cr concentrations.

THERAPEUTIC APPROACH

Use dietary therapy to stabilize blood sugar. Reactive hypoglycemia is not a disease, but a complex set of symptoms caused by faulty carbohydrate metabolism induced by inappropriate diet.

- **Diet:** avoid all simple, processed, and concentrated carbohydrates and food choices with high glycemic load. Emphasize complex-carbohydrate, high-soluble fiber foods: legumes and low-glycemic vegetables. Small meals may stabilize blood sugar more easily. Avoid alcohol (see the chapter on diabetes).
- **Supplements:**
  - High-potency vitamin-mineral that includes the following:
    - **Cr:** 200 to 400 mcg q.d.
    - **Fiber:** Several grams several times per day
- **Exercise:** graded exercise program appropriate to patient's fitness level and interest that elevates heart rate to at least 60% of maximum for 30 minutes three times a week.

Glucose Tolerance Test Response Criteria

Diagnosis	Response
Normal	No elevation greater than 200 mg
	Less than 200 mg at the end of first hour
	Less than 140 mg at the end of second hour
	Never lower than 20 mg below fasting
Flat	No variation more than ±20 mg from fasting value
Prediabetic	More than 140 mg at the end of second hour
Diabetic	≥200 mg at the end of the second hour
Reactive hypoglycemia	A normal 2- or 3-hour response curve followed by a decrease of 20 mg or more from the fasting level during the final hours
Probable reactive hypoglycemia	A normal 2- or 3-hour response curve followed by a decrease of 10-20 mg from the fasting level during the final hours
Flat hypoglycemia	An elevation of 20 mg or less followed by a decrease of 20 mg or more below the fasting level
Prediabetic hypoglycemia	A 2-hour response identical to the prediabetic response but showing a hypoglycemic response during the final 3 hours
Hyperinsulinism	A marked hypoglycemic response with a value of less than 50 mg during the third, fourth, or fifth hour

Glucose-Insulin Tolerance Test Criteria

Pattern	Response
Pattern 1	Normal fasting insulin 0-30 units. Peak insulin at 0.5-1 hr. The combined insulin values for the second and third hours are less than 60 units. This pattern is considered normal.
Pattern 2	Normal fasting insulin. Peak at 0.5-1 hour with a delayed return to normal. Second and third hour levels between 60 and 100 units usually are associated with hypoglycemia and considered borderline for diabetes; values greater than 100 units considered definite diabetes.
Pattern 3	Normal fasting insulin. Peak at second or third hour instead of 0.5-1 hour. Definite diabetes.
Pattern 4	High fasting insulin. Definite diabetes.
Pattern 5	Low insulin response. All tested values for insulin less than 30. If this response is associated with elevated blood sugar levels, it probably indicates insulin-dependent DM (juvenile pattern).

Hypoglycemia Questionnaire

	No	Mild	Moderate	Severe
Crave sweets	0	1	2	3
Irritable if a meal is missed	0	1	2	3
Feel tired or weak if a meal is missed	0	1	2	3
Dizziness when standing suddenly	0	1	2	3
Frequent headaches	0	1	2	3
Poor memory (forgetful) or concentration	0	1	2	3
Feel tired an hour or so after eating	0	1	2	3
Heart palpitations	0	1	2	3
Feel shaky at times	0	1	2	3
Afternoon fatigue	0	1	2	3
Vision blurs on occasion	0	1	2	3
Depression or mood swings	0	1	2	3
Overweight	0	1	2	3
Frequently anxious or nervous	0	1	2	3
Total				

Scoring: <5, hypoglycemia is not likely a factor; 6-15, hypoglycemia is a likely factor; >15, hypoglycemia is extremely likely.

Oral Hypoglycemic Drugs

- Chlorpropamide (Diabinese)
- Glipizide (Glucotrol)
- Glibenclamide, glyburide (DiaBeta, Micronase)
- Tolazamide (Tomlins)
- Tolbutamide (Orinase)
- Metformin (Glucophage)
- Thiazolidinediones: pioglitazone (Actos) or rosiglitazone (Avandia)
- Acarbose (Precose, Glucobay)
- Glimepiride (Amaryl)
- Gliclazide (Gen-Gliclazide)
- Nateglinide (Starlix)
- Repaglinide (Prandin)

Hypothyroidism

DIAGNOSTIC SUMMARY

- Depression
- Difficulty losing weight
- Dry skin
- Headaches
- Lethargy or fatigue
- Memory problems
- Menstrual problems
- Hyperlipidemia
- Recurrent infections
- Sensitivity to cold
- Thinning of head hair
- Voice changes

GENERAL CONSIDERATIONS

Hypothyroidism affects virtually all cells and body functions. Severity of symptoms in adults ranges from mild (not detectable with standard blood tests [subclinical hypothyroidism]) to severe, which can be life-threatening (myxedema).

- Low thyroid hormone and elevated thyroid-stimulating hormone (TSH) levels indicate defective thyroid hormone synthesis —called *primary hypothyroidism.*
- Low TSH and low thyroid hormone: pituitary gland is responsible for low thyroid function—called *secondary hypothyroidism.*
- Normal blood thyroid hormone and TSH plus low functional thyroid activity (low basal metabolic rate) suggest *cellular hypothyroidism,* involving impaired cellular conversion of thyroxine (T_4) to triiodothyronine (T_3).

From 1% to 4% of the adult population have moderate to severe hypothyroidism. Another 10% to 12% have mild hypothyroidism. The rate of hypothyroidism increases steadily with advancing age. The rate of hypothyroidism is 25% of adults and much higher in the elderly.

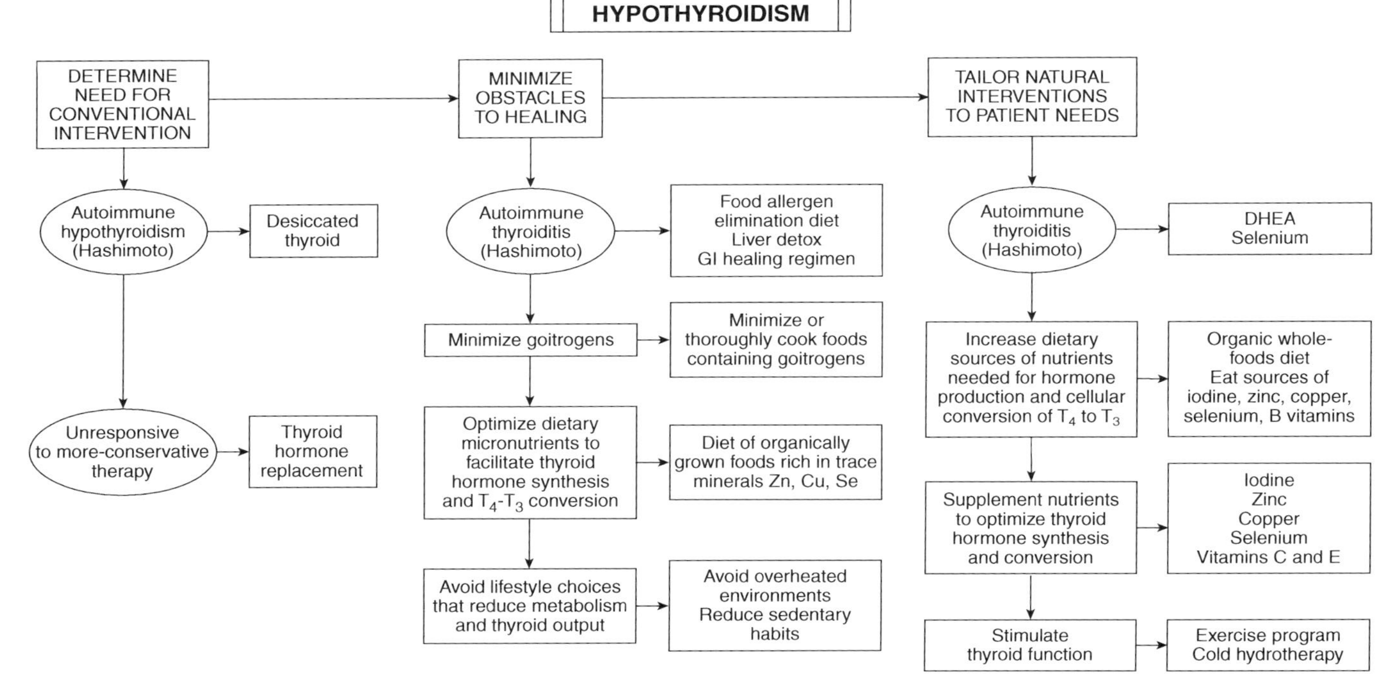
HYPOTHYROIDISM
DETERMINE NEED FOR CONVENTIONAL INTERVENTION
Autoimmune hypothyroidism (Hashimoto)
Desiccated thyroid
Unresponsive to more-conservative therapy
Thyroid hormone replacement
MINIMIZE OBSTACLES TO HEALING
Autoimmune thyroiditis (Hashimoto)
Food allergen elimination diet
Liver detox
GI healing regimen
Minimize goitrogens
Minimize or thoroughly cook foods containing goitrogens
Optimize dietary micronutrients to facilitate thyroid hormone synthesis and T_4-T_3 conversion
Diet of organically grown foods rich in trace minerals Zn, Cu, Se
Avoid lifestyle choices that reduce metabolism and thyroid output
Avoid overheated environments
Reduce sedentary habits
TAILOR NATURAL INTERVENTIONS TO PATIENT NEEDS
Autoimmune thyroiditis (Hashimoto)
DHEA
Selenium
Increase dietary sources of nutrients needed for hormone production and cellular conversion of T_4 to T_3
Organic whole-foods diet
Eat sources of iodine, zinc, copper, selenium, B vitamins
Supplement nutrients to optimize thyroid hormone synthesis and conversion
Iodine
Zinc
Copper
Selenium
Vitamins C and E
Stimulate thyroid function
Exercise program
Cold hydrotherapy

Causes of Hypothyroidism

- **Overt hypothyroidism:** 95% of all cases of overt hypothyroidism are primary. The most common cause in the past was iodine deficiency. The thyroid gland cells add iodine to amino acid tyrosine to create thyroid hormones. Iodine deficiency leads to hypothyroidism and/or enlarged thyroid gland (goiter).
  - **Goiters** affect 200 million people worldwide. All but 4% are caused by iodine deficiency. Iodine deficiency is rare in industrialized countries because of iodized table salt. Prolonged thyrotropin (TSH) elevation can lead to thyrocyte hypertrophy, manifesting as a goiter. Goiters regress as thyrotropin is suppressed but in rare cases may require surgical resection.
  - **Nodules** can form within the gland during or independent of output dysfunction. On palpation, 20% of adults have nodules; on random screening by ultrasound, 50% of the population have them. Main clinical relevance: 5% of nodules may be cancerous.
  - **Dietary goitrogens**—foods block iodine use: *Brassica* plants (turnips, cabbage, mustard greens, radishes, broccoli, Brussels sprouts, kale, rutabagas, cauliflower, horseradishes), cassava root, soybean, peanuts, pine nuts, millet. Cooking usually inactivates goitrogens.
  - Thyroid surgery and ablation.
  - Postpartum hypothyroidism, a transient form that affects 5% to 10% of women in the United States.
  - Lack of thyroid hormone–releasing hormone (THRH) from the hypothalamus, called *tertiary hypothyroidism.*
  - **Environmental goitrogens:** perchlorate, iodine in excess of 1000 mcg/day, fluoride, and mercury. Medicines that induce goiters and suppress thyroid function: amiodarone, carbamazepine, lithium, potassium iodine, phenobarbitone, phenytoin, and rifampin.
  - **Autoimmune disease:** the most frequent cause of clinical hypothyroidism in the United States is Hashimoto's thyroiditis.

Hashimoto's Thyroiditis

This disorder involves antibodies that bind to thyroid peroxidase enzyme, thyroglobulin, and TSH receptors and inhibit hormone synthesis. Antibodies may also bind to adrenal glands, pancreas, and acid-producing cells (parietal cells) of the stomach. Hashimoto's thyroiditis is a histologic diagnosis, but it can be assumed with signs of autoimmune thyroid disease, including the following:

- Serum antibodies against thyroid proteins—thyroglobulin (TG) or thyroperoxidase (TPO); however, 10% to 15% of patients can be antibody-negative.
- Diffuse enlargement of the gland detected by palpation, ultrasound, or computed tomography
- Diffuse iodine uptake and glandular enlargement on radioiodine uptake scan

After histologic assessment via biopsy, fine-needle aspiration, or thyroidectomy, the typical findings are cellular infiltration of immune cells—lymphocytes. Variables that predict Hashimoto's thyroiditis are family history of any thyroid disease and exposure to environmental triggers. Certain toxins are taken up via the sodium iodide symporter and concentrated in thyroid follicles, where they generate free radicals that activate immune responses and sensitize immune cells to thyroid proteins. Chemicals that correlate with Hashimoto's thyroiditis include iodine (in excess or when intake increases significantly), perchlorate, fluoride, lithium, mercury, bisphenol A (BPA), Teflon. Autoimmune thyroid disease can exist without serum hypothyroidism, but patients progress to hypothyroidism. Hashimoto's disease elevates risk of other autoimmune diseases.

- **Subclinical hypothyroidism:** TSH is elevated (or simply near the top of the normal range) and serum thyroid hormone levels are normal. The body compensates for decreased thyroid function by increasing TSH. Causes include mild autoimmune thyroid destruction, drug or surgical interventions and, functionally, decreased cellular conversion of T_4 to the more-active T_3. Earliest stages of hypothyroidism can precede serum abnormalities by several years and manifest with mild fatigue or depression. Advanced stages, rare at present, manifest with life-threatening myxedema coma. Degrees of severity range from early, mild deficiency not detectable with standard blood tests (hypothyroid syndrome) to severe deficiency—life-threatening myxedema. Subclinical hypothyroidism is relatively common, affecting 2% to 7% of adults. It is linked to increased risk for cardiovascular disease. Thyroid disease without overt laboratory findings is *hypothyroid syndrome,* defined by the following clinical findings:
  - — Hypothyroid symptoms
  - — Absence of other explanatory diseases

— Possible functional thyroid abnormalities—basal body temperature (BBT) and Achilles reflex testing

The presence of one or more of the following objective findings helps confirm the diagnosis:

— Suboptimal blood levels

— Abnormal antibody studies

— Abnormal ultrasound findings

— Abnormal findings on fine-needle aspiration of the thyroid

Most patients with hypothyroid syndrome may have early Hashimoto's disease, although some may have impaired thyroid hormone synthesis or conversion related to nutritional deficiencies or environmental toxins.

- **Functional hypothyroidism:** thyroid activity is measured by functional test (Barnes test) rather than solely by blood thyroid hormone levels. Incidence is 25%. Functional tests show greater incidence of low thyroid than blood tests; blood tests measure T_4, which accounts for 90% of hormone secreted; but T_3 (made by cells from T_4) has four times the activity of T_4. If cells cannot convert, the person has normal blood levels of the hormone yet is functionally thyroid deficient. Blood tests for T_3 miss low thyroid function in 50% of patients. Measuring thyroid effects on the body is better; measure resting metabolic rate controlled by thyroid gland. BBT is a good way of assessing basal metabolic rate. Some physicians look for high reverse T_3/T_4 ratio as evidence of this condition.

DIAGNOSTIC CONSIDERATIONS

BBT (temperature of body at rest) and Achilles reflex time (reflexes are slowed in hypothyroidism) are old indicators of dysfunction. Routine blood tests may not be sensitive enough to diagnose milder, most common forms of hypothyroidism. BBT is the most sensitive functional test of thyroid function. To distinguish autoimmune Hashimoto's thyroiditis and other nonautoimmune subclinical and functional conditions, use TSH, antithyroid peroxidase, and antithyroglobulin antibody tests. Suspect Wilson's disease with low BBT and high reverse T_3/T_4 ratio.

Clinical Symptomatology

- **Psychological:** the brain is sensitive to low thyroid hormone levels. Depression, weakness, and fatigue are the first symptoms of hypothyroidism. Later, hypothyroid persons have difficulty concentrating and are extremely forgetful.

- **Metabolic:** hypothyroidism decreases the rate of use of fat, protein, and carbohydrate. Moderate weight gain and sensitivity to cold weather (cold hands or feet) are common. Cholesterol and triglycerides are increased in even mildest hypothyroidism, increasing the risk of atherosclerosis and cardiovascular disease. Hypothyroidism increases capillary permeability and slows lymphatic drainage, causing swelling of tissue (edema).
- **Endocrine:** hormonal complications are loss of libido in men and menstrual abnormalities in women. Women have prolonged and heavy menses, with a shorter menstrual cycle. Infertility is problematic; miscarriages, premature deliveries, and stillbirths are common. Rarely does a pregnancy result in normal labor and delivery in the overtly hypothyroid woman. Adrenal dysfunction is a common comorbidity with primary and secondary hypothyroidism. Patients with thyroid antibodies are more likely to possess adrenal cortex antibodies. Cortisol secretion can be increased to compensate for low T_3.
- **Skin, hair, and nails:** dry, rough skin covered with fine superficial scales. Hair is coarse, dry, and brittle. Hair loss can be quite severe and is diffuse and uniform as opposed to patchy. Nails become thin and brittle with transverse grooves.
- **Psychological:** the brain is sensitive to hypothyroidism. Depression with weakness and fatigue are first symptoms; later, difficulty concentrating and extreme forgetfulness.
- **Muscular and skeletal:** muscle weakness and joint stiffness are predominant features. Some patients have muscle and joint pain and tenderness.
- **Cardiovascular:** predisposition to atherosclerosis and myocardial infarction from induced hyperlipidemia and increased homocysteine and C-reactive protein. Hypothyroidism can also cause hypertension, reduce function of heart, and reduce heart rate.
- **Other manifestations:** shortness of breath, constipation, and impaired kidney function. Patients with dermatitis herpetiformis have significantly increased abnormalities of thyroid function tests, with significant hypothyroidism being the most common abnormality.

Diagnostic Considerations

- Before blood testing, diagnosis was based on "functional" tests—BBT (temperature of the body at rest) and Achilles reflex time (reflexes are slowed in hypothyroidism). Normal BBT is 97.6°F to 98.2°F. BBT is not just an indicator of thyroid status, as it is affected by adrenal function, body composition, activity level, menstrual status, immune function, and so on. It has little specificity but can be used as an indicator within a complete clinical evaluation.

- **Wilson's temperature syndrome (WTS):** hypothyroid symptoms despite normal thyroid laboratory results as a result of excessive conversion of T_4 into reverse T_3 (rT_3) within cell membrane, so that laboratory tests are not reflective of serum T_3 or rT_3. T_4 accounts for 90% of hormone secretion by the thyroid; T_4 is converted by cells into T_3, which is four times more active. If cells cannot convert T_4 to T_3, a person can have normal levels in the blood yet be thyroid deficient. There is currently little support for this hypothesis in medical literature or any way of accurately assessing conversion; serum T_3 or rT_3 levels do not correlate with intracellular levels. Closest known correlate: euthyroid sick syndrome (ESS), which involves abnormal thyroid function test results during nonthyroidal illness (NTI), without preexisting hypothalamic-pituitary and thyroid gland dysfunction. Serum T_3 may be low, and rT_3 may be elevated. During metabolic crises, the body can alter peripheral conversion of T_4 to slow metabolic processes beneficially. This effect is transient, 3 weeks or shorter, and resolves spontaneously. Wilson claims that if ascending and descending doses of compounded sustained-release T_3 are taken, the positive feedback loop from excess rT_3 is broken and cells form T_3 again as needed. During these cycles, doses of T_3 as high as 100 mcg are used without overt hypothyroidism, exceeding the typical full replacement dose for adults lacking endogenous thyroid secretion by more than twofold. This protocol carries risk; some fatalities occurred. Nonetheless, there are a significant number of integrative medicine practitioners reporting success with this protocol.

Clinical Assessment

A clinical score based on the Colorado Thyroid Disease Prevalence Study simplifies symptom evaluation in suspected cases. Many patients with symptoms do not have clinical hypothyroidism defined by overly strict definition of severely elevated TSH and low T_4. Best indicators for hypothyroidism are the following:

- Symptoms: impairment of hearing, diminished sweating, constipation, paresthesia, hoarseness, weight gain, dry skin

- Physical signs: slow movements, periorbital puffiness, delayed ankle reflex, coarse skin, cold skin

Laboratory Evaluation

Testing helps confirm diagnosis and refute other causes. When clinically indicated, thyroid screening ideally includes a marker of thyroid regulation (TSH), markers of thyroid output (free T_4, free T_3), and markers of thyroid inflammation (thyroid microsomal antibody; TPO antibody; antithyroglobulin antibody). The American Thyroid Association recommends TSH screening every 5 years beginning at age 35. Laboratory diagnosis is based on results of total T_4, free T_4, T_3, and TSH levels.

- Normal value of serum thyroid hormone
  - T_4: 4.8 to 13.2 mg/dL
  - Free T_4: 0.9 to 2 ng/dL
  - T_3: 80 to 220 ng/dL
  - TSH: 0.35 to 5.50 μIU/mL

Diagnosis is straightforward in overt cases. In subclinical cases, diagnosis is less clear. Benefit of treatment in the absence of symptoms is debated. Elevated TSH with normal T_4 suggests subclinical state. Accepted normal range for TSH is quite broad: 0.35 to 5.50 μIU/mL (conventional approach does not treat unless TSH is above 10 μIU/mL).

Laboratory Findings in Thyroid Disease

Disease	Primary Hypothyroidism	Secondary Hypothyroidism	Tertiary Hypothyroidism	Peripheral Hypothyroidism
THRH	High to normal	High	Low to normal	Normal to high
TSH	High	Normal to low	Low to normal	Normal to high
Free T_4	Low	Low	Low	Normal
Free T_3	Low to normal	Low to normal	Low to normal	Low
Reverse T_3	Normal	Normal	Low to normal	Normal to high

T_3, triiodothyronine; T_4, thyroxine; THRH, thyroid hormone–releasing hormone; TSH, thyroid-stimulating hormone.

Patients with a combination of subclinical hypothyroidism and objective signs of autoimmune thyroiditis can benefit from TSH reduction. This can be achieved through diet and lifestyle changes and possible thyroid replacement therapy.

THERAPEUTIC CONSIDERATIONS

Although conventional diagnostic model might be too restrictive, relying solely on symptoms or BBT to determine who needs treatment often leads to many attempts ending in side effects and no benefits. If these are the sole factors for determining dose increases, many patients will end up on dangerous supraphysiologic doses. Adult patients at full physiologic doses (2 to 2.5 gr) who have TSH scores below 1.0 might be receiving maximal improvement from thyroid treatment. Because superphysiologic doses speed rate of T_4 degradation, further increases will not yield lasting benefit. Also, chronically suppressed TSH raises risk of dementia, atrial fibrillation, and osteoporosis. Patients with hypothyroid syndrome have a positive clinical response to thyroid treatment when they have all of the following characteristics:

- Objective signs of early Hashimoto's—positive serum antibodies or abnormalities on thyroid anatomy during examination or ultrasound.
- Pertinent hypothyroid symptoms—Colorado study.
- Suboptimal thyroid blood levels. TSH above 2.5 raises likelihood of Hashimoto's and hypothyroid symptoms.

Patients with less-sensitive symptoms—overweight, depression, or poor libido—who the aforementioned three criteria will respond poorly to thyroid treatment, even if they demonstrate low BBT or delayed Achilles tendon reflex.

Diet and Food Allergy

A clear correlation exists among autoimmunity, intestinal permeability, and food allergy. Roughly 2% of patients with celiac disease have overt autoimmune thyroid disease. Serologic autoantibody markers become undetectable 6 months after a gluten-free diet is started. Use an elimination diet and/or detoxification regimen (*Textbook*, "Food Allergies") to decrease antigen load, strengthen gut integrity, and normalize autoantibody activity in autoimmune thyroid patients.

Physiologic and Hormonal Considerations

Thyroxine-binding globulin (TBG) from the liver transports thyroid hormones, including 75% of circulating T_4. Factors increasing TBG include excess estrogens (as in pregnancy, oral estrogens of birth control pills and hormone replacement therapy), tamoxifen for breast cancer, and liver diseases. High TBG reduces free thyroid

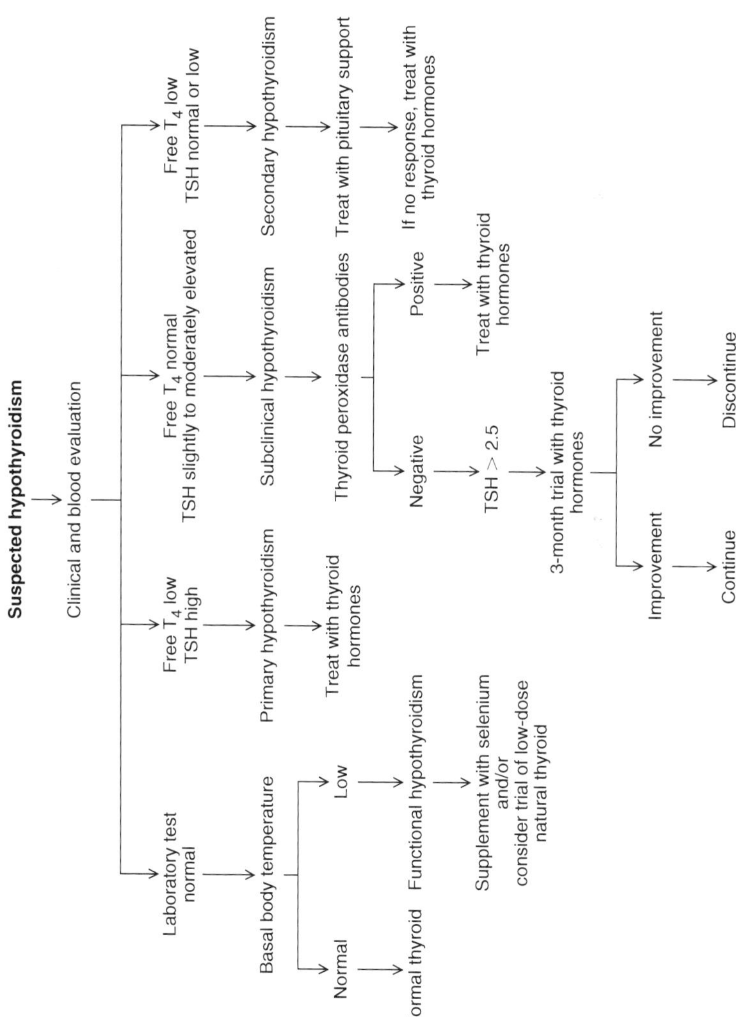
Suspected hypothyroidism
Clinical and blood evaluation
Laboratory test normal
Free T_4 low TSH high
Free T_4 normal TSH slightly to moderately elevated
Free T_4 low TSH normal or low
Basal body temperature
Normal
Normal thyroid
Low
Functional hypothyroidism
Supplement with selenium and/or consider trial of low-dose natural thyroid
Primary hypothyroidism
Treat with thyroid hormones
Subclinical hypothyroidism
Thyroid peroxidase antibodies
Negative
TSH > 2.5
3-month trial with thyroid hormones
Improvement
Continue
No improvement
Discontinue
Positive
Treat with thyroid hormones
Secondary hypothyroidism
Treat with pituitary support
If no response, treat with thyroid hormones

hormone availability, worsening hypothyroidism. Depending on clinical picture, consider moderating estrogen excess by decreasing intake of oral estrogens or using nonoral regimens to bypass the liver first pass and/or helping liver metabolism of estrogens.

Nutritional Considerations

Nutritionally support the thyroid gland with key nutrients required for synthesis of thyroid hormone. Avoid goitrogens.

- **Iodine, tyrosine, and goitrogens:** thyroid hormones are made from iodine and the amino acid tyrosine. The recommended daily allowance for iodine in adults is quite small: 150 mcg. Average intake of iodine in the United States is more than 600 mcg q.d. Too much iodine inhibits hormone synthesis. The only function of iodine in the body is thyroid synthesis. Dietary levels or iodine supplements should not exceed 600 mcg q.d. for any length of time. Goitrogens combine with iodine, making it unavailable to thyroid. Cooking inactivates goitrogens. Goitrogenic foods should not be eaten in excess.
- **Vitamins and minerals:**
  - — Zinc (Zn), vitamin E, and vitamin A function together to manufacture thyroid hormone. A deficiency of any of these reduces the amount of active hormone produced. Low Zn level is common in the elderly, as is hypothyroidism.
  - — Riboflavin (B_2), niacin (B_3), pyridoxine (B_6), and vitamin C are necessary for hormone synthesis.
  - — Zn, copper (Cu), and selenium (Se) are required cofactors for iodothyronine iodinase enzyme converting T_4 to T_3. Each form requires a different trace mineral. Supplementation with Zn reestablishes normal thyroid function in Zn-deficient hypothyroid patients even though serum T_4 is normal.
  - — Areas of the world where Se is deficient have a greater incidence of thyroid disease. Se deficiency does not decrease conversion of T_4 to T_3 in thyroid or pituitary, but it does decrease conversion of T_4 to T_3 in peripheral cells. People with Se deficiency have elevated T_4 and TSH. Se supplements decrease T_4 and TSH and normalize thyroid activity. Se decreases thyroid antibodies in thyroid autoimmunity. Se is deficient in 50% of the population's diets. Se deficiency induces low cellular thyroid activity despite normal or elevated hormone.
- Antioxidants (vitamin C, vitamin E, *Curcuma longa* [turmeric] extract) increase thyroid function in animal studies, with

decreased abnormal thyroid weight changes, less suppression of T_4 and T_3, and attenuated increases in cholesterol. Thyroid hormone abnormalities correlated with decreased glutathione in testicular tissues. No human studies exist to corroborate these findings; consider these safe components in an anti-inflammatory antioxidant regimen.

Exercise

Exercise stimulates thyroid secretion and increases tissue sensitivity to thyroid hormone. Many health benefits of exercise may result from improved thyroid function. Exercise is especially important in dieting overweight hypothyroid patients. A consistent effect of dieting is decreased metabolic rate as the body strives to conserve fuel. Exercise prevents decline in metabolic rate in response to dieting.

Thyroid Hormone Replacement

If more-conservative measures fail, exogenous thyroid hormones are necessary. Several preparations are available, each with advantages and disadvantages. Conventional treatment: oral tetraiodothyronine/l-evothyroxine sodium (T_4). Levothyroxine preparations are bioidentical to human T_4 and readily absorbed. The half-life of T_4 is 7 days; once-daily administration is adequate. For maximum and consistent absorption, take thyroid hormones at least ½ hour before food and beverages other than water. Morning administration is preferred, to mimic circadian thyroid cycle.

Titrate dose to reduce TSH to normal range and to elevate T_4 to normal.

- Common starting dose: 50 mcg (0.05 mg)
- Common ending doses: 88 to 137 mcg for women and 100 to 150 mcg for men

Some patients remaining clinically hypothyroid may poorly deiodinate levothyroxine (T_4) into T_3. Give oral T_3 to these patients. One is liothyronine (Cytomel). T_3 is well absorbed orally and easily bound by many nutrients. T_3 half-life is 2½ days; once-daily administration still works. Commonly used doses are 5 or 10 mcg daily.

Naturopathic physicians prefer natural desiccated thyroid (NDT), complete with all thyroid hormones—T_4, T_3, T_2, amino acids, and micronutrients (0.2% iodine per tablet). Normal tissue levels of T_4 and T_3 are achieved only with infusion of T_4 and T_3, not by T_4 alone. Many patients treated with desiccated thyroid tend to feel better.

- **Preparations containing only T_4** (Synthroid, Levothroid): advantages include consistent potency and prolonged duration of action. T_3 is rarely used alone; it is four times more potent with shorter duration of action than T_4.
- **Desiccated thyroid:** advantage is that it provides T_4 and T_3, plus relevant amino acids and micronutrients. Drawback: it lacks consistency of potency. By United States Pharmacopoeia standard, these preparations must contain at least 85% and not more than 115% of labeled amount of T_4 and at least 90% and not more than 110% for T_3; labeled amount is 38 mg T_4 and 9 mg T_3 per grain (65 mg).
- **Synthetic mixtures of T_4 and T_3 (Liotrix, Thyrolar)**: in similar ratios provide consistency that whole NDT lacks.
- **Equivalencies** (1 thyroid unit) for thyroid agents based on clinical response:
  - — 100 mcg of T_4 (e.g., Synthroid)
  - — 20 to 25 mcg T_3 (e.g., Cytomel)
  - — 1 grain desiccated thyroid
  - — 12.5 mcg T_4 plus 50 mcg T_4 (e.g., Thyrolar)

  (Note: 0.5 thyroid units would be equal to 50% of the values shown in the list.)
- **Food fiber:** may interfere with absorption and bioavailability of oral thyroid supplements.
- **Lifestyle and diet changes:** implement along with hormone replacement to improve lipid profile.

THERAPEUTIC APPROACH

Natural treatment strategies are tailored to specifics of pathologic condition: autoimmunity, Wilson's syndrome, or subclinical or overt hypothyroidism.

Treatments for Autoimmune Hypothyroidism (Hashimoto's Disease)

- **Thyroid replacement:** normalizes thyroid hormone levels and suppresses thyroid activity, decreasing autoimmune processes. Use desiccated or synthetic thyroid in high enough doses to decrease TSH to at or near zero. Some literature reports that TSH values of 0.1 μIU/mL or lower are linked to atrial fibrillation and bone density loss but not additional fracture. Desiccated thyroid stimulates blocking antibodies to antithyroid antibodies and acts as decoy for thyroid antibodies. Some patients recover from Hashimoto's disease after extended thyroid treatment and no longer need replacement. Some patients may not benefit from desiccated thyroid (adverse reaction to antigenic thyroid substances). Use synthetic thyroid promptly. Use frequent TSH and antibody tests to verify suppression of thyroid activity and monitor autoimmunity. Caveat: early in Hashimoto's disease, hyperthyroidism often occurs. In this case replacement is contraindicated.

- **Diet and lifestyle:** food elimination, detoxification, and gut healing options may ameliorate root factor of antigenic autoimmunity.
- **Other recommendations:**
  — Dehydroepiandrosterone (DHEA) is beneficial in autoimmunity. Clinical studies used high doses (100 to 200 mg q.d.), but consider much lower physiologic range of 5 to 10 mg q.d. or 10 to 20 mg q.d. in women and men, respectively. Side effects of high doses: hirsutism and acne. Start at low level; increase slowly and monitor DHEA blood levels and clinical symptoms of excess androgens. Effects of long-term DHEA are unknown; use with caution, particularly in patients at risk for hormone-dependent cancers.
  — Se at 200 mcg q.d. for Hashimoto's disease, especially in patients with high titers of anti–thyroid peroxidase antibodies.

Treatments for Nonautoimmune Overt or Subclinical Hypothyroid Disorder

- **Diet:** low in goitrogens. Organic foods are richer in trace minerals needed for thyroid hormone production and activation. When eaten, these foods must be cooked to break down goitrogens. Eat sources of iodine: sea fish, sea vegetables (kelp, dulse, arame, hijiki, nori, wakame, kombu), iodized salt. Eat sources of Zn: seafood (oysters), beef, oatmeal, chicken, liver, spinach, nuts, seeds. Cu sources: liver, organ meats, eggs, yeast, beans, nuts, seeds. B vitamin sources: yeast, whole grains, liver. Se source: unshelled Brazil nuts.
- **Supplements:**
  — Zn: 20 to 30 mg elemental Zn q.d. (picolinate)
  — Cu: 1 to 2.5 elemental Cu mg q.d.
  — Se: 200 to 400 mcg elemental Se q.d.

— Vitamin C: 1 to 3 g q.d. in divided doses
— Vitamin E: 200 to 400 IU q.d. (mixed tocopherols)

- **Thyroid hormones:** begin at levels ranging from 0.5 to 2 thyroid units (see earlier) q.d. based on patient's size and serum hormone levels. Reevaluate BBT, TSH, T_4, T_3, and free T_4 4 to 6 weeks later. Treatment goal: normalize BBT and serum hormone levels. After stabilizing dose, periodically evaluate based on individual needs or at least annually. In subclinical hypothyroidism, limit dose to 0.5 thyroid units daily for first 3 months. Administer hormones on empty stomach to increase absorption. Avoid taking thyroid concurrently with other medicines and supplements (especially iron) that affect absorption. Once-daily administration gives stable increases in hormone levels. Dose during pregnancy: increased because estrogens increase serum TBG. Monitor carefully during pregnancy. Dose requirements increase by 30% to 50% during pregnancy and return to prepregnancy levels after delivery.
- **Exercise, physical therapy, lifestyle:** invigorating water sports, avoidance of overheated environments, and cold hydrotherapy can stimulate thyroid function.

Infectious Diarrhea

DIAGNOSTIC SUMMARY

- Increased bowel movement frequency (usually more than three bowel movements per day)
- Increased stool liquidity
- Abdominal pain
- Sense of fecal urgency
- Fecal incontinence
- Perianal discomfort
- Possible blood and/or mucus in stool

GENERAL CONSIDERATIONS

Clinical syndromes of diarrheal disease are acute watery diarrhea, bloody diarrhea, and persistent diarrhea. Features include daily stool production of more than 250 g containing 70% to 95% water. More than 14 L of fluid may be lost daily in severe cases. Dysentery is defined by low volume, pain, and bloody stool. Diarrheal illness commonly causes morbidity and mortality. Intestinal infection is most common cause of diarrhea worldwide, killing 3 to 4 million persons annually, most of whom (2 million) are preschool children. Ninety percent of acute cases are mild, self-limited, and responsive within 5 days to simple rehydration or antidiarrheal agents.

INFECTIOUS AGENTS AND SYMPTOMS

Categories of etiologic pathogens are viral, bacterial, and parasitic. Diarrhea arises from inhibition of intestinal absorption, increased secretion, and inflammatory response to promote secretory and exudative response.

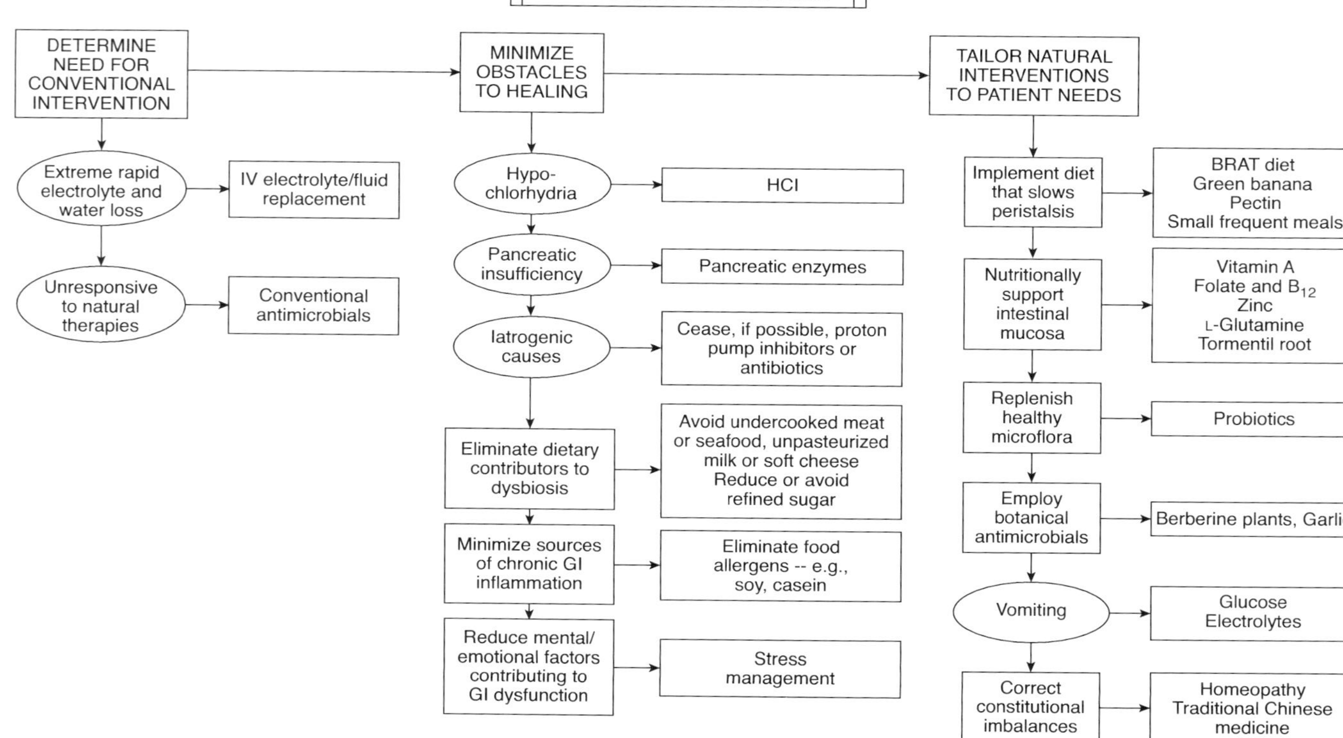
INFECTIOUS DIARRHEA
DETERMINE NEED FOR CONVENTIONAL INTERVENTION
Extreme rapid electrolyte and water loss
IV electrolyte/fluid replacement
Unresponsive to natural therapies
Conventional antimicrobials
MINIMIZE OBSTACLES TO HEALING
Hypo-chlorhydria
HCl
Pancreatic insufficiency
Pancreatic enzymes
Iatrogenic causes
Cease, if possible, proton pump inhibitors or antibiotics
Eliminate dietary contributors to dysbiosis
Avoid undercooked meat or seafood, unpasteurized milk or soft cheese
Reduce or avoid refined sugar
Minimize sources of chronic GI inflammation
Eliminate food allergens -- e.g., soy, casein
Reduce mental/emotional factors contributing to GI dysfunction
Stress management
TAILOR NATURAL INTERVENTIONS TO PATIENT NEEDS
Implement diet that slows peristalsis
BRAT diet
Green banana
Pectin
Small frequent meals
Nutritionally support intestinal mucosa
Vitamin A
Folate and B12
Zinc
L-Glutamine
Tormentil root
Replenish healthy microflora
Probiotics
Employ botanical antimicrobials
Berberine plants, Garlic
Vomiting
Glucose
Electrolytes
Correct constitutional imbalances
Homeopathy
Traditional Chinese medicine

Viral Agents

In healthy adults, clinical manifestation is acute, self-limited gastroenteritis. Twenty-five different types of bacteria and protozoa can cause an identical clinical syndrome; more than 75% of diarrhea-associated cases of gastroenteritis are caused by viruses. Suspect viruses when vomiting is prominent, incubation period is longer than 14 hours, entire illness is over in less than 72 hours, no warning signs of bacterial infection are present (high fever, bloody diarrhea, severe abdominal pain, more than six stools per 24 hours), and no epidemiologic clues can be gleaned from the history (e.g., travel, sexual contact, antibiotic use).

- **Rotavirus:** ubiquitous agent of acute, dehydrating diarrhea in children that causes more than 800,000 annual deaths of young children in developing countries. Disease is seasonal (in the United States it begins in autumn and ends in spring in the southwest and northeast). Transmission is by the fecal-oral route, including person to person. Virions infect villous enterocytes of the small intestine, causing watery diarrhea, fever, and vomiting.
- **Parvovirus (Norwalk virus):** caliciviruses (Norwalk-like viruses or small, round-structured viruses) cause 66% of 13.8 million cases of food-related illnesses in the United States annually. Suspect these viruses when acute gastroenteritis sweeps a semiclosed community (e.g., family, school, residential home, hospital, ship, dormitory). Transmission is by contaminated food or water or person to person. Sources of outbreaks include well water, raspberries, lunchmeat, oysters. Symptoms are nausea and vomiting, diarrhea, abdominal cramping, headache, low-grade fever, malaise, myalgias.
- **Cytomegalovirus:** is present latently in most people from birth or from sexual or parenteral exposure. It emerges from latency as a result of strong allergenic or antigenic stimulation of the immune system or severe immunodeficiency. Viral activity in the bowel wall triggers gastrointestinal disease in AIDS, transplantation, and cancer chemotherapy.
- **Epstein-Barr virus (EBV):** almost all adults are infected by age 20 years. It infects B cells and persists for life because B cells proliferate indefinitely. Proliferation is controlled by virus-specific cytotoxic T lymphocytes. EBV causes diarrhea in immunocompromised patients.

Bacterial Agents

- ***Escherichia coli:*** four varieties of diarrheagenic *E. coli* are enterotoxigenic, enterohemorrhagic, enteroinvasive, enteroadherent.

In North America the most prominent is the enterohemorrhagic serotype *E. coli* O157:H7. Transmission is by contaminated ground beef. Incubation period is 1 to 8 days. Symptoms are abdominal cramping and diarrhea—mild, moderate, or severe. Bowel movements begin as loose and watery, eventually with gross blood. Some patients (children) develop life-threatening hemolytic uremic syndrome, characterized by triad of hemolytic anemia, renal failure, and thrombocytopenia.

- ***Campylobacter jejuni:*** native intestinal flora of many mammals. Transmission is by contaminated, improperly cooked meat, unpasteurized dairy, and contaminated water. Incubation period is 1 to 7 days after ingestion. Symptoms include fever, headache, and malaise followed by diarrhea and abdominal cramps within 1 to 2 days. Stools are watery to bloody. *Campylobacter* enterocolitis is usually acute and self-limited over 7 to 10 days. Rarely relapses, complications, severe disease, and death may occur.
- ***Clostridium difficile:*** most common cause of infectious diarrhea in hospitalized patients, especially the elderly. It can be catalyzed by antibiotics.
- ***Salmonella (Enterobacteriaceae):*** has 2200 known serotypes (*Salmonella enteritidis* in 85% of all *Salmonella* cases in the United States; *Salmonella* Typhi and *Salmonella* Paratyphi, which are responsible for typhoid fever). Transmission is by contaminated food. Symptoms of nontyphoid salmonellosis include fever; gastroenteritis-related diarrhea; localized infections of the gastrointestinal tract, endothelium, pericardium, meninges, lungs, joints, bones, urinary tract, or soft tissues. Typhoidal symptoms include gradual onset of fever, headache, arthralgias, pharyngitis, constipation, anorexia, and abdominal discomfort.
- ***Shigella (Enterobacteriaceae):*** ingesting as few as 10 organisms may cause clinical disease. Transmission is by contaminated food or water, person to person, and flies. Incubation period is 1 to 4 days. Symptoms in adults are nonbloody diarrhea with or without fever, gripping abdominal pain, urgency, relief with defecation. Episodes may increase, with mucus and blood in stool. Mild cases often spontaneously resolve in 4 to 8 days; 3 to 6 weeks may be necessary in severe cases.
- ***Yersinia enterocolitica (Enterobacteriaceae):*** one of the less-frequent causes of bacterial enterocolitis in North America. Transmission is by fecally contaminated food or water and contaminated blood products. Incubation is 4 to 7 days. Symptoms are watery to bloody diarrhea. *Yersinia* invades lymphoid tissues,

causing mesenteric lymphadenitis that mimics acute appendicitis. Resolution is 1 to 4 weeks, but complicating septicemia may develop in patients with underlying disease.
- ***Laribacter hongkongensis:*** a novel genus and species first isolated recently from blood and empyema pus of cirrhotic patient with bacteremic empyema thoracis. It was also identified in six diarrhea patients in Hong Kong and Switzerland.

Parasitic Agents

Diarrheal diseases caused by parasites (protozoa, helminths) are the greatest single worldwide cause of illness and death. Poor sanitation in undeveloped nations, worldwide travel, and migration to the United States are the most common cause of spread.

- ***Giardia lamblia:*** most frequent cause of parasitic enteritis in the United States, with history of recent hiking and drinking out of streams.
- **Waterborne infection:** in developed nations, from domestic water contaminated with cysts of *Giardia intestinalis* and *Cryptosporidium parvum.*
- **Other diarrhea-linked parasites:** *Entamoeba histolytica, Microsporidia,* Cystoisospora belli, *Strongyloides* species.
- **Symptoms:** abdominal pain, cramping, explosive diarrhea, but not in every case. They can be milder. Some cases of irritable bowel syndrome, indigestion, and poor digestion are caused by parasites. Parasites are an unsuspected cause of chronic illness and fatigue.

LABORATORY DIAGNOSIS

- Tests include bacterial cultures using selective media, detection of pathogen-specific genes using polymerase chain reaction, electron microscopy and antigen detection for viruses, and direct examination with or without special stains for protozoa.
- Microbial cause is identified in only 50% of patients. In descending order, the most commonly identified pathogens are *C. jejuni, Salmonella, Shigella, E. coli* O157:H7.
- Important independent variables predictive of positive stool culture in adult patients with clinical picture of infectious diarrhea: month of presentation, fever, duration of abdominal pain at presentation, and requirement of intravenous (IV) fluid therapy. Neither a history of bloody diarrhea nor persistent diarrhea is associated with positive stool culture.

- Consider testing if patient is febrile or has bloody stool. With visible blood present in stool, one third of cases were caused by Shiga toxin–producing *E. coli* O157:H7.
- Ova and parasite testing has very low yield in most cases; run only when diarrheal illness has persisted for longer than 7 days.

THERAPEUTIC CONSIDERATIONS

Conventional Medicines

- Antibiotics and opiates are appropriate in certain cases but adversely affect gastrointestinal motility. Resistance to antimicrobials, with risk of worsened illness (hemolytic uremic syndrome with Shiga toxin–producing *E. coli* O157:H7), complicates antimicrobial and antimotility drug use, especially in children.
- Selective antibiotics treat traveler's diarrhea, shigellosis, and *Campylobacter.*
- Bismuth salts (e.g., Pepto-Bismol) for travel abroad; they coat the intestinal lining and help prevent infection.
- Antibiotic therapy benefits in salmonellosis and *E. coli* O157:H7 remains unclear.
- Avoid antimotility agents in bloody diarrhea, especially for *E. coli* O157:H7, which could increase risk of subsequent hemolytic uremic syndrome. In selected at-risk populations, vaccines, including oral typhoid vaccine and cholera vaccine (available only outside the United States), are recommended.
- 5-HT_2 and 5-HT_3 receptor antagonists, calcium-calmodulin antagonists, and alpha-receptor agonists may avoid adverse affects on gastrointestinal motility.

Underlying and Predisposing Factors

Host factors that predispose to illness include the following:

- Poor digestive function, including low stomach acid and/or achlorhydria and inadequate pancreatic enzymes. Hydrochloric acid and pancreatic enzymes may be advisable.
- Immunoglobulin A (IgA) antibodies discourage epithelial adherence of pathogens. Depressed secretory IgA weakens gastrointestinal immunity. Decreased intestinal motility, caused by chronic stress and high sugar intake, allows microbes to fester. Food allergy or sensitivity encourages recurrent infectious diarrhea.

- Some pharmaceuticals increase susceptibility to infectious diarrhea: proton pump inhibitors, antifolate drugs, and antibiotics. Hospitalized patients taking proton pump inhibitors have increased risk of *C. difficile* diarrhea. Drug inhibition of stomach acid allows pathogens and undigested food to reach intestines without proper processing. Broad-spectrum antibiotics are associated with diarrhea. Antibiotics disrupt local bowel flora, allowing pathogens to flourish (see section Probiotics: Lactobacillus and Saccharomyces).

Hydration and Electrolyte Balance

- Keep diarrhea patient well hydrated; ensure electrolyte replenishment, especially in children.
- Signs of dehydration: decreased or absent urination, decreased skin turgor, dry tongue.
- Rehydrate with solutions of glucose, sodium, and potassium.
- IV rehydration: severe dehydration with weight loss of more than 10% or unconsciousness.

Diet

- Prevention: avoid undercooked meat or seafood, unpasteurized milk, and soft cheese.
- BRAT diet (binding foods that slow peristalsis) helps decrease gastrointestinal motility: bananas, white rice, apples, plain white toast or bread, and tea.
- Larger, less-frequent meals are more taxing to gastrointestinal digestive and absorptive capacities, prolong diarrhea, advance colonization by hemolytic enteropathogenic *E. coli,* and prolong shedding of rotavirus. Dividing same nutrient intake into small, equal portions eaten at regular intervals produces less-severe response.
- Traditional preparations for diarrhea (carrot soup, rice) are absorbent and reduce stool output and duration of diarrhea but may not diminish loss of water and electrolytes.
- Green banana and pectin contain nondigestible dietary precursors to colonic short-chain fatty acids. Treatment with cooked green banana reduces intestinal permeability. Pectin produces similar results. In male infants, commonly allergenic soy- and casein-based diets were not helpful in alleviating persistent diarrhea; yogurt and broken-down amino acid formulas were helpful in encouraging reduction in stool output and duration of diarrhea.
- For vomiting patients, small amounts of glucose can help.

Supplements

- **Vitamin A:** 60 mg can reduce incidence of persistent diarrhea in children without changing duration or average stool frequency. Children who are not breastfed have shorter duration of diarrhea. Mean number of stools passed, proportion of episodes lasting more than 14 days, and percentage of children passing watery stools were lower in those treated with vitamin A.
- **Folic acid and B_{12}:** low levels of folic acid and vitamin B_{12} correlate with increased susceptibility to diarrhea. Folate deficiency promotes malabsorption because of altered structure of intestinal mucosal cells—inflammation, atrophy, erosion, flattening of villi, lymphatic ectasia, and focal fibrosis. Antifolate chemotherapeutic drugs (methotrexate) induce folate and B_{12} deficiency, triggering diarrhea. Supplements reduce toxicity and abolish treatment-related deaths without affecting drug efficacy. Gastrointestinal disturbances (diarrhea) reduce availability of folate and B_{12} to pregnant mother and fetus, increasing risk of birth defects. One or more episodes of periconceptional diarrhea increase risk of neural tube defect, independent of fever, obesity, maternal age, maternal birthplace, income, prior unproductive pregnancy, and dietary plus multivitamin folate intake. Regardless of cause of diarrhea, ensure proper folic acid and B_{12} nutrition in women likely to conceive and pregnant women. Be aware that large amounts of folic acid can mask nerve damage associated with vitamin B_{12} deficiency.
- **Zinc (Zn):** diarrhea is a clinical manifestation of Zn deficiency. Zn has antimicrobial effect on enteric pathogens (*Salmonella* Typhi, *Salmonella, E. coli, Enterobacter, Shigella, Staphylococcus albus, Streptococcus pyogenes, Vibrio cholerae*) and may be a tool to treat diarrhea. Zn absorption occurs throughout the small intestine, not only in the duodenum, jejunum, and ileum. Many illnesses noted to cause chronic diarrhea (celiac disease, cystic fibrosis) entail malabsorption of Zn. Dietary sources of Zn include meat, fish, and human milk. Acrodermatitis enteropathica (skin lesions, chronic diarrhea, recurring infections) is related to intestinal malabsorption of Zn and is treated with pharmacologic doses of oral Zn. Factors influencing Zn absorption are dietary fiber and phytates (in soy, wheat bran, peas, carob, brown rice), which inhibit absorption; picolinic and citric acid facilitate it. Citric acid is the ligand linked to high bioavailability of Zn in human milk. *Caution:* Some dietary treatments for persistent postenteritis diarrhea (eliminating cow's milk, increasing fiber, using carob powder, using soy formula for infants) can

contribute to Zn deficiency and promote persistence of diarrhea itself. Supplement Zn during diarrhea.

- **L-Glutamine:** most abundant amino acid in blood and major fuel of intestinal mucosal cells; readily available in diet and synthesized in body. Supplementation improves metabolism of mucosa, stimulating regeneration. Glutamine prevents mucosal damage and decreases bacterial leakage across mucosal membranes, after damage, by stimulating repair. Applicability: enhancing repair of mucosal injury by infections, toxic agents, malnutrition, or chemotherapy- or radiation-induced enteritis. Glutamine enhances sodium and water absorption in animal models of infectious diarrhea. At dose of 0.3 g/kg/day, glutamine shortens duration of diarrhea in children. Even at high doses, it is without side effects and is well tolerated. Typical dose is 1000 mg t.i.d. (*Textbook,* "Glutamine").

Probiotics: *Lactobacillus* and *Saccharomyces*

- Species: *Lactobacillus acidophilus* and *Bifidobacterium bifidum* (plus *Lactobacillus casei, Lactobacillus fermentum, Lactobacillus salivarius, Lactobacillus brevis*). (*Textbook,* "Probiotics.")
- Probiotics protect against acute diarrheal disease and treat or prevent infectious diarrhea: rotavirus, *C. difficile,* traveler's diarrhea. They may prevent future nosocomial rotaviral gastroenteritis with immune-modulating effect of increasing number of cells secreting IgA.
- *Lactobacillus* species inhibit *E. coli* O157:H7 but not *Salmonella* in refrigerated storage.
- Children are especially susceptible to infectious diarrhea and its sequelae. Supplementing formula with *B. bifidum* and *Streptococcus thermophilus* dramatically reduces risk of developing diarrhea and rotavirus shedding. Probiotics may provide protective effects similar to breast milk to prevent infection. *Lactobacillus rhamnosus* may reduce risk of nosocomial diarrhea and rotavirus gastroenteritis in children.
- *Saccharomyces boulardii (Saccharomyces cerevisiae)* is a nonpathogenic probiotic yeast helpful in diarrhea of *C. difficile* affecting the elderly. Vancomycin is conventional treatment in severe cases. But *S. boulardii,* alone or in combination with vancomycin, is effective for recurrent infection. Fungemia and sepsis are rare complications of *S. boulardii* in immunocompromised patients, and *S. boulardii* may be contraindicated. Daily adult dose is 1 g in divided doses (500 mg b.i.d.) for 4 or more weeks.

- Probiotics reduce the risk of antibiotic-induced diarrhea and reduce hospital stay from diarrhea. *L. acidophilus* corrects increase of gram-negative bacteria after broad-spectrum antibiotics, which occurs with any acute or chronic diarrhea. Mixture of *B. bifidum* and *L. acidophilus* inhibits lowering of fecal flora induced by ampicillin and maintains equilibrium of intestinal ecosystem.
- Use of *L. acidophilus* during antibiotic therapy may prevent reductions of friendly bacteria and/or superinfection with antibiotic-resistant flora. Dose is 15 to 20 billion organisms. Take probiotics as far away from antibiotics as possible.
- Antibiotics should be used only when benefits outweigh risks; adjunctive therapy may decrease untoward effects of antibiotics on gastrointestinal system.
- Choose only high-quality, laboratory-tested probiotics.

Botanical Medicines

Berberine-Containing Plants

- Goldenseal *(Hydrastis canadensis)*, barberry *(Berberis vulgaris)*, Oregon grape *(Berberis aquifolium)*, and goldthread *(Coptis chinensis)* contain broad-spectrum antibiotic alkaloid berberine, effective against bacteria, protozoa, and fungi, including *Candida albicans.*
- Berberine's action against some pathogens is stronger than that of common antibiotics. Berberine prevents overgrowth of yeast. Berberine has remarkable antidiarrheal activity in even severe cases of cholera, amebiasis, giardiasis, *E. coli, Shigella, Salmonella, Klebsiella,* and chronic candidiasis.
- Dose is based on berberine content. Standardized extracts are preferred. Dose (t.i.d.):
  - — Dried root or as infusion (tea): 2 to 4 g
  - — Tincture (1:5): 6 to 12 mL (1.5 to 3 tsp)
  - — Fluid extract (1:1): 2 to 4 mL (0.5 to 1 tsp)
  - — Solid (powdered dry) extract (4:1 or 8% to 12% alkaloid content): 250 to 500 mg
  - — Note: Dose recommendations for berberine are 25 to 50 mg t.i.d. or daily up to 150 mg for adults. For children, dose is based on body weight. Daily dose: 5 to 10 mg berberine/kg (2.2 pounds) body weight.
- Berberine and berberine-containing plants are nontoxic at recommended doses, but avoid during pregnancy. Higher doses may interfere with B vitamin metabolism.

***Potentilla tormentilla* (Tormentil Root)**

- Contains more than 15% tannic acid, an astringent to treat infectious diarrhea, shorten rotavirus diarrhea, and decrease requirement for rehydration solutions.
- Dose in children: 3 drops tormentil root extract per year of age t.i.d. until diarrhea ends or for a maximum of 5 days.
- Dose for adults: 60 drops of tincture b.i.d.
- Powdered herb may be more effective. Dose: ¼ tsp b.i.d. for adults.

***Allium sativum* (Garlic)**

- Garlic affects DNA and RNA synthesis and is being investigated as an antibiotic.
- In vitro antimicrobial sensitivity is confirmed for *E. coli, Shigella* species, *Salmonella* species, and *Proteus mirabilis.*
- Gram-negative diarrheagenic pathogens from stool samples are highly sensitive to garlic. Few tested intestinal pathogens are resistant to garlic.

Other Antiparasitic Botanicals

Future studies should evaluate potential benefits and toxicities of these antiparasitic herbs: *Artemisia absinthium* (wormwood), *Dysphania ambrosioides* (wormseed), *Curcuma longa* (turmeric), *Phytolacca decandra* (pokeweed, pokeroot), *Juglans* species (black and white walnut), and *Tanacetum vulgare* (tansy). Curcumin protects against castor oil– and carrageenan-induced diarrhea in rat models. The Brazilian *Ocimum selloi* essential oil reduces severity and frequency of diarrhea produced by castor oil and also reduces transit time in mice. A Thai herbal formula, Pikutbenjakul—containing *Piper longum, Piper sarmentosum, Piper interruptum, Plumbago indica,* and *Zingiber officinale*—is effective in vitro against some *Vibrio* species, *Salmonella, Shigella, E. coli,* and *Staphylococcus aureus.* Human clinical trials are lacking.

THERAPEUTIC APPROACH

Natural treatments can manage most cases of non–life-threatening diarrhea. Diarrhea itself is an eliminative function that clears toxins and should not be completely suppressed. Chronic diarrhea and diarrhea causing extreme or rapid electrolyte and water loss may require conventional interventions. Maintain hydration and electrolyte balance, especially in children younger than 5 years.

Address the following underlying factors:

- Low stomach and pancreatic output; depressed IgA.
- Eliminate iatrogenic causes (proton pump inhibitors and antibiotics) if possible.

- Reduce refined sugar.
- Eliminate food allergens.
- Reduce and manage stress.

Monitor closely by standard laboratory methods (e.g., repeat multiple stool samples 2 weeks after initiation of therapy).

Diet: BRAT diet to discourage large volume loss in infectious diarrhea. Green banana and pectin fiber might be useful. Yogurt may be helpful. Very small frequent meals, hourly if possible, with glucose administered in case of vomiting. Avoid soy, casein, and other known allergenic foods.

Nutritional Supplements

The following doses are for adults unless otherwise indicated:

- **Vitamin A:** 60 mg q.d. in children; up to 50,000 international units (IU) q.d. for 1 to 2 days for adults with infections. Beware doses above 10,000 IU q.d. in pregnant women.
- **Folic acid:** 1 mg q.d.
- **Vitamin B_{12}** (methylcobalamin): 600 to 1000 mcg q.d.
- **Zinc picolinate:** 30 mg elemental Zn q.d.
- **L-Glutamine: 1000 mg t.i.d**
- ***Lactobacillus species* and *Bifidobacterium species:*** 6 to 10 billion colony-forming units (CFUs) b.i.d. To prevent antibiotic-induced diarrhea: at least 15 to 20 billion organisms. Take as far away from antibiotic as possible. In children younger than 6 years with antibiotic-induced diarrhea, give probiotic every day of antibiotic administration and continue for 1 week after discontinuing antibiotic.
- ***S. boulardii:*** for *C. difficile* specifically. Daily adult dosage: 1 g q.d. in divided doses (500 mg b.i.d.) for at least 4 weeks. Can be used adjunctively with vancomycin.

Botanicals

- **Berberine:** 25 to 50 mg t.i.d. or daily dose up to 150 mg. For children, dose is based on body weight: 5 to 10 mg berberine/kg (2.2 pounds) body weight.
- **Tormentil:** 60 drops tincture b.i.d. or powdered herb: ¼ tsp b.i.d. Children: 3 drops tormentil root extract per year of age t.i.d. until discontinuation of diarrhea, or maximum of 5 days.

Infertility, Female

DIAGNOSTIC SUMMARY

- Inability to conceive a child after 12 months of regular unprotected intercourse (at least twice weekly) with the same male partner and in the absence of male causes.

GENERAL CONSIDERATIONS

- See table "Causes of Female Infertility."
- Factors in women contribute to 50% of infertility cases as primary (30%) and combined (20%) factor. In United States, one in seven couples experience this condition. After 12 months, intervention is recommended. Initiate earlier intervention for women older than 35. After age 35, women need comprehensive review and discussion about natural or assisted conception owing to age-related concerns.

Causes of Female Infertility

Ovulation disorders (40%)	Aging
	Diminished ovarian reserve
	Endocrine disorder (e.g., hypothalamic amenorrhea, hyperprolactinemia, thyroid disease, adrenal disease)
	Polycystic ovary syndrome
	Premature ovarian failure
	Tobacco use
Tubal factors (30%)	Obstruction (e.g., history of pelvic inflammatory disease, tubal surgery)
Endometriosis (15%)	

Continued

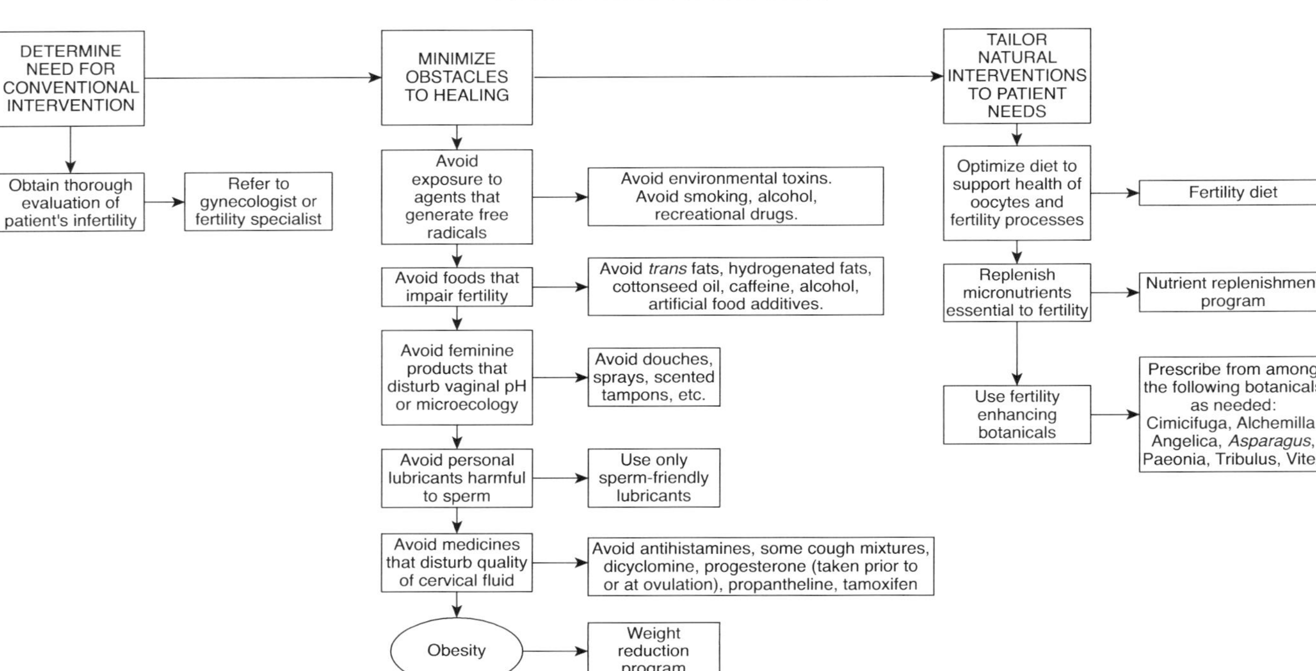
INFERTILITY, FEMALE
DETERMINE NEED FOR CONVENTIONAL INTERVENTION
Obtain thorough evaluation of patient's infertility
Refer to gynecologist or fertility specialist
MINIMIZE OBSTACLES TO HEALING
Avoid exposure to agents that generate free radicals
Avoid environmental toxins. Avoid smoking, alcohol, recreational drugs.
Avoid foods that impair fertility
Avoid trans fats, hydrogenated fats, cottonseed oil, caffeine, alcohol, artificial food additives.
Avoid feminine products that disturb vaginal pH or microecology
Avoid douches, sprays, scented tampons, etc.
Avoid personal lubricants harmful to sperm
Use only sperm-friendly lubricants
Avoid medicines that disturb quality of cervical fluid
Avoid antihistamines, some cough mixtures, dicyclomine, progesterone (taken prior to or at ovulation), propantheline, tamoxifen
Obesity
Weight reduction program
TAILOR NATURAL INTERVENTIONS TO PATIENT NEEDS
Optimize diet to support health of oocytes and fertility processes
Fertility diet
Replenish micronutrients essential to fertility
Nutrient replenishment program
Use fertility enhancing botanicals
Prescribe from among the following botanicals as needed: Cimicifuga, Alchemilla, Angelica, Asparagus, Paeonia, Tribulus, Vitex

Causes of Female Infertility—cont'd

Other (approximately 10%)	
Uterine or cervical factors (>3%)	Congenital uterine anomaly
	Fibroids
	Endometrial polyps
	Poor-quality or low-quantity cervical mucus (caused by smoking, infection); hostility of mucus (sperm antibodies)
	Uterine synechiae or adhesions (Asherman's syndrome)

Data from Jose-Miller A, Boyden JW, Frey KA. Infertility. *Am Fam Physician.* 2007;75:849-858.

- Fertility reflects general well-being. We are constructed to pass on the best genetic information; the optimal ages for reproduction are 18 to 35 years for females and 16 to 40 years for males.
- Delaying pregnancy contributes to number of childless couples. Women have optimal fertility before age 30 to 31 years. After age 31, probability of conception declines rapidly, which can be partly overcome by continued insemination for additional cycles. Probability of adverse pregnancy increases beyond age 31. Thereafter, fertility decreases, with acceleration toward age 40. In women, fertility remains stable until age 30, producing more than 400 pregnancies per 1000 exposed women per year. By age 45, fertility rate is only 100 pregnancies per 1000 exposed women.
- By age 40 to 41, half of women lose capacity for reproduction. Reproductive aging is ovarian aging—decreasing quantity and quality of pool of follicles preserved in ovaries.

What is needed for normal conception:

- Viable sperm—motility, morphology, count, DNA integrity
- Sperm transport through male genital tract and deposition in female genital tract near cervix during sexual intercourse
- Normal oocyte (ovulation) by ovaries
- Sperm and oocyte transport within female genital tract to site of fertilization in fallopian tube
- Penetration of sperm into oocyte, fertilization, development of pre-embryo, and its transport to and implantation in uterus

Fecundity is a couple's chance of conception in a single menstrual cycle.

- Normal monthly success rate for couples trying to conceive naturally at age 25 is 25% and decreases with increasing age of the woman. Male fertility declines with age as seen in semen abnormalities.

- Probability of fecundity is calculated to determine monthly chance of conception, including variables for persons. Clinical presentation may suggest blatant fertility impediments (e.g., genetic abnormality), or each partner may have minor health issues that combine into major impediments.

Integrative Infertility Treatment

Assisted Reproductive Technologies and Naturopathy

- Of U.S. infants, 4.6% were a result of ovulation treatments not involving assisted reproductive technologies (ARTs).
- ART treatments account for 1.2% of total U.S. live births, 16% of U.S. twins, 38% of U.S. triplets or higher-order live-born infants.
- Recommend the following safe, integrated treatment:
  - — Before in vitro fertilization (IVF) cycle, a 3- to 4-month preconception program for both partners to ensure proper nutritional status and detoxification to optimize successful outcome.
  - — Identify and eliminate contributing factors that may hinder success of IVF cycle.
  - — Address preexisting conditions during 3 to 4 months preconception.
- During an IVF cycle, maintain open professional communication with fertility specialist to prevent interactions. Encourage dietary and lifestyle improvements; but nutritional and/or herbal prescriptions must be made with consideration regarding potential negative interactions with IVF drugs. Individualize all prescriptions.
- After IVF and conception, modify treatment to support pregnancy, focusing on miscarriage prevention in first trimester and adjusting as pregnancy continues.

Optimizing Natural Fertility

- Assess key variables: ovulation detection and timing and frequency of intercourse.
- Before diagnosing infertility, encourage couples to attempt conception for 12 months of unprotected properly timed intercourse. Reduce time period if female is older than 35.
- A couple's fertility is highest in first few months of unprotected sex and declines gradually thereafter. If no conception within first 3 months, fecundity decreases. Couples likely to conceive do so in a few short cycles. If not, other impediments may be present.
- Encourage couples to attempt conception during fertile window. A recently ovulated egg will survive for only a few hours

(maximum of 24 hours); however, sperm can survive for up to 5 to 6 days in estrogen-supported, fertile-quality cervical fluid. The fertile window is 6-day interval ending on day of ovulation. Fertile-quality cervical fluid protects sperm from acidic pH of the vagina and provides a nutritive survival medium.

- Misconception: frequent ejaculations decrease male fertility. Semen profiles remain normal even with daily ejaculation. Abnormalities in sperm (e.g., oligozoospermia, lowered sperm count, and poor motility) may be improved with more frequent (daily) ejaculation.

Ovulation Detection

Fertility charting incorporates consideration of basal body temperature (waking temperature) and changes in both cervical fluid and cervical position.

Waking temperature is a hindsight measurement that confirms ovulation occurrence. It is able to assist only in *predicting* ovulation once a woman is aware of her cyclic changes. It is used to confirm the luteal shift to progesterone and is beneficial for assessing the lengths of the follicular and luteal phases. It is also used to assess progesterone stability in the luteal phase to support implantation and pregnancy; it can also confirm anovulatory cycles. Progesterone causes the endometrium to support the implantation of a fertilized ovum. It also causes temperature to rise perceptibly, typically 0.4°F (0.2°C). Temperature is best taken via oral assessment immediately on waking after a minimum of 6 hours of unbroken sleep.

Fertile-quality cervical fluid is produced 3 to 5 days before ovulation in response to increasing estrogen levels before the luteinizing hormone (LH) surge. Sperm can theoretically survive for 5 to 6 days in the presence of fertile-quality cervical fluid. The role of cervical fluid is multifaceted; it buffers the pH of the vagina to provide a hospitable environment for sperm survival; provides a medium for sperm to swim in on their journey through the female reproductive system; provides nutritional supplementation for sperm survival; and acts as a lubricant to increase sexual pleasure and increase frequency of intercourse, thus providing more opportunities for conception. Assessment should be conducted from the vagina (inserting a finger into the vaginal opening and extracting fluid for assessment) rather than relying on toilet paper or underwear changes.

Cervical position assessment is the most controversial of self-assessments, with reproductive specialists often discrediting its value. This is because the position of the cervix is affected by numerous variables, including the timing of bowel movements. The cervical tissue is responsive to fluctuations in estrogen and produces physical and tangible changes when ovulation is approaching. Signs of fertility include softening, opening of the cervical os, increased wetness from cervical fluid, and a lengthening of the vaginal canal as the cervix shortens away from the vaginal opening. Signs of infertility include a closed os, hardening, shortening, and dryness.

Urine-based ovulation testing detects the LH surge that occurs before ovulation, typically 24 to 36 hours before ovulation. Testing can produce false-positive results and is inadvisable in women with polycystic ovary syndrome (PCOS) or other, similar conditions because of LH increase in these populations. In addition, because sperm require an optimal 2 days' travel time, detection of the LH surge can often be too late to optimize conception. It is therefore advisable to make sure that all variables are synchronistic rather than isolated. Also, in some women the LH surge is shorter (12 hours or less). This can occur in those with hyperprolactinemia and other conditions that interfere with follicle-stimulating hormone (FSH) or LH secretion from the anterior pituitary. In these women it is advisable to encourage LH testing twice a day (i.e., morning and night), because they can often "miss" the surge.

Saliva assessment testing and tools base their justification on the premise that with increasing estrogen fluctuations, changes in cervical fluid are synchronistic with other fluid media including saliva. Fertility potential is detected by the presence of a ferning pattern in the saliva (viewed by microscopy) suggestive of a synchronicity in cervical fluid changes that enable sperm travel. This method is inappropriate for older patients owing to natural estrogen reductions and is also not optimal for hypothyroid patients because of the relationship between estrogen and thyroid function. In addition, caution with patients experiencing estrogen displacement, such as those with fibroids and/or endometriosis, is advisable.

DIAGNOSTIC CONSIDERATIONS

Female Reproductive Assessment

- Some of these assessments may require referral to a fertility specialist, gynecologist, or endocrinologist; however, primary care provider must elucidate a full history and assess causative or contributing factors.
- Screen with queries listed in tables "Fertility Assessment", "Stage 1 Investigations" and "Stage 2 Investigations"

Fertility Assessment

Assessment	Elaboration and Explanation
Age	What are the ages of the couple?
Fertility history	How long have they been trying to conceive, and have they ever conceived previously (together or separately)? Do they have any idea why they have not been able to conceive?
Sexual history	Potential sexually transmitted disease exposure, symptoms of genital inflammation (e.g., vaginal discharge, dysuria, abdominal pain, fever)
Medical history	Genetic disorders, endocrine disorders, history of pelvic inflammatory disease
Medication history	Hormone therapy, contraceptive pills, psychotropics, nonsteroidal anti-inflammatory drugs (NSAIDs)
Surgical history	Prior surgeries (e.g., previous reproductive or genitourinary surgery)
Contraception	When it was ceased and the likely speed of its reversibility
Fertile times	Whether the couple engage in regular intercourse during fertile times

Fertility Assessment—cont'd

Assessment	Elaboration and Explanation
Lifestyle factors	Diet, exercise, alcohol, smoking cessation, recreational drug use, caffeine, environmental toxin screen
Prior paternity	Previous fertility
Psychosexual issues	Interference with conception
Pubertal development	Poor progression can suggest underlying reproductive issue; initial query regarding age of menarche and secondary sexual characteristics to eliminate Turner's syndrome and the like
Physical examination	Breast formation Galactorrhea Genitalia (e.g., patency, development, masses, tenderness, discharge) Signs of hyperandrogenism (e.g., hirsutism, acne, clitoromegaly) Body mass index and waist-to-hip ratio to assess weight impact

Modified from Hechtman L. Clinical naturopathic medicine. Sydney, New South Wales, Australia: Elsevier; 2011.

Stage 1 Investigations

Assessment	Timing in Cycle	Justification
Follicle-stimulating hormone (FSH)	Day 3	Stimulates follicle development. High levels can indicate menopause or declining fertility; query primary ovarian failure. Useful to assess ratio of FSH to luteinizing hormone to ensure that hormone status is optimal. Eliminates primary ovarian failure.
Luteinizing hormone (LH)	Day 3 or preovulation (day 13)	Triggers ovulation when surges; excessive levels may indicate polycystic ovary syndrome (PCOS). Useful to assess ratio of LH to FSH to ensure hormone status is optimal.
17-OH progesterone (P4) (17-hydroxyprogesterone)	Day 21 (7 days post-ovulation)	Evaluates adequacy of progesterone, confirms ovulation. Eliminates luteal phase defect.
Prolactin (PRL)	Any day	Inhibits ovarian production of estrogen; inhibitory role with progesterone if high; stimulates production of breast milk.
Estradiol (E2)	Day 3	Stimulates egg maturation and endometrial maturation for implantation; responsible for fertile quality cervical fluid.

Continued

Stage 1 Investigations—cont'd

Assessment	Timing in Cycle	Justification
Testosterone (TT), free androgen index (FAI), androstenedione	Any day	Eliminate PCOS or testosterone dominance.
Sex hormone-binding globulin (SHBG)	Any day	Evaluates if concentration of SHBG is affecting the amount of testosterone available to body tissues.
Transvaginal ultrasound	Day 7	Evaluates follicle maturation, ovulation, endometrial thickness, and character. General assessment of pelvic organs for diagnosing abnormalities of the uterus and ovaries. Assesses thickness and appearance of endometrium to be followed. Enables antral follicle count.
Beta-human chorionic gonadotropin (beta-HCG)	Any day	Eliminates pregnancy and tumor.
Antimüllerian hormone (AMH)	Any day	Assesses ovarian reserve (best when combined with antral follicle count through ultrasound).
General Health Screen		
Complete blood count (CBC), urea electrolytes and creatine (UEC), liver function tests (LFTs), iron studies, thyroid-stimulating hormone (TSH), urinary iodine (24-hour or morning spot), serum zinc and copper (including ratio), ceruloplasmin red cell folate, serum vitamin B_{12}, homocysteine, (25-OH-D), fasting glucose, cholesterol profile, celiac screen, Pap smear	Not applicable (NA)	General health assessments to eliminate other abnormalities.
General Prepregnancy Screen		
Blood group and agglutinins, infectious disease screening, rubella immunity	NA	General prepregnancy assessments.

Stage 1 Investigations—cont'd

Assessment	Timing in Cycle	Justification
Cervical Swab and Urinalysis		
Bacterial culture, screen for sexually transmitted infections	NA	Assess for infective pathogen compromising fertility. General urinalysis to eliminate underlying infection or abnormality. Urogenital infections have been found to play a part in the genesis of miscarriage and infertility; however, patients may be unaware of their presence owing to the asymptomatic nature of many infections. Screening for a range of genitourinary infections is necessary in preconception care to detect possible infection and thus barriers to conception. The most common and essential infections that require screening include the following: • Primary genitourinary tract infections: *Chlamydia trachomatis, Ureaplasma urealyticum, Mycoplasma hominis, Neisseria gonorrhoeae* • Secondary genitourinary tract infections: *Gardnerella vaginalis,* group B *Streptococcus,* beta-hemolytic *Streptococcus, Staphylococcus aureus, Staphylococcus milleri*
Other Fertility Assessments		
Waking temperature, cervical fluid assessment, cervical position assessment, ovulation testing (urine), ovulation testing (saliva)	Various	Assessment and interpretation of self-directed assessments (if used). See box "Ovulation Detection" for further discussion.
Other Considerations		
Salivary hormone screen, including reproductive and adrenal	NA	Salivary screen provides an advantage over blood levels in yielding significantly greater accuracy for interpretation of findings. The adrenal hormone profile determines adrenal function and may help to determine the presence or extent of acute and/or chronic mental and/or physical stress. Prolonged stress has been shown to have suppressive effects on the fertility of both the male and the female. Of importance, it is likely to have a profound impact on gonadotropin release (FSH, LH).

Continued

Stage 1 Investigations—cont'd

Assessment	Timing in Cycle	Justification
Nutrient and toxic element screening	NA	Assessment of toxic elements including aluminum, arsenic, cadmium, lead, and mercury is crucial so that these can be eliminated as causative or contributing factors. It is widely accepted that excessive exposure to heavy metals has detrimental effects on fertility and must therefore be assessed and remedied during the preconception period.
Environmental screen	NA	Other environmental assessments including those that check for porphyrins, polychlorinated biphenyls (PCBs), chlorinated pesticides, volatile solvents, phthalates, parabens, and other toxins. These should also be considered owing to their deranging effects on reproductive function, endocrinology, gamete development, and thus embryologic potential.

Modified from Hechtman L. Clinical naturopathic medicine. Sydney, New South Wales, Australia: Elsevier; 2011.

Stage 2 Investigations

Assessment	Timing in Cycle	Justification
	Not applicable (NA)	Indicated if thyroid function appears compromised, ovulation potential is reduced, or patient appears to have implantation issues.
Sperm antibodies (serum)	NA	Determines whether antibodies are present against the partner's sperm. If blood results are positive, cervical mucus sperm antibodies may be required.
Laparoscopy, hysteroscopy, and salpingoscopy	Before ovulation	Inspection of uterotubal junctions. Diagnosis and treatment of pelvic diseases (endometriosis) or adhesions. Hysteroscopy complements hysterosalpingography (HSG) in revealing pathology that disturbs the shape of the endometrial cavity, especially intrauterine adhesions, submucosal fibroids, and endometrial polyps. These can be diagnosed with HSG, but hysteroscopy is required to locate the pathology accurately and treat it accordingly.

Stage 2 Investigations—cont'd

Assessment	Timing in Cycle	Justification
HSG with or without selective salpingogram (if indicated)	Day 7	Vaginal examination and injection of radiographic fluid into the uterus and fallopian tubes on x-ray study. Determines whether fallopian tubes are clear and uterine cavity is normal.
Clomid challenge test	Day 3, FSH and estradiol Day 10, FSH	Determines ovarian reserve and if pregnancy can occur before assisted reproductive techniques are implemented.
Curettage or endometrial biopsy	Day 26 (just before menses are expected)	Reveals the tissue structure of the endometrium. Estimates normal ovulation based on timing. Not advised regularly because of risk of scarring.
Other	NA	If all results show no abnormality or if the patient is older than 38 years, the clinician is advised to consider a number of miscarriage assessments to improve outcome, because a number of these assessments are associated with implantation failure as well as miscarriage (see Table "Miscarriage Screen")

Modified from Hechtman L. Clinical naturopathic medicine. Sydney, New South Wales, Australia: Elsevier; 2011.

COMPLICATIONS

Miscarriage

- Incidence is as high as one in four pregnancies. Although 25% of pregnancies result in miscarriage, less than 5% of women experience two consecutive miscarriages; only 1% experience three or more.
- Recurrent pregnancy loss is distinct from infertility, defined by two or more failed pregnancies. When cause is unknown, each loss merits careful review to determine whether specific evaluation is indicated. Although consensus is to evaluate after three or more losses, the naturopathic paradigm recommends reviewing all patients after the first and more comprehensively after the second or subsequent miscarriages.
- Risk of miscarriage is highest immediately after implantation; 50% of all fertilized eggs do not survive, resulting in a normal (or slightly late) period. This is termed "unnoticed miscarriage," not acknowledged by the woman who is unaware of pregnancy.

Classic Causes of Miscarriage

- Genetic or chromosomal: 60% of early miscarriages.
- Age: after age 40, one third of pregnancies end in miscarriage.
- Hormonal abnormalities: luteal phase deficiencies (low progesterone) are the most common cause. This can relate to hyperprolactinemia.
- Metabolic abnormalities: poorly controlled blood sugar levels or diabetes mellitus; polycystic ovary syndrome (PCOS) increases risk.
- Uterine abnormalities: distortion of uterine cavity causes 15% to 20% of miscarriages.
- Antiphospholipid syndrome: causes 3% to 15% of losses.
- Thrombophilia: increased risk of thrombosis and consequent increased risk of pregnancy loss, especially second half of pregnancy.
- Male factors: abnormal sperm DNA (see chapter on Male Infertility).
- Unexplained: no explanation found in 50% to 75% of couples.

Unexplained Causes of Miscarriage

- When causes of miscarriage are unexplained, naturopathy can provide the most beneficial care.

Miscarriage Screen

Assessment	Justification	Interpretation
On Presentation: at Any Time in the Ovarian (Menstrual) Cycle		
General health screen including complete blood count (CBC), liver function tests (LFTs), fasting glucose, blood group, and agglutinins chemistry panel	General medical checkup.	Various; assess for compounding factors.

Miscarriage Screen—cont'd

Assessment	Justification	Interpretation
Red cell folate, serum vitamin B_{12}	Unsuspected folate deficiency; if low, test fasting serum homocysteine.	Folate supplementation in vitamin B_{12} deficiency masks pernicious anemia and the risk of subacute spinal cord degeneration. Red blood cells (RBCs) and serum are not definitive assessment tools for these nutrients. Additional assessments may be warranted.
Fasting homocysteine	Elevations can correlate with vitamins B_9 and B_{12} findings, presence (or absence) of MTHFR polymorphism, and coagulation or vascular abnormalities.	Treat as indicated with high doses of vitamins B_6, B_9, and B_{12}. Correlate findings with vitamins B_9 and B_{12} and MTHFR status.
Thyroid function tests (TFTs)	Although mild hypothyroidism is strongly associated with anovulation, even mild hyperthyroidism is strongly associated with miscarriage.	It is important to keep all TFT values well within normal limits: avoid even slightly excessive thyroid replacement in cases of hypothyroidism.
Antithyroglobulin antibodies (anti-TG Abs), thyroperoxidase antibodies (TPO Abs), thyroid-stimulating hormone (TSH) receptor antibodies	The presence of thyroid antibodies can occur with normal TFT results (especially TPO Abs) and is strongly correlated with a first-trimester miscarriage.	Miscarriage is increased in the presence of any of the thyroid Abs directly correlating with immune modulation requirements of gestation (i.e., implantation and throughout the first trimester at individual increments).
Fasting plasma glucose	Assess for preclinical diabetes. If fasting plasma glucose is raised, assess insulin and hemoglobin A_{1c} (HbA_{1c}) (with or without glucose tolerance test [GTT]) and assess for polycystic ovary syndrome (PCOS) factors.	Miscarriage is increased in overt diabetes and PCOS.
Serum testosterone, free androgen index, sex hormone- binding globulin (SHBG), with or without androstenedione	Screen for PCOS. If results are positive, confirm with day 7 ultrasound.	Miscarriage is more likely to occur because of disordered follicular development and oocyte function.

Continued

Miscarriage Screen—cont'd

Assessment	Justification	Interpretation
Serum gliadin antibodies (immunoglobulin G [IgG], IgA), serum IgA levels and antibodies to tissue transglutaminase or endomysial antibodies. If the patient is already on a low-gluten or gluten-free diet, referral for celiac gene screen is advisable. Note that it is only 95% accurate, and a negative reading is not conclusive.	Asymptomatic celiac disease an occasional (though not unequivocal) cause of unexplained infertility or repeated miscarriage. Underdiagnosed in young adult women (population prevalence 1:250 and satisfies World Health Organization [WHO] criteria for population screening).	Confirmation is via small bowel biopsy needed for diagnosis; however, this will require consumption of gluten for 3 months. Objective clinical opinion is required to warrant this necessity in the fertility context. Note that missing celiac disease in a woman with otherwise unexplained reproductive dysfunction might prove embarrassing if later it manifests more classically. Classic presentation may include marked anemia and/or general nutritional deficiencies.
Pregnancy infection screen (rubella, hepatitis B, hepatitis C+, human immunodeficiency virus [HIV], toxoplasmosis, cytomegalovirus [CMV], Epstein-Barr virus [EBV])	Each infection can correlate with miscarriage eventualities (dependent on each infection and timing in pregnancy).	As indicated with each assessment.
Serum copper, serum zinc, and ceruloplasmin	Wilson's disease, a rare copper storage disorder, can manifest in young women with repeated miscarriage before other symptoms and signs develop (liver disease, Kayser-Fleischer rings, cerebral dysfunction).[21] Screen for high copper and ceruloplasmin levels; confirm with elevated 24-hour urinary copper excretion (and then liver biopsy). In assessing zinc status, a 1:1 zinc/copper ratio should be observed. Zinc supplementation can then be calculated on an as-required basis.	Population prevalence is approximately 1:30,000 (in any ethnic group); *ATP7B* mutant gene carrier frequency is approximately 1:90; more than 100 mutations are known, and affected people are usually compound heterozygotes. Possible mechanism: raised copper levels in uterine secretions compromising mitochondrial function in the conceptus. In addition, raised copper levels are antagonistic to zinc absorption and will warrant supplementation. Depending on copper reading, treatment with copper-binding agents may be required and has been shown to reverse pregnancy losses.

Miscarriage Screen—cont'd

Assessment	Justification	Interpretation
Prolactin and beta-human chorionic gonadotropin (beta-HCG)	Assess impact of these hormonal levels on pregnancy sustenance and achievement.	Address as indicated; typically, hormonal modulation is required to ensure that hormone levels are optimal for each stage of pregnancy (and preconceptionally).
Karyotype, peripheral blood (both partners)	Assess for balanced chromosomal translocation in either partner. If an imbalance is detected, not only are couples prone to conceive embryos with unbalanced translocations, but their unstable meiotic spindles also make otherwise unremarkable aneuploidies more common.	Referral for genetic counseling to estimate unbalanced chromosomal segregation patterns and initiate preimplantation genetic diagnosis (PGD) if required.
Hysterosalpingogram	To assess tubal patency and fallopian tube structure.	Address as relevant.
Antinuclear antibody, anticardiolipin antibody (IgM, IgG), lupus inhibitor or anticoagulant, IgA	Screening for the antiphospholipid syndrome, either secondary to systemic lupus erythematosus (SLE) or, more commonly but often less aggressively, primary.	Laboratory testing for anticardiolipin antibody is not well standardized and interpretations of isolated elevations are difficult. SLE necessitates referral to immunologist or rheumatologist. Treatment of definite cases is through allopathic means with low-molecular-weight heparin, vaginal progesterone (immunosuppressive locally), corticosteroids, and occasionally plasmapheresis. Naturopathic means include immune modulation, blood coagulation normalization, and dietary modification to support appropriate immune and hematologic systems.

Continued

Miscarriage Screen—cont'd

Assessment	Justification	Interpretation
CA 125	Presence does not automatically confirm cancer; however, it can correlate with cancerous conditions, endometriosis, or proliferative disorders.	In instances of endometriosis can indicate increased development, poor management, or contributing factors to miscarriage.
Anti-Tj[a] antibody (anti-PP_1P^k hemolysin)	Rare but well described.	Plasmapheresis and immunoglobulin replacement during pregnancy can enable term delivery.
Thrombophilia screen	Protein S, protein C, activated protein C (APC) resistance, antithrombin III.	Protein S deficiency: second trimester miscarriage increase × 7.4. Protein C deficiency: less convincing. APC resistance: first trimester × 2.1, second trimester 3 3.317.
Thrombophilia polymerase chain reaction (PCR) testing (DNA assessments)	Test for Factor V Leiden, prothrombin *G20210A*, *MTHFR C677T*, and *A1298C*.	Meta-analysis reports the following increased risks of miscarriage with homozygosity: Factor V Leiden: first trimester × 2.1, second trimester × 3.3. Prothrombin G20210: first trimester × 2.3, second trimester × 2.3. MTHFR alleles (increase miscarriage risk with elevated homocysteine): × 4.3 (if controlled with adequate folate may actually protect against miscarriage and intrauterine growth retardation). The naturopathic model also acknowledges the impact of MTHFR on folate metabolism and its subsequent effects on ensuring that DNA replication within each cell (including the cells of the fetus) is consistent. In addition, folate is responsible for a number of other roles in the body. Therefore an MTHFR abnormality can correlate with a number of other health concerns regardless of homocysteine status.

Miscarriage Screen—cont'd

Assessment	Justification	Interpretation
Antimüllerian hormone (AMH)	Reduced levels may indicate failing ovarian reserve. Increased levels can indicate PCOS.	Interpretation is controversial; however, in instances of reduced AMH, refer to fertility specialist and possibly concurrent assisted reproductive technologies.
Day 2 of the Menstrual Cycle		
Serum follicle-stimulating hormone (FSH), luteinizing hormone (LH), estradiol (E2) Note: ovulation tracking over two cycles is advisable (E2, LH, and P4)	Reduced oocyte numbers: serum FSH >11 U/L PCOS: suspected when LH/FSH (U/L) >2:1 In either case, E2 >200 pmol/L indicates more-severe condition. Correlate any findings with a day 7 ultrasound.	Low oocyte numbers: risk of early menopause; in vitro fertilization (IVF) may be indicated if also infertile. PCOS: requires additional treatment changes; incidence correlates highly with increased miscarriage risk.
Day 7 of the Menstrual Cycle (or Estimated 1 Week before Ovulation)		
Transvaginal Ultrasound		
Uterine assessment	Normal endometrium is >5 mm thick and echolucent (thick echogenic endometrium means hyperplasia or polyp; if it is thin, consider endometritis). Assess for fibroid or diagnose other uterine abnormalities.	Treat specific to findings (e.g., thin endometrium will require progesterone support; thick endometrium will respond to uterine tonics, such as herbal medicines) and antioxidant regulation. For fibroid-specific treatment (*Textbook,* "Uterine Fibroids").
Ovarian assessment	Follicles present in the ovary indicate the typical number of eggs achievable: many peripheral follicles indicate PCOS; few follicles can indicate premenopause (or oopause).	If PCOS, low follicle numbers, or endometriotic cyst, specialist management is indicated, possibly including IVF.

Continued

Miscarriage Screen—cont'd

Assessment	Justification	Interpretation
Vaginal and cervical swabs and culture (cervical swabs are often indicated for the most accurate interpretation)	Vaginosis, either *Gardneralla vaginalis* or other organismal overgrowth, with loss of *Lactobacillus.* Primary genitourinary infections: *Chlamydia trachomatis, Ureaplasma urealyticum, Mycoplasma hominis, Neisseria gonorrhoeae* Secondary genitourinary infections: *G. vaginalis,* group B *Streptococcus,* beta-hemolytic *Streptococcus, Staphylococcus aureus, Staphylococcus milleri*	Urogenital infections have been found to play a part in the genesis of miscarriage and infertility; however, patients may be unaware of their presence because of the asymptomatic nature of many infections. Midtrimester (and later) pregnancy losses can occur after internal cervical os becomes covered by growing sac, at 13 weeks. Vaginal flora modulation is required. Herbal douches, probiotic supplementation, and in some instances, antibiotic treatment.
7 Days after Ovulation (Typically Days 21-28)		
Serum progesterone (P4)	Screen for ovulation confirmation	If <35 nmol/L, consider further investigation confirming ovulation Support progesterone cascades as required.
12 Days after Ovulation (Premenstrual Phase)		
Premenstrual endometrial biopsy for dating	Check integrated action of almost 2 weeks of progesterone on decidualizing the endometrium; confirm progesterone falling to low level and negative beta-HCG day before test. Extremely time-critical investigation: usefulness lost if performed in midluteal phase.	Often deficient stromal decidualization in disorders of ovulation (adjust treatment as indicated if present). A deficiency can also indicate endometrial atrophy (which can be untreatable) or, rarely, a molecular defect; in these two cases, gestational surrogacy may be the only treatment option. Best screen for rare molecular bases for decidualization failure causing implantation failure.

Miscarriage Screen—cont'd

Assessment	Justification	Interpretation
Premenstrual endometrial biopsy for lymphocyte (T-cell) subsets on immunocytochemistry (with adjunct T-cell subsets in blood)	Specialist laboratories can look for relative abundance of peripheral natural killer (NK) cells (CD57+) versus normal uterine (CD56+) NK cells in relation to T cell numbers	If unfavorable, consider vaginal progesterone during early pregnancy. Relevance of findings is conflictual. Naturopathic treatment measures are adapted to modulate the immune response in relevant instances.

Data from Jansen R, Gee A. Testing for miscarriage. *O&G Mag.* 2008;10(2):48-52.

THERAPEUTIC CONSIDERATIONS

Supporting Female Fertility

- Naturopathic treatment cannot address all variables (e.g., genetic factors or physical impediments); however, it can attenuate conditions.
- Assess fairly and holistically: previous pregnancy, duration of infertility, age of partner, severity of present pathology, and other factors. Example: For a woman in her 40s, late in her window of fertility, initiate integrative care with reproductive endocrinology and infertility (REI) or fertility specialist, because ART is likely to be required.
- **Summary of possible approaches:**
  - — Treatable conditions: blatant deficiencies or disease processes that require interventions to improve natural fertility. Patients respond well to preconception program of detoxification.
  - — Untreatable subfertility: some factors may be beyond naturopathic resolution. Refer for ART or IVF.
  - — Untreatable female sterility: mature patients, genetic disorders, or previous conditions that compromise fertility. Adoption or donor oocytes are the only possibilities.

Naturopathic Preconception Treatment

- Encourage a program that correlates with final stages of gamete development (oocytes). Women are born with all of their oocytes. Treatment options are limited to remedy primordial stage of development (unless modify epigenetic factors are modified).
- Follicle development takes 120 days; therefore, prescribe preconception care within this time period. The provider can influence other stages of oocyte development (secondary → antral → graafian). Optimizing oocyte environment during development

and improving patient's general health supports development of oocytes.

- Principles of preconception approach: attenuate preexisting conditions; optimize nutritional status; detoxify the body; and encourage healthy holistic approach to parenting.
- Nutritional repletion is required throughout preconception and may require higher doses to optimize nutritional status.
- A healthy body is a fertile one. The body is primed to pass genetic material only when the environment and conditions are optimal. If survival is evolutionarily compromised, fertility is hindered. Encourage couples to participate in treatment for 3 to 4 months to address all genetic and epigenetic variables.
- Co-treatment of both persons in a couple will produce best outcome; 65% of couples who had previously undergone multiple IVF cycles conceived within 2 years of preconception therapy.
- Most fertility patients incorporate several treatment options concurrently. Point out scope of all treatments; discuss protocols openly to foster collaborative approach and reduce adverse interactions.

Fertility-Damaging Factors

Age

Older age is the biggest preventable cause of infertility; 20% of women wait until after age 35 to begin families as a result of contraception, careers, marrying at older ages, high divorce rates, financial security, or lack of realization that fertility declines rapidly after age 35. Regardless of a woman's health, age-related changes cannot be prevented or modified. The age of oocytes is fixed. Considerations regarding effects of age on fertility include the following:

- **Ovarian function:** women are born with all the oocytes they will ever have—300,000 follicles remaining at menarche. Women lose 20 to 30 follicles each cycle. Of the oocytes remaining at puberty, 360 to 400 of these will mature over 30 years and be released, with the remainder lost in each cycle. The rest undergo atresia degeneration.
- **Ovarian reserve:** declines with each cycle as a result of natural loss of eggs and declining quality of remaining eggs, which become "poor responders" to follicle-stimulating hormone (FSH) and luteinizing hormone (LH), thus shortening menstrual cycles. Young women may have reduced ovarian reserve because of smoking, family history of premature menopause, or ovarian surgery, or even without known risk factors.

- **Genetic abnormalities:** aging increases risk of neonatal genetic abnormalities. As a female ages, risk for child with Down syndrome and total chromosomal abnormalities increases dramatically.
- **Miscarriage risk:** older oocytes increase risk of miscarriage.

Weight Balance

Body fat percentage should be 20% to 25% to support fertility and gestation. Less than 17% induces anovulation. It can take as long as 2 years to restore regular conception, even after body fat has been replenished. Women with body mass index (BMI) below 19 and irregular or absent menses should gain weight. Obesity poses a risk for infertility; its impact is more comprehensive than that of underweight, and the necessary treatment is easier to prescribe. Obesity affects reproductive function as follows:

- **Ovulation potential:** ovulation returns with modest weight loss; 90% of obese women resume ovulation if they lose more than 5% of pretreatment weight; and 30% conceive. In very obese women, these statistics are higher for pregnancy rates than expected from a single IVF cycle. This recommendation is crucial and encouraging for obese women.
- **IVF outcome:** success rate of ART is reduced in obese women—IVF success is reduced by 25% to 50%. IVF centers are reluctant to perform fertility treatment on women with a BMI above 35; they recommend BMI of 30 before treatment.
- **Miscarriage:** risk of first trimester miscarriage is 12% to 15% in normal-weight women younger than age 37. The rate of recurrent miscarriage increases fourfold in obese women.
- **Birth defects:** newborns of obese women have three times the risk of neural tube and structural heart defects. Folic acid at normal dose is less effective in preventing neural tube defects, so high-dose supplementation is required. It is always beneficial to calculate nutrient requirements based on patient weight, using Clark's rule:

  Dose = ([Patient weight in lb]/[150 lb]) × Standard dose

- **Pregnancy complications:** more common in obese women (gestational diabetes is six times more common); pregnancy-induced hypertensive diseases are more common (gestational hypertension and preeclampsia). Complications increase risk of premature delivery and/or need for cesarean section. The babies of obese women have heavier birth weights (fetal macrosomia), increasing

risk of traumatic vaginal delivery. There is a higher complication rate for cesarean and vaginal deliveries (e.g., excessive blood loss, thromboembolic disease, and postoperative infection).
- **Pregnancy outcomes:** increasing BMI doubles risk of stillbirth.
- **The newborn:** increased risk of being overweight as an adult and increased likelihood of weight-related diseases.

IMMUNOLOGIC CONSIDERATIONS

Because optimal production of gametes requires healthy immune response, any deviation from "normal" can affect outcomes. A number of miscarriage factors (e.g., implantation factors) relate to autoimmune diseases. Stabilizing and modulating immune response is a key objective of treatment. The immune system must "switch itself off" at conception, at implantation, and at key stages in first trimester. Consider the following crucial variables:
- **Environmental factors:** industrial and agricultural toxins adversely affect male and female fertility. Radiation, heavy metals, and chemicals cause oxidative damage to DNA, harming female fertility. Xenoestrogens have disturbed female reproductive physiologic behavior. Makeup, fragrances, hair dyes, nail polishes, and so on can have negative impact on reproductive function and hormone cascades. Reduce such exposures, specifically within preconception window and during first trimester, when embryogenesis and placentogenesis are paramount. Gestational exposure to carcinogens and endocrine disruptors affects more than one generation. Chemicals known to induce phenotypic effects in unexposed generations include alloxan, cyclophosphamide, orthoaminoasotoluol, benzpyrene, diethylstilbestrol, and vinclozolin.
- **Sleep irregularities:** shift work negatively affects regularity of the menstrual cycle and reproductive function and increases risk of adverse pregnancy outcome. Women wishing to achieve pregnancy must normalize their cycles and optimize and regulate sleep patterns.
- **Smoking:** both active and passive cigarette smoking adversely affect pregnancy rates and long-term ovarian function. Smokers are more likely to have premature menopause; smoking is a readily avoidable cause of infertility. Smoking reduces fertility by increasing thickness of the ovum's zona pellucida, increasing difficulty for a sperm to penetrate and fertilize the ovum. Smoking ages oocytes prematurely by 10 years. Recommend

immediate smoking cessation coupled with systematic antioxidant therapy. Smoking decreases ovarian vascularization, reduces oocyte maturation, and induces premature ovarian aging (premature menopause) and increased risk of miscarriage.
- **Caffeine:** avoid caffeine during preconception period and during pregnancy. Caffeine increases time to conception and is linked with endometriosis and increased risk of spontaneous abortion. Caffeine increases dopamine production, which in turn stimulates progesterone secretion, thus inhibiting production of prolactin (antagonistic and regulatory interrelationship between progesterone and prolactin). Any prolactin abnormality, excess or deficiency, affects fertility negatively. One caffeinated beverage daily can temporarily reduce conception. Caffeine increases early follicular estrogen levels and interferes with adrenal function and cortisol secretion. Caffeine's diuretic effects increase loss of nutrients beneficial to fertility. Quantity of coffee directly correlates with pregnancy rates.
- **Alcohol:** alcohol intake is linked to miscarriage; excessive alcohol is linked to hyperprolactinemia, adverse effects on oocyte retrieval, and lower chance of subsequent pregnancy in IVF; 50% reduction in conception with intake of just one drink weekly during a menstrual cycle. Alcohol produces negative effects on blastocyst development and implantation; increases estrogen levels, causing a subsequent reduction in FSH secretion and suppressing folliculogenesis, leading to anovulation and infertility. Recommend cessation of alcohol intake during preconception period. Fetal abnormalities are linked to alcohol intake during pregnancy.
- **Marijuana:** contains cannabinoids, which impair signaling pathways, alter hormonal regulation, and interfere with timing of implantation. Marijuana may cause ovulatory abnormalities and disrupt ovarian function. It also harms the developing fetus.

NUTRITIONAL CONSIDERATIONS

The Fertility Diet

Dietary modulation improves ovulation, conception, and health of the newborn. The "high-fertility diet and lifestyle" includes the following:
- Less *trans* fatty acids and more monounsaturated fats
- Less animal protein and more vegetable protein

- High-fiber, low-glycemic carbohydrates
- High-fat dairy products (they reduce risk of anovulatory infertility by 50%)
- Sources of nonheme iron (Fe)
- Multivitamin
- Less coffee, tea, and alcohol
- Vigorous physical activity for 30 minutes or more daily
- No smoking

Women who follow this diet and lifestyle are likely to have the following characteristics:

- Less likely to have long menstrual cycles
- Recent user of oral contraceptives
- Weight balance: BMI of 20 to 25

Mediterranean diet increases chance of successful pregnancy in those undergoing IVF or intracytoplasmic sperm injection (ICSI). High content of B vitamins (vitamin B_6) combined with high intake of vegetable oils may be a factor responsible for positive outcome.

Arginine

Arginine is a precursor of nitric oxide synthesis and is required for angiogenesis, embryogenesis, fertility in general, and hormone secretion. It is required for replication of cells and essential for oocyte development and embryo formation. Arginine supplementation (oral at 16 g/day) improves ovarian response, endometrial receptivity, and pregnancy rates. Arginine research has assessed too small a sample of women to allow definitive conclusions. Further research is needed during ART procedures.

Carnitine

Carnitine transports fatty acids into mitochondria. A deficiency reduces energy production. Mitochondria are crucial to oocyte development, acceptance of spermatozoa, and subsequent embryogenesis. It is mRNA within the oocyte that requires power of mitochondria to allow conception to occur. Carnitine is indicated for women experiencing implantation issues and/or aging oocytes. Carnitine may protect oocytes, reducing damage to oocyte cytoskeleton and mitigating embryo apoptosis induced by incubation in peritoneal fluid of patients with endometriosis. Although peritoneal fluid strongly affects endometriosis, it helps regulate endometrial lining production and implantation factors. Human studies are needed.

Antioxidants

- Compared with male fertility, little evidence supports specific antioxidants for female infertility. Consensus: antioxidants and good diet improve fertility in women. Patients on vitamin therapy, compared with controls, are less likely to develop preeclampsia and more likely to have multiple pregnancies. Holistic, effective vitamin prescriptions will have a positive effect on female fertility.
- Transgenerational epigenetic effects are physiologic and behavioral (intellectual) transfer of information across generations. Modification of chromosomes passing to future generations via gametes is part of transgenerational genetic or epigenetic inheritance.
- Oocytes are vulnerable to environmental influences and epigenetic environmental influences from patient's mother and grandmother.
- Oxidative stress is detrimental to female fertility by increasing time to conception; decreasing fertilization rates; decreasing oocyte penetration function and viability; decreasing implantation; and increasing loss of implantation.
- Oocyte requires regular antioxidant supply to reduce oxidative damage from current conditions and historical (transgenerational) exposure. During conception, mRNA uses antioxidant reserves to address DNA fragmentation or oxidation from sperm and oocyte. Conception and subsequent travel of embryo through fallopian tube to implantation generate free radical damage. Oxidative stress hinders optimal fertility.
- **Alpha-lipoic acid:** in both lipid- and water-soluble forms, Alpha-lipoic acid is a powerful antioxidant in all human cells. It assists in chelating heavy metals, minimizing risk of cellular damage, and regenerating other antioxidants—vitamins C and E, coenzyme Q10 (CoQ10), and glutathione.
- **Vitamin A:** powerful antioxidant assisting in cellular growth and differentiation, crucial for embryogenesis and placentogenesis; required for gene expression and cellular differentiation in organogenesis, embryonic development, immunity, regulatory functions, integrity of epithelial tissue, and health of cilia in fallopian tubes. It works with zinc (Zn); deficiency of Zn is linked with infertility, miscarriage, and cleft palate. It is a cofactor of 3-beta-dehydrogenase in steroidogenesis (estrogen production), and deficiencies may impair enzyme activity. Low vitamin A is linked to anovulation; plasma levels are low in women who

habitually miscarry. Supplementation during pregnancy is inadvisable because of the potential for congenital abnormalities. However, supplementation in preconception period is strongly advised. Lipid solubility and liver high storage capacity indicate keeping prescriptions below 10,000 international units (IU) per day. Cross-placental transfer occurs primarily with lipid-soluble nutrients; thus cessation of vitamin A supplementation is advisable immediately before conception attempts. Alternative: carotenoids (beta-carotene) have lower toxic potential; they support ovarian oocyte and follicular maturation. However, 15% to 25% of whites are unable to convert beta-carotene to vitamin A.

- **CoQ10 (ubiquinone, ubidecarenone, ubiquinol):** endogenous fat-soluble antioxidant involved in intracellular adenosine triphosphate (ATP) production. It is a cofactor in oxidative stress respiration for the citric acid cycle and is essential for development of cells in maturation process. It is endogenously produced from tyrosine in a 17-step process that requires riboflavin (B_2), niacinamide (B), pantothenic acid (B_5), pyridoxine (B_6), cobalamin (B_{12}), folic acid (B_9), vitamin C, tetrahydrobiopterin, and trace elements as cofactors. Patients who are hyperthyroid and hypothyroid require additional CoQ10 because tyrosine is a CoQ10 building block. There are no clinical trials assessing effects of CoQ10 on reproductive outcome. However, CoQ10 is an important ingredient in culture media in IVF setting and crucial component to mimic various reproductive fluids incorporated in natural conception. Its therapeutic efficacy is irrefutable. Dietary sources are inadequate; supplementation is essential. Select the active ubiquinol form. Oocytes are at greater risk of oxidative damage in the zona pellucida, preventing acrosome reaction with sperm (fertilization). Receptivity of the zona pellucida is strongly correlated with antioxidant status of oocytes; CoQ10 is most specific antioxidant for this application. CoQ10 requirements are higher for women older than 35 or women undergoing ART procedures owing to the increased oxidative effect on the oocyte.
- **Vitamin C:** primary water-soluble antioxidant. It protects folic acid and vitamin E from oxidation and improves fertility outcomes in women with luteal-phase defects. Ovaries are primary sites of ascorbic acid accumulation. Midcycle change of retention and excretion of ascorbic acid is a biomarker of ovulation. Vitamin C is crucial for collagen biosynthesis, growth and repair of ovarian follicles, and development of the corpus luteum. It

may facilitate luteal steroidogenesis and maturation of the preovulatory follicle and reduce the risk of preeclampsia when taken concurrently with vitamin E. Deficiency increases risk of miscarriage, spontaneous rupture of membranes, and brain tumors in offspring. Vitamin C is best co-prescribed with bioflavonoids, which strengthen capillaries, preventing miscarriage and breakthrough bleeding during pregnancy.

- **Vitamin E:** powerful plant-derived, lipid-soluble antioxidant essential for fertility and reproduction. It exists in eight different isomers. D-Alpha-tocopherol is the most biologically active form for conception. It maintains health of ovaries, reduces PMS symptoms, relieves benign breast disease, and ameliorates menstrual migraine, indicating regulation of hormonal activity. Vitamin E may benefit infertile women by reducing scar formation (e.g., keloid scarring when applied topically)—hence its usefulness in endometriosis or complex reproductive conditions (e.g., Asherman's syndrome). Infertile women with endometriosis have relatively lower vitamin E and increased lipid peroxidation. Antioxidant capacity is compromised in infertile women.
- **Selenium (Se):** powerful antioxidant with immune-modulating properties. Supplementation reduces risk of miscarriage, especially with thyroid autoantibodies. Indication: thyroid autoimmunity (e.g., thyroperoxidase [TPO] antibodies). Several thyroid hormone synthesizing enzymes are selenoproteins. Se supports the immune system and the coagulation system. Se decreases TPO antibodies in euthyroid subjects and increases quality of life. It also decreases TPO antibodies in hypothyroid patients treated with T_4. Low Se is linked to first-trimester miscarriage and recurrent miscarriage.
- **Zn:** cofactor for 200 enzymes (e.g., production of nucleic acids in DNA and RNA). Zn has specific antioxidant properties for reproductive organs and protects oocytes from free radicals. It facilitates reproduction, ovulation, fertilization, and development of oocytes. Deficiency may alter synthesis or secretion of FSH or LH. Deficiency may produce abnormal ovarian development, increased risk of miscarriage, or increased risk of teratogenicity. It is the single most important nutrient for preconception and pregnancy and is disrupted by oral contraceptives or copper intrauterine devices. Caution: excessive intake of Zn can be detrimental; base dosage on assessments and clinical findings. During preconception, Zn enhances fertility and supports healthy pregnancy and delivery. Poor maternal Zn status is

linked to low birth weight, premature delivery, complications of labor and delivery, and congenital anomalies. Zn requirements increase during pregnancy. Monitor patients carefully. Supplementing 25 mg from 19 weeks' gestation has increased birth weight. Zn induces a 14% reduction in premature deliveries.

- **B-complex vitamins:** provide synergistic benefits given as a group. Specific needs: folate for methylenetetrahydrofolate reductase (MTHFR), polymorphisms; B_6 in luteal-phase defects or progesterone insufficiency. B-complex deficiencies are linked to fetal abnormalities—neural tube defects, neonatal or perinatal death, low birth weight, and miscarriage. Alcohol, carbohydrate-rich diets, and oral contraceptives increase requirements for B vitamins. Couples need additional B vitamins to prepare for conception. Stress increases requirements and contributes to difficulty conceiving.
- **Vitamin B_1 (thiamine):** stabilizes membranes of newly generated neuronal cells during embryogenesis and slows cell death. It supports plasma membrane transformation of uterine epithelial cells during pregnancy. Deficiency is linked to altered cellular differentiation and proliferation and disrupted hormonal processes, increasing risk of miscarriage. Taken preconceptionally in combination with B_3 and B_6, it may prevent oral facial clefts.
- **Vitamin B_2 (riboflavin):** crucial for energy production, antioxidant defense, and many enzyme systems dependent on B vitamins. Insufficiency alters estrogen and progesterone levels, causing irregular menstruation. Supplementation often addresses menstrual difficulties, irregular menses, premenstrual syndrome (PMS), and infertility. Deficiency impairs embryonic growth and cardiac development and is linked to low birth weight and risk of congenital heart defects.
- **Vitamin B_6 (pyridoxine):** required for metabolism of amino acids, lipids, pathways of gluconeogenesis, and synthesis of neurotransmitters during periconception. It is required for the synthesis of prostaglandins; it helps B_9 and B_{12} regulate homocysteine. Elevated homocysteine is linked to infertility, recurrent spontaneous miscarriage, and poor oocyte and embryo qualities in patients with PCOS who are undergoing assisted reproduction. B_6 helps reduce elevated prolactin, support luteal-phase defects by increasing progesterone, increase influx of magnesium into myometrium, improve absorption of Zn, and prevent preeclampsia, toxemia, and infarction of the placenta. Serum B_6 is often low in hyperemesis gravidarum and is linked to gestational diabetes.

- **Vitamin B_9 (folic acid):** required for healthy DNA and RNA synthesis, protein synthesis, and regulation of gene expression. Supplement for 3 months any woman planning pregnancy to prevent neural tube defects; but it must be supplemented for the first 28 days of gestation to achieve this goal. Most women are unaware of pregnancy status until confirmed after 14 days. Folate supplementation decreases incidence of ovulatory infertility and supports oocyte quality and maturation. Inadequate folate elevates homocysteine and adversely alters DNA methylation and oocyte and early embryo quality. Folate deficiency– induced hyperhomocysteinemia poses risk for placenta-mediated diseases—preeclampsia, spontaneous abortion, and placental abruption.
- **Vitamin B_{12} (cyanocobalamin):** B_9 (folate) and B_{12} work together to ensure uniform, regulated replication of DNA and RNA. Folate and B_{12} levels decline during pregnancy. Supplement B_{12} and folate together to avoid the presence of one masking deficiency of the other. Low maternal B_{12} is linked to threefold risk of neural tube defects. B_{12} deficiency correlates with infertility and recurrent spontaneous miscarriage. Pregnancy occurs after correction of deficiency. B collaborates with B_6, folate, vitamin C in controlling homocysteine.
- **Vitamin D:** main functions include calcium (Ca) homeostasis; modeling of bone (mother and child); immune activation; cell differentiation, proliferation, and growth. Active form: 1,25-dihydroxyvitamin D_3. It regulates transcription and function of genes of placental invasion, normal implantation, and angiogenesis. Vitamin D is a powerful immune modulator for autoimmunity that affects fertilization, implantation, and increased risk of miscarriage. There are vitamin D receptors in immune cells. Vitamin D may have receptors on the oocyte zona pellucida and the sperm head. Theory: the acrosome reaction with the zona pellucida is enabled by vitamin D. It is engaged in acceptance of the sperm by the oocyte; vitamin D receptors act as gatekeepers to enable immune regulation and thus prevent rejection. Maternal vitamin D deficiency might be an independent risk factor for preeclampsia and infertility.
- **Ca:** required for oocyte maturation, fertilization, and bone formation of mother and child. It protects against preeclampsia, reducing risk by 50%, which supports the prescription of Ca for all preconceptional women whose dietary intake is inadequate.

- **Iodine:** preconceptionally minimizes risk of thyroid-related disorders and/or mental retardation in infants, commonly seen in offspring of deficient mothers. Low iodine negatively affects development of the fetal central nervous system; deficiency can hinder conception. Iodine is integral to triiodothyronine (T_3) and thyroxine (T_4) hormones affecting ovulation. Deficiency may induce miscarriage, stillbirth, mental retardation, and cretinism (deaf mutism and spasticity). Thyroid autoimmunity is higher among infertile women than among fertile women and increases the rate of miscarriage. Subclinical hypothyroidism may lead to ovulatory dysfunction and adverse pregnancy outcomes. Assess thyroid (and iodine) status for infertile males and females. A diagnosis of hypothyroidism based on thyroid-stimulating hormone (TSH) values in isolation may not suffice to diagnose mild to moderate iodine deficiency in pregnant women. Assess urinary iodine status with a morning spot urine test, a 24-hour urinary excretion test, or iodine/creatinine ratio.
- **Fe:** required for formation of red blood cells, transport of oxygen to tissues via hemoglobin, nucleic acid metabolism; acts as cofactor for enzyme systems. To avoid hemochromatosis, assess patients thoroughly before prescribing. Address this deficiency preconceptionally to help prevent Fe deficiency during pregnancy. Fe supplements can lower risk of ovulatory infertility. Study the patient's Fe profile and ensure that all components are within normal ranges, aiming to achieve serum ferritin stores of 80 ng/mL before conception, and saturation of higher than 30%. Assess a full Fe study profile: ferritin can be elevated because of inflammation, giving a false sense of Fe repletion. Some women cannot take Fe supplements during the first trimester because of aggravation of nausea.
- **Magnesium (Mg):** involved in cell signaling and energy production. Spontaneous abortion is linked to low plasma Mg. Those experiencing stress regarding fertility benefit from both Mg and B-vitamin supplements. Stress impairs fertility; results include miscarriage and failed pregnancy.
- **Essential fatty acids (EFAs):** omega-3 fatty acids help maintain lipid bilayers in all cell membranes and serve as precursors for anti-inflammatory prostaglandin synthesis. In preventing miscarriage, omega-3s (4 g/day providing 795 mg of docosahexaenoic acid [DHA] and 1190 mg of eicosapentaenoic acid [EPA]) improve velocity of blood flow in uterine arteries in women with recurrent miscarriage resulting from impaired uterine perfusion. Supplementing omega-3s improves endometrial

function and is vital for women with endometriosis or endometrial insufficiency. Omega-3s may help reduce spontaneous preterm births from intrauterine inflammation.

- **Probiotics:** alterations in vaginal microflora and subsequent genital and intrauterine infections are linked to reproductive failure and adverse pregnancy outcomes—preterm labor, miscarriage, and spontaneous preterm birth. During the first half of pregnancy, women with altered vaginal bacteria have four times the overall rate of spontaneous preterm birth.

Botanical Medicines

- ***Cimicifuga racemosa* (black cohosh; *Actaea racemosa*):** shows promise assisting fertility. In women who were not responding to clomiphene citrate, adding black cohosh at 120 mg daily increased pregnancy rates.
- **Alchemilla vulgaris (lady's mantle):** astringent beneficial for menorrhagia or frequent early miscarriage. Its tannins display antihemorrhagic properties. Traditional prescribing used it to halt bleeding and heal wounds (internal or external). *A. vulgaris* is used to treat female reproductive problems such as menstrual disorders, to prevent miscarriage, and to aid conception.
- ***Angelica sinensis* (dong quai):** traditional Chinese herbal medicine with gentle warming action. It nourishes blood, restores the body's natural balance, and serves as a female tonic, including for amenorrhea. It increases uterine tone and relaxes uterine musculature. Active constituents: ligustilide (essential oil component) and ferulic acid. Animal studies reveal that it regulates prostaglandin synthesis and experimentally induced inflammatory responses resulting from prostaglandin release. It regulates thromboxane A_2, which promotes blood clotting. Prescribe it for women with compromised fertility who also have blood disorders, menorrhagia, and reproductive inflammatory responses (e.g., endometriosis). Key point: fertilization and implantation are inflammatory events. *A. sinensis* is an antimiscarriage botanical serving to promote and sustain conception. It has spasmolytic effects on the uterus in dysmenorrhea. It eases pelvic blood flow, relieving pelvic congestion and pain. It is traditionally combined with *Paeonia lactiflora* and *Ligusticum wallichii* for menstrual pain aggravated by cold. *A. sinensis* is a relaxing blood mover, improving uterine circulation, normalizing the endometrial lining, and supporting implantation.

- ***Asparagus racemosa*** **(shatavari):** Ayurvedic botanical renowned for effects on the female reproductive tissues. It is an aphrodisiac, promoting strength and enhancing sexual appetite, preventing miscarriage, and supporting fertility. It exerts estrogenic effects. Few clinical studies exist; however, in Ayurveda this herb has been used safely over long periods of time, even during pregnancy and lactation.
- ***Chamaelirium luteum*** **(false unicorn root):** restricted herb owing to its threatened status from excessive wildcrafting. Prescribe other botanicals containing similar steroidal saponins (e.g., *Dioscorea villosa* [wild yam]). Prescribe *C. luteum* if the clinical objective is not achieved. The combination of *Asparagus racemosa* (shatavari) and *D. villosa* (wild yam) may be a better choice because of synergistic action rhizomes function as a uterine tonic; prescribed to remedy any imbalance or symptom in female reproductive organs. Historical use was for repeated and successive miscarriages. It was used for uterine displacement with threatened abortion, combined with *Viburnum prunifolium* to optimize this effect. It was applied to regulate ovarian function, highly indicated for menstrual issues in the first half of the cycle. It is an ovarian amphoteric because it regulates and normalizes ovarian function. The mechanism of action is unknown; however, it contains steroidal saponins, converted through digestion into the sapogenin diosgenin, which affects ovarian function via action on the hypothalamic-pituitary axis.
- ***P. lactiflora*** **(white peony):** traditional Chinese herb for effects on female reproductive organs. It is used in the formulation Dong-Quai-Shao-Yao-San for treating ovulatory disorders and to promote fertility. Another formulation, Unkei-To (traditional Japanese combination of shakuyaku [Paeonia radix, P. lactiflora Pallas] and keihi [cinnamomi cortex, *Cinnamomum cassia* Blume]) stimulates ovulatory process and human granulosa cells in vitro. This formulation promotes steroidogenesis, cytokine secretion, 17-beta-estradiol secretion, and progesterone secretion in highly luteinized granulosa cells obtained from IVF patients.
- ***Tribulus terrestris*** **(tribulus):** male tonic, but used to treat female reproductive disorders, even infertility. It has FSH-stimulating properties at the start of the menstrual cycle, initiating ovulation and improving conception rates. However, it lacks research substantiation. Expect to see marked increase in cervical

fluid within a few days. This increase precedes ovulation and supports conception. For delayed or absent ovulation, it regulates the ratio of FSH to LH. Tribulus improves fertility, libido, release of cervical fluid, mood, and patient confidence in fertility.

- ***Vitex agnus-castus* (chaste tree):** beneficial for anovulatory cycles, hyperprolactinemia, hypothalamic dysfunction, hypothalamic-pituitary-ovarian (HPO) axis modulation, and promotion of a regular and normal menstrual cycle. It is beneficial in PMS. It alleviates symptoms of latent hyperprolactinemia, with lower-than-normal progesterone secretion and normal to mildly elevated prolactin. Thus *Vitex* addresses menstrual disorders—typical PMS symptoms, altered menstrual cycle lengths, and amenorrhea. Causative factor: alteration in hypothalamic pituitary axis. *V. agnus-castus* corrects menstrual irregularities—amenorrhea when caused by latent hyperprolactinemia—by inhibiting prolactin secretion via competitively binding to dopamine D_2 and opioid receptors (dopaminergic effect).

THERAPEUTIC APPROACH

General Measures

- Avoid exposure to free radicals.
- Identify and eliminate environmental hazards—pesticides, solvents, heavy metals, other toxins.
- Use effective stress-reduction techniques and psychological counseling.
- Avoid cigarette smoking, alcohol, and recreational drugs.
- Avoid douches, vaginal sprays, scented tampons, or other feminine products that change vaginal pH and disturb vaginal microecology.
- Ensure healthy BMI (20% to 25%).
- Avoid medications that affect quality of cervical fluid (e.g., antihistamines, some cough mixtures, dicyclomine, progesterone [taken before or at ovulation], propantheline, tamoxifen).
- Avoid personal lubricants (except sperm-friendly types).

Diet

- Encourage principles of the fertility diet.
- Avoid dietary free radicals, saturated fats, hydrogenated oils, *trans* fatty acids, and cottonseed oil.

- Increase dietary antioxidant vitamins, carotenes, and flavonoids (dark vegetables and fruits) and EFAs (nuts and seeds).
- Recommend daily 8 to 12 servings of vegetables and 1 to 2 servings of fresh fruits.
- Optimize protein intake from vegetarian and organic animal sources.
- Ensure optimal hydration: 30 mL/2.2 lb (1 kg)
- Eliminate caffeine, alcohol, sugar, and artificial substances (preservatives, colorings, additives).
- Encourage sufficient EFA intake: half a cup of raw nuts or seeds, cold-pressed oils, and sustainably farmed fish (from organic sources).

Nutritional Supplements

Implement nutritional repletion program:

- Vitamin A: 3000 to 5000 IU q.d.[a]
- Vitamin B_1 (thiamine): 50 to 100 mg q.d.
- Vitamin B_2 (riboflavin): 50 mg q.d.
- Vitamin B_3 (niacin): 50 to 200 mg q.d.
- Vitamin B_5 (pantothenic acid): 50 to 200 mg q.d.
- Vitamin B_6 (pyridoxine): 50 to 250 mg q.d.
- Vitamin B_9 (folic acid): 800 to 5000 mcg q.d. (dependent on MTHFR status and homocysteine levels)
- Vitamin B_{12} (cyanocobalamin): 800 to 5000 mcg q.d. (reflecting vitamin B_9 with a 1:1 ratio where possible)
- Vitamin C: 1000 to 4000 mg q.d. in divided doses
- Vitamin D_{3b}: 1000 to 5000 IU q.d. (decrease to 1000 IU/day in summer and 2000 IU/day in winter when repleted)[b]
- Vitamin E (mixed tocopherols and tocotrienols): 500 to 1000 IU q.d.
- Vitamin Kc: 2 to 75 mg q.d.[c]
- Beta-carotene: 10 to 30 mg q.d.
- CoQ10: 100 to 300 mg q.d. in divided doses
- Ca: 1000 to 1500 mg q.d.
- Chromium: 100 to 1000 mcg q.d.[d]
- Copper: 2 to 4 mg q.d.[e]
- Iodine: 200 to 400 mcg q.d. (decrease to 200 mcg/day when repleted)[f]
- Fe: 10 to 100 mg q.d.
- Magnesium: 500 to 1000 mg q.d.
- Se: 150 to 300 mcg q.d.
- Zn: 40 to 80 mg q.d. (decrease to 25 mg q.d. when repleted)

- Total omega-3 EFAs: 1000 to 5000 mg q.d.
- DHA: 400 to 700 mg q.d.
- EPA: 800 to 1000 mg q.d.
- Total omega-6 EFAs: 1000 to 2000 mg q.d.
- Evening primrose oil: 1000 to 1500 mg q.d.
- L-Arginine: 3000 to 10,000 mg q.d.
- L-Carnitine: 1000 to 4000 mg q.d.
- Probiotics (mixed strains): 25 to 50 billion q.d.

---

a. Retinol equivalents (REs) are now used: 1 mcg RE = 1 mcg retinol = 6 mcg beta-carotene = 12 mcg other carotenoids. Avoid during pregnancy. Ensure that prescription is based on need because of fat solubility and potential for placental transfer in second trimester. Monitor dose carefully. Alternatively, beta-carotene may be a more appropriate prescription.
b. Prescribe based on pathology results.
c. Consider prescription in instances of coagulation disorders. Monitor closely to ensure no drug interaction is present.
d. Dose dependent on blood sugar level control and weight requirements. Calculate based on patient's weight.
e. Avoid in instances of Wilson's disease (assess before prescription) and ensure that prescription is recommended only when Zn/copper ratio is considered.
f. Assessment before prescription is essential to determine dose; should only be conducted when thyroid function values can be reviewed.

Botanical Medicines

- *C. racemosa* (black cohosh)
  - Fluid extract (1:2): 2 to 4 mL (0.5 to 1 tsp) three times daily
  - Extracts equivalent to dry herbal medicine: 42.25 mg/day
- *A. vulgaris* (lady's mantle)
  - Fluid extract (1:1): 40 to 85 mL/day
- *A. sinensis* (dang gui)
  - Fluid extract (1:1): 2 to 4 mL (0.5 to 1 tsp) three times a day
- *Asparagus racemosa* (shatavari)
  - Fluid extract (1:1): 2 to 4 mL (0.5 to 1 tsp) three times a day
- *P. lactiflora* (white peony)
  - Fluid extract (1:1): 2 to 4 mL (0.5 to 1 tsp) three times a day

- *T. terrestris* (Tribulus)
  - Standardized extract, equivalent to dried herb (aerial parts of leaf), standardized to contain furostanol saponins as protodioscin 12.22 mg/L, 9 to 36 g/day.
- *V. agnus-castus* (chasteberry)
  - The usual dose of chasteberry extract (often standardized to contain 0.5% agnuside) in tablet or capsule form is 175 to 225 mg/day. If using the liquid extract, the typical dose is 2 to 4 mL/day (½ to 1 tsp/day).

Infertility, Male

DIAGNOSTIC SUMMARY

- Inability to conceive child after 12 months of regular unprotected sexual intercourse (at least twice weekly) with the same female partner and in the absence of female causes
- Sperm abnormalities confirmed by two properly performed semen analyses of sperm count, morphology, motility, or other aspects

GENERAL CONSIDERATIONS

- In the United States 18% of couples have difficulty conceiving a child. In one third of cases the man is responsible; in another third both are responsible; in another third the woman is responsible. Six percent of men aged 15 to 50 years are infertile.
- Most male infertility reflects abnormal sperm count (oligospermia) or quality. Natural barriers in the female reproductive tract allow only 40 of 20 million ejaculated sperm to reach the vicinity of the egg. The number of sperm in ejaculate correlates strongly with fertility. In 90% of oligospermia cases, the reason is deficient sperm production; in 90% of these cases the cause of decreased sperm formation is unidentified—known as *idiopathic oligospermia* or *azoospermia.* Azoospermia is the complete absence of living sperm in semen.
- Worldwide recent, dramatic decline in fertility appears unrelated to national socioeconomic status; however, deferred childbearing and improved contraception are factors. In the United States some patients will require assisted reproductive technologies (ARTs) to conceive.
- General rule: three in five couples conceive within 6 months of trying; one in four take 6 months to a year. Conception taking more than a year suggests a problem.

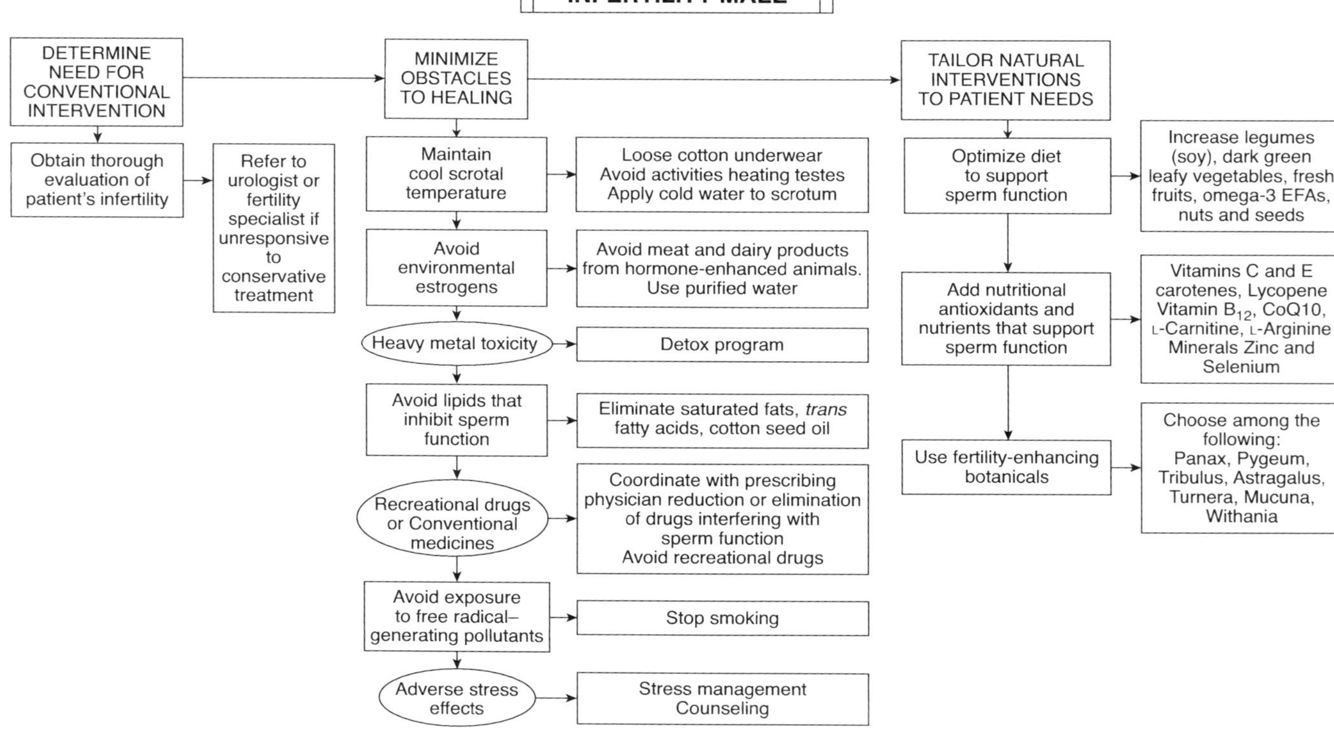
INFERTILITY MALE
DETERMINE NEED FOR CONVENTIONAL INTERVENTION
Obtain thorough evaluation of patient's infertility
Refer to urologist or fertility specialist if unresponsive to conservative treatment
MINIMIZE OBSTACLES TO HEALING
Maintain cool scrotal temperature
Loose cotton underwear
Avoid activities heating testes
Apply cold water to scrotum
Avoid environmental estrogens
Avoid meat and dairy products from hormone-enhanced animals.
Use purified water
Heavy metal toxicity
Detox program
Avoid lipids that inhibit sperm function
Eliminate saturated fats, *trans* fatty acids, cotton seed oil
Recreational drugs or Conventional medicines
Coordinate with prescribing physician reduction or elimination of drugs interfering with sperm function
Avoid recreational drugs
Avoid exposure to free radical–generating pollutants
Stop smoking
Adverse stress effects
Stress management
Counseling
TAILOR NATURAL INTERVENTIONS TO PATIENT NEEDS
Optimize diet to support sperm function
Increase legumes (soy), dark green leafy vegetables, fresh fruits, omega-3 EFAs, nuts and seeds
Add nutritional antioxidants and nutrients that support sperm function
Vitamins C and E
carotenes, Lycopene
Vitamin B_{12}, CoQ10,
L-Carnitine, L-Arginine
Minerals Zinc and Selenium
Use fertility-enhancing botanicals
Choose among the following:
Panax, Pygeum, Tribulus, Astragalus, Turnera, Mucuna, Withania

- **Primary infertility** exists when pregnancy has never occurred despite regular unprotected intercourse for a year or more.
- **Secondary infertility** exists if, despite achieving past pregnancy (which may or may not have led to childbirth), a couple is unable to conceive again despite a year or more of regular unprotected intercourse.
- **Unexplained infertility** occurs in 5% to 10% of couples. Assessments find no apparent cause. Inquiry into causation is complicated by poor investigation or the lack of current assessment strategies. Attempt to elucidate answers by taking a holistic view in assessing patients to produce positive outcomes.
- Fertility reflects general health and well-being and can indicate latent or undiagnosed genetic abnormalities or other etiologic considerations. Conduct comprehensive, holistic review.
- **Spermatogenesis:** sperm are produced by repeated divisions of cells in small, coiled tubules within the testes at a rate of 100 million daily. Each spermatogenic cycle consists of six stages, and five cycles are required to produce one mature sperm. From the beginning of stem cell division to the appearance of mature sperm in semen takes 72 to 76 days. Anything the male experiences during spermatogenesis can affect mature sperm regardless of his health at time of examination. Factors include illness, toxicity, trauma, nutritional status. Sperm spend 2 to 10 days passing through the epididymis, maturing en route for swimming and penetrating oocytes. At the beginning of ejaculation, sperm are transported from the tail of the epididymis via the vas deferens to the urethra. The seminal vesicles, prostate gland, and Cowper's glands secrete most of the volume of semen to deliver sperm during ejaculation. Semen volume: less than 5% from the two epididymides; 60% from seminal vesicles; 30% from prostate gland. Average normal semen volume ejaculating every 2 days is 3 mL. Average sperm concentration is 85 million/mL. During ejaculation, sperm and prostatic fluid are ejected first; seminal vesicle fluid follows. Seminal vesicle fluid coagulates, causing lumpy, gel-like appearance. Liquefaction occurs after 20 minutes, when gel disappears.

DIAGNOSTIC CONSIDERATIONS

Andrology Assessments

- **Semen analysis (SA):** primary basis of assessment; snapshot of male fertility and reflects male's general health in preceding

72 to 76 days. Semen quality can vary among samples. Diagnosis is not achieved until abnormality is confirmed by two separate investigations. Two or three semen analyses are needed, several weeks apart, to gauge accurate average semen quality. Sperm count can be adversely affected by illness—fever—which may temporarily suppress sperm count for several months. In this case, delay SA. In-clinic collection versus at-home collection: carefully consider laboratory guidelines (abstinence timing, lubricant use) and standard of andrology laboratory facility.

- Overall, male fertility is declining. The greatest difference can be denoted by reviewing morphology, owing to differing criteria and percentage scales. SA can be done by a number of assessments as follows:
  - General SA: assesses motility, morphology, concentration, volume, appearance, and so on
  - Sperm chromatin integrity test: determines level of DNA damage to sperm
  - Immunobead test: assesses antibodies against sperm
  - Semen culture: screens for infection
  - Retrograde ejaculatory testing: identifies retrograde semen flow or obstruction if SA yields extremely low count
  - Trial wash: assesses sperm factors and determines whether in vitro fertilization (IVF) or intracytoplasmic sperm injection (ICSI) is more appropriate; conducted before IVF and/or ICSI procedures
  - Microsurgical epididymal sperm aspiration (MESA), testicular sperm extraction (TESE), or percutaneous epididymal sperm aspiration (PESE): extracts sperm from testicles by specialized procedure when sperm count is low or absent or if ejaculation is not possible

Semen Terminology

Aspermia	An absence of semen despite male orgasm.
Azoospermia	A complete absence of sperm (spermatozoa) in the semen.
Oligozoospermia	Reduced number of normal motile sperm cells (spermatozoa) in the ejaculate (compared with azoospermia, which means no sperm in the ejaculate). It includes laborious terms such as *asthenozoospermia, teratozoospermia,* and *oligoasthenoteratozoospermia.*
Teratozoospermia	Sperm with abnormal morphology.

Semen Terminology

Necrospermia	Death of sperm.
Oligoasthenoteratozoospermia	A long name that indicates low count, weak motility, and abnormal morphology.

Male Reproductive Assessment

- Assess male patient thoroughly to determine general and fertility health.
- Refer to fertility specialist, urologist, or endocrinologist if needed.
- Elucidate full history and assess causative or contributing factors.

Fertility Assessment

Assessment	Elaboration and Explanation
Age	What ages are the couple?
Fertility history	How long have they been trying to conceive, and have they ever conceived previously (together or separately)? Do they have any idea why they have not been able to conceive?
Sexual history	Sexually transmitted infection (STI) screen: potential sexually transmitted disease exposure, symptoms of genital inflammation (e.g., urethral discharge, dysuria)
Medication history	Use of medications such as sulfasalazine (Azulfidine), methotrexate, colchicine, cimetidine (Tagamet), spironolactone (Aldactone)
Surgical history	History of surgery such as previous genitourinary surgery
Contraception	When it was ceased and the likely speed of its reversibility
Fertile times	Whether the couple engage in regular intercourse during fertile times
Lifestyle factors	Diet, exercise, alcohol, smoking cessation, recreational drug use, environmental toxin screen
Prior paternity	Previous fertility
Psychosexual issues (erectile, ejaculatory)	Interference with conception

Continued

Fertility Assessment

Assessment	Elaboration and Explanation
Pubertal development	Poor progression suggests underlying reproductive issue
A history of undescended testes	Risk factor for infertility and testicular cancer
Previous genital infection (STI) or trauma	Risk of testis damage or obstructive azoospermia
Symptoms of androgen deficiency	Indicative of hypogonadism
Previous inguinal, genital, or pelvic surgery	Testicular vascular impairments, damage to vasa, ejaculatory ducts, ejaculation mechanisms
Medications, drug use	Transient or permanent damage to spermatogenesis
General health (diet, exercise, smoking)	General health screen

Physical Examination

Assessment	Elaboration and Explanation
General examination	Acute or chronic illness, nutritional status. Assess for varicocele, testicular size, and other genital factors. Testes: Small testes suggest spermatogenic failure. Presence of vas deferens: may be congenitally absent. Epididymides: thickening or cysts may suggest previous infection and resultant obstructive problems. Varicoceles: detected when patient is standing, coughing, or performing Valsalva maneuver. Penis: assessed for abnormalities (e.g., Peyronie's disease) that may interfere with intercourse.
Degree of virilization assessment	Assess for signs of virility. Signs of androgen deficiency (e.g., increased body fat, decreased muscle mass, decreased facial and body hair, small testes, Tanner stage below 5).
Prostate examination	Assess if history suggests prostatitis or a sexually transmitted infection.

Endocrinologic Assessments

Assessment	Justification for Assessment
Follicle-stimulating hormone (FSH) Progesterone (P4) Prolactin (PRL) Luteinizing hormone (LH) Total testosterone, free testosterone	Assessment to ensure that hormonal status is optimal to eliminate hormonal abnormalities. *Testosterone:* is often normal (8-27 nmol/L) even in men with significant spermatogenic defects. Some men with severe testicular problems display a fall in testosterone levels and rise in serum LH. These men should undergo evaluation for androgen deficiency. The finding of low serum testosterone and low LH suggests a hypothalamic-pituitary problem (e.g., prolactinoma; serum prolactin levels required). *FSH:* elevated levels are seen when spermatogenesis is poor (primary in testicular failure); in normal men, the upper reference value is approximately 8 international units (IU) per liter. In azoospermic men, 14 IU/L strongly suggests spermatogenic failure; 5 IU/L suggests obstructive azoospermia; a testis biopsy may be required to confirm that diagnosis.
Sex hormone–binding globulin (SHBG)	Evaluates if concentration of SHBG is affecting the amount of testosterone available to body tissues.
DHEA-S, cortisol	Additional hormone levels should be reviewed on an individual basis, including a full adrenal profile if the impact of stress is considered relevant.

Other Assessments

Assessment	Justification
General Health Assessments	
CBC, blood type Standard blood chemistries 25(OH)D_3	General health assessments to eliminate other abnormalities.
Fasting glucose Cholesterol profile General sexually transmitted infection (STI) screen	

Continued

Other Assessments

Assessment	Justification
Thyroid-stimulating hormone (TSH) and urinary iodine (24-hour or morning spot)	Check thyroid function and iodine status.
Urinalysis or swab	
Infection screen	General urinalysis to eliminate underlying infection or abnormality. Urogenital infections have been found to play a part in the genesis of miscarriage and infertility. Most patients are unaware of their presence owing to the asymptomatic nature of these infections. The most common infections that require screening include *Chlamydia trachomatis, Ureaplasma urealyticum, Mycoplasma hominis,* and *Neisseria gonorrhoeae.*
Advanced Fertility Assessments	
Karyotyping and subsequent genetic testing	Advanced fertility assessments if previous results show no abnormality or if infertility remains unexplained. World Health Organization (WHO) guidelines suggest that peripheral blood karyotyping analysis can be diagnostically helpful. Abnormal genotype may be present in up to 12% of azoospermic men and 4% of oligospermic men. Cystic fibrosis screening is recommended for azoospermia if due to congenital bilateral absence of the vas deferens (CBAVD). Optional screening for Y-chromosome microdeletion if sperm count is <5 million/mL.
Scrotal (testicular) ultrasonography	History of undescended testes or concern regarding testicular cancer.
Transrectal ultrasonography	If ejaculatory duct obstruction suspected.
MTHFR C677T MTHFR 1298C Prothrombin G20210A Factor V Leiden Selenium assay Fasting homocysteine	Indicated in instances of miscarriage, unexplained infertility, marked sperm abnormalities, or implantation issues.
Other Considerations	

Other Assessments—cont'd

Assessment	Justification
Nutrient and toxic element screening	Assessments of toxic elements, including aluminum, arsenic, cadmium, lead, and mercury, are crucial so as to eliminate them as causative or contributing factors. It is widely accepted that excessive exposure to heavy metals has detrimental effects on fertility and must therefore be assessed and remedied during the preconception period.
Environmental impact	Other environmental assessments, including those that assess porphyrins, polychlorinated biphenyls (PCBs), chlorinated pesticides, volatile solvents, phthalates, parabens, and other toxins. These should also be considered because of their deranging effects on reproductive function, endocrinology, and gamete development and thus embryologic potential.

THERAPEUTIC CONSIDERATIONS

Ensure thorough, comprehensive assessment. Determine whether issue can be effectively treated: genetic factors or physical impediments require additional interventions.

- **Treatable conditions:** one in eight infertile men has a treatable condition whose resolution can allow natural conception.
- **Untreatable subfertility:** three quarters of infertile men have sperm in semen, but in abnormally low numbers. Pregnancies may occur, but at low rates. Naturopathic intervention may address infertility factors or offer referral for ARTs or IVF.
- **Untreatable male sterility:** one in nine infertile men has no sperm in semen or testes and cannot be treated. Sperm-producing cells in testes either never developed or were irreversibly destroyed.

Develop preconception program for both prospective parents. Preconception treatment arises from view that final stages of gamete production can be modified and influenced. Final stages of spermatogenesis last 72 to 76 days. Improving sperm environment and optimizing general well-being may support sperm development.

Nutrition status throughout sperm developmental can influence outcome. Concept: nutrient repletion is highly applicable to fertility. Nutritional interventions are required for at least 3 months to resolve deficiencies. Structure treatment to include all health concerns and optimize general health. The most favorable fertility occurs when health is optimal, to pass on genetic material only when the conditions are at their best. If survival from an evolutionary perspective is compromised, fertility will be hindered. Everything a person eats, drinks, experiences, or is exposed to will influence fertility. Encourage couples to participate in treatment for 3 to 4 months to properly address all genetic and epigenetic variables affecting the gamete.

SA is the most widely used test of male fertility potential. Semen is analyzed for concentration of sperm and sperm quality. Sperm count and quality in the male population has deteriorated over the last few decades. Men now supply 40% of the number of sperm per ejaculate compared with 1940 levels.

Causes of Male Infertility

Deficient sperm production

Ductal obstruction

- Congenital defects
- Postinfectious obstruction
- Cystic fibrosis
- Vasectomy

Ejaculatory dysfunction

- Premature ejaculation
- Retrograde ejaculation

Disorders of accessory glands

- Infection
- Inflammation
- Antisperm antibodies
- Coital disorders
- Defects in technique
- Premature withdrawal
- Erectile dysfunction

POSSIBLE CAUSES OF FALLING SPERM COUNTS

Increased scrotal temperature

- Tight-fitting clothing and briefs
- Varicoceles more common

Environmental
- Increased pollution
- Heavy metals (e.g., lead, mercury, arsenic)
- Organic solvents
- Pesticides

Dietary
- Increased saturated fats
- Reduced intake of fruits, vegetables, and whole grains
- Reduced intake of dietary fiber
- Increased exposure to synthetic estrogens

Environmental, dietary, and lifestyle changes in recent decades interfere with a man's ability to manufacture sperm. As sperm counts have declined, the line differentiating infertile and fertile men has been reduced progressively from 40 million/mL to 5 million/mL. Quality is more important than quantity; a high sperm count is meaningless if the percentage of healthy sperm is not also high.

Normal Spermatogenesis

Criteria	Value
Volume	1.5-5.0 mL
Density	>20 million sperm/mL
Motility	>30% motile
Normal forms	>60%

If most sperm are abnormally shaped or nonmotile, the man is infertile despite normal sperm concentration. Low sperm count does not always mean a man is infertile.

Causes of Temporary Low Sperm Count

- Increased scrotal temperature
- Infections, common cold, flu
- Increased stress
- Lack of sleep
- Overuse of alcohol, tobacco, or marijuana
- Many prescription drugs
- Exposure to radiation
- Exposure to solvents, pesticides, and other toxins

Conventional SA: must be interpreted with caution. Functional tests are indicated, especially when screening couples for IVF.

Postcoital test: measures ability of sperm to penetrate cervical mucus after intercourse.

Hamster egg penetration test: human sperm can, under appropriate conditions, penetrate hamster eggs. Fertile males have a range of penetration of 10% to 100%; penetration of less than 10% indicates infertility. This test predicts fertility in 66% of cases compared with 30% for conventional SA.

Antisperm antibodies: those produced by men attack the tail of sperm, impeding motility and penetration of cervical mucus. Antibodies produced by women attack the head. Antibodies in semen are a sign of past or current infection in the male reproductive tract.

THERAPEUTIC CONSIDERATIONS

- Standard medical treatment of oligospermia is effective when the cause is known (increased scrotal temperature, chronic infection of male sex glands, pharmaceuticals, endocrine disturbances such as hypogonadism and hypothyroidism), but 90% of cases are idiopathic. Azoospermia caused by ductal obstruction is surgically correctable.
- Rational approach is to enhance factors promoting spermatogenesis. Sperm formation is linked to scrotal temperature and nutritional status. Eat a healthy diet and use nutritional factors: antioxidants, essential fats and oils, zinc (Zn), vitamin B_{12}, carnitine, arginine. Avoid dietary sources of estrogens. Use botanicals that increase sperm counts and glandular therapy.

Improving Sperm-Controlling and Sperm-Damaging Factors

First steps to improve sperm counts, morphology, and function: control factors that damage or impair sperm formation (see box).

- Scrotal temperature
- Estrogen and xenoestrogen exposure
- Heavy metals
- Radiation
- Cigarettes, alcohol, illicit drugs
- Obesity
- Infection

Scrotal Temperature

Normal temperature is 94°F to 96°F. Above 96°F, sperm production is inhibited or halted. Mean scrotal temperature is higher in infertile men than in fertile men. Reducing scrotal temperature may be enough to make them fertile. Best methods are to avoid tight-fitting underwear, tight jeans, and hot tubs. Avoid performing exercises that raise scrotal temperature while wearing synthetic fabrics, tight shorts, or tight bikini underwear, such as rowing machines, simulated cross-country ski machines, treadmills, and jogging.

- Allow testicles to hang free to recover from heat buildup. Wear boxer-type underwear.
- Apply cold shower or ice to scrotum. Use "testicular hypothermia device" or "testicle cooler," which must be worn daily during waking hours. It is fairly comfortable and easy to conceal.
- Rule out varicocele, which can increase temperatures high enough to inhibit sperm production and motility. Surgical repair may be necessary, but try scrotal cooling first.

Genitourinary Infections

Genitourinary infections play a major role in many cases. Many infections are asymptomatic. Antisperm antibodies are good indicators of chronic infection. A wide range of microbes can infect the male genitourinary system.

- *Chlamydia* is the most common and serious and a major cause of acute nonbacterial prostatitis and urethritis. Symptoms are pain or burning on urination or ejaculation. More serious is *Chlamydia* infection of the epididymis and vas deferens; scarring and blockage can occur. Antibiotics are essential—tetracyclines and erythromycin. Because *Chlamydia* organisms live within host cells, total eradication is difficult. Chronic infections can be asymptomatic. Twenty-eight percent to 71% of infertile men have evidence of chlamydial infection. Antibiotics typically provide only limited improvements in sperm count and quality, but isolated cases of tremendous improvement after antibiotics have occurred. Both partners should take the antibiotic, but only if evidence of chronic infection is present. Antisperm antibodies may indicate chronic *Chlamydia* infection. In the absence of a positive culture, rectal ultrasonography and anti-*Chlamydia* antibodies confirm diagnosis.

Avoiding Estrogens

- The "virtual sea of estrogens" in the environment increases exposure to estrogens during fetal development and reproductive years. This is a major cause of increased disorders of development and function of the male sexual system.
- Avoiding hormone-fed animal and milk products is important for male sexual vitality, especially in oligospermia and hypotestosteronemia.

- Estrogens have been detected in drinking water and are harmful to male sexual vitality. These are presumably recycled synthetic estrogens (birth control pills), which are more potent because they do not bind to sex hormone–binding globulin. Use purified water. Avoid bottled water owing to bisphenol A content of plastic bottles.
- Weakly estrogenic xenobiotics (polychlorinated biphenyls, dioxin, dichlorodiphenyltrichloroethane) resist biodegradation and are recycled in the environment and interfere with spermatogenesis.
- Greatest impact is during fetal development. Estrogens inhibit multiplication of Sertoli cells, the number of which is directly proportional to the number of sperm produced. Sertoli cell multiplication occurs during fetal life and before puberty under control of follicle-stimulating hormone (FSH). Estrogens inhibit FSH secretion, causing a reduced number of Sertoli cells and reduced sperm counts.
- **Fiber:** a low-fiber, high-fat diet is linked to higher levels of estrogens because estrogens excreted in bile are reabsorbed because they are not being bound by fiber.
- **Phytoestrogens:** if testosterone is low or marginal or if estrogens are elevated, milled flaxseed and legumes (beans), especially soy foods, may be of benefit. Milled flaxseed is our best source of lignan precursors to mammalian lignan phytoestrogens. Soy is a good source of isoflavonoid phytoestrogens. Phytoestrogens have 0.2% of estrogen activity of estradiol. Mammalian lignans and isoflavones bind to estrogen receptors. Their weak estrogenic action is antiestrogenic, preventing binding of endogenous estrogen to receptors. Phytoestrogens may reduce effects of estrogens by stimulating production of sex hormone–binding globulin, which binds estrogens.
- **Phytosterols:** milled flaxseed, soy, other legumes, nuts, and seeds are good sources of phytosterols that aid steroid hormone synthesis, including testosterone.

Environmental Toxins

- Linked to increasing testicular cancer rates, testicular dysgenesis syndrome (TDS), cryptorchidism, and hypospadias.
- Pathogenesis may depend on timing and nature of xenobiotic attack and genetic background on which factors are acting.
- Take into account patient's polymorphism profile for proteins involved in detoxification—cytochrome p450s and glutathione-*S*-transferases.

- Novel industrial complex chemicals are reproductive toxicants, capable of impairing fertility and inducing developmental abnormalities in the embryo, including errors in normal sexual differentiation. They can generate damage passed down the generations via genetic or epigenetic means.
- Paternal smoking: generates spermatozoa with DNA damage from oxidative stress. Children arising from damaged DNA have increased incidence of childhood cancer. DNA damage in the germ line impairs well-being of future generations. Discourage exposure to cigarette smoke.

Exposure Route

Environmental toxins may exert germ line genetic or epigenetic effects via several potential routes of exposure:

1. Women exposed to xenobiotics during pregnancy, disrupting normal differentiation of germ line in the fetus.
2. Women exposed to toxicants may transmit xenobiotics to offspring via breast milk.
3. Because of acquired toxicity, men may contribute adverse effects on integrity of DNA in the male germ line.

Toxicity Assessment

Specific areas to consider include the following:

- Full occupational exposure review
- Nonoccupational exposure

- Area where couple lives
- Age of couple's home
- Ages of carpet, floor coverings, floorboards
- Renovations—when, what, and how
- Type of heating and air conditioning
- Indoor or outdoor pesticides
- Attached garage
- Blinds, curtains
- Cleaning products
- Pool, spa, sauna
- Pets—type, medicines, foods
- Food sources
- Water source
- Others

- Recommend avoidance of other exposures—renovation materials, cleaning products, personal toiletries, new furniture, new carpet or cabinets, plastics, gas, chemical gases, and so on. Organic, environmentally sound, sustainable practices are safest.
- Men who work in occupations that may affect fertility must wear protective clothing and follow all occupational health and safety guidelines.

Heavy Metals

Sperm are susceptible to damage by heavy metals (lead, cadmium, arsenic, mercury). Hair mineral analysis is indicated for all men with oligospermia.

Radiation: Cell Phones

Cell phones operate at 400- and 2000-MHz frequency bands and emit radiofrequency electromagnetic waves (EMWs). Cordless phones use 900-MHz, 1.9-GHz, 2.4-GHz, and 5.8-GHz bands. Reports of adverse effects of radiofrequency EMWs on the brain, heart, endocrine system, and DNA are common. They are implicated in DNA strand breaks. Relationship between cell phone use and male infertility remains unclear. Harmful EMWs may interfere with spermatogenesis, thereby decreasing sperm quality and motility. Cell phones decrease sperm count, motility, viability, and normal morphology, with decline worsening as cell phone use increases. Use of cell phones more than 4 hours daily causes a 25% drop in sperm count and only 20% of remaining sperm are normal.

Cigarettes, Alcohol, and Illicit Drugs

- **Cigarette smoking:** source of oxidants linked to decreased sperm counts and motility and higher frequency of abnormal sperm. Heavy smokers produce 20% less sperm. Cigarette smoking accelerates sperm DNA damage; smoking cessation is the quickest treatment to reverse the trend. When a sperm head enters an oocyte during conception, oocyte mRNA attempts to defragment sperm DNA and provide antioxidant support. Improvements to sperm occur before any oocyte maintenance. Only after sperm issues have been addressed can oocyte mRNA antioxidant potential address oocyte deficiency, oxidative process, or DNA (or chromosomal) abnormality. If the man is a heavy smoker, there are insufficient reserves to repair damage for both gametes. The oocyte fails, resulting in either fertilization deficits, lack of implantation, or embryo abnormalities, thus initiating early miscarriage or impaired long-term health and fertility of the child. The woman's surveillance does not allow compromised embryo to mature. Active or passive smoking is linked to reduced fertility and infant health. Smoking impairs sperm respiration, affecting mitochondrial function and causing reduced sperm motility and semen quality.

- **Alcohol intake:** excessive alcohol intake diminishes sperm function. Encourage avoidance during preconception period to ensure optimal sperm parameters.
- **Marijuana and other recreational drugs:** A known fertility toxicant, marijuana contains *cannabinoids,* which impair signaling pathways, alter hormonal regulation, and complicate timing issues during embryo implantation. Cannabinoids inhibit mitochondrial respiration of sperm, reduce testosterone production, decrease sperm motility, compromise sperm morphology, and decrease sperm capacitation and acrosome reactions.

Obesity

- Obese men have lower sperm counts (up to 50%), reduced sperm motility, reduced spermatogenesis, increased sperm DNA fragmentation, and increased erectile dysfunction. Extra-abdominal obesity increases scrotal temperature.
- Cause: reduced total and free testosterone relative to the level of obesity. Estrogens, increased owing to aromatization of androgens in adipose tissue, induce negative feedback on gonadotropin production, thereby reducing FSH. FSH decline reduces testosterone production and spermatogenesis.
- Excess body fat and sedentary lifestyle elevate testicular temperature, impairing spermatogenesis.

Infections and Infertility

- Infections in genitourinary tract—epididymis, seminal vesicles, prostate, bladder, and urethra—can cause infertility. They can be asymptomatic. Antisperm antibodies or abundant debris in semen can indicate chronic infection absent other clinical findings.
- A wide range of bacteria, viruses, and so on can infect the male genitourinary system.

Diet

- **Essential fatty acids (Eva's):** surrounding entire sperm is "shield" of EFAs—protecting structure, enabling continuity of movement, and safeguarding genome. Assess dietary intake: avoid *trans,* hydrogenated, rancid, and oxidized fats; cotton oils; and excessive saturated fats. EFAs ensure sperm fluidity and flexibility, regulating acrosome reaction, sperm-oocyte fusion, and sperm-oocyte fertilization. Cottonseed contains gossypol, which inhibits sperm function and is being studied for a "male birth control pill." Minimize long-chain saturated fats in meat. Supplement long-chain omega-3 fatty acids for sperm motility. Excessive omega-6/omega-3 ratio in seminal fluid decreases sperm concentration, motility, and morphology in idiopathic oligoasthenoteratozoospermia. Restrict omega-6 cooking oils—soy, corn, and safflower. Omega-3 dose: 1000 to 2000 mg eicosapentaenoic acid (EPA) plus docosahexaenoic acid (DHA) daily. Add: as raw nuts and seeds; cold-pressed monounsaturated olive oil; avocados; wild, sustainably harvested fish.

- **Protein:** entire sperm depends on protein status of the male. Insufficient protein impairs sperm morphology and motility. Assess protein statue via laboratory assessments (total protein status) and dietary calculation. Standard calculation: 0.8 to 1.2 g protein per 2.2 pounds (1 kg) body weight. Sedentary lifestyle: 0.8 g protein. Active lifestyle: 1.2 g protein.
- **Hydration:** dehydration enhances coagulation of semen and concentration levels of toxins. Water intake calculation: 30-mL/2.2-pound (1-kg) rule. For example, a 176-pound (80-kg) patient should drink 2.4 L pure water daily with additional intake for dehydration, exercise, and alcohol or caffeine intake.

Nutritional Supplements

- Antioxidant supplementation in subfertile men improves outcomes of live births and pregnancy rates for subfertile couples undergoing ART cycles. Subfertile men have lower levels of antioxidants in their semen than fertile men. Levels of reactive oxygen species (ROSs) are higher in infertile sperm compared with healthy controls.
- ROSs cause fertility problems by (1) damaging sperm membrane, impairing sperm motility and ability to break down oocyte membrane (zona pellucida); (2) altering sperm DNA.
- All antioxidants are concentrated in the head of the sperm to varying degrees. Encourage combination products to ensure greatest antioxidant potential. Antioxidants protect DNA within sperm head and reduce workload of oocyte mRNA. Optimizing oxidant status supports survival and longevity of sperm and enables them to detect signals from ovulated oocyte.
- Free radical or oxidative damage to sperm is the major cause of idiopathic oligospermia in many cases. Free radicals are abundant in semen of 40% of infertile men.

- Three factors combine to render sperm susceptible to free radical damage: (1) high membrane concentration of polyunsaturated fatty acids, (2) active generation of free radicals, and (3) lack of defensive enzymes.
- Health of sperm depends on antioxidants. Men exposed to increased levels of free radicals are more likely to have abnormal sperm and sperm counts. Sperm are sensitive to free radicals, which depend on integrity and fluidity of the cell membrane for proper function. Improper membrane fluidity activates enzymes that impair motility, structure, and viability of sperm. The major determinant of membrane fluidity is concentration of omega-3 polyunsaturated fatty acids (alpha-linolenic acid [ALA], EPA, DHA), which are susceptible to free radical damage.
- Sperm have low superoxide dismutase and catalase to neutralize free radicals and generate free radicals abundantly to break through barriers to fertilization.
- **Vitamin C:** vitamin C protects sperm DNA. Ascorbate is much higher in seminal fluid compared with other body fluids, including blood. Low dietary vitamin C is likely to lead to infertility. Smoking reduces vitamin C throughout the body. Sperm quality in smokers improves with ascorbate supplementation. Nonsmokers benefit from vitamin C as much as smokers.
- Sperm become agglutinated when antibodies bind to them. Antibodies to sperm are linked to chronic genitourinary tract or prostatic infection. When more than 25% of sperm are agglutinated, fertility is unlikely. Vitamin C reduces percentage of agglutinated sperm. Vitamin C is very effective in treating male infertility because of antibodies against sperm.
- **Vitamin E:** is the main antioxidant in sperm membranes. Free radicals lead to peroxidation of phospholipids in sperm mitochondria, making sperm immotile. It inhibits free radical damage to polyunsaturated fatty acids, enhances ability of sperm to fertilize egg in vitro, and decreases malondialdehyde in sperm pellet suspensions. Supplementation is indicated on the basis of its physiologic effects alone. It exerts more-beneficial effects on sperm counts or motility at higher doses (600 to 800 international units [IU] q.d.) and in combination with selenium (Se; 100 to 200 mcg q.d.). Vitamin E may also benefit couples undergoing IVF. Vitamin E (200 mg/day for at least 3 months) improves IVF rate of fertile normospermic males with low fertilization rates after 1 month of treatment, possibly by reducing lipid peroxidation. Benefits are also seen in ICSI: vitamin E helps prevent DNA fragmentation.

- **Vitamin A, beta-carotene, lycopene:** vitamin A is required for cellular growth and differentiation, gene expression and cellular differentiation, immunity, regulatory functions, and epithelial tissue integrity. It is essential for health of testes and for sperm production. Low vitamin A linked to abnormal semen parameters and loss of spermatogenesis as a result of degeneration of germ cells, which is restored once vitamin A is given. Beta-carotene levels are reduced in immune-infertile men. Intake can increase sperm concentration and motility. Lycopene may be even more useful than beta-carotene. Lycopene is present in high concentrations in testes and seminal plasma; levels are decreased in infertile men. In idiopathic nonobstructive oligozoospermia, asthenozoospermia, and teratozoospermia, 2 mg lycopene b.i.d. for 3 months improved sperm concentration by 22 million/mL, motility by 25%, and morphology by 10%.
- **Se:** antioxidant involved in testosterone synthesis, sperm maturation, and motility. It increases sperm motility and assists production of spermatozoa. Sperm's capsular selenoprotein is critical to the stability and motility of mature sperm. Se is part of glutathione peroxidase antioxidant system, vital for spermatogenesis, and protects sperm from ROSs. Depletion of mitochondrial glutathione peroxidase impairs sperm quality and structural integrity in midpiece of spermatozoa, leading to infertility. The tail of the sperm relies on adequate Se status to maintain its whip-like action. Without sufficient Se, sperm are unable to swim in the right direction or may display marked immotility, thus preventing oocyte location and fusion. Se (200 mcg/day) in combination with antioxidant *N*-acetylcysteine (600 mg/day) improves semen parameters in men with idiopathic oligoasthenoterato-spermia-plasma over 6.5 months, with improved sperm count, motility, and morphology. Parameters revert back to baseline in two spermatogenesis cycles if supplementation is halted.
- **Zn:** found in high concentrations within prostate, testes, and semen (2.5 mg Zn is lost per ejaculate). Zn is most critical trace mineral for male sexual function—works in hormone metabolism, sperm formation, and sperm motility. Zn is involved in transcription of RNA, replication of DNA, and synthesis of protein, all of which are crucial for reproduction and fertility. Zn protects against free radical damage and ROSs. Zn deficiency in males can lead to gonadal dysfunction and idiopathic male infertility and impotence. Zn deficiency decreases testosterone and sperm counts. Zn levels are much lower in

infertile men with oligospermia. Zn status correlates with sperm count and improvements in morphology and motility. Zn influences motility and the head-neck connection of sperm; it also helps stabilize sperm membranes and chromatin. Zn exerts antimicrobial effect on seminal plasma, helpful relative to sperm antibodies or underlying genitourinary infection. Zn supplementation (60 mg elemental Zn q.d. for 45 to 50 days) is indicated for oligospermia with low testosterone levels. Results of one study showed Zn supplements increased testosterone and sperm counts in men with infertility for longer than 5 years and resulted in impregnation of female partners. Zn deficiency is increasing worldwide depending on soil content. Owing to negative effects of excess copper, check serum Zn and copper status. Recommended daily allowance is 15 mg. Sources include whole grains, legumes, nuts, and seeds. Supplement dose: 45 to 60 mg q.d.

- **B vitamins (folic acid and vitamin B_{12}):** folic acid and vitamin B_{12} are concentrated within head of sperm for sperm generation and survival. Folate and B_{12} support DNA and RNA synthesis, protein synthesis, and regulation of gene expression. They help ensure that DNA within the sperm head is structured appropriately and that DNA replicates identically. Both facilitate spermatogenesis, which relies on DNA synthesis for germ cell growth and rapid division. Low folate in seminal plasma is linked to increased sperm DNA damage. B_{12} deficiency is linked to reduced sperm count and motility. High bodily B_{12} turnover necessitates supplementation, especially for sperm counts below 20 million/mL or motility rate below 50%. Recommend both folate and B_{12} together to avoid the masking of a deficit in one by supplementing only the other.
- **L-Carnitine** (Crn): is vital to long-chain fatty acid metabolism. It works synergistically with coenzyme Q10 (CoQ10). Crn is an antioxidant with greatest amount of clinical research for treating male infertility. It is essential for transporting fatty acids into mitochondria; deficiency decreases fatty acid levels in mitochondria and reduces energy production. Crn helps supply energy to testicles and spermatozoa. Fertile men have greater amount of carnitine in seminal samples than infertile men. Carnitine levels are high in epididymis and sperm. Epididymis gets most of its energy from fatty acids, as do sperm during transport through epididymis. After ejaculation, sperm motility correlates with carnitine content; the higher the carnitine content, the more

motile are the sperm. Carnitine deficit impairs sperm development, function, and motility. With 3000 mg L-carnitine q.d. for 4 months in patients with poorest sperm motility, motile sperm increased from 19.3% to 40.9% and sperm with rapid linear progression increased from 3.1% to 20.3%. Optimal dose: 1000 mg t.i.d.

- **Alpha-lipoic acid:** powerful antioxidant with lipid and water solubility. It assists in chelation of heavy metals regardless of storage site. It regenerates other antioxidants—vitamins C and E, CoQ10, and glutathione. Alpha-lipoic acid may act as a shield for sperm, forming a protective barrier around the midpiece, first attacked by free radicals, (aqueous layer) and within the structure itself (lipid layer). Consider Alpha-lipoic acid for patients with high DNA fragmentation. Alpha-lipoic acid improves sperm motility and viability, minimizes DNA damage, and protects against inflammatory bacterial lipopolysaccharides.
- **CoQ10:** concentrated in head and midpiece (neck) of sperm. It is the most crucial and powerful antioxidant in sperm because of its role in mitochondrial energy release. It may promote motility, foster sperm survival, and provide energy for sperm's travel to the oocyte. As fat-soluble antioxidant and free radical scavenger, CoQ10 helps maintain cell membrane integrity. It is specific for health of all new spermatozoa. CoQ10 in seminal fluid and sperm helps to maintain sperm motility. Decreased levels are found in the seminal plasma and spermatozoa of males with idiopathic and varicocele-associated asthenospermia.
- **L-Arginine:** required for replication of cells and essential in sperm formation. Nitric oxide synthase (NOS) converts L-arginine into nitric oxide, which protects sperm from lipid peroxidase damage. L-Arginine required for angiogenesis, spermatogenesis, and hormone secretion. L-Arginine may improve sperm count and motility. Stress decreases levels of arginine in sperm production pathways. It may be an effective treatment of male infertility. The critical determinant is the level of oligospermia; if counts are below 20 million/mL, arginine is less beneficial. Dosage: 4 or more g q.d. for 3 months. Reserve it for use after other nutritional measures have been tried. Prelox, a combination of 80 mg/day of pycnogenol and 3 g/day of L-arginine aspartate, improves semen parameters in idiopathic infertility after 4 weeks. It also increased ejaculate volume, concentration, number of sperm, percentage of vital sperm, and percentage of sperm with good progressing

motility. It decreases percentage of immotile sperm. L-Arginine stimulates activity of endothelial NOS, leading to enhanced motility of sperm.

Botanical Medicines

- ***Panax ginseng* (Chinese or Korean ginseng):** *Panax* is effective in male infertility. *Panax* promotes growth of testes, increases sperm formation and testosterone levels, and increases sexual activity and mating behavior in studies with animals. *Panax* enhances nitric oxide production, which helps regulate capacitating process of sperm and acrosome reaction. Thus *Panax* improves fertilization sperm motility. Ginsenosides influence hypothalamic-pituitary-testicular axis, modulating stress-induced infertility or lowered testosterone from insufficient dehydroepiandrosterone (DHEA) synthesis. *Panax* may increase testosterone levels and sperm counts. Panax can be used for oligospermia, even with varicocele, and for improvement of erection and libido.
- ***Pygeum africanum:*** improves fertility if diminished prostatic secretion plays significant role. It increases prostatic secretions and improves composition of seminal fluid by increasing total seminal fluid, alkaline phosphatase, and protein. It is most effective if alkaline phosphatase activity is reduced (<400 IU/ cm^3) with no evidence of inflammation or infection (no white blood cells or immunoglobulin A [IgA]). Lack of IgA in semen is a good indicator of potential clinical success. It improves capacity to achieve erection in patients with benign prostatic hypertrophy or prostatitis as determined by nocturnal penile tumescence. (Benign prostatic hypertrophy and prostatitis often are linked to erectile dysfunction and other sexual disturbances.)
- ***Tribulus terrestris:*** Ayurvedic tonic and aphrodisiac; used in European folk medicine to increase sexual potency. Chief constituent: protodioscin, a steroidal saponin. Correct sourcing of *Tribulus* is critical to ensure its effectiveness. All scientific data and clinical outcomes are based on a leaf extract from Bulgaria, highest in protodioscin. Sources form other nations or plant parts may be less effective. In animal studies, *Tribulus* increased sex hormones (e.g., testosterone) and improved nitric oxide synthesis; however, these results have not been observed in some human studies. Explanation: differences in extract and plant parts and the fact that studies included healthy males

with normal testosterone. *Tribulus* enhances male fertility by increasing sperm count, viability, and libido; however, study results are unclear.

- ***Astragalus membranaceus:*** increases motility of sperm in semen. *Astragalus* increases motility of sperm in semen and motility of washed sperm, relevant to those seeking ART treatment.
- ***Turnera diffusa* (damiana):** traditionally used for "its positive aphrodisiac effects, acting energetically on the genitourinary organs of both genders where it was highly indicated for sexual weakness and debility." It is a stimulant tonic of sexual organs, especially during "enfeeblement of the central nervous system." It is especially beneficial for sexual debility, erectile difficulty, and depression. Human studies are lacking. In male rats: damiana facilitates sexual behavior in rats with sexual dysfunction, reduces ejaculation latency, produces a restorative effect in sexual exhaustion, and hastens recovery. It suppresses aromatase activity, perhaps increasing levels of testosterone.
- ***Mucuna pruriens*** (velvet bean): Ayurvedic medicine for endurance against stress, resistance against infection, retardation of aging process, and improvement of male sexual function; it alleviates psychogenic impotence and unexplained infertility. *M. pruriens* seed powder helps fight stress-mediated poor semen quality. It is a restorative and invigorating tonic and aphrodisiac in infertile subjects. Mechanism: regulation of steroidogenesis and resulting improvements in semen quality. It improves testosterone, luteinizing hormone (LH), dopamine, adrenaline, and noradrenaline levels in infertile men and reduces FSH and prolactin (PRL). Sperm count and motility were also improved in infertile men.
- ***Withania somnifera*** *(Withania):* has antistress and adaptogenic effects. At a dose of 5 g powdered root daily, *Withania* inhibited lipid peroxidation and improved sperm count and motility. It increased serum testosterone and LH and reduced follicle FSH and PRL, all beneficial effects in infertile men.

THERAPEUTIC APPROACH

Refer to a urologist or fertility specialist for complete evaluation. Encourage detoxification program at start of treatment to optimize spermatogenesis. Optimize nutrition (antioxidants and Zn). Identify and eliminate environmental pollutants. Use fertility-enhancing botanicals. Avoid xenobiotics, pollutants, and toxicants.

- **General measures:**
  - — Maintain scrotal temperature at 94°F to 96°F.
  - — Avoid exposure to free radicals.
  - — Identify and eliminate environmental pollutants.
  - — Stop or reduce, in coordination with prescribing physicians, all drugs (antihypertensives, antineoplastics [cyclophosphamide], and anti-inflammatories [sulfasalazine]),
  - — Avoid cigarette smoking and recreational drugs.
- **Stress-reduction techniques** and psychological counseling, if needed
- **Dietary measures:**
  - — Avoid dietary free radicals, saturated fats, hydrogenated oils, *trans* fatty acids, and cottonseed oil.
  - — Increase legumes (soy for phytoestrogens and phytosterols), dietary antioxidant vitamins, carotenes, and flavonoids (dark-colored vegetables and fruits), EFAs, and Zn (nuts and seeds).
  - — Eat 8 to 10 servings of vegetables, 2 to 4 servings of fresh fruits, and half a cup of raw nuts or seeds daily.
  - — Optimize protein intake from vegetarian and organic animal sources.
  - — Optimize hydration: 30-mL/2.2-pound (1 kg) daily.
  - — Eliminate caffeine, alcohol, sugar, artificial substances (preservatives, colorings, additives).
  - — Ensure sufficient EFA intake: raw nuts and seeds, organic cold-pressed monounsaturated and omega-3 oils, wild and sustainably farmed fish.
- **Nutritional supplements:**
  - — High-potency multiple vitamin-mineral q.d.
  - — Fish oil: 1000 to 2000 mg combined EPA plus DHA
  - — Vitamin C: 500 to 1000 mg t.i.d.
  - — Vitamin E: 200 to 400 IU q.d. (mixed tocopherols)
  - — Beta-carotene: 15,000 to 30,000 IU q.d. (mixed carotenoids)
  - — Folic acid: 400 mcg q.d.
  - — Vitamin B_{12} (methylcobalamin): 1000 mcg q.d.
  - — Zn: 30 to 60 mg elemental Zn q.d. (picolinate)
  - — Se: 200 to 400 mcg q.d.
  - — Lycopene: 2 mg q.d.
  - — CoQ10: 200 to 400 mg q.d.

— L-Carnitine: 2000 to 3000 mg q.i.d.
— L-Arginine: 2000 to 4000 mg q.d.

- **Botanical medicines:**

Choose one or more of the following:

- *P. ginseng* (Korean ginseng)
  — High-quality crude ginseng root: 1.5 to 2 g q.d. (standardized extract containing at least 10.5 mg/mL ginsenosides with Rg1/Rb1 greater than or equal to 0.5 by HPLC), 1 to 6 mL q.d.
- *P. africanum (Pygeum)*
  — Standardized extract (standardized to 14% content of sterols): 100 to 200 mg q.d. in divided doses
- *T. terrestris* (tribulus)
  — Standardized extract, equivalent to dried herb (aerial parts of leaf), standardized to contain furostanol saponins as protodioscin 12.22 mg/L g, 9 to 36 g q.d.
  — Fluid extract (2:1): 7 to 21 mL q.d.
- *A. membranaceus (Astragalus)*
  — Doses administered q.d. to t.i.d. as follows:
  — Dried root (or as decoction or as powder in capsules or tablets): 1 to 2 g
  — Tincture (1:5): 2 to 4 mL
  — Fluid extract (1:1): 1 to 2 mL solid (dried powdered) extract (standardized to contain 0.5% 4-hydroxy-3-methoxy isoflavone): 100 to 150 mg
- *T. diffusa* (damiana)
  — Dried leaves or as tea: 2 to 4 g q.d.
  — Fluid extract (1:2): 3.0 to 6.0 mL q.d.
  — Dried powdered extract (4:1): 500 to 1000 mg q.d.
- *M. pruriens* (velvet bean)
  — Dose equivalent to 5 g q.d. of powdered dried seed
- *W. somnifera (Withania)*
  — Dose equivalent to 5 g of the powdered root per day
  — Dried powdered extract (root and leaves), 125 to 250 mg/day (standardized to contain 8% withanolide glycoside conjugates and 32% oligosaccharides)
  — Fluid extract (2:1): containing a minimum of 4.0 mg/mL of withanolides, 2.5 to 5.0 mL q.d.

Inflammatory Bowel Disease

DIAGNOSTIC SUMMARY

Crohn's Disease

- Abdominal pain—can be localized anywhere in the abdomen
- Complicated by intestinal obstruction, abscesses, fistulas, strictures, perianal disease
- Intermittent diarrhea or constipation, low-grade fever, weight loss
- Frequently misdiagnosed as irritable bowel syndrome; time to diagnosis—8 years
- Diagnostic modalities: serologies, ileocolonoscopy, capsule endoscopy
- Radiographic evidence: abnormality of terminal ileum is characteristic
- Stools: high in lactoferrin and calprotectin—noninvasive inflammatory markers
- Genetic predisposition, environmental trigger (e.g., infection, medications), chronic full-thickness patchy intestinal inflammation
- Risk of digestive tract cancer higher than in general population

Ulcerative Colitis

- Bloody diarrhea with cramps in lower abdomen
- Mild abdominal tenderness, weight loss, fever
- Involves only the colon; distinguishing point from Crohn's disease (CD), which can involve any portion of the alimentary tract
- Inflammation is superficial and continuous
- Diagnosis is confirmed by radiography and sigmoidoscopy
- Risk of colon cancer increased after 10 years of disease and universal distribution throughout colon
- Genetic predisposition, triggers similar to those of CD

GENERAL CONSIDERATIONS

Definition

Inflammatory bowel disease (IBD) is a general term for a group of chronic inflammatory disorders of the bowel. The two major

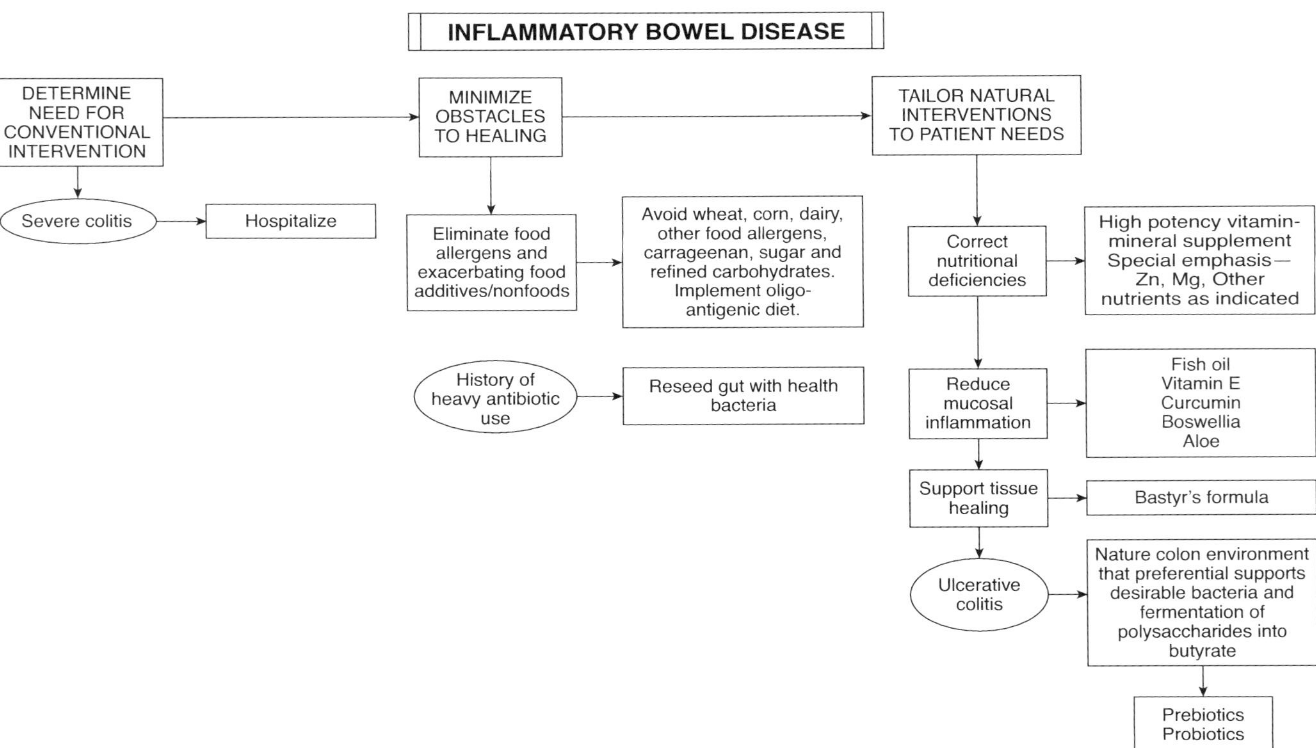
INFLAMMATORY BOWEL DISEASE
DETERMINE NEED FOR CONVENTIONAL INTERVENTION
Severe colitis
Hospitalize
MINIMIZE OBSTACLES TO HEALING
Eliminate food allergens and exacerbating food additives/nonfoods
Avoid wheat, corn, dairy, other food allergens, carrageenan, sugar and refined carbohydrates. Implement oligo-antigenic diet.
History of heavy antibiotic use
Reseed gut with health bacteria
TAILOR NATURAL INTERVENTIONS TO PATIENT NEEDS
Correct nutritional deficiencies
High potency vitamin-mineral supplement Special emphasis— Zn, Mg, Other nutrients as indicated
Reduce mucosal inflammation
Fish oil
Vitamin E
Curcumin
Boswellia
Aloe
Support tissue healing
Bastyr's formula
Ulcerative colitis
Nature colon environment that preferential supports desirable bacteria and fermentation of polysaccharides into butyrate
Prebiotics
Probiotics

categories are CD and ulcerative colitis (UC). IBD is characterized by recurrent inflammatory involvement of specific intestinal segments, resulting in diverse clinical manifestations.

- **CD:** lesions are a granulomatous inflammatory reaction throughout entire thickness of bowel wall. In 40% of cases, granulomas are either poorly developed or totally absent. May involve buccal mucosa, esophagus, stomach, duodenum, jejunum, ileum, and colon. Rectal biopsies during flexible sigmoidoscopy or colonoscopy often reveal granulomas at this site. CD of small intestine is called *regional enteritis;* colon involvement is called *Crohn's disease of the colon* or *granulomatous colitis* (only a portion of patients develop granulomatous lesions).
- **UC:** lesions are a nonspecific inflammatory response limited to colonic mucosa and submucosa. Well-developed granuloma formation does not occur.

Common features shared by CD and UC include the following:

- Colon is frequently involved in CD and invariably involved in UC.
- Although rarely, patients with UC and total colon involvement may develop "backwash ileitis"; both conditions may cause changes in small intestine.
- Patients with CD often have close relatives with UC and vice versa.
- When no granuloma is present in CD of the colon, the two lesions may resemble each other clinically and pathologically.
- Many epidemiologic similarities exist between CD and UC: age, race, sex, and geographic distribution.
- Both conditions are associated with similar extraintestinal manifestations.
- The two conditions have etiologic parallels.
- Both conditions are associated with increased frequency of colonic carcinoma.

Etiology

UC is more common. The incidence of UC in Western Europe and the United States is six to eight cases per 100,000, and prevalence is 7 to 150 cases per 100,000. The incidence of CD is two cases per 100,000, and prevalence is 20 to 40 per 100,000. The incidence of CD is increasing in Western cultures. IBD may occur at any age but most often from ages 15 to 35 years. Women are affected slightly more frequently than men. Whites are affected two to five times more frequently than African Americans or Asian Americans. Jews have threefold to sixfold higher incidence compared with non-Jews. Theories about etiology of IBD include the following:

- **Genetic predisposition:** supported by ethnic distribution of incidence and multiple members of a family having CD or UC in 15% to 40% of cases.
- **Infectious cause:** the idea that a transmissible agent is responsible for IBD is a hotly debated subject. Viruses (rotavirus, Epstein-Barr virus, cytomegalovirus, and an uncharacterized RNA intestinal cytopathic virus) and mycobacteria continue to be favored candidates. Gastrointestinal (GI) infections with *Aeromonas* bacteria (*Aeromonas sobria* and *Aeromonas hydrophila*) and *Candida albicans* can initiate and perpetuate colitis. Test all IBD patients for these infections at start of and during course of illness. Other candidates include pseudomonas-like organisms, enteric anaerobes, *Chlamydia,* and *Yersinia enterocolitica.*
- **Antibiotic exposure:** before the 1950s, CD was found in selected groups with strong genetic component. Since then, a rapid increase has occurred in developed countries and countries that previously had virtually no reported cases. CD has spread like an epidemic. Wherever antibiotics are used early and in large quantities, the incidence of CD is now quite high. An infectious agent may be a normal intestinal organism suddenly producing immunostimulatory toxins or becoming invasive after sublethal doses of antibiotics that induce flora to become stronger in virility and numbers and more capable of producing toxins. Other drugs implicated as etiopathogenic include nonsteroidal anti-inflammatory agents (NSAIDs) and isotretinoin (Accutane).
- **Immunologic derangements in IBD:** whether causal of IBD or secondary to it remains unclear. Current evidence indicates that derangements are secondary to disease process.
- Dietary factors:
  - CD is increasing in cultures consuming a Western diet. It is virtually nonexistent in cultures consuming a primitive diet. People who have CD habitually eat more refined sugar and chemically modified fats and fast food and less raw fruit and vegetables, omega-3–rich foods, and dietary fiber than do healthy people (122 g sugar daily versus 65 g daily). Corn flakes have been linked to CD; they are high in refined carbohydrates and derived from common allergen (corn).
  - UC is not linked to refined carbohydrates. Food allergy is overlooked by conventional medicine.

— Reduced intake of omega-3 oils and increased intake of omega-6 oils are linked to growing rise of CD in Japan. Genetics of the Japanese are relatively homogenous; therefore the increased incidence is from incorporation of Western foods. CD is strongly correlated with increased dietary total fat, animal fat, omega-6 fatty acids, animal protein, milk protein, and ratio of omega-6 to omega-3 fatty acids. CD is less correlated with total protein and not correlated with fish protein. CD is inversely correlated with vegetable protein. Increased animal protein is the strongest independent factor, followed by increased ratio of omega-6 to omega-3 fatty acids.

- **Miscellaneous factors:** mental and emotional stress can promote exacerbation of IBD. Thus stress management techniques may prove useful for some patients.

THERAPEUTIC CONSIDERATIONS

Control of Causative Factors

- **Natural history of CD:** many patients undergo spontaneous remission, 20% at 1 year and 12% at 2 years. "Success" of placebo therapy rises dramatically. In patients having no history of steroid therapy, 41% attained remission after 17 weeks; 23% of this group continued in remission after 2 years, compared with 4% of group with history of steroid use. Once remission is achieved, 75% of patients continue in remission at the end of 1 year and up to 63% by 2 years, regardless of maintenance therapy used. The key is achieving remission, which, once attained, can be maintained by conservative nondrug therapy.
- **Eicosanoid metabolism:** prostaglandins are greatly increased in colonic mucosa, serum, and stools of IBD patients. Increased synthesis of lipoxygenase products, leukotrienes, and monohydroxyeicosatetraenoic acid by neutrophils amplifies inflammation and causes smooth muscle contraction. Release of lipoxygenase products is promoted by activation of alternative complement pathway. Sulfasalazine inhibits cyclooxygenase and neutrophil lipoxygenase and inhibits degranulation of mast cells. Corticosteroids inhibit phospholipase A_2, blocking release of arachidonic acid from membrane phospholipids. Natural flavonoid polyphenols (e.g., quercetin, curcumin, resveratrol) interact with these enzymes. Formation of inflammatory compounds is decreased by reducing dietary omega-6

rich foods (corn, meat, and dairy) and increasing omega-3 fatty acids (small wild cold-water ocean fish), containing eicosapentaenoic acid (EPA) and docosahexaenoic acid (DHA). Fish oil supplements (2.7 to 5.1 g total omega-3 oils daily) prevent or delay relapses in CD and UC.

- **Mucin defects in UC:** mucins are high-molecular-weight, carbohydrate-rich glycoproteins responsible for viscous and elastic characteristics of secreted mucus. Alterations in mucin composition and content in colonic mucosa are noted in UC. Factors include a dramatic decrease in mucous content of goblet cells (proportional to severity of disease) and decrease in major sulfomucin subfraction. These abnormalities are not found in CD. Mucin content of goblet cells returns to normal during remission, but sulfomucin deficiency does not. Specific components of sulfomucin and the cause of its lower level are unknown. Mucin abnormalities are a major factor in increased risk of colon cancer in these patients. Many herbs effectively used to treat UC are demulcents, agents that soothe irritated mucous membranes and promote secretion of mucus.
- **Intestinal microflora** (*Textbook,* "Bacterial Overgrowth of the Small Intestine" and "Comprehensive Digestive Stool Analysis"): include 400 distinct species. Fecal flora of patients with IBD contain higher numbers of gram-positive anaerobic coccoid rods and *Bacteroides vulgatus,* a gram-negative rod. These alterations in fecal flora are not from disease. Alterations in metabolic activity of bacteria are more important than alterations in number of bacteria. Specific bacterial cell components may promote lymphocyte cytotoxic activity against colonic epithelial cells. Early research is showing some response to fecal transplants, supporting the concept that microflora imbalance plays an important role in the underlying pathophysiology.
- **Carrageenans:** sulfated polymers of galactose and D-anhydrogalactose extracted from red seaweeds (*Eucheuma spinosum* or *Chondrus crispus*) have been used to induce IBD in animals. They are used by the food industry as stabilizing and suspending agents (e.g., in ice cream, cottage cheese, milk chocolate) because of their ability to stabilize milk proteins. No correlation has been proven between human consumption of carrageenan and development of UC. Differences in intestinal bacterial flora probably are responsible for discrepancy: germ-free animals do not display carrageenan-induced damage. A bacterium linked

to facilitating carrageenan-induced damage in animals is a strain of *B. vulgatus* found in much higher concentrations (six times as high) in fecal cultures of patients with IBD. Carrageenan is metabolized into nondamaging components in most human beings, but people with overgrowth of *B. vulgatus* may be at risk. Avoid carrageenan.

- **Aspirin and intestinal permeability:** first-degree relatives of CD patients had a 110% increase in intestinal permeability after acetylsalicylic acid (ASA) compared with an increase of 57% in control subjects. Thirty-five percent were hyperresponders. Familial permeability defect is a significant predisposing factor for CD because leaky gut is linked to increased incidence of food allergy and absorption of intestinal toxins (*Textbook,* "Food Allergy").
- **Endotoxemia and alternative complement pathway:** endotoxemia is linked to CD and UC. Endotoxemia-induced activation of alternative complement pathway could explain extra-GI manifestations of IBD. Whole-gut irrigation significantly reduces endotoxin pool in the gut and has a beneficial antiendotoxinemic effect. Colonic irrigation may offer similar benefit. Colonic irrigation during acute inflammatory flare is contraindicated.

Extraintestinal Manifestations

More than 100 disorders are systemic complications of IBD. The most common extraintestinal lesion (EIL) in adults is arthritis (25% of patients).

- **Arthritis:** the more-common form is peripheral arthritis that affects knees, ankles, and wrists. Arthritis is more common in patients with colon involvement. Severity of symptoms is proportional to disease activity. Arthritis may primarily affect the spine, with low back pain and stiffness and eventual limitation of motion. This EIL occurs mainly in men with human leukocyte antigen (HLA) HLA-B27 and resembles ankylosing spondylitis. It may antedate bowel symptoms by several years. A consistent underlying factor in progression of ankylosing spondylitis and IBD is likely.
- **Skin manifestations:** seen in 15% of patients. Lesions include erythema nodosum, pyoderma gangrenosum, and aphthous ulcerations. Recurrent aphthous stomatitis occurs in 10% of patients.
- **Liver:** serious liver disease (sclerosing cholangitis, chronic active hepatitis, cirrhosis) affects 3% to 7% of patients with IBD from

increased endotoxin load. Liver enzyme abnormalities indicate need for hepatoprotection from *Glycyrrhiza glabra* (licorice), *Silybum marianum* (milk thistle), catechin, and curcumin.
- **Other common EILs:** thrombophlebitis; finger clubbing; ocular manifestations (episcleritis, iritis, and uveitis); nephrolithiasis; cholelithiasis; and, in children, failure to grow, thrive, and mature normally.

Malnutrition

Nutritional complications of IBD have a great influence on morbidity (and mortality).

Protein-calorie malnutrition and associated weight loss are prevalent in 65% to 75% of IBD patients. Malabsorption arises from extensive mucosal involvement of small intestine and resection of segments of small intestine. Fat malabsorption causes a loss of calories and fat-soluble vitamins and minerals. Ileum involvement or resection causes vitamin (especially B_{12}) and bile acid malabsorption, and cathartic effect of bile acids on colon causes chronic watery diarrhea. Expect electrolyte and trace mineral deficiency from chronic diarrhea, plus calcium (Ca) and magnesium (Mg) deficiency from chronic steatorrhea. Loss of plasma proteins across damaged and inflamed mucosa may exceed the ability of the liver to replace plasma proteins. Chronic blood loss causes iron (Fe)–depletion anemia. Drugs used to treat IBD (corticosteroids and sulfasalazine) increase nutritional needs.

Causes of Malnutrition in Inflammatory Bowel Disease

- Decreased oral intake:
  - Disease-induced (pain, diarrhea, nausea, anorexia)
  - Iatrogenic (restrictive diets without supplementation)
- Malabsorption:
  - Decreased absorptive surface from disease or resection
  - Bile salt deficiency after resection
  - Bacterial overgrowth
  - Drugs (e.g., corticosteroids, sulfasalazine, cholestyramine)
- Increased secretion and nutrient loss:
  - Protein-losing enteropathy
  - Electrolyte, mineral, and trace mineral loss in diarrhea
- Increased use and increased requirements:
  - Inflammation, fever, infection
  - Increased intestinal cell turnover

- **Corticosteroids** are known to do the following:
  - Stimulate protein catabolism
  - Depress protein synthesis
  - Decrease the absorption of Ca and phosphorus
  - Increase the urinary excretion of ascorbic acid, Ca, potassium (K), and zinc (Zn)
  - Increase blood glucose, serum triglycerides, and serum cholesterol
  - Increase the requirements for vitamin B_6, ascorbic acid, folate, and vitamin D
  - Decrease bone formation
  - Impair wound healing
- **Sulfasalazine** has been shown to do the following:
  - Inhibit the absorption and transport of folate
  - Decrease serum folate and Fe
  - Increase the urinary excretion of ascorbic acid

Nutritional Consequences of Chronic Inflammatory and/or Infectious Disease

Protein requirement may be increased. Elevated sedimentation rate signifies increased protein breakdown and synthesis. IBD requires 25% more protein than usual recommended allowance.

Prevalence of Nutritional Deficiencies

Nutritional deficiencies are quite high in hospitalized patients with IBD. Hospitalized patients have a greater incidence of nutritional deficiencies than do outpatients (more-severe condition). Ambulatory patients with CD also display nutrient deficiencies: Fe, B_{12}, folate, Mg, K, retinol, ascorbate, vitamin D, Zn, vitamin K, copper, niacin, and vitamin E. Assume that most patients have micronutrient deficiency. Deficiency often is subclinical and only detected by laboratory investigation. Use therapeutic-potency vitamin supplements of at least five times the recommended daily allowance. Several minerals may need supplementing at similar levels. Dietary treatment is either elemental or elimination diet.

- **Elemental diet:** effective nontoxic alternative to corticosteroids as a primary treatment of acute IBD. It contains all essential nutrients: protein as predigested or free-form amino acids. It provides nutritional improvement, alters fecal flora, and serves as allergy elimination diet. The main drawback is unpalatability and hyperosmolality (causing diarrhea). Hospitalization is often required for satisfactory administration, and relapse is common when patients resume normal eating. Elimination diet may be acceptable alternative for acute flare-up of IBD, especially in chronic cases of IBD.

- **Elimination (oligoantigenic) diet:** elimination is the primary therapy for chronic IBD. The most common offending foods are wheat and dairy. Alternative approach is to determine actual allergens by laboratory methods—measure reactions mediated by immunoglobulin G (IgG) and IgE. Then avoid allergens or use rotary diversified diet (*Textbook,* "Food Reactions" and "Rotation Diet: A Diagnostic and Therapeutic Tool").

Minerals

- **Zn:** deficiency occurs in 45% of patients with CD because of low dietary intake, poor absorption, and excess fecal losses. Many complications of CD may result from Zn deficiency: poor healing of fissures and fistulas, skin lesions (acrodermatitis), hypogonadism, growth retardation, retinal dysfunction, depressed cell-mediated immunity, chronic diarrhea, and anorexia. Many patients are unresponsive to oral or intravenous Zn because of a defect in tissue transport. Zn picolinate may improve intestinal absorption and tissue transport. Patients with pancreatic insufficiency may show no improvement. Zn citrate may also be appropriate alternative. Make every attempt to ensure adequate tissue stores because disease activity correlates with Zn deficiency. Use parenteral administration as needed.
- **Mg:** deficiency is prevalent in IBD. Poor correlation exists between serum levels (frequently normal) and intracellular levels (commonly decreased). Low intracellular Mg causes weakness, anorexia, hypotension, confusion, hyperirritability, tetany, convulsions, and electrocardiographic or electroencephalographic abnormalities, which are responsive to parenteral Mg supplementation. Administer daily intravenous dose of 200 to 400 mg elemental Mg if patient is unresponsive to oral supplements. IBD may require intravenous route because of cathartic action of Mg and poor absorption in patients with short bowel. Oral supplement: Mg chelates (e.g., citrate, aspartate) are preferred over inorganic Mg salts (e.g., chloride, oxide).
- **Fe:** Fe-deficiency anemia is frequent in IBD from chronic gut blood loss. Serum ferritin is the most useful index of Fe status. Ferritin level above 55 ng/mL indicates adequate Fe reserves. Ferritin level below 18 ng/mL indicates Fe deficiency. Improve

absorption with supplemental vitamin C rather than direct Fe supplements because Fe promotes intestinal infection.

- **Ca:** risk of Ca deficiency is from the loss of absorptive surfaces, steatorrhea, corticosteroids, and vitamin D deficiency.
- **K:** diarrhea is linked to K^+ and other electrolyte deficiencies. Symptoms of K^+ deficiency are rare in IBD patients, but levels are below optimum. Correcting K^+ deficiency reduces rates of surgical complications.

Vitamins

- **Vitamin A:** low serum retinol occurs in 20% of patients with CD, correlated with activity of disease. Vitamin A affects metabolism and differentiation of intestinal epithelial mucosa; increases the number of goblet cells, production of mucins, and secretion of mucus; and restores normal barrier function. Vitamin A may be useful in CD, but long-term trials (at 50,000 international units [IU] b.i.d.) found no benefit in the majority of CD cases. Certain patients may respond to vitamin A. Zn supplements often normalize vitamin A metabolism because Zn is a component of retinol-binding protein.
- **Vitamin D:** deficiency is common in IBD, particularly in patients with other signs of nutritional deficiency from decreased absorption of 25-hydroxyvitamin D. This deficit increases risk of metabolic bone diseases (osteoporosis and osteomalacia). Vitamin D supports proper immune regulation. It influences T-regulatory cell function and dampens proinflammatory cytokines produced in animal models of IBD. Clinical studies using vitamin D at supraphysiologic doses are under way.
- **Vitamin E:** deficiency can occur in IBD with presenting symptoms including bilateral visual field scotomata, generalized motor weakness, broad-based gait with marked ataxia, brisk reflexes, bilateral Babinski response. Vitamin E inhibits leukotriene formation and reduces free radical damage.
- **Vitamin K:** deficiency results in formation of abnormal prothrombin (deficient in gamma-carboxyglutamic acid), common in patients with IBD. It also contributes to osteoporosis and osteopenia common in CD patients. Best laboratory test for early vitamin K deficiency before lowered serum levels occur is incomplete gamma carboxylation of serum proteins osteocalcin and prothrombin. Incomplete carboxylation of osteocalcin and coronary artery disease arise from vitamin K deficiency by

unknown mechanisms. The test is called PIVKA II (protein in absence of vitamin K carboxylation) by Quest Diagnostics via LabCorp, designer specialty laboratories.

- **Folic acid:** low serum levels occur in 25% to 64% of cases. Sulfasalazine interferes with folate-dependent enzymes and intestinal folate transport system. Deficiency promotes malabsorption from altered structure of intestinal mucosa; cells have rapid turnover (1 to 4 days) versus red blood cells (3 to 4 months). Deficiency affects these cells earlier than red blood cells. Testing CD patients for elevations in serum homocysteine or single nucleotide polymorphisms (SNPs) for enzymes involved in methylation of folate (e.g., methyl tetrahydrofolate reductase) may be diagnostic for early detection of aberrant folate metabolism in CD patients.
- **Vitamin B_{12}:** B_{12} absorption and terminal ileal disease and/or resection are significantly correlated. Abnormal Schilling test results are seen in 48% of patients with CD. When ileal resection exceeds 90 cm, Schilling test result is abnormal in all patients and never improves. If the length of resection is less than 60 cm or if extent of inflammatory lesion is less than 60 cm, adequate absorption may occur.
- **Ascorbic acid:** low vitamin C intake is common in patients with IBD, particularly those on low-fiber diet. Serum and leukocyte ascorbic acid is much lower in patients with CD than in matched control subjects. Vitamin C is important to prevent fistulas. Patients with fistulas have lower ascorbic acid levels than those without.
- **Antioxidant defenses:** increased oxidative stress and decreased antioxidant defenses in mucosa are hallmarks of IBD, with associated protein and DNA oxidative damage. IBD patients have serum and mucosal deficiencies in antioxidant defenses—selenium-dependent glutathione peroxidase and copper-zinc superoxide dismutase, along with cofactors for these enzyme systems (Zn and copper), ascorbate, vitamin E, and vitamin A.
- **High-potency multiple vitamin-mineral formula:** absolutely essential in IBD, with additional antioxidants to manage increased oxidative stress and decreased antioxidant defenses in mucosa. Two primary antioxidants in the human body are vitamins C (aqueous phase) and E (lipid phase).
- Vitamin E (mixed tocopherols with 40% gamma-tocopherol): 400 to 800 IU q.d.
- Vitamin C (ascorbic acid): 1000 to 3000 mg q.d.

Botanical Medicines

- **Curcumin:** turmeric spice from the root of *Curcuma longa,* in the ginger family, and traditional Ayurvedic medicine. Major chemical constituents are curcuminoids (curcumin). Curcumin may be an intracellular signaling agent, similar to green tea polyphenols as an inhibitor of nuclear factor kappa B (NF-κB), and leads to downstream regulation and inhibition of proinflammatory genes and cytokines. It also modulates other cytokines and signaling pathways—iNOS, MMP-9, TNF-α, JNK, p38, AKT, JAK, ERK, and PKC. In murine colitis models, curcumin induced clinical and histopathologic improvement and decreased inflammatory cytokine production. At a dose of 1 g b.i.d., curcumin provided clinical improvement and decreased rate of relapse. It also has an excellent safety profile.
- ***Boswellia:*** Ayurvedic herb *Boswellia serrata* (Indian frankincense) contains boswellic acids, which inhibit leukotriene biosynthesis in neutrophilic granulocytes by noncompetitive inhibition of 5-lipoxygenase. At a dose of 350 mg t.i.d., *Boswellia* gum resin was as effective as sulfasalazine (1000 mg t.i.d.) in reducing symptoms or laboratory abnormalities of active UC. A proprietary *Boswellia* extract, H15, was as effective as mesalazine in improving symptoms of active CD.
- **Quercetin:** plant flavonoids are natural biologic response modifiers. Quercetin is the most pharmacologically active flavonoid. Many enzymes affected by quercetin are involved in release of histamine and other inflammatory mediators from mast cells, basophils, neutrophils, and macrophages; in the migration and infiltration of leukocytes; and in smooth muscle contraction. Quercetin antagonizes calmodulin. When Ca is bound to calmodulin, it activates enzymes involved in cyclic nucleotide metabolism, protein phosphorylation, secretory function, muscle contraction, microtubule assembly, glycogen metabolism, and Ca flux. Quercetin interacts directly with calmodulin and Ca channels. Quercetin and other flavonoids potently inhibit mast cell and basophil degranulation. It inhibits receptor-mediated Ca influx, inhibiting primary signal for degranulation. It is also active when Ca channel mechanism is not operative; therefore other mechanisms are also involved. It inhibits inflammatory processes of activated neutrophils by membrane stabilization, antioxidant effect (prevents production of free radicals and inflammatory leukotrienes), and inhibition of hyaluronidase (preventing breakdown of collagen). Its membrane-stabilizing effect

prevents mast cell and basophil degranulation and decreases neutrophil lysosomal enzyme secretion. Quercetin inhibits eicosanoid metabolism by inhibiting phospholipase A_2 and lipoxygenase. The net result is the reduction in formation of leukotrienes. Excess leukotrienes are linked to asthma, psoriasis, atopic dermatitis, gout, possibly cancer, and IBD. Leukotrienes C_4, D_4, and E_4 (comprising slow-reacting substances of anaphylaxis) are 1000 times as potent as histamine in promoting inflammation. Leukotrienes cause vasoconstriction (increasing vascular permeability) and other smooth muscle contractions and promote white blood cell chemotaxis and aggregation. Reducing leukotrienes has strong anti-inflammatory effects in IBD.

- ***Aloe vera:*** *Aloe vera* gel has a dose-dependent inhibitory effect in vitro on production of prostaglandin E_2 and (at high doses) interleukin-8 (IL-8) by human colonic epithelial cells. Oral *Aloe vera* gel at 100 mL b.i.d. for 4 weeks produced a clinical response in 30% of UC patients. Aloe also reduced histologic activity, and with few side effects. (*Aloe vera* gel is used as a laxative.) Acemannan, an extract concentrated to a mucopolysaccharide (MPS) concentration of 30% of solid weight, reduces symptoms and indexes of inflammation in UC.
- **Bastyr's formula** (modified Robert's formula):
  - — *Althea officinalis* (marshmallow root): demulcent, soothing to mucous membranes
  - — *Baptisia tinctoria* (wild indigo): used for GI infections
  - — *Echinacea angustifolia* (purple coneflower): antibacterial that normalizes immune system (*Textbook,* "Echinacea Species [Narrow-Leafed Purple Coneflower]")
  - — *Geranium maculatum:* a GI hemostatic
  - — *Hydrastis canadensis* (goldenseal): inhibits growth of many enteropathic bacteria (*Textbook,* "Hydrastis canadensis [Goldenseal] and Other Berberine-Containing Botanicals")
  - — *Phytolacca americana* (poke root): used for healing ulcerations of intestinal mucosa
  - — *Symphytum officinale* (comfrey): anti-inflammatory; promotes tissue growth and wound healing
  - — *Ulmus fulva* (slippery elm): demulcent
- **Other ingredients:** cabbage powder heals GI ulcers (*Textbook,* "Peptic Ulcer—Duodenal and Gastric"). Pancreatin assists digestive process (*Textbook,* "Pancreatic Enzymes"). Niacinamide has anti-inflammatory effects. Duodenal substance heals GI ulcers.

Composition of Bastyr's Formula

- Eight parts A. officinalis
- Four parts B. tinctoria
- Eight parts E. angustifolia
- Eight parts G. maculatum
- Eight parts H. canadensis
- Eight parts P. americana
- Eight parts U. fulva
- Eight parts cabbage powder
- Two parts pancreatin
- One part niacinamide
- Two parts duodenal substance

Butyrate Enemas in Ulcerative Colitis

Short-chain fatty acids (SCFAs) and colon function: SCFAs (acetate, propionate, and butyrate) are colon end products of bacterial carbohydrate fermentation. They function as primary energy sources for luminal colon cells, especially distal segments. Decreased levels or use of SCFAs impairs cellular energetics, suggesting a major role in UC. Enemas providing SCFAs (butyrate only at 80 to 100 mmol/L or SCFA combinations with acetate 60 mmol/L, propionate 25 mmol/L, and butyrate 40 mmol/L) displayed excellent preliminary results in a well-designed double-blind study. Butyrate and SCFA enemas may prove useful adjuncts for UC.

Prebiotics

- Nondigestible food ingredients that stimulate growth or modify metabolic activity of intestinal bacteria that can improve health of human host.
- Criteria of classification as prebiotic: (1) remains undigested and unabsorbed during passage through upper GI tract; (2) acts a selective substrate for growth of specific strains of beneficial bacteria (lactobacilli or bifidobacteria) instead of all colon species.
- Examples: bran, psyllium husk, milled flaxseed, chia seed, resistant (high amylose) starch, inulin (polymer of fructofuranose), lactulose, and various natural or synthetic oligosaccharides (short-chain complexes of sucrose, galactose, fructose, glucose, maltose, or xylose).
- Effect: increase fecal water content, relieving constipation.
- Bacterial fermentation of prebiotics yields SCFAs (e.g., butyrate). Oat bran at 60 g/day (supplying 20 g of fiber), given to UC

patients, increased fecal butyrate by 36%, and abdominal pain improved.

- Fish oil plus fructo-oligosaccharides (FOS) and xanthan gum reduced glucocorticoid dose needed in steroid-dependent UC.
- Japanese germinated barley foodstuff (GBF) containing hemicellulose-rich fiber, given at 20 to 30 g/day, increased stool butyrate, decreased active disease, and prolonged remission in inactive disease.
- Mixture of *Bifidobacterium longum* and inulin-derived FOS for 1 month as monotherapy for UC improved sigmoidoscopic appearance, histology, and biochemical indexes of tissue inflammation.

Probiotics in Crohn's Disease

Probiotics are beneficial yeast and bacteria ingested for therapeutic benefit. Overall, patients with UC do not benefit from probiotics during active flare disease; but probiotics remarkably benefit maintaining remissions. Study results are inconsistent with all strains of probiotics for CD overall.

THERAPEUTIC MONITORING AND EVALUATION

- **Fecal calprotectin:** protein secreted into intestinal lumen in direct proportion to inflammation. Calprotectin in stool samples is a sensitive and specific noninvasive assessment tool for inflammatory status in IBD and for distinguishing IBD from other noninflammatory GI conditions (e.g., irritable bowel syndrome).
- **CD activity index (CDAI):** a monitoring tool providing uniform clinical parameters to be assessed with consistent numeric index for recording results. CDAI is calculated by adding eight variables (*Textbook*, Appendix 3). Subjective and objective information is included. A form (*Textbook*, Appendix 3) is given to patients for completion at home. Calculation of disease activity is determined. CDAI scores below 150 indicate better prognosis than higher scores. CDAI is a very useful way to monitor progress.
- **Monitoring of the pediatric patient:** achieving normal growth and development is quite difficult. Growth failure occurs in 75% of pediatric patients with CD and 25% in those with UC. Evaluate at least twice yearly: pertinent history, clinical anthropometry, Tanner staging, and appropriate laboratory testing (see accompanying box). Use aggressive nutritional program including supplements (enteral or parenteral methods) with doses adjusted as appropriate. CDAI is not as accurate in monitoring disease in children as in adults. Lloyd-Still and Green clinical

scoring system for IBD in children: divided into five major divisions (maximal score is in parentheses): general activity (10), physical examination and clinical complications (30), nutrition (20), radiographs (15), laboratory (25). Elevated scores (scores in the 80s) represent good status, whereas scores in the 30s and 40s represent severe disease.

MONITORING OF THE PEDIATRIC PATIENT WITH INFLAMMATORY BOWEL DISEASE

History

- Appetite, extracurricular activities
- Type and duration of inflammatory bowel disease, frequency of relapses
- Severity and extent of ongoing symptoms
- Medication history

3-Day Diet Diary

Physical Examination

- Height, weight, arm circumference, triceps skinfold measurements
- Loss of subcutaneous fat, muscle wasting, edema, pallor, skin rash, hepatomegaly

Laboratory Tests

- Complete blood count and differential, reticulocyte and platelet counts, sedimentation rate, urinalysis
- Serum total proteins, albumin, globulin, and retinol-binding protein
- Serum electrolytes, calcium, phosphate, ferritin, folate, carotenes, tocopherol, and vitamin B_{12}
- Leukocyte ascorbate, magnesium, and zinc
- Creatinine height index, blood urea nitrogen/creatinine ratio

THERAPEUTIC APPROACH

- IBD is life-threatening, requiring emergency treatment in some patients. A small percentage of patients with severe colitis may have severe exacerbations requiring hospitalization (more common in patients with UC): fever of 101°F or higher; profuse, constant, loose, bloody stools; anorexia, apathy, and prostration. Abdominal signs may be normal but physical examination reveals distended abdomen, tympany, absent bowel sounds, and

even rebound tenderness. IBD is typically a chronic disease requiring long-term therapy and follow-up.
- Identify and remove all factors initiating or aggravating inflammation (e.g., food allergens, carrageenan).
  — Follow diet maximizing macronutrients and micronutrients and minimizing aggravating foods and nonfood substances.
  — Use nutritional supplements to correct deficiencies in a broad-based individualized nutritional supplement plan; critical components are Zn, Mg, folate, and vitamin A.
  — Reduce inflammatory process and promote healing of damaged mucosa.
  — Use botanical medicines to promote healing and normalize intestinal flora.
- **Diet:** eliminate all allergens, wheat, corn, dairy, and carrageenan-containing foods. Select foods high in complex carbohydrates and fiber, low in sugar and refined carbohydrates. Fiber is poorly tolerated in CD with luminal narrowing, whereas complex carbohydrates are prebiotic for healthful enteric flora and helpful for UC.
- **Supplements:**
  — Multivitamin and mineral supplement with trace mineral cofactors for antioxidant systems
  — Mg: 200 mg elemental Mg q.d.
  — Zn picolinate or carnosine: 50 mg elemental Zn q.d.
  — Vitamin E: 400 to 800 IU q.d. mixed tocopherols with approximately 40% concentration of gamma-tocopherol
  — Fish oil: 3 g q.d. of combined EPA plus DHA
  — Probiotic (*Lactobacillus* and *Bifidobacterium* species): minimum of 5 to 10 billion colony-forming units q.d.
  — Prebiotics (e.g., inulin, fructose oligosaccharides): 5 g q.d.
  — SCFA enemas (60 mL of 80 to 100 mmol/L) nightly for left-sided colitis
- **Botanical medicines:**
  — Curcumin from turmeric *(C. longa):* 1000 b.i.d. to t.i.d. before meals
  — *Boswellia* extract: equivalent to 400 mg boswellic acids t.i.d.
  — *Aloe vera:* choose one of the following:
    - *Aloe vera* gel: oral preparations—100 mL q.d.
    - *Aloe vera* juice: a variety of different preparations types and concentrations make accurate dose recommendations difficult. They can be consumed orally as a beverage or tonic.
    - Acemannan: 400 to 800 mg q.d.
  — Bastyr's formula: 2 or 3 "00" capsules with each meal

Insomnia

DIAGNOSTIC SUMMARY

- Difficulty falling asleep (sleep-onset insomnia)
- Frequent or early awakening (maintenance insomnia)

GENERAL CONSIDERATIONS

Insomnia is an extremely common complaint with many causes.

Causes of Insomnia*

Sleep-Onset Insomnia	Sleep-Maintenance Insomnia
Anxiety or tension	Depression
Environmental change	Environmental change
Emotional arousal	Sleep apnea
Fear of insomnia	Nocturnal myoclonus
Phobia of sleep	Hypoglycemia
Disruptive environment	Parasomnias
Pain or discomfort	Pain or discomfort
Caffeine	Drugs
Alcohol	Alcohol

*The boundary between the categories is not entirely distinct.

- Up to 30% of the population experience insomnia. A total of 12.5% of the adult population uses prescribed anxiolytics or sedative hypnotics. Half of these drugs, especially benzodiazepines, are prescribed by primary care physicians.
- Psychological factors account for 50% of insomnia cases evaluated in sleep laboratories and are closely associated with affective disorders (see the chapter on affective disorders). Cognitive therapy is often indicated and can improve sleep quality.

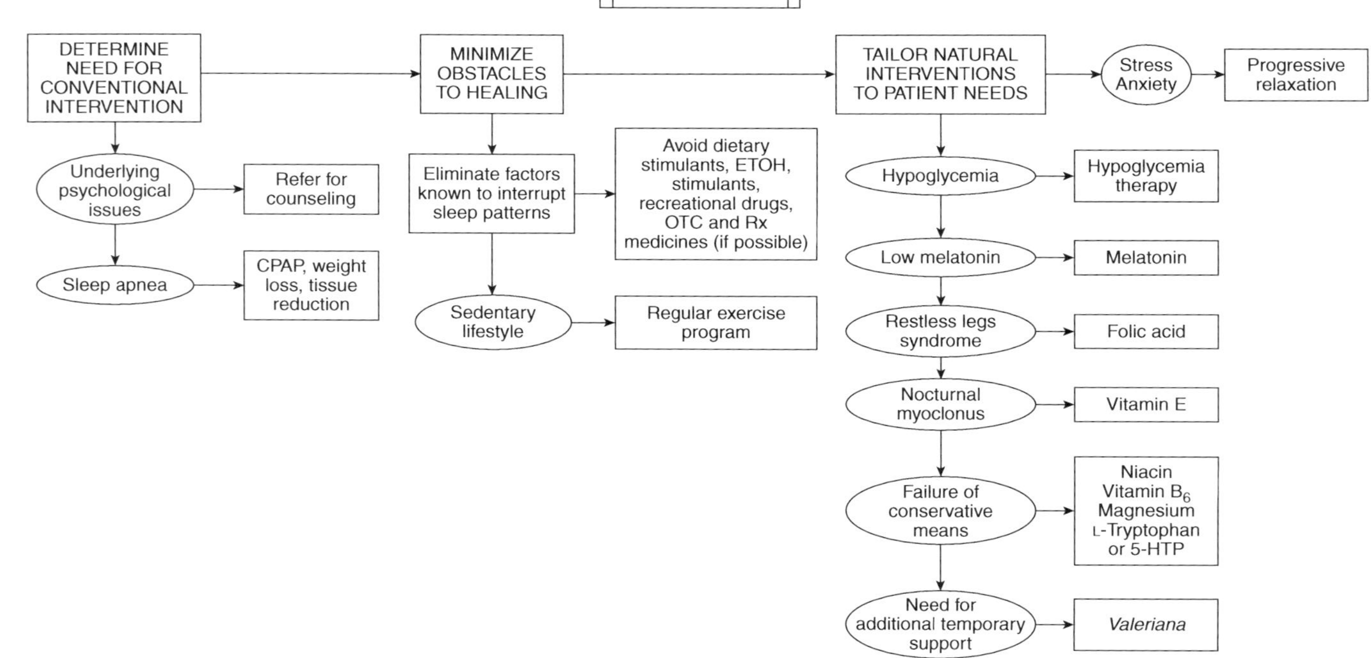
INSOMNIA
DETERMINE NEED FOR CONVENTIONAL INTERVENTION
Underlying psychological issues
Refer for counseling
Sleep apnea
CPAP, weight loss, tissue reduction
MINIMIZE OBSTACLES TO HEALING
Eliminate factors known to interrupt sleep patterns
Avoid dietary stimulants, ETOH, stimulants, recreational drugs, OTC and Rx medicines (if possible)
Sedentary lifestyle
Regular exercise program
TAILOR NATURAL INTERVENTIONS TO PATIENT NEEDS
Stress Anxiety
Progressive relaxation
Hypoglycemia
Hypoglycemia therapy
Low melatonin
Melatonin
Restless legs syndrome
Folic acid
Nocturnal myoclonus
Vitamin E
Failure of conservative means
Niacin
Vitamin B_6
Magnesium
L-Tryptophan or 5-HTP
Need for additional temporary support
Valeriana

- Insomnia may be a presenting symptom for a more-serious condition. Conduct thorough history taking and examination; elicit details on recreational, prescription, and nonprescription drug use plus dietary and beverage history to identify stimulants or other agents known to interfere with sleep—thyroid preparations, oral contraceptives, beta-blockers, marijuana, alcohol, coffee, tea, chocolate.
- Consider and rule out narcolepsy and sleep apnea syndromes.

Sleep Apnea

- Sleep apnea is the most common type of sleep-disordered breathing. It is characterized by brief interruptions of breathing during sleep, with snoring between apnea episodes (not everyone who snores has this condition) or choking sensations. Frequent sleep interruptions prevent deep, restorative sleep, causing excessive daytime sleepiness and early morning headache.
- An estimated 18 million Americans have sleep apnea.
- Associated issues: daytime fatigue, irregular heartbeat, hypertension, myocardial infarction, stroke, loss of memory function, other intellectual deficits.
- Patient usually is unaware and incredulous when told. Sleep partner notes heavy snoring or interrupted breathing.
- Definitive diagnosis: sleep disorder specialist in a sleep laboratory.
- Cause is excess fatty tissue accumulated in airway, causing it to be narrowed, leading to heavy snoring, periods of no breathing, and frequent arousals (causing abrupt changes from deep sleep to light sleep). Ingestion of alcohol and sleeping pills increases the frequency and duration of breathing pauses in people with sleep apnea. In some cases sleep apnea occurs even if no airway obstruction or snoring is present. This form of sleep apnea is called *central sleep apnea* and is caused by a loss of perfect control over breathing by the brain. In both obstructive and central sleep apnea, obesity is the major risk factor and weight loss is the most important aspect of long-term management. People with sleep apnea have periods of anoxia (oxygen deprivation of the brain) with each apneic episode, which ends in arousal and a reinitiation of breathing. Seldom does the individual with sleep apnea awaken enough to be aware of the problem. However, the combination of frequent periods of oxygen deprivation (20 to several hundreds of times per night) and the greatly disturbed sleep can greatly diminish quality of life and lead to serious problems.

The most common treatment of sleep apnea is the use of nasal continuous positive airway pressure (CPAP). In this treatment the patient wears a mask over the nose during sleep, and pressure from an air blower forces air through the nasal passages. The air pressure is adjusted so that it is just enough to prevent the throat from collapsing during sleep. The pressure is constant and continuous. Nasal CPAP prevents airway closure while in use, but apnea episodes return when CPAP is stopped or used improperly. Surgery for reducing soft tissue in the throat or soft palate should be used only as a last resort because often it does not work and can make the condition worse. Laser-assisted uvulopalatoplasty is a highly promoted surgical option. In this procedure, lasers are used to surgically remove excessive soft tissue from the back of the throat and from the palate. This procedure initially works well in approximately 90% of those with sleep apnea, but within 1 year the apnea in many people is the same or even worse than before because of scar tissue that inevitably occurs.

Normal Sleep Patterns

- Normal sleep patterns repeat themselves on a 24-hour cycle, of which sleep constitutes one third. Sleep tends to decrease with age, but whether this is normal is unknown. A 1-year-old baby requires 14 hours of sleep, a 5-year-old 12 hours, and adults 7 to 9 hours. Women require more sleep than men; the elderly sleep less at night but doze more during day than younger adults.
- Two distinct types of sleep (based on eye movement and electroencephalographic recordings): rapid eye movement (REM) and non-REM sleep.
  - **REM sleep:** eyes move rapidly and dreaming takes place; when people are awakened during non-REM sleep, they report they were thinking about everyday matters but rarely report dreams.
  - **Non-REM sleep:** four stages graded 1 to 4 according to the level of electroencephalographic activity and ease of arousal. As sleep progresses, it deepens and brainwave activity is slower until REM sleep, when the brain suddenly becomes much more active. In adults, the first REM cycle is triggered 90 minutes after going to sleep and lasts 5 to 10 minutes; electroencephalographic patterns return to non-REM for another 90-minute sleep cycle.
- Each night most adults have five or more sleep cycles; REM periods grow progressively longer as sleep continues. The last

sleep cycle may produce a REM period lasting an hour. Non-REM sleep lasts 50% of a 90-minute sleep cycle in infants and 80% in adults. With aging, in addition to less REM sleep, people tend to awaken at transition from non-REM to REM sleep.

Importance of Adequate Sleep

- Growth hormone (GH), the anabolic antiaging hormone, is secreted during sleep. It stimulates tissue regeneration, liver regeneration, muscle building, breakdown of fat stores, and normalization of blood sugar regulation, as well as helping to convert fat to muscle. Small amounts are secreted during the day, but most secretion occurs during sleep.
- Sleep is the antioxidant for the brain; free radicals are removed during this time. It is required to minimize neuronal damage from free radical accumulation during waking. Chronic sleep deprivation accelerates aging of the brain. Animal research has shown that prolonged sleep deprivation causes neuronal damage.

Therapeutic Considerations

Uncover causative psychological and physiologic factors; counseling and/or stress reduction techniques (biofeedback, hypnosis) are indicated in many cases.

- **Exercise:** regular physical exercise improves sleep quality; perform in the morning or early evening, not before bedtime, and at moderate intensity; 20 minutes of aerobic exercise at a heart rate 60% to 75% of maximum (220 minus age in years).
- **Progressive relaxation:** based on simple procedure of comparing tension with relaxation; patient is taught what it feels like to relax by comparing relaxation with muscle tension. Muscle is first asked to contract forcefully for 1 to 2 seconds and then give way to feeling of relaxation; procedure goes progressively through all muscles of the body, and eventually deep state of relaxation results. Start with contracting facial and neck muscles, then upper arms and chest, then lower arms and hands, abdomen, buttocks, thighs, calves, and feet; repeat two or three times or until asleep.
- **Nocturnal glucose levels:** increased nocturnal blood glucose volatility is a major cause of sleep-maintenance insomnia. A drop in blood glucose promotes awakening by release of glucose regulatory hormones (epinephrine, glucagon, cortisol, and GH). Rule out hypoglycemia in maintenance insomnia (*Textbook*, "Hypoglycemia").

Serotonin Precursor and Cofactor Therapy

Serotonin is the initiator of sleep; synthesis of central nervous system serotonin depends on tryptophan.

- **L-Tryptophan:** has modest effect on insomnia with dramatic relief in some patients; it is more effective in sleep onset and less effective in sleep maintenance. An advantage of L-tryptophan over over-the-counter (OTC) drugs and prescription drugs is absence of significant distortions of normal sleep processes, whether given once for a prolonged period or during withdrawal. Doses below 2000 mg are ineffective. L-Tryptophan enhances melatonin synthesis and reduces sleep latency, but in normal individuals the effects are at odds with serotonin, reducing REM and increasing non-REM sleep. Some of L-tryptophan's sleep effects do not involve serotonin or melatonin. Effects of L-tryptophan can be negated by kynurenine pathway—partially inhibited by niacin (30 mg), enhancing effects of L-tryptophan. Sleep actions of L-tryptophan are cumulative; a few nights are often necessary for L-tryptophan to start working. It should be used for at least 1 week to gauge effectiveness in chronic insomnia. L-Tryptophan does exert good sleep-promoting effects with single administration (e.g., insomnia that occurs while sleeping in an unfamiliar place); high-dose L-tryptophan (4 g) during the day can promote sleep. High tryptophan-containing foods during the day may contribute to daytime sleepiness; an evening meal high in tryptophan relative to competing amino acids may promote sleep.
- **5-Hydroxytryptophan (5-HTP):** is one step closer to serotonin than L-tryptophan. It is not dependent on transport system for entry into the brain; it produces dramatically better results than L-tryptophan in promoting and maintaining sleep. It increases REM sleep (by 25%) and increases deep sleep stages 3 and 4 without increasing total sleep time. Sleep stages reduced to compensate for increases are non-REM stages 1 and 2, the least important stages. 5-HTP dose for sleep promotion is 100 to 300 mg 30 to 45 minutes before retiring; start with lower dose for at least 3 days before moving up.
- **Cofactors for serotonin synthesis:** vitamin B_6, niacin, and magnesium are given with tryptophan to ensure conversion to serotonin; other amino acids compete for transport into the central nervous system across the blood-brain barrier, and insulin increases tryptophan uptake by the central nervous system. Avoid protein consumption near administration, and take with

a carbohydrate source (fruit or fruit juice). Niacin has sedative effect, probably from a peripheral dilating action and shunting of tryptophan toward serotonin synthesis.

- **Melatonin:** modestly effective in inducing and maintaining sleep in children and adults, in those with normal sleep patterns and those with insomnia. Sleep effects of melatonin are apparent only if melatonin levels are low; melatonin is not like sleeping pill or 5-HTP; it produces a sedative effect only when melatonin levels are low. Normally, just before retiring, melatonin secretion rises; melatonin supplement is effective as a sedative only when the pineal gland's own production of melatonin is low. It is most effective for insomnia in elderly, in whom low melatonin is common; dose is 3 mg at bedtime. No serious side effects at this dose, but melatonin supplementation could disrupt normal circadian rhythm.

Restless Legs Syndrome and Nocturnal Myoclonus

Restless legs syndrome (RLS) and nocturnal myoclonus (NM) are significant causes of insomnia.

- RLS is characterized during waking by the irresistible urge to move legs; almost all affected patients have NM.
- NM is a neuromuscular disorder with repeated contractions of one or more muscle groups, typically of the leg, during sleep. Each jerk lasts less than 10 seconds. The patient is unaware of myoclonus and only reports frequent nocturnal awakenings or excessive daytime sleepiness; questioning sleep partner reveals myoclonus.
- If patient has family history of RLS (one third of patients), high-dose folic acid (35 to 60 mg q.d.) is helpful but requires a prescription. The Food and Drug Administration limits the amount per capsule to 800 mcg. RLS is common in patients with malabsorption syndromes.
- If no family history, measure serum ferritin, which is the best measure of iron (Fe) stores; low Fe is linked to RLS. Serum ferritin is reduced in RLS patients compared with controls; serum Fe, B_{12}, folate, and hemoglobin do not differ; treatment with Fe (ferrous sulfate) at a dose of 200 mg t.i.d. for 2 months reduced symptoms. Fe deficiency, with or without anemia, is a contributor to RLS in the elderly, and Fe supplements can produce significant improvement.
- Low serum ferritin has been found in psychiatric patients experiencing akathisia (from the Greek word meaning "can't sit

down"). Akathisia is a drug-induced agitation caused by antidepressants selective serotonin re-uptake inhibitors; the level of Fe depletion correlates with severity of akathisia. If serum ferritin is below 35 mg/L, try 30 mg Fe bound to succinate or fumarate b.i.d. between meals; if this therapy causes abdominal discomfort, try 30 mg with meals t.i.d.
- For NM and muscle cramps at night, magnesium (250 mg at bedtime) and/or vitamin E (400 to 800 international units [IU] mixed tocopherols q.d.) may help; if patient is older than 50 years, *Ginkgo biloba* extract (80 mg t.i.d.) may also be used.

Botanicals with Sedative Properties

- *Valeriana officinalis* root
  — Most clinical research; improves sleep quality and sleep latency (time required to fall asleep); as effective in reducing sleep latency as small doses of barbiturates or benzodiazepines. Although these drugs also increase morning sleepiness, valerian usually reduces morning sleepiness.
- *Passiflora incarnata*
- *Humulus lupulus*
- *Scutellaria lateriflora*
- *Matricaria chamomilla*

THERAPEUTIC APPROACH

Treatment should be as conservative as possible; treat psychological factors. Foremost, eliminate factors known to disrupt normal sleep patterns: stimulants (e.g., coffee, tea, chocolate, coffee-flavored ice cream), alcohol, hypoglycemia, stimulant-containing herbs (e.g., *Ephedra,* guarana), marijuana and other recreational drugs, numerous OTC medications, prescription drugs. If this approach fails, use more-aggressive measures; once normal sleep pattern is established, supplements and botanicals should be slowly decreased. If the patient has RLS, add 5 to 10 mg q.d. folic acid; for NM use 400 IU natural vitamin E q.d.

- **Lifestyle:** regular exercise program that elevates heart rate 60% to 75% of maximum for 20 min q.d.
- **Supplements:** taken 45 minutes before bedtime:
  — Niacin: 100 mg (decrease dose if uncomfortable flushing interferes with sleep induction)
  — Vitamin B_6: 50 mg

- — Mg: 250 mg elemental Mg
- — Tryptophan: 3 to 5 g, or 5-HTP 100 to 300 mg
- — Melatonin: 3 mg (timed release may be better for some patients)
- **Botanical medicines:** taken 45 minutes before bedtime:
  - — *V. officinalis* root: dried root (or as tea), 2 to 3 g; tincture (1:5), 4 to 6 mL (1 to 1.5 tsp); fluid extract (1:1), 1 to 2 mL (0.5 to 1 tsp); dried powdered extract (0.8% valerenic acid), 150 to 300 mg

Intestinal Protozoan Infestation and Systemic Illness

GENERAL CONSIDERATIONS

- Gastrointestinal tract is largest organ of immune surveillance, home to two thirds of the total lymphocyte population.
- Regulatory T cells respond to protozoan infestation; parasitic infestation may alter immune response environment, affecting systemic responses, including allergy and autoimmunity. Systemic immunologic reactivity may occur without digestive complaints.

Protozoa

Giardia Species

- Giardiasis may provoke asthma, urticaria, arthritis, and uveitis, presumably by inducing immunologic hypersensitivity.
- Urticaria from *Giardia* is linked to specific anti-*Giardia* immunoglobulin E (IgE) not found in patients with intestinal symptoms only.
- IgE production is linked to increased activity of vascular and intercellular adhesion molecules. *Giardia* may provoke systemic illness through malabsorption or protein loss, which can occur without diarrhea. Iron deficiency, low carotene and folate levels, and abnormal absorption of vitamin A, folic acid, and vitamin B_{12} can result from chronic giardiasis, even in patients who appear well nourished.
- Giardiasis may induce small intestinal bacterial overgrowth and jejunal candidiasis.
- *Giardia lamblia* can be vector for double-stranded RNA viruses.
- Common chief complaint: chronic fatigue.

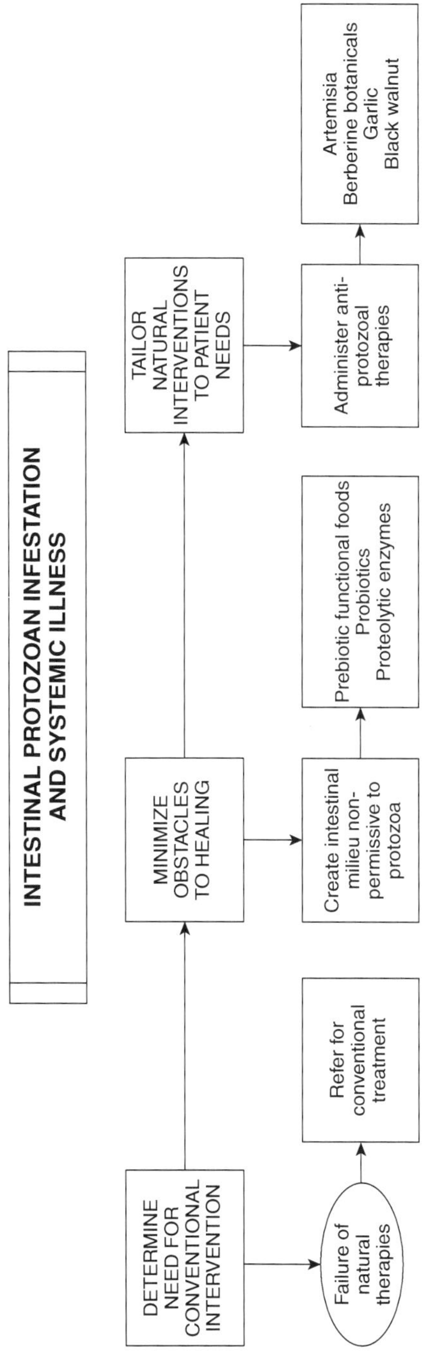
INTESTINAL PROTOZOAN INFESTATION AND SYSTEMIC ILLNESS
DETERMINE NEED FOR CONVENTIONAL INTERVENTION
MINIMIZE OBSTACLES TO HEALING
TAILOR NATURAL INTERVENTIONS TO PATIENT NEEDS
Failure of natural therapies
Refer for conventional treatment
Create intestinal milieu non-permissive to protozoa
Prebiotic functional foods
Probiotics
Proteolytic enzymes
Administer anti-protozoal therapies
Artemisia
Berberine botanicals
Garlic
Black walnut

Systemic Symptoms of Patients with Chronic Fatigue Immune Dysfunction Syndrome

Symptom	With Giardiasis (%) (n = 63)	Without Giardiasis (%) (n = 157)
Depression	61	41
Muscle weakness	46	19
Headache	41	36
Sore throat	41	11
Lymphadenopathy	36	8
Arthralgia	36	27
Myalgia	34	18
Flulike symptoms	34	6
Poor exercise tolerance	30	10

Modified from Galland L, Lee M, Bueno H, et al. *Giardia lamblia* infection as a cause of chronic fatigue. *J Nutr Med.* 1990;2:27-32.

- Symptoms: myalgia, muscle weakness, flulike feelings, sweats, adenopathy, previous diagnosis of chronic fatigue immune dysfunction syndrome (CFIDS).
- Cure results: clearing of fatigue and related "viral" symptoms (myalgia, sweats, flulike feelings).
- Association between intestinal protozoa and chronic fatigue without prominent digestive complaints is common; 80% of patients with diagnosis of CFIDS infected with protozoan *Blastocystis hominis* showed improved fatigue after treatment that cleared protozoa from stool specimens.
- Infestation with *B. hominis* shows several patterns of urticaria: acute, chronic, and pressure induced.

Entamoeba histolytica

- Chronic *E. histolytica* infection is linked to autoimmune phenomena (e.g., antibodies to colonic epithelial cells and ulcerative colitis after cure of amebic colitis).
- Extraintestinal autoimmune reactions to intestinal amebiasis: antiphospholipid antibody syndrome with deep vein thrombosis and pulmonary embolism and symmetrical polyarthritis mimicking rheumatoid arthritis.
- Symptoms: diarrhea, polyarthritis, and circulating antinuclear antibodies.

- Amebic arthritis: parasitic rheumatism, an inflammatory polyarthropathy produced by circulating antigen-antibody complexes.
- Reiter's syndrome (arthritis, uveitis, and urethritis) is a complication of infection with *Cryptosporidium* and *Cyclospora.*
- *Cyclospora cayetanensis* has provoked Guillain-Barré syndrome, a severe autoimmune neuropathy.
- *E. histolytica* contains a soluble lectin that is mitogenic for T lymphocytes. Activation of helper T cells by this lectin may induce replication of human immunodeficiency virus (HIV) in vivo.
- Infection with *E. histolytica* and other parasites may promote acquired immunodeficiency syndrome (AIDS) in HIV-infected patients (e.g., Kaposi's sarcoma among homosexual men).
- Although influence of treating intestinal protozoan infection on course of HIV infection has not been studied, treatment of intestinal helminth infestation decreased HIV viral load among African patients with AIDS.
- Synergism between intestinal parasites and other lymphotropic retroviruses explains pathogenesis of Burkitt's lymphoma and adult T-cell leukemia and/or lymphoma.

DIAGNOSTIC CONSIDERATIONS

- Usually diagnosed with stool examination; however, stool may fail to contain identifiable parasites even at height of acute giardiasis.
- Option: empiric natural therapy for intestinal parasites in high-risk groups—immigrants from Asia, Middle East, sub-Saharan Africa, Eastern Europe, Latin America, Caribbean; similarly for chronically ill patients at high risk for parasitic infection because of residence, travel, sexual practices, or context in which illness occurred.

THERAPEUTIC CONSIDERATIONS

Artemisia annua (Sweet Annie or Qinghao)

- Most extensively studied antiprotozoan botanical.
- *A. annua* yields lactone artemisinin (qinghaosu), the basis for new class of antimalarial compounds widely used in Asia and Africa.

- Artemisinin has antiprotozoan effects owing to its content of endoperoxides and killing of parasites via oxidation. Its activity in treating simian malaria is enhanced by coadministration of cod liver oil and diminished by coadministration of vitamin E.
- Artemisinin has low toxicity. It stimulates macrophages that respond to protozoan infestation.
- Artemisinin may induce abortion if given during pregnancy.

Berberine

- The alkaloid berberine from roots of several plant species—*Berberis aquifolium* (Oregon grape), *Hydrastis canadensis* (goldenseal) root, and *Coptis chinensis* (goldthread).
- Berberine has protostatic and protocidal activity against *E. histolytica, G. lamblia,* and *B. hominis.* It is beneficial in treating giardiasis in children.

Allium sativum and *Juglans nigra*

- *A. sativum* (garlic) and *J. nigra* (black walnut) are antimicrobials.
- Allicin inhibits growth of *E. histolytica* in culture.
- Human studies on efficacy of garlic and black walnut in treatment of protozoan infections are lacking.

Intestinal Bacterial Milieu

- Intestinal bacterial milieu affects protozoan infestation, especially for colonic organisms such as *E. histolytica.*
- Pathogenic strains of *E. histolytica* are able to evade lysis by both classic and alternative pathways of complement. Intestinal bacteria such as *Escherichia coli* are necessary for complement resistance and for amebic virulence.
- Ingested bacteria lower redox potential within parasites and allow amebas to escape destruction by oxidative enzymes.
- One can reversibly change zymodeme patterns of *E. histolytica* isolates from nonpathogenic to invasive by culturing amebas with gut flora of patients who have either invasive disease or no symptoms.
- Optimal treatment of protozoan infection requires not only antimicrobial substances but also strategies aimed at enhancing function of intestinal resistance factors—secretory IgA and phagocyte function—and creating a bacterial milieu that is not parasite friendly.

Irritable Bowel Syndrome

DIAGNOSTIC SUMMARY

- Functional disorder of the large intestine with no evidence of accompanying structural defect.
- Characterized by some combination of the following:
  - — Abdominal pain
  - — Altered bowel function, constipation, or diarrhea
  - — Hypersecretion of colonic mucus
  - — Dyspeptic symptoms (flatulence, nausea, anorexia)
  - — Varying degrees of anxiety or depression
- Synonyms include nervous indigestion, spastic colitis, mucous colitis, intestinal neurosis.
- Splenic flexure syndrome is a variant of irritable bowel syndrome (IBS) in which gas in bowel leads to pain in lower chest or left shoulder.
- Many patients with IBS also have extraintestinal symptoms—sexual dysfunction, fibromyalgia, dyspareunia, urinary frequency and urgency, poor sleep, menstrual difficulties, lower back pain, headache, chronic fatigue, and insomnia—which increase in number with severity of IBS.
- In some cases, extraintestinal manifestations—restless legs syndrome (RLS), migraine headaches, chronic fatigue, irritable bladder syndrome, and dyspareunia.

GENERAL CONSIDERATIONS

IBS is the most common gastrointestinal (GI) disorder in general practice, accounting for 30% to 50% of all referrals to gastroenterologists. Many people with IBS never seek medical attention. Fifteen percent of the population have IBS symptoms; women predominate 2:1 (men do not report symptoms as often). The cause is attributed to physiologic, psychological, and dietary factors. IBS often is a diagnosis of exclusion, but clinical judgment is needed to determine extent of diagnostic process. Detailed history and physical examination can eliminate vagueness in diagnosing IBS.

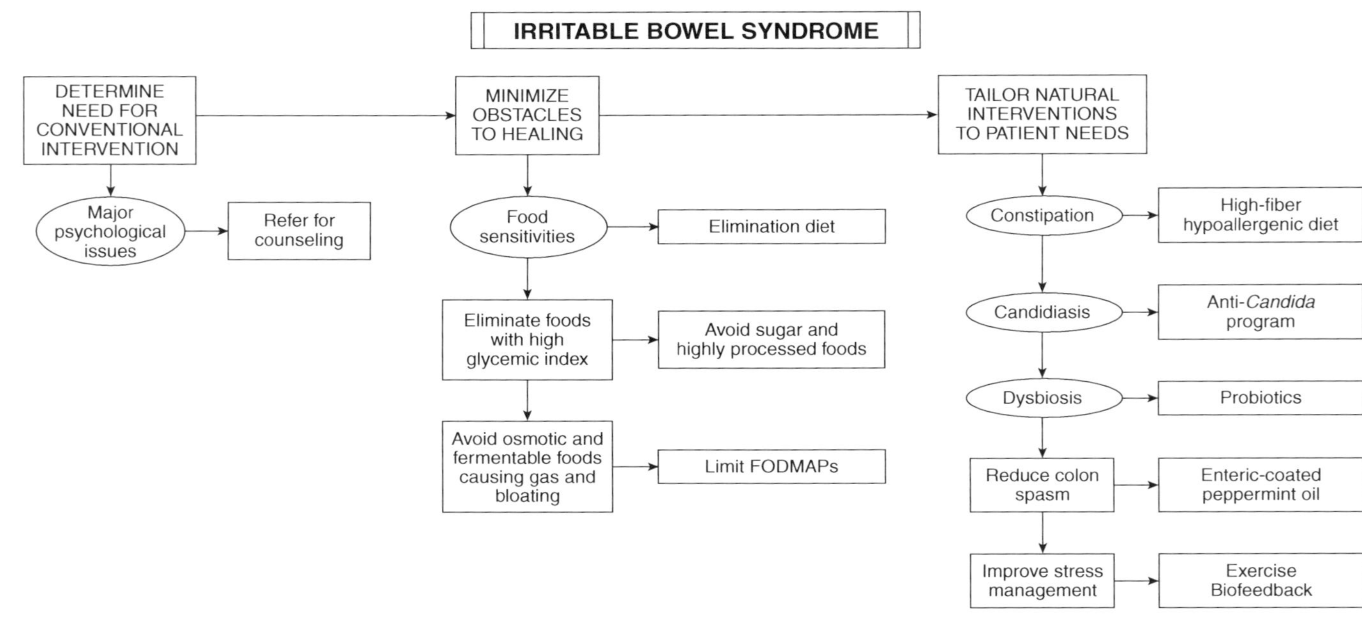
IRRITABLE BOWEL SYNDROME
DETERMINE NEED FOR CONVENTIONAL INTERVENTION
Major psychological issues
Refer for counseling
MINIMIZE OBSTACLES TO HEALING
Food sensitivities
Elimination diet
Eliminate foods with high glycemic index
Avoid sugar and highly processed foods
Avoid osmotic and fermentable foods causing gas and bloating
Limit FODMAPs
TAILOR NATURAL INTERVENTIONS TO PATIENT NEEDS
Constipation
High-fiber hypoallergenic diet
Candidiasis
Anti-*Candida* program
Dysbiosis
Probiotics
Reduce colon spasm
Enteric-coated peppermint oil
Improve stress management
Exercise
Biofeedback

Distention, relief of pain with bowel movements, and onset of loose or more-frequent bowel movements with pain correlate best with diagnosis of IBS. Comprehensive stool and digestive analysis (*Textbook,* "Comprehensive Digestive Stool Analysis 2.0") with special attention to dysbiosis, complete blood count, erythrocyte sedimentation rate, thyroid stimulating hormone, free thyroid triiodothyronine (T_3) hormone level, celiac testing (antiendomysial antibody test), and serum protein concentration are necessary to determine diagnosis. If diarrhea is the predominant symptom, consider pan-endoscopy with duodenal, colonic, and terminal ileal biopsies autoimmune conditions, such as celiac disease, inflammatory bowel disease, lymphocytic colitis, and collagenous colitis. If food allergy is suspected, consider stool testing for eosinophilic cationic protein. If no discernible cause is identified, screening for fecal occult blood and flexible sigmoidoscopy are indicated in patients younger than 50 years and colonoscopy in patients older than 50 years.

CONDITIONS THAT CAN MIMIC IRRITABLE BOWEL SYNDROME

- Gastrogenic dietary factors: excessive tea, coffee, carbonated beverages, simple sugars
- Infectious enteritis: amebiasis, giardiasis
- Inflammatory bowel disease
- Lactose intolerance
- Laxative abuse (An easy test exists to rule out this possibility: add a few drops of sodium hydroxide [NaOH] solution to stool specimen. Most laxatives contain phenolphthalein, causing the stool to turn red.)
- Intestinal candidiasis
- Disturbed bacterial microflora as a result of antibiotic or antacid use
- Malabsorption diseases: pancreatic insufficiency, celiac disease
- Metabolic disorders: adrenal insufficiency, diabetes mellitus, hyperthyroidism
- Mechanical causes (e.g., fecal impaction)
- Diverticular disease
- Neoplasm

THERAPEUTIC CONSIDERATIONS

Four major treatments to consider: (1) increasing dietary fiber, (2) eliminating allergic or intolerable foods, (3) controlling psychological components, and (4) peppermint oil for spastic colon (*Textbook,* "Food Reactions," "Irritable Bowel Syndrome," and "Role of Dietary Fiber in Health and Disease").

Additional considerations: (5) acupuncture for pain modulation and motility regulation; (6) melatonin as stress adaptogen and mood stabilizer and for promotion of restful sleep; (7) possible silent triggers of IBS—small intestinal bacterial overgrowth (SIBO), intestinal dysbiosis, and food allergies; (8) dietary FODMAPs (fermentable oligosaccharides, disaccharides, monosaccharides, and polyols), which may promote IBS and should be limited.

- **Dietary fiber:** patients with constipation are more likely to respond to dietary fiber than are those with diarrhea. Food allergy has been ignored in studies of fiber. Wheat bran is usually contraindicated because food allergy is a significant factor in IBS. Fiber from fruit and vegetables, rather than cereals, is more beneficial in some patients. In certain cases, especially diarrhea cases, fiber may aggravate diarrhea. Cooked vegetables in small quantities at first may be most helpful (*Textbook,* "Role of Dietary Fiber in Health and Disease"). Partially hydrolyzed guar gum (PHGG), from the ancient guar plant *Cyamopsis tetragonolobus* of India and Pakistan, is a natural, water-soluble fiber that decreases frequency of IBS symptoms—flatulence, abdominal spasms, and tension. At a dose of 5 g q.d., PHGG works well for altered intestinal motility and is easy to use because of its nongelling properties, unlike unhydrolyzed gum.
- **Food allergy:** the type of food sensitivity most significant in IBS is nonimmunologic—food intolerance rather than food allergy (*Textbook,* "Food Allergy"). Two thirds of patients with IBS have food intolerances. Foods rich in carbohydrates and fats, coffee, alcohol, and hot spices are problematic. The most common allergens are dairy (40% to 44%) and grains (40% to 60%). The reaction arises from prostaglandin synthesis or immunoglobulin G (IgG) rather than IgE mediation; thus skin tests and IgE radioallergosorbent test are poor indicators of intolerances. Enzyme-linked immunosorbent assay (ELISA) ACT or ELISA IgE/IgG_4 may be a better indicator. Many sensitivities are undetectable by current laboratory procedures. Elimination diets can give marked clinical improvement. Many patients with IBS have associated symptoms of vasomotor instability (palpitation, hyperventilation, fatigue, excessive

sweating, headache) consistent with food allergy or intolerance reactions.

- **Sugar:** meals high in refined sugar contribute to IBS and SIBO by decreasing intestinal motility. A rapid rise in blood sugar slows GI tract peristalsis. Glucose is primarily absorbed in the duodenum and jejunum; hence the message affects this portion of GI tract most strongly; the duodenum and jejunum become atonic.
- **Dietary FODMAPs:** short-chain carbohydrates that are osmotically active and fermentable by intestinal bacteria yielding gases—hydrogen or carbon dioxide—causing abdominal bloating. FODMAPs include oligosaccharides (e.g., fructans, chains of fructose with one glucose molecule on the end). Minimal amounts of fructans are absorbed in human intestine, and they may interfere with absorption of fructose, thus aggravating fructose malabsorption. Foods rich in fructans are wheat, onions, and artichokes; less-problematic fructan foods are asparagus, leeks, garlic, chicory roots, and chicory-based coffee substitutes. Fructans with more than 10 molecules of fructose in a chain are termed *inulins,* and those with fewer than 10 fructose molecules are termed *fructo-oligosaccharides* or *oligofructoses.* Fructans cause problems mainly in fructose malabsorption. Galactans (e.g., stachyose and raffinose) are chains of fructose with one galactose molecule on the end. The main foods rich in galactans are legumes (soy, beans, chickpeas, lentils), cabbage, and Brussels sprouts. Three of four IBS patients respond well to restriction of FODMAP intake. Breath hydrogen testing helps identify which sugars behave as FODMAPs in each person.
- **Disaccharides:** lactose (milk sugar) is found in dairy products, chocolate, sweets, beer, preprepared soups and sauces, and other foods. Lactose is poorly absorbed by individuals with lactose intolerance, SIBO, and small intestinal inflammation (Crohn's disease, celiac disease).
- **Monosaccharides:** fructose (fruit sugar) foods: honey, dried fruits (prunes, figs, dates, raisins), apples, pears, sweet cherries, peaches, agave syrup, watermelon, and papaya. High-fructose corn syrup is added to commercial foods and drinks. Excessive fructose intake causes symptoms even in healthy people, especially in those with fructose malabsorption or SIBO.
- **Polyols:** "sugar alcohols" (artificial sweeteners in commercial foods and drinks). Sorbitol is used in "sugar-free chewing gum" and "low-calorie foods" and occurs naturally in stone fruits (peaches, apricots, plums). Xylitol naturally appears in some

berries. Polyols may cause bloating or diarrhea in healthy children and in persons with fructose malabsorption or SIBO. Other polyols (e.g., mannitol, isomalt, arabitol, erythritol, glycol, glycerol, lactitol, and ribitol) may be problematic in individuals with fructose malabsorption and SIBO.

Nutritional Supplements

- **Probiotics:** dietary supplements containing live microorganisms that, when ingested, exert beneficial effects. Commonly used and studied species: *Lactobacillus, Bifidobacterium,* and *Saccharomyces boulardii.* Association between IBS and SIBO is established. Successful treatment of SIBO with antibiotics improves IBS symptoms. *Bifidobacterium infantis* 35624 has improved all IBS symptoms except stool frequency and consistency, coinciding with normalized proinflammatory cytokine profile (elevated interleukin-10 [IL-10]/IL-12 ratio). Daily administration of 108–colony-forming unit (CFU) dose of *B. infantis* given for 4 weeks improves abdominal pain and global symptom assessment scores. In pediatric IBS, *Lactobacillus* GG reduced frequency of pain. However, in IBS, placebo response is quite high in many studies. Probiotic mixture containing *Lactobacillus rhamnosus* GG, *L. rhamnosus* LC705, *Bifidobacterium breve* Bb99, *Propionibacterium freudenreichii,* and *Propionibacterium shermanii* JS, taken by IBS patients over 6 months, improved total symptom scores (abdominal pain, distention, flatulence, and borborygmi). VSL#3 in IBS with bloating reduced flatulence during treatment and retarded colonic transit. Fermented milk containing *Bifidobacterium animalis, Streptococcus thermophilus,* and *Lactobacillus bulgaricus* in constipation-predominant IBS improved quality-of-life discomfort score and bloating.
- **L-Tryptophan:** this amino acid and its derivative 5-hydroxytryptophan (5-HTP) are considered for IBS because of their relation to serotonin, the neurotransmitter produced in the digestive tract and brain. Because comorbidity of psychiatric conditions (depression or anxiety) correlates highly with IBS, modulation of serotonin pathway with tryptophan seems indicated and needs further investigation. Although IBS lacks reliable biologic markers, IBS disease state is viewed as a disorder of the brain-gut axis, involving both central and peripheral serotonergic systems. Altered tryptophan metabolism and indoleamine 2,3-dioxygenase (IDO) activity are hallmarks of many stress-related disorders. The kynurenine pathway of tryptophan degradation may link

these findings to low-level immune activation in IBS. IDO, the immunoresponsive enzyme that degrades tryptophan along this pathway, is abnormally high in IBS. Males with IBS degrade tryptophan owing to higher IDO activity, identifying kynurenine pathway as a potential source of biomarkers. This degradation suggests need for supplementation of tryptophan or 5-HTP.

Botanical Medicines

- **Enteric-coated volatile oils:** peppermint oil and similar volatile oils inhibit GI smooth muscle action in laboratory animals and human beings. Peppermint oil reduces colonic spasm during endoscopy; enteric-coated peppermint oil is used to treat IBS.
  - — Enteric coating is necessary because menthol and other monoterpenes in peppermint oil are rapidly absorbed, limiting effects to upper intestine and causing relaxation of cardiac esophageal sphincter with esophageal reflux and heartburn.
  - — Symptoms reduced: abdominal pain and distention, stool frequency, borborygmi, flatulence. Transient hot or burning sensation in rectum on defecation (unabsorbed menthol) is noted in some patients.
  - — Dose: 0.2 mL b.i.d. between meals. Improves rhythmic contractions of intestinal tract and relieves intestinal spasm.
  - — Effective against *Candida albicans.* Overgrowth of *C. albicans* may be an underlying factor in cases unresponsive to dietary advice and in patients consuming large amounts of sugar. Nystatin (600,000 international units [IU] q.d. for 10 days) given to patients unresponsive to elimination diet produced dramatic improvement.
  - — Safe and effective in children with moderate pain from IBS.

  Robert's formula: has a long history of use in this condition (see chapter on peptic ulcers).

  Tibetan herbal formula Padma Lax: effective for constipation-predominant IBS. It may cause loose stools in some patients, which is easily remedied by lowering the dose.

  Asian medicines: individualized therapies with Chinese herbal medicines, acupuncture, and Ayurvedic herbal preparations improve bowel and global symptoms and recurrence rate.

Miscellaneous Considerations

- **Psychological factors:** mental and/or emotional problems (anxiety, fatigue, hostile feelings, depression, sleep disturbances) are reported by almost all patients with IBS. Symptom severity and frequency correlate with psychological factors. Anxiety predicts a high degree of food-related symptoms in IBS. Poor sleep quality increases symptom severity.

- **Theories linking psychological factors to IBS:** (1) Learning model: when exposed to stressful situations, some children learn to develop GI symptoms to cope with stress. (2) IBS is a manifestation of depression, chronic anxiety, or both. Individuals with IBS have higher anxiety and more feelings of depression. (3) IBS is either secondary to bowel disturbances (malabsorption) or the result of common etiologic factors (stress, food allergy, or candidiasis).
- **Increased colonic motility during stress:** occurs in normal subjects and patients with IBS. This accounts for increased abdominal pain and irregular bowel functions seen in IBS and normal subjects during emotional stress. Those with IBS may have difficulty adapting to life events. Psychotherapy (relaxation therapy, biofeedback, hypnosis, counseling, or stress management training) reduces symptom frequency and severity and enhances results of conventional treatment of IBS. Hypnosis, practiced at home with use of computer audio files, reduces fasting colonic motility and rectal sensitivity. Anxiolytic drugs (tranquilizers, antispasmodics, antidepressants) have not yielded effective results.
- **Physical medicine:** increasing physical exercise is helpful; daily leisurely walks markedly reduce symptoms.

THERAPEUTIC APPROACH

IBS is a multifactorial disease requiring consideration and integration of many factors: dietary fiber, determination and elimination of food allergies and intolerances, stress reduction, and exercise. Peppermint oil and Robert's formula temporarily ameliorate symptoms. Because diagnosis is made by exclusion, careful diagnostic workup is always indicated.

- **Diet:** increase fiber-rich foods (*Textbook,* "Role of Dietary Fiber in Health and Disease"). Eliminate allergenic foods, refined sugar, highly processed foods, and FODMAPs.
- **Supplements:**
  — Probiotic supplement that includes *Lactobacillus* and *Bifidobacterium* species: 2 to 12 billion live organisms q.d.

- **Botanical medicine:**
  - — Enteric-coated volatile oil preparations (peppermint oil): 0.2 to 0.4 mL b.i.d. between meals.
- **Exercise:** take daily, leisurely 20-minute walks.
- **Counseling:** advise patient on developing effective stress reduction program. Biofeedback is particularly useful for IBS patients.

Kidney Stones

DIAGNOSTIC SUMMARY

- Usually asymptomatic.
- Diagnosed adventitiously or by acute symptoms of urinary tract. Excruciating intermittent radiating pain to groin area originating in flank or kidney.
- Nausea, vomiting, abdominal distention.
- Chills, fever, and urinary frequency if infection is present.

GENERAL CONSIDERATIONS

- In the past, stone formation occurred almost exclusively in the bladder; today most stones form in upper urinary tract. Ten percent of all men have kidney stones (KSs) during their lifetime. Annual incidence is 0.1% to 6.0% of the general population. Males have a 3:1 ratio in formation of KSs compared with females, except in sixth decade, when incidence falls in men but rises in women—a trend toward gender equivalence. Incidence is steadily increasing, paralleling rise in other diseases linked to a Western diet (e.g., ischemic heart disease, cholelithiasis, hypertension, diabetes).
- In the western hemisphere, KSs usually are composed of calcium (Ca) salts (75% to 85%), uric acid (5% to 8%), or struvite (10% to 15%).
- Mutations in genes can lead to hypercalciuria, excess urinary excretion of oxalate, cystine, and uric acid.
- Incidence varies geographically, reflecting environmental factors, diet, and components of drinking water.
- Men are affected more than women. Most patients are older than 30 years.
- Human urine is supersaturated with Ca oxalate, uric acid, and phosphates. They remain in solution because of pH control and secretion of inhibitors of crystal growth.
- Primary and secondary metabolic diseases can cause KSs; they must be ruled out early in the clinical process (e.g., hyperparathyroidism, cystinuria, vitamin D excess, milk-alkali syndrome,

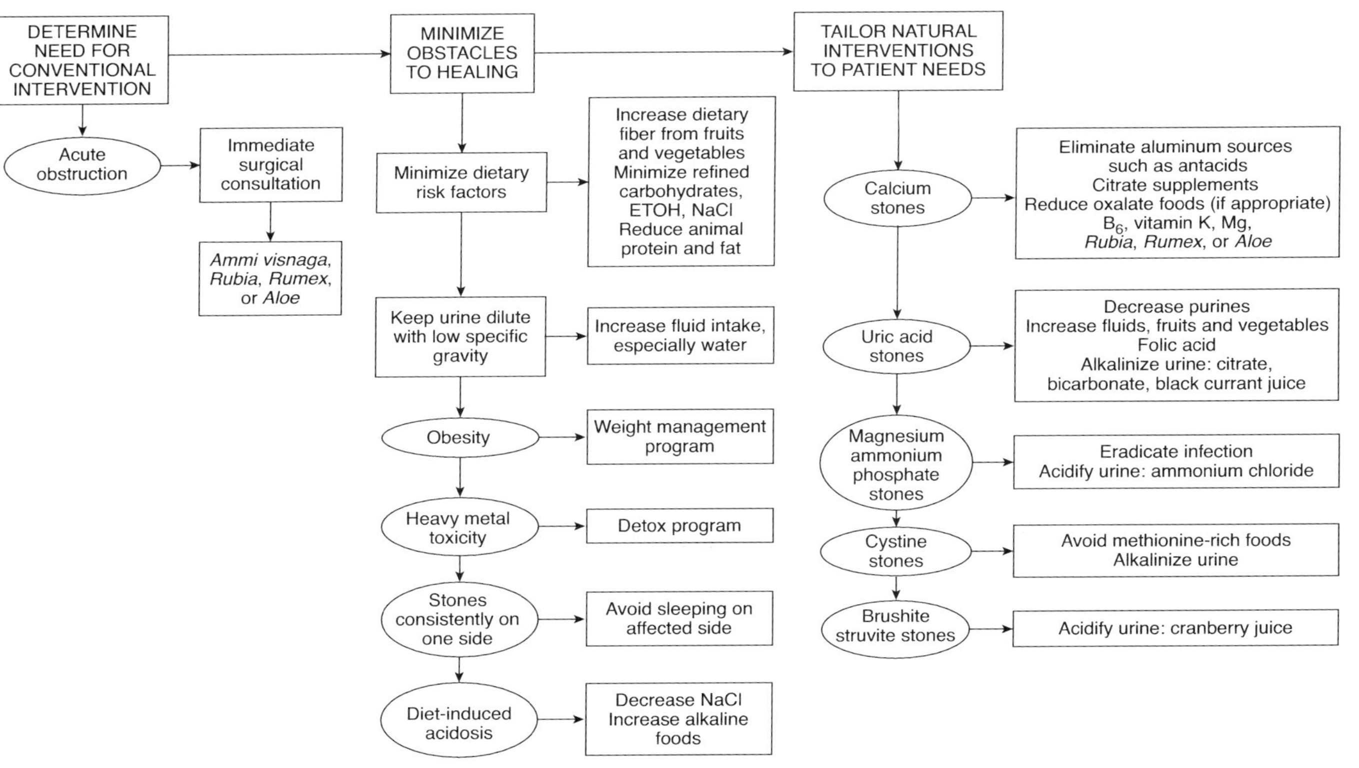
KIDNEY STONES
DETERMINE NEED FOR CONVENTIONAL INTERVENTION
Acute obstruction
Immediate surgical consultation
Ammi visnaga, Rubia, Rumex, or Aloe
MINIMIZE OBSTACLES TO HEALING
Minimize dietary risk factors
Increase dietary fiber from fruits and vegetables
Minimize refined carbohydrates, ETOH, NaCl
Reduce animal protein and fat
Keep urine dilute with low specific gravity
Increase fluid intake, especially water
Obesity
Weight management program
Heavy metal toxicity
Detox program
Stones consistently on one side
Avoid sleeping on affected side
Diet-induced acidosis
Decrease NaCl
Increase alkaline foods
TAILOR NATURAL INTERVENTIONS TO PATIENT NEEDS
Calcium stones
Eliminate aluminum sources such as antacids
Citrate supplements
Reduce oxalate foods (if appropriate)
B_6, vitamin K, Mg,
Rubia, Rumex, or Aloe
Uric acid stones
Decrease purines
Increase fluids, fruits and vegetables
Folic acid
Alkalinize urine: citrate, bicarbonate, black currant juice
Magnesium ammonium phosphate stones
Eradicate infection
Acidify urine: ammonium chloride
Cystine stones
Avoid methionine-rich foods
Alkalinize urine
Brushite struvite stones
Acidify urine: cranberry juice

destructive bone disease, primary oxaluria, Cushing's syndrome, sarcoidosis).

DIAGNOSTIC CONSIDERATIONS

Conditions favoring stone formation include the following:

- **Factors increasing concentration of stone crystalloids:** reduced urine volume (dehydration) and increased excretion of stone constituents
- **Factors favoring stone formation at normal urinary concentrations:** urinary stasis, pH changes, foreign bodies, reduction of normal substances that solubilize stone constituents

Causes of Excessive Excretion of Relatively Insoluble Urinary Constituents

Constituent	Cause of Excess Excretion	Laboratory Findings
Calcium	(>250 mg/day excreted)	Low serum PO_4
	Absorptive hypercalciuria	30%-40% of all stone
	Renal hypercalciuria (renal tubular acidosis)	formers
	Primary hyperparathyroidism	High serum parathyroid
	Hyperthyroidism	hormone
	High vitamin D intake	High urinary cAMP
	Excess intake of milk and alkali	High serum calcium
	Aluminum salt intake	High $1,25\text{-}(OH)_2D_3$
	Destructive bone disease	Low serum phosphate
	Sarcoidosis	High $1,25\text{-}(OH)_2D_3$
	Prolonged immobility	High NaCl in urine
	Methoxyflurane anesthesia	Low urinary pH
	Excessive dietary acidity	Decreased urinary citrate
Oxalate	Familial oxaluria	Rare
	Ileal disease, resection, or bypass	Vitamin B_6 deficiency or
	Steatorrhea	abnormal oxalate me-
	High oxalate intake	tabolism
	Ethylene glycol poisoning	
	Vitamin C excess (extremely unlikely)	
Uric acid	(<750 mg/day excreted)	Rapid cell destruction
	Gout	
	Idiopathic hyperuricosuria	
	Excess purine intake	
	Anticancer drugs	
	Myeloproliferative disease	
	Excessive dietary acidity	
Cystine	Hereditary cystinuria	

$1,25\text{-}(OH)_2D_3$, 1,25-dihydroxyvitamin D_3; cAMP, cyclic adenosine monophosphate; NaCl, sodium chloride; PO_4, phosphate.

Physical Changes in the Urine and Kidney

Condition	Possible Cause
Increased concentration	Dehydration Stasis Obstruction Foreign-body concretions
Urinary pH	Low—uric acid, cystine High—calcium oxalate and PO_4
Infection	Proteus—struvite
Uricosuria	Crystals of uric acid initiate precipitation of calcium oxalate from solution
Nuclei for stone formation	Cells, bacteria, blood clots, and other materials initiate precipitation Sponge kidney
Deformities of kidney	Horseshoe kidney Caliceal obstruction or defect

PO_4, phosphate.

Chemical and Physical Characteristics of Urinary Stones

Composition	Crystal Name	Frequency (%)	X-ray Appearance	Urine Characteristics	Crystal Characteristics
Calcium oxalate	Whewellite	30-35	Opaque	Nonspecific	Small, hempseed or mulberry shaped, brown or black
Calcium oxalate plus calcium phosphate		30-35	Opaque	pH >5.5	Small, hempseed or mulberry shaped, brown or black
Calcium phosphate	Apatite	6-8	Opaque	pH >5.5	Staghorn configuration, light in color
Magnesium ammonium phosphate	Struvite Triple phosphate	15-20	Opaque	pH >6.2 Infection	Staghorn configuration, light in color
Uric acid		6-10	Translucent	pH <6.0	Ellipsoid, tan or red-brown
Cystine		2-3	Opaque	pH <7.2	Multiple, faceted, maple syrup color

THERAPEUTIC CONSIDERATIONS

- **Stone composition:** diagnosing the type of stone is critical to therapy. Evaluate the following to determine stone composition if one is not available for analysis: (1) diet; (2) underlying metabolic or disease factors; (3) serum and urinary Ca, uric acid, creatinine, and electrolyte levels; (4) urinalysis results; (5) urine culture findings.

Dietary Factors

- **Ca-containing stones are Ca oxalate, Ca oxalate mixed with Ca phosphate, or (very rarely) Ca phosphate alone.** High incidence of Ca stones in affluent societies is linked to a diet low in fiber and high in refined carbohydrates, alcohol, animal protein, fat, high-Ca food, vitamin D–enriched food, soft drinks, and fructose. Dietary factors induce hyperuricemia, hypercalciuria, and stone formation, building a cumulative effect.
- Vegetarians have a decreased risk of developing stones. Among meat eaters, those eating more fresh fruits and vegetables have a lower incidence of stones. Using bran supplements and changing to whole-wheat bread lower urinary Ca.
- **Dietary factors in acidifying or alkalinizing urine:** depending on stone type, the ability to alter urine pH may help treat and prevent stones. Cranberry juice decreases urine pH and increases oxalic acid excretion and relative supersaturation for uric acid. Blackcurrant juice increases urine pH, excretion of citric acid, and oxalic acid loss. Blackcurrant juice may treat or prevent uric acid stones by alkalizing urine. Cranberry juice acidifies urine and may treat brushite and struvite stones and urinary tract infections.
- **Water:** increased fluid intake to decrease urine supersaturation. Increasing urine volume decreases stone prevalence. Consuming more than 2 L of water per day to achieve urine output of more than 2.5 L/day lowers KS recurrence risk by 60%. Avoid using other beverages as water substitutes.
- **Sodium (Na) and salt:** high Na intake reduces renal tubular reabsorption of Ca, increasing Ca excretion in urine. High-Na diet increases urine pH and may reduce urine citrate. Stone formers may be sensitive to calciuric effect of Na. Patients with idiopathic Ca stones treated with Na restriction (60 mmol/day) and high fluid intake exhibited reduction of 100 mmol of urinary Na with a reduction of 64 mg/day in urinary Ca; 30% of patients

achieved normal urine Ca. Other results are conflicting. Nevertheless, reducing dietary Na remains a recommendation for most patients with a history of KS.

- **Fructose:** sports drinks' content of citrate should increase urine citrate excretion and urine pH, protecting against Ca and uric acid stones. However, high Na content, promoted as boosting "rehydration," might increase urine Ca excretion. In addition, ingesting large amounts of sucrose and fructose may increase Ca excretion. Fructose, in corn syrup that sweetens sports drinks and sodas, is linked to hyperuricemia, metabolic syndrome, and stones.
- **Citrate:** inhibits aggregation and growth of Ca oxalate and Ca phosphate crystals. In the past, dietary interventions to increase citrate involved lemonade and orange juice. The results with lemonade are conflicting. Avoid grapefruit juice: women drinking 8 oz daily increased risk of stones by 44%.
- **Oxalates:** hyperoxaluria is a metabolic risk factor for KSs. Dietary oxalate may contribute 80% of urine oxalate. Low-oxalate diet benefit patients with hyperoxaluria. Dietary Ca can minimize intestinal oxalate absorption. In men with recurrent Ca oxalate stones, reduction in oxalate excretion and incidence of recurrent stones arose from a normal-Ca (1200 mg/day), low–animal-protein, low-salt diet compared with a low-Ca diet (400 mg/day).

Dietary Recommendations for Patients with High Urine Oxalate

- **Low-oxalate diet:** ultimate goal is to reduce oxalic acid excreted in urine. People with recurrent KSs absorb more dietary oxalates compared with the normal 3% to 8% of intake. Low-oxalate diet: less than 50 mg of oxalate daily. Oxalate content in foods can vary twofold to fifteenfold depending on climate, soil, state of ripeness, or part of the plant ingested.
- **Alkaline diet:** diet-induced acidosis has been shown in recent research to be the strongest predictor of Ca oxalate and uric acid stones. Excessive consumption of acid-forming foods, such as those containing amino acids rich in sulfur, causes increased breakdown of bone resulting in increased excretion of Ca in the urine. In addition, one of the adaptations is decreased urinary excretion of citrate because it is conserved to balance acid; however, because it is a key factor in solubilizing Ca oxalate, this results in increased stone formation. Excessive consumption of salt also

causes increased urinary acidity, perhaps by decreasing excretion of ammonium compounds. Excessive acidity also increases risk of urate stones owing to increased excretion of uric acid by the kidneys as part of the adaptation to decrease body acidity.

- **Weight and carbohydrate metabolism:** excess weight and insulin insensitivity induce hypercalciuria and higher risk. After glucose ingestion, urinary Ca rises along with decreased phosphate reabsorption. Low plasma phosphate stimulates 1,25-dihydroxycholecalciferol (active vitamin D) production, increased intestinal absorption of Ca, and hypercalciuria. Sucrose and other simple sugars cause exaggerated increase in urinary Ca oxalate in 70% of recurrent KS formers.
- **Gut flora:** oxalate homeostasis depends in part on the colon anaerobic bacterium *Oxalobacter formigenes.* Its absence (from prolonged antibiotic use) predisposes idiopathic Ca oxalate KSs from increased hyperoxaluria and Ca-oxalate stone formation. *O. formigenes* therapy repopulates gut and reduces urinary oxalate after oxalate load, thereby reducing Ca oxalate stone formation. Supplementing deficient persons may protect against future KSs.

Nutrients

- **Magnesium (Mg) and vitamin B_6:** Mg-deficient diet accelerates renal tubular Ca deposition in rats. Mg increases solubility of Ca oxalate and inhibits precipitation of Ca phosphate and Ca oxalate. Low urinary Mg/Ca ratio is an independent risk factor in stone formation. Supplemental Mg alone prevents recurrences. Use of Mg plus vitamin B_6 has even greater effect. Induced B_6 deficiency in rats produces oxaluria and Ca oxalate lithiasis (prevented by Mg supplementation).
- **Pyridoxine (vitamin B_6):** reduces endogenous production and urinary excretion of oxalates. Patients with recurrent oxalate stones show abnormal erythrocyte glutamate pyruvate transaminase (EGPT), erythrocyte glutamic- oxaloacetic transaminase (EGOT), urinary glutamic-pyruvic acid transaminase (UGPT), and urinary glutamic-oxaloacetic transaminase (UGOT) activation levels, indicating clinical insufficiency of B_6 and impaired glutamic acid synthesis. Levels normalize after 3 months of treatment.
- **Glutamic acid:** decreased glutamic acid (from B_6 deficiency or other reasons) is linked to KSs; increased glutamic acid in urine reduces Ca oxalate precipitation. Glutamic acid supplementation

in rats reduces incidence of calculi but may be superfluous with adequate vitamin B_6.

- **Ca:** Ca restriction enhances oxalate absorption and stone formation absorption. Ca supplements reduce oxalate excretion. KS risk is higher in persons with lowest daily Ca intakes compared with those with highest. Ca supplementation (300 to 1000 mg q.d.) may be preventive. However, postmenopausal women with no KS history have exhibited a 17% increased risk of stones after consuming 1000 mg of Ca carbonate plus 400 international units (IU) of vitamin D daily. Postmenopausal women may respond differently to Ca carbonate compared with younger women and men for unknown reasons. This study contradicts others indicating that vitamin D can be taken by postmenopausal women who are not stone formers and who are vitamin D insufficient without fear of an increased risk of KS.
- **Citrate:** low urinary citrate excretion is a risk factor for nephrolithiasis. Urinary Ca rises in patients taking Ca citrate, but citrate reduces urinary saturation of Ca oxalate and Ca phosphate. It retards nucleation and crystal growth of Ca salts. Potassium and Na citrate for recurrent Ca oxalate are quite effective; they cease stone formation in 90% of patients. Mg citrate may offer the greatest benefit. In people with a history of Ca stones and low urinary citrate, potassium citrate reduced frequency of stone formation. Mg citrate offers greatest benefit. Mg citrate slows growth of brushite crystals, nucleation rate, and supersaturation of urine. In addition, because Mg competes with Ca in binding oxalates in both gut and urine, ratio of Mg to Ca in urine is used in estimating stone risk. In one study, five of eight patients with oxalate stones experienced complete dissolution of their stones after 6 months of treatment.
- **Vitamin K:** urinary glycoprotein inhibitor of Ca oxalate monohydrate growth requires posttranscription carboxylation of glutamic acid to form gamma-carboxyglutamic acid. Vitamin K is essential for this carboxylation. Impairment of glutamic acid formation or vitamin K deficiency reduces this glycoprotein. Vitamin K in green leafy vegetables may be one reason vegetarians have a lower incidence of KSs.
- **Uric acid metabolism:** dietary purine intake is linearly related to rate of urinary uric acid excretion. Hyperuricosuria is a causative factor in recurrent Ca oxalate stones. High supplemental folic acid promotes purine scavenging and xanthine oxidase

inhibition, decreasing excretion of uric acid (see the chapter on gout). Higher urine pH also helps with uric acid solubility; however, manipulation of urine pH is complex because it is affected not only by diet and hydration but also by weight and body mass index (BMI). Higher BMI is linked to lower urine pH. Weight management, when indicated, may benefit patients with uric acid stones or low urine pH; but long-term benefits are unknown.

Botanicals

- Few clinical trials involve medicinal herbs for KS, and those are poorly designed. We focus here on traditional use of botanicals.
- Anthraquinones isolated from *Rubia* (madder root), *Cassia* (senna), and *Aloe* species bind Ca and reduce growth of urinary crystals when used in oral doses lower than laxative dose. *Rubia tinctura, Rumex* (yellow dock), *Rheum* (rhubarb), *Polygonum aviculare, Aloe, Senna, Frangula alnus,* and *Mitchella repens* (squaw vine) are sources of anthraquinones, which are used to prevent formation and, during acute attacks, reduce the size of stones.
- Furanocoumarin-containing herb *Ammi visnaga* (khella) is unusually effective at relaxing the ureter and allowing stone to pass. Ca channel–blocking capabilities act primarily on the ureters. Atropine and papaverine have similar, but less active, smooth muscle–relaxing effects. *Peucedanum, Leptotania, Ruta graveolens* (rue, bitterwort), and *Hydrangea* contain similar furanocoumarins promoting smooth muscle relaxation, justifying historic uses in KSs.
- **Eupatorium purpureum (gravel root):** name implies traditional use for urinary stones ("gravel"). Eclectic natural medicine physicians considered it mildly astringent, stimulant, and tonic with specific action on urinary organs and power to dissolve concretions.
- **Spasmolytic herbs:** KS pain comes in part from spasm in ureters. Spasmolytic herbs control ureteral spasm, whereas diuretic herbs push small stones through ureters slowly and tolerably. Application of these herbs depends on tradition in the absence of scientific data.
  - *A. visnaga* (khella) fruit: used also for angina pectoris and acute asthma
  - Lobelia
  - *Piscidia piscipula* (Jamaican dogwood) bark
  - *Gelsemium*

— Western pasque flower
— *Hyoscyamus niger* (henbane) herb: even stronger anticholinergic antispasmodic, like belladonna but with affinity for genitourinary tract.
— *Orthosiphon grandiflorus:* in patients with history of nephrolithiasis and radiographic stones present, *O. grandiflorus* extract at 2.5 g in tea b.i.d. and Na potassium citrate at 5 to 10 g t.i.d. for 18 months were equally effective at reducing stone size in 1 year, with far fewer adverse effects with the herb.
— *Phyllanthus niruri:* inhibits Ca oxalate crystallization in vitro. It dissolves stones in vivo and may be diuretic. At 450 mg of extract t.i.d. for 3 months, there was a reduction of hypercalciuria but no real effect on calculus elimination or calculus size.

Lifestyle

- **Sleep position:** patients with recurrent renal calculi often have calculi on the same side. Sleep posture may affect renal hemodynamics. The side of the stone is identical to dependent sleep side in 76% of cases, with positive predictive values of right and left side-down posture for ipsilateral stones of 82% and 70%, respectively.
- **Stress:** events of intense emotional impact with apprehension and distress, for at least 1 week in duration, increase risk of KS formation. These events may encourage loss of litholytic urinary constituents (Mg, citrate). Sympathetic fight-or-flight response may increase vasopressin, causing more-hypertonic urine.

Miscellaneous

- **Hair mineral analysis:** heavy metals (mercury, gold, uranium, and cadmium) are nephrotoxic. Cadmium (elevated serum cadmium) increases incidence of KSs.
- **Vitamin C and oxalate stones:** in persons who are not on hemodialysis and do not have recurrent KSs, severe kidney disease, or gout, high-dose vitamin C will not cause KSs. Vitamin C up to 10 g q.d. has no effect on urinary oxalate levels. However, the form of vitamin C used can be important. A large percentage of people—regardless of KS history, age, gender, and race—who ingest 1000 to 2000 mg of ascorbic acid for short periods experience hyperoxaluria to some degree. Vitamin C with metabolites (Ester-C), compared with ascorbic acid, induces less 24-hour oxalate excretion. Ester-C might be more beneficial for

stone formers; however, beneficial effects of Ester-C are still controversial.

- **Inositol hexaphosphate (phytic acid or IP_6):** a naturally occurring compound in whole grains, cereals, legumes, seeds, and nuts that is known for antineoplastic activity. Inadequate intake may increase Ca oxalate in urine, predisposing to urolithiasis. The use of 120 mg daily of IP_6 reduced, within 15 days, formation of Ca oxalate crystals in urine of people with KS history. It has proven effective against four types of KSs.

THERAPEUTIC APPROACH

Accurately differentiate stone types. Recognize and control underlying metabolic diseases or structural abnormalities of the urinary tract. The goal is to prevent recurrence. Dietary management is effective, inexpensive, and free of side effects. Specific treatment is determined by type of stone.

Possible interventions include the following:

- Reducing urinary Ca
- Reducing purine intake
- Avoiding high oxalate–containing foods
- Increasing foods with a high Mg/Ca ratio
- Increasing vitamin K–rich foods

For all types of stones, increase urine flow with increased intake of water to dilute urine. Maintain specific gravity below 1.015 and daily urinary volume of at least 2000 mL. If stones occur on one side only, avoid sleeping on that side. Consider stress reduction techniques and counseling for patients with stones and a history of significant stress.

Acute Obstruction

Surgical removal or lithotripsy may be necessary.

- *A. visnaga* (khella) extract (12% khellin content): 250 mg t.i.d.
- *R. tinctura, Rumex crispus* (yellow dock), or *Aloe vera* at below-laxative doses

Calcium Stones

- **Diet:** increase fiber, complex carbohydrates, and green leafy vegetables. Decrease simple carbohydrates and purines (meat, fish, poultry, yeast). Increase high Mg/Ca ratio foods (barley, bran, corn, buckwheat, rye, soy, oats, brown rice, avocado, banana, cashew, coconut, peanut, sesame seed, lima beans, potato).

If stones are oxalate, reduce oxalate foods (black tea, cocoa, spinach, beet leaves, rhubarb, parsley, cranberry, nuts). Limit dairy products.

- **Supplements:**
  — Vitamin B_6: 25 mg q.d.
  — Vitamin K: 2 mg q.d.
  — Mg: 600 mg q.d. in divided doses.
  — Ca: 300 to 1000 mg q.d.
- **Botanicals:** use any of the following in a dose below the laxative effect:
  — *R. tinctura*
  — *R. crispus*
  — *Aloe vera*
- **Miscellaneous:** avoid aluminum compounds and alkalis.

Uric Acid Stones

- **Diet:** decrease dietary purines (listed previously); ensure adequate water intake (room temperature or warmer) and a high alkali load with plenty of fruits and vegetables.
- **Supplements:** folic acid at 5 mg q.d.
- **Miscellaneous:** alkalinize urine with citrate, bicarbonate, blackcurrant juice.

Magnesium Ammonium Phosphate Stones

- Eradicate infection (*Textbook,* "Immune Support").
- Acidify urine: ammonium chloride (100 to 200 mg t.i.d.).

Cystine Stones

- **Diet:** avoid methionine-rich foods (eggs, soy, wheat, dairy products [except whole milk], fish, meat, lima beans, garbanzo beans, mushrooms, and all nuts except coconut, hazelnut, and sunflower seeds).
- **Miscellaneous:** alkalinize urine; optimal pH is 7.5 to 8.0.

Brushite and Struvite Stones

- Acidify urine: cranberry juice.

Leukoplakia

DIAGNOSTIC SUMMARY

- Adherent white patch or plaque appearing anywhere on oral mucosa.
- Asymptomatic until ulceration, fissuring, or malignant transformation.
- Diagnosis confirmed by biopsy.

GENERAL CONSIDERATIONS

Leukoplakia is the clinical term for a white plaquelike lesion anywhere on the oral mucosa. It is a reaction to irritation (cigarette smoking, tobacco, betel nut chewing) and early sign in human immunodeficiency virus (HIV) infection. It most frequently occurs in men aged 50 to 70 years. In 90% of cases, it represents epithelial hyperkeratosis and hyperplasia. In 10% of cases epithelial dysplasia also is present; these lesions are considered precancerous.

Oral cancer is a common malignant neoplasm; 50,000 new cases and 12,000 deaths occur in the United States alone each year. Survival rates with chemotherapy, radiation, and surgery are unchanged in the past few decades. Prevent death by preventing occurrence with abstinence from tobacco and increased intake of antioxidants.

THERAPEUTIC CONSIDERATIONS

Remove all irritants. Electrodesiccation, cryosurgery, and proteolytic enzymes have not yielded predictably favorable results. Photodynamic therapy, vitamin A, beta-carotene, and lycopene have clinical resolution rates higher than 50%.

- **Vitamin A and beta-carotene:** clinically effective for leukoplakia. The micronucleus test is a useful indicator of cancerous tendency of epithelial cells, giving immediate information on genotoxic damage. Micronuclei are formed during chromatid or chromosomal breakage; the rate of formation is linked to

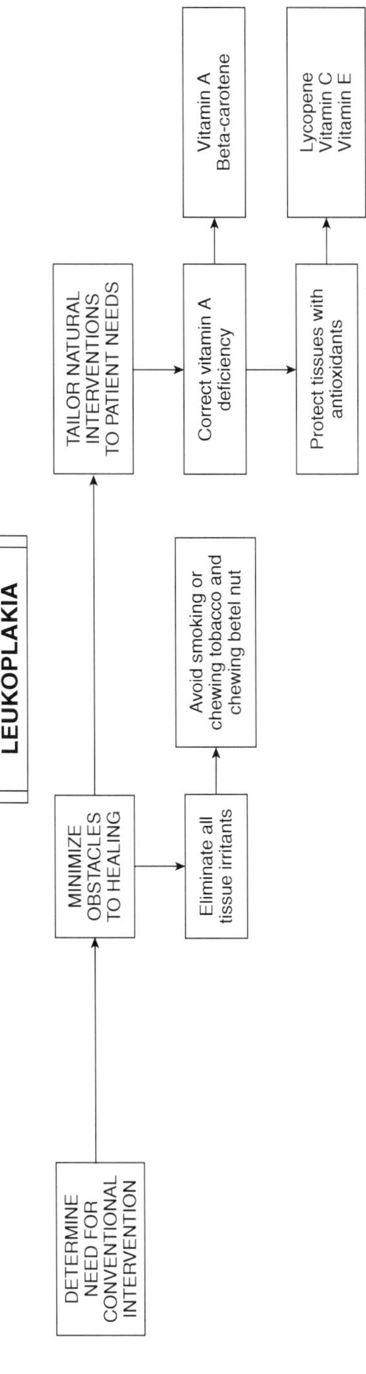
LEUKOPLAKIA
DETERMINE NEED FOR CONVENTIONAL INTERVENTION
MINIMIZE OBSTACLES TO HEALING
Eliminate all tissue irritants
Avoid smoking or chewing tobacco and chewing betel nut
TAILOR NATURAL INTERVENTIONS TO PATIENT NEEDS
Correct vitamin A deficiency
Vitamin A
Beta-carotene
Protect tissues with antioxidants
Lycopene
Vitamin C
Vitamin E

oral carcinogenesis. It is a good predictor of cancer, which takes years to develop recognizable signs. Beta-carotene is quite effective in decreasing the mean proportion of cells with micronuclei on buccal mucosa in Asian betel nut and tobacco chewers. (Subjects continued to chew betel nut and tobacco during the study.) Evidence documenting the protective effect of carotenoids and retinoids against epithelial cancers is overwhelming (*Textbook,* "Beta-carotene and Other Carotenoids"). An inverse relationship exists between serum retinol and carotene levels and cancer incidence; this holds true for oral carcinomas. Studies on leukoplakia used very high but effective retinol doses (150,000 to 900,000 international units [IU] q.d.). Beta-carotene is as effective as retinol in decreasing micronuclei, with a much higher therapeutic index. (*Note:* Vulvar leukoplakia is responsive to retinol and perhaps beta-carotene.) Head-to-head comparative study found an advantage with retinol. Homogeneous leukoplakia and smaller lesions respond better than did nonhomogeneous and larger lesions. No major toxicities were observed even with prolonged vitamin A supplementation.

- **Lycopene:** the carotenoid lycopene administered over 5 months displayed no difference in clinical response with doses of 8 mg lycopene b.i.d. versus 4 mg b.i.d. Histologic assessment was better after 8 mg.
- **Other antioxidants:** vitamin E (alpha-tocopherol 400 IU b.i.d. for 24 weeks) produces a 65% response rate. Use a combination of antioxidants (including mixed tocopherols rather than just one of the eight isomers) to accommodate their interactions and limitations. A combination of vitamin C (1000 mg q.d.), beta-carotene (30 mg q.d.), and vitamin E (400 mg q.d.) gives encouraging results.
- **Curcumin:** shows promising in vitro chemopreventive properties for leukoplakia.

THERAPEUTIC APPROACH

Leukoplakia is caused by a combination of excessive carcinogenic irritation and marginal or low levels of vitamin A. Eliminate all sources of irritation. The main irritants are tobacco smoking and chewing, betel nut chewing, and ultraviolet exposure. Establish optimal vitamin A, beta-carotene, and antioxidant levels.

Supplements

- **Vitamin A:** 5000 IU q.d.
- **Beta-carotene:** 30 to 90 mg q.d.
- **Lycopene:** 8 mg b.i.d.
- **Vitamin C:** 1000 to 3000 mg q.d.
- **Vitamin E:** 400 IU q.d. (mixed tocopherols).

Lichen Planus

DIAGNOSTIC SUMMARY

- Inflammatory, pruritic disease of skin and mucous membranes described by the six *P*s: pruritic, polygonal, planar (flat-topped), purple papules, and plaques.
- Primary common complaint: intense pruritus; can occur without pruritus.
- **History:** pruritus (can be severe); rash or skin eruption.
- **Physical examination:** skin lesions are flat topped, violaceous to purple, polygonal or oval papules from 1 to 10 mm wide with edges that are sharply defined and shiny. Lesions may be grouped, linear (Koebner phenomenon), annular, or disseminated when generalized. White lines (Wickham striae) are possible. Use handheld lens; apply clear oil over lesion to intensify visibility of Wickham striae. In dark-skinned patients appears as postinflammatory hyperpigmentation. Lesion location: flexor surfaces of wrists, lumbar region, eyelids, shin, scalp, glans penis, mouth, but may occur anywhere. An uncommon presentation is plaque-size lesions. Location is on nails and hair follicles, with dystrophic changes and scarring.
- **Oral lesions:** inflammation and leukohyperkeratoses generating reticulated, white puncta or papules and lines in a lacelike pattern. Plaques may occur. Inflammation may cause erosions with blisters. Location is on buccal mucosa; bilateral in nearly all patients on tongue, lips, and gingiva. Skin lesions occur in 10% to 60% of oral cases.
- **Other locations:** genitalia; papular, annular, or erosive lesions on penis, scrotum, labia majora, labia minor, and vagina. On the scalp, atrophic skin and scarring alopecia; on the nails, destruction of nail fold and nail bed with longitudinal splintering.
- **Biopsy:** if doubt exists or if blisters, plaques, or erosions occur in the oral form.

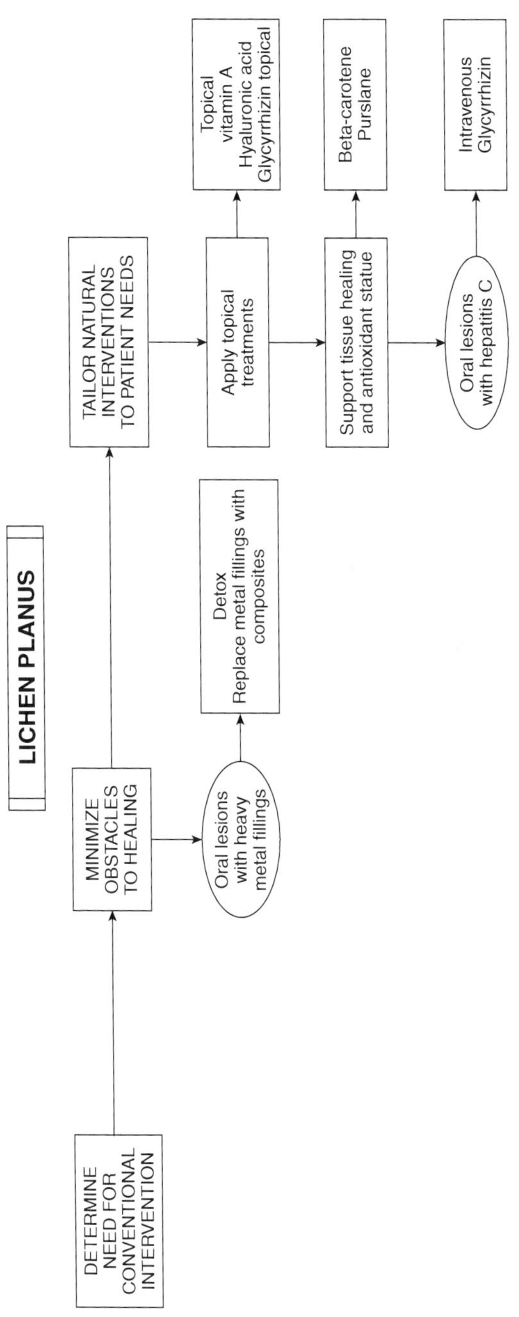
LICHEN PLANUS
DETERMINE NEED FOR CONVENTIONAL INTERVENTION
MINIMIZE OBSTACLES TO HEALING
Oral lesions with heavy metal fillings
Detox
Replace metal fillings with composites
TAILOR NATURAL INTERVENTIONS TO PATIENT NEEDS
Apply topical treatments
Topical vitamin A
Hyaluronic acid
Glycyrrhizin topical
Support tissue healing and antioxidant statue
Beta-carotene
Purslane
Oral lesions with hepatitis C
Intravenous Glycyrrhizin

GENERAL CONSIDERATIONS

Lichen planus (LP) is an inflammatory, pruritic disease of the skin and mucous membranes and can be generalized or localized. Characteristic features include distinctive purplish, flat-topped papules (discrete or coalescent into plaques) on the trunk and flexor surfaces.

- **Epidemiology:** higher prevalence of hepatitis C virus infection in patients with LP, but a pathogenic relation has not been established. LP affects women more than men. Age of onset is 30 to 60 years. Hypertrophic LP is more common in African Americans.
- **Variants:**
  - **Hypertrophic:** large, thick plaques on foot and shins; more common in African-American men. Hypertrophic lesions may become hyperkeratotic rather than smooth.
  - **Follicular:** individual keratotic-follicular papules and plaques leading to cicatricial alopecia. Graham Little syndrome is a complex of spinous follicular lesions, any LP, and cicatricial alopecia.
  - **Vesicular:** vesicular or bullous lesions within or independent of lesions. Direct immunofluorescence reveals bullous pemphigoid; patients have bullous pemphigoid immunoglobulin G (IgG) autoantibodies.
  - **Actinicus:** papular lesions in sun-exposed areas (e.g., dorsum of hands and arms).
  - **Ulcerative:** therapy-resistant ulcers (soles) requiring skin grafting.
  - **Oral or mucous membranes:** reticular, hyperkeratotic, erosive, plaque type, atrophic, bullous types
- **Etiology:** often unknown. Drugs, metals, or infection (hepatitis C virus) resulting in alteration of cell-mediated immunity may play a role. Human leukocyte antigen–associated genetic susceptibility predisposes some patients. Immunoglobulins (IgM, IgA, IgG) and complement (C3) are at dermal-epidermal junction in 95% of lesions. Lesions can occur with certain drugs, graft-versus-host disease reactions, and dermatomyositis and as cutaneous manifestations of malignant lymphoma. Immune factor involved: cell-mediated processes.
- **Incidence:** six per 1000 dermatology patients, or 4.4 per 1000 people in the United States per year. Oral LP is the most common cause of oral white lesions, occurring in 0.5% to 1% of dental patients. Oral LP occurs alone or with skin lesions.

- **Onset:** acute or insidious. Lesions remain for months to years. Lesions are asymptomatic or mildly to severely pruritic; they are more painful on mucous membranes and worse with ulceration.
- **Course of oral LP:** chronic from months to years; two thirds of cases undergo spontaneous resolution within 1 year. Recurrence is uncommon (less than 20% of patents). Mucous membrane cases have course that is much more prolonged, but 50% remit in 2 years. Incidence of oral squamous cell carcinoma in patients with oral LP is increased by 5%. LP-like eruptions can occur from graft-versus-host disease and dermatomyositis and as cutaneous manifestations of malignant lymphoma and certain drugs.
- **Possible causative medicines:** most common are gold, antimalarial agents, penicillamine, thiazide diuretics, beta-blockers, nonsteroidal anti-inflammatory drugs, quinidine, and angiotensin-converting enzyme inhibitors. Interval between taking an offending agent and developing lichenoid drug eruptions ranges from 10 days to several years.

THERAPEUTIC CONSIDERATIONS

The underlying mechanism of LP is unknown. The immune system's role is evidenced by the presence of IgM (possibly IgA, IgG) and complement at the dermal-epidermal junction in 95% of LP lesions; certain drug eruptions and graft-versus-host reactions in bone marrow transplant recipients mimic LP. Primary immune factor is cell-mediated processes. Activated T-helper (Th) cells in early lesions target basal cells, which may have antigenic alterations. Ts cells predominate in older lesions.

- **Dental amalgams:** oral LP is more resistant to therapy than are skin lesions. Dental amalgams are linked to oral LP. Replacing mercury amalgam fillings with alternative substances dramatically improves chronic lichenoid reactions. The greatest effect is noted with gold crowns versus palladium-based crowns. If gold crowns are present, have the patient patch tested for gold allergy; consider removal if positive. (*Note:* Many patch test–negative patients still respond to amalgam removal.) However, for positive patch-test reactions to mercury, replacement of amalgam fillings can lead to improvement in nearly all patients.
- **Photodynamic therapy:** a case report showed LP of the penis resistant to steroids (and initially diagnosed as intraepidermal

carcinoma). Photodynamic therapy was preceded by topical 5-aminolevulinic acid (20%) ointment (4 hours before treatment). Irradiate with a Paterson-Whitehurst lamp (Paterson Institute, Christie Hospital, Manchester, United Kingdom) at center wavelength of 630 and rectangular pass band of 27 nm. Dose gradually increased to 50 J/cm^2 at fluence rate of 55 mW/cm^2 to prevent edema and phimosis. Treatment was repeated after 6 weeks. Lesions completely resolved after another 4 weeks, with no recurrence at 6 months. Biopsy: mild changes identifying condition as LP. Photodynamic therapy with medium-dose ultraviolet A1 has successfully treated ulcerative LP of feet.

Supplements and Botanical Medicines

Correction of deficiencies in vitamins B_1 and B_6 has provided clinical and subjective improvement in the majority of patients treated, but did not produce complete remission of lesions.

Vitamin A and Beta-carotene

- Topical retinoic acid (0.1% in petroleum jelly base) applied three times a day over a 3-week period to hypertrophic LP of the palms or soles caused irritation because of the frequency of application. When applied every other day two or three times per day, it induced regression after 2 to 3 weeks. A slight recurrence arose after 3 to 4 months.
- Topical retinoic acid 0.05% was not as effective as fluocinolone acetonide 0.1% applied q.i.d. to various stages of oral LP.
- Small doses of vitamin A acid locally applied produced improvement or regression in hypertrophic LP of the palms or soles in a small number of patients.
- Retinaldehyde gel 0.1% applied to oral LP resulting in 6% disappearance and 82% improvement of lesions, confirmed by downregulation of filaggrin and CK-10 as markers of terminal differentiation.
- In LP of the penis or anal region, applying 0.1% retinoic acid in Orabase overnight and 10 mg (33,330 international units [IU]) of oral retinoic acid t.i.d. or q.i.d. for 3 days to 3 weeks improved or resolved all cases.
- Patients with mucosal dysplasia (leukoplakia, LP, erythroplasia, leukokeratosis) are low-normal for serum vitamin A, beta-carotene, and *cis*-retinoic acid. Of 18 patients receiving beta-carotene (30 mg q.i.d.), one deteriorated, nine remained stable, and eight

improved (six completely). The addition of isotretinoin (Accutane) 10 mg t.i.d. caused three stable patients to improve. Response to treatment was much higher in smokers (30 pack-years or more) than in nonsmokers.

- Vitamin A can be applied with folic acid in an adhesive base (Orabase).

Synthetic Retinoids

Topical 0.1% 13-*cis*-retinoic acid for 8 weeks resolved physiologic cell morphology in oral LP. Both 0.05% and 0.18% isotretinoin might improve atrophic-erosive oral LP.

Glycyrrhizin

Of nine patients with oral LP and hepatitis C receiving intravenous glycyrrhizin (40 mL 0.2% solution of glycyrrhizin q.d. for 4 consecutive weeks), six improved clinically. They had only mildly raised alanine aminotransferase and aspartate aminotransferase levels. (*Note:* Scientific Botanicals *Glycyrrhiza* SE is standardized to 17% glycyrrhizin. A comparable oral dose is 500 mg solid extract.)

Aloe vera

In women's vulval LP with erosive and ulcerative lesions, topical *Aloe* gel clinically improved lesions 50% after 8 weeks.

Hyaluronic Acid

In erosive oral LP, topical 0.2% hyaluronic acid (HA) preparation for 28 days reduced soreness scores for up to 4 hours after application. It also reduced size of erosive and ulcerated areas after 28 days. Consider very frequent applications for more clinical benefit.

Purslane

In oral LP, 235 mg solid extract of purslane daily for 3 months can produce partial or complete clinical improvement.

THERAPEUTIC APPROACH

Because the cause of LP is undetermined, curative approaches are unclear. For oral lesions and significant metal-based fillings, consider heavy metal detoxification and replacement of metal fillings.

Supplements

Topical Treatments

Apply q.i.d.

- **Vitamin A (0.1% solution):** May cause inflammation and mildly increase pain temporarily.
- **HA gel**
- *Aloe vera* **gel**
- **Glycyrrhizin** topical application

Oral Treatments

- **Vitamin A:** 33,330 IU t.i.d. or q.i.d. for 3 days to 3 weeks while monitoring liver enzymes; *or* use **beta-carotene** 30 mg q.i.d.
- **Purslane:** 235 mg dried herb q.d.

Intravenous Treatments (Lichen Planus with Hepatitis C)

- **Glycyrrhizin:** 40 mL of 0.2% solution q.d. for 4 consecutive weeks.

Macular Degeneration

DIAGNOSTIC SUMMARY

- Progressive visual loss caused by degeneration of the macula.
- Ophthalmologic examination may reveal spots of pigment near macula and blurring of macular borders.

GENERAL CONSIDERATIONS

The macula is the area of the retina where most images focus and the portion of the retina responsible for fine vision. Macular degeneration (MD) is the leading cause of severe visual loss in the United States and Europe in persons aged 55 years and older; it is second to cataracts as the leading cause of decreased vision in persons older than 65 years.

- **Major risk factors:** smoking, aging, atherosclerosis, and hypertension. Degeneration results from free radical damage. Decreased blood and oxygen supply to the retina are a harbinger of MD.
- **Other factors:** region of chromosome 10 may be linked to age-related macular degeneration (ARMD) but the diversity in phenotype and late onset of disease complicate feasibility of linkage. Higher birth weight and lower head circumference/birth weight ratio are associated with increased risk.

Types of Age-Related Macular Degeneration

In either form, patients experience blurred vision. Straight objects appear distorted or bent. A dark spot appears near or around the center of the visual field. While the patient is reading, parts of words are missing. The two types of ARMD are as follows:

- **Atrophic "dry" ARMD:** 80% to 95% of people with ARMD have the dry form. Primary lesions are atrophic changes in retinal pigmented epithelium (RPE) (innermost layer of retina). Cells of RPE gradually accumulate, throughout life, sacs of cellular debris (lipofuscin)—remnants of degraded molecules from damaged RPE or phagocytized rod and cone membranes. Progressive lipofuscin engorgement of RPE cells extrudes tissue

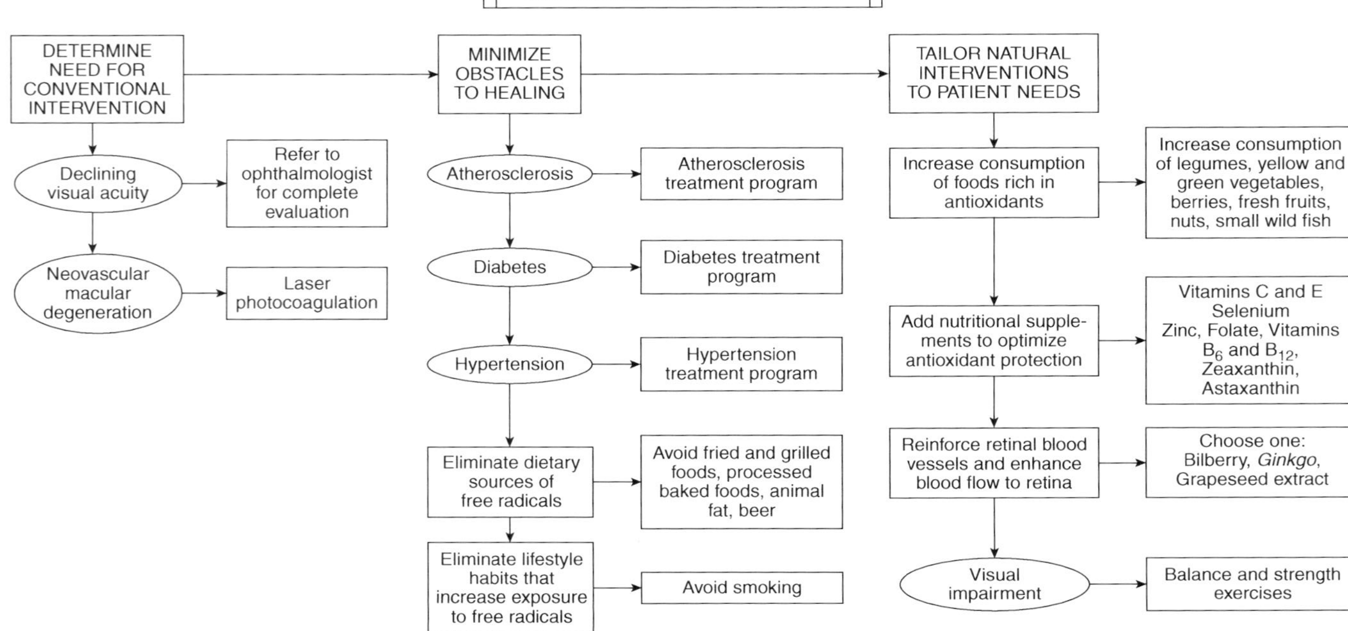
MACULAR DEGENERATION
DETERMINE NEED FOR CONVENTIONAL INTERVENTION
Declining visual acuity
Refer to ophthalmologist for complete evaluation
Neovascular macular degeneration
Laser photocoagulation
MINIMIZE OBSTACLES TO HEALING
Atherosclerosis
Atherosclerosis treatment program
Diabetes
Diabetes treatment program
Hypertension
Hypertension treatment program
Eliminate dietary sources of free radicals
Avoid fried and grilled foods, processed baked foods, animal fat, beer
Eliminate lifestyle habits that increase exposure to free radicals
Avoid smoking
TAILOR NATURAL INTERVENTIONS TO PATIENT NEEDS
Increase consumption of foods rich in antioxidants
Increase consumption of legumes, yellow and green vegetables, berries, fresh fruits, nuts, small wild fish
Add nutritional supplements to optimize antioxidant protection
Vitamins C and E
Selenium
Zinc, Folate, Vitamins B_6 and B_{12},
Zeaxanthin,
Astaxanthin
Reinforce retinal blood vessels and enhance blood flow to retina
Choose one:
Bilberry, *Ginkgo*,
Grapeseed extract
Visual impairment
Balance and strength exercises

components (hyaline, sialomucin, cerebroside). Hallmark excrescences beneath RPE seen on ophthalmoscopic examination are called *drusen.* The formation of drusen results from free radical damage similar to that of cataracts. However, decreases in nutrient, blood, and oxygen supply to the retina are harbingers of developing drusen and subsequent MD. The disease progresses slowly and only central vision is lost; peripheral vision remains intact. Total blindness from dry ARMD is rare. No standard medical treatment exists.

- **Neovascular "wet" ARMD:** neovascular form affects 5% to 20% of those with ARMD. It involves growth of abnormal blood vessels and can be treated effectively in the early stages with laser photocoagulation. The disease rapidly progresses to a point at which surgery is ineffective; perform surgery as soon as possible. Wet ARMD is treated effectively in early stages with laser photocoagulation therapy. Antiangiogenics or anti–vascular endothelial growth factor (anti-VEGF) agents are also used. These drugs can cause regression of abnormal blood vessels and improvement of vision when injected directly into the vitreous humor of the eye. The injections are repeated monthly or bimonthly. Examples of these agents: ranibizumab (Lucentis), bevacizumab (Avastin), and pegaptanib (Macugen).

THERAPEUTIC CONSIDERATIONS

Treatment for wet form is laser photocoagulation. New treatments include photodynamic therapy with photosensitive drugs (verteporfin) and low-powered laser and low-dose radiation.

Treating the dry form and preventing the wet form involve antioxidants and natural substances that correct underlying pathophysiology—free radical damage and poor oxygenation of macula. For example, tobacco smoking increases risk of ARMD by two to three times that of nonsmokers. Risk does not return to control rate until after 15 years of being smoke free.

There is a strong genetic component. Strong family history may offer most convenient screening method. Higher birth weight and lower head circumference/birth weight ratio are associated with higher risk. Reduce risk factors for atherosclerosis; increase dietary fresh fruits and vegetables and use nutritional and botanical antioxidants.

Reducing and Preventing Atherosclerosis

Atherosclerosis is a risk factor for MD. In subjects younger than 85 years, plaques in carotid bifurcation indicate 4.7-fold increased prevalence of MD; lower extremity atherosclerosis indicates a 2.5 times greater risk (see the chapter on atherosclerosis).

- **Dietary fruits and vegetables:** dietary factors mirror those that prevent other chronic degenerative diseases (e.g., atherosclerosis). A diet rich in fruits and vegetables offers a lower risk for ARMD by increasing intake of antioxidants (e.g., vitamins C and E, zinc [Zn], and selenium). Non–provitamin A carotenes lutein, zeaxanthin, and lycopene and flavonoids are more protective against ARMD than traditional nutritional antioxidants. The macula (and central portion, the fovea) owes its yellow color to high concentrations of lutein and zeaxanthin, which prevent oxidative damage to the retina and protect against MD. Individuals with lycopene in the lowest quintile are twice as likely to have ARMD. Persons with lowest plasma concentrations of zeaxanthin have a 2.0 odds ratio for risk of ARMD. Risk was increased in people with lowest plasma lutein plus zeaxanthin and with lowest lutein, but neither of these relations was statistically significant.
- **Animal fat:** intake of animal fat and processed baked goods carried a twofold increased risk of progression of ARMD. Higher fish intake lowers risk of progression in individuals with lower linoleic acid intake. Nuts are protective. Egg yolks are an excellent source of bioavailable lutein and zeaxanthin but increase low-density lipoprotein by 8% to 11%. Other studies found no change in cholesterol in healthy volunteers with moderate egg consumption and that only those with concomitant high plasma cholesterol and triglycerides were subject to hyperlipidemic increases when eating foods with dietary cholesterol, such as eggs.
- **Omega-3 fats:** long-chain omega-3 fatty acids reduce incidence of ARMD and are inversely associated with 12-year progression to ARMD.
- **Alcohol:** moderate red wine consumption decreases MD risk. Red-purple foods contain protective anthocyanin antioxidants. Avoid beer because it increases drusen accumulation and risk of exudative MD.
- **Nutritional supplements:** antioxidants (vitamin C, selenium, beta-carotene, vitamin E) are important for treatment and prevention. Combinations are better than any single nutrient alone because none alone accounts for impaired antioxidant status in

ARMD. Decreased antioxidant status reflects decreases in combinations of nutrients. Exemplary specific daily research doses of antioxidants and Zn: 500 mg vitamin C, 400 international units (IU) vitamin E (mixed tocopherols), 15 mg beta-carotene (equivalent to 25,000 IU of vitamin A), 80 mg of Zn as Zn oxide, and 2 mg copper as cupric oxide.

- **Antioxidant preparations:** progression of dry ARMD was halted (but not reversed) with a commercial antioxidant combination. Another antioxidant containing beta-carotene, vitamins C and E, Zn, copper, manganese, selenium, and riboflavin was able to maintain or improve visual acuity in these patients.
- **B vitamins:** a combination of folic acid (2.5 mg q.d.), pyridoxine hydrochloride (50 mg q.d.), and cyanocobalamin (1 mg q.d.) given for 7.3 years reduced manifestation of ARMD in female patients with high cardiovascular risk, by 34% to 41%.
- **Lutein**: the Lutein Antioxidant Supplementation Trial studying atrophic ARMD found that patients receiving lutein (10 mg) alone or in combination with other vitamins and minerals in a broad-spectrum formula had improved mean eye macular pigment optical density, Snellen equivalent visual acuity, and contrast sensitivity. In patients with early-stage nonadvanced ARMD and visual acuity at or equal to 0.2 logarithm of the minimum angle of resolution, a carotenoid-antioxidant combination—vitamin C (180 mg), vitamin E (30 mg), Zn (22.5 mg), copper (1 mg), lutein (10 mg), zeaxanthin (1 mg), and astaxanthin (4 mg) daily for 12 months—induced a positive response.
- **Zn:** essential in metabolism of retina; the elderly have a high risk for Zn deficiency. Supplementing 200 mg q.d. Zn sulfate (80 mg elemental Zn) reduces visual loss. Age-Related Eye Disease Study used 500 mg vitamin C, 400 IU vitamin E, 15 mg beta-carotene, 80 mg Zn (Zn oxide), and 2 mg copper (cupric oxide) to reduce risk of development of advanced ARMD. Researchers recommended combination of Zn and antioxidants for patients older than 55 years at risk for ARMD. These results were not confirmed in a study of wet ARMD. Zinc monocysteine (ZMC) given to ARMD patients at 25 mg b.i.d. for 6 months improved visual acuity and contrast sensitivity. Macular light-flash recovery time shortened by 2.1 to 3.6 seconds at 3 months and at 6 months by 7.2 to 7.4 seconds.
- **Flavonoid-rich extracts:** *Vaccinium myrtillus* (bilberry), *Ginkgo biloba,* and *Vitis vinifera* (grapeseed) are beneficial in preventing and treating ARMD. These excellent antioxidants improve

retinal blood flow and function. They can halt progressive visual loss of dry ARMD and may even improve visual function. Bilberry extracts standardized to 25% anthocyanidins are most useful. *Vaccinium* anthocyanosides have very strong affinity for RPE, the functional portion of retina affected by ARMD, reinforcing collagen structures of the retina and preventing free radical damage. *G. biloba* extract (24% *Ginkgo* flavon glycoside and 6% terpenoids) is a better choice if patient also has signs of cerebrovascular insufficiency. Grapeseed extract is most useful with photophobia or poor night vision.
- **Exercise:** may not play a role in reversing or preventing ARMD, but strength and balance training can minimize risk of falling in visually impaired patients.

THERAPEUTIC APPROACH

Prevention or treatment at an early stage is most effective. The treatment for wet form of ARMD is laser photocoagulation as soon as possible. For the dry form, use antioxidants and promote retinal blood flow. Refer any patient 55 years or older with visual loss to an ophthalmologist for complete evaluation, especially if visual loss is progressing rapidly. Investigate and treat underlying diabetes and/or hypertension (see the chapters on diabetes mellitus and hypertension).

- **Diet:** avoid fried and grilled foods and other sources of free radicals; animal fat; processed baked goods; beer. Increase legumes (high in sulfur-containing amino acids), yellow and green vegetables (carotenes), flavonoid-rich berries (blueberries, blackberries, cherries), vitamin E– and vitamin C–rich foods (fresh fruits and vegetables), nuts, and small wild fish. Moderate red wine intake is advised for those without contraindications to alcohol.
- **Supplements:**
  — Vitamin C: 1 g t.i.d.
  — Vitamin E: 200 to 400 IU q.d. (mixed tocopherols)
  — Selenium: 200 to 400 mcg q.d.
  — Zn: 30 mg q.d.
  — Folic acid: 800 mcg q.d. (activated folates better if available)
  — Pyridoxine hydrochloride: 50 mg q.d.
  — Vitamin B_{12}: 800 mcg q.d.
  — Lutein: 10 to 15 mg q.d.
  — Zeaxanthin: 1 to 2 mg q.d.
  — Astaxanthin: 4 to 6 mg q.d.

- **Botanical medicines (choose one):**

Choose one of the following extracts:

— *G. biloba* extract (24% *Ginkgo* heterosides): 120 to 240 mg q.d.

— *V. myrtillus* (bilberry) extract (25% anthocyanidin content): 120 to 240 mg/day

— Grapeseed extract (95% procyanidolic oligomer content): 150 to 300 mg q.d.

- **Exercise:** balance training and strength exercises, especially for those who are visually impaired.

Maldigestion

This chapter provides an overview of digestive dysfunction and ways to improve digestion. For specific digestive tract disorders (e.g., irritable bowel syndrome, peptic ulcers, inflammatory bowel disease, celiac disease), see the chapters devoted to those topics. For information on various laboratory procedures for evaluation of digestive function (e.g., comprehensive digestive stool analysis, intestinal permeability assessment, small intestinal bacterial overgrowth breath test), see Section 2 of the *Textbook*.

THERAPEUTIC CONSIDERATIONS

Indigestion

- The term *indigestion* is often used by patients to describe feelings of abdominal gaseousness, fullness, heartburn, early satiety, loss of appetite, and postprandial fullness (bloating).
- Use of antacids to treat indigestion raises gastric pH above 3.5, inhibiting action of pepsin, the enzyme involved in protein digestion that can be irritating to the stomach. Although raising pH can reduce symptoms, it also impairs protein digestion and mineral disassociation. Change in pH can adversely affect gut microbial flora by allowing pathogenic organisms to pass through the normally antimicrobial acid stomach and promoting overgrowth of *Helicobacter pylori.* Most nutrition-oriented physicians believe that lack of acid, not excess, is true culprit in most patients with indigestion.

Reflux Esophagitis

Most people use antacids to relieve reflux esophagitis. However, reflux esophagitis is most often caused by overeating and other factors, not excessive acid. Common causes include the following:

- Obesity
- Cigarette smoking
- Chocolate
- Fried foods

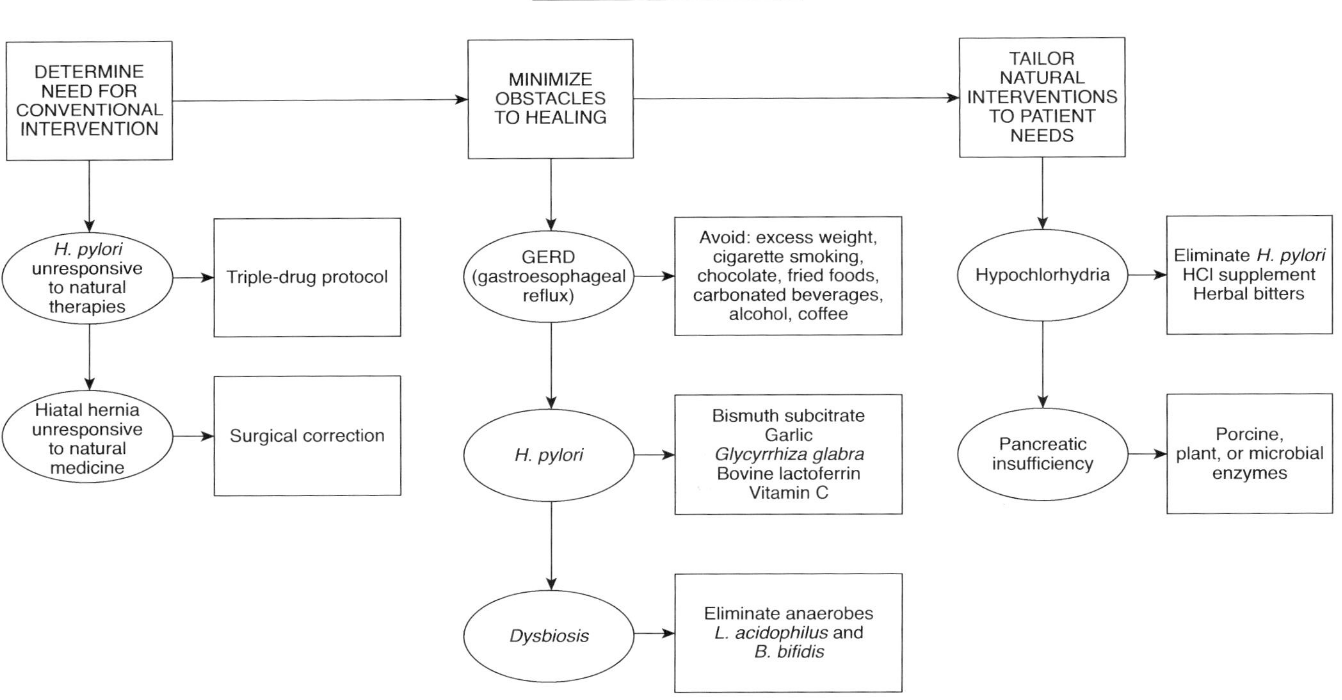
MALDIGESTION
DETERMINE NEED FOR CONVENTIONAL INTERVENTION
MINIMIZE OBSTACLES TO HEALING
TAILOR NATURAL INTERVENTIONS TO PATIENT NEEDS
H. pylori unresponsive to natural therapies
Triple-drug protocol
Hiatal hernia unresponsive to natural medicine
Surgical correction
GERD (gastroesophageal reflux)
Avoid: excess weight, cigarette smoking, chocolate, fried foods, carbonated beverages, alcohol, coffee
H. pylori
Bismuth subcitrate
Garlic
Glycyrrhiza glabra
Bovine lactoferrin
Vitamin C
Dysbiosis
Eliminate anaerobes
L. acidophilus and B. bifidis
Hypochlorhydria
Eliminate H. pylori
HCl supplement
Herbal bitters
Pancreatic insufficiency
Porcine, plant, or microbial enzymes

- Carbonated beverages
- Alcohol
- Coffee

These factors either increase intra-abdominal pressure or decrease tone of esophageal cardiac sphincter. Chronic heartburn is also a sign of a hiatal hernia. Although 50% of people older than 50 years have hiatal hernias, only 5% of patients with hiatal hernias experience reflux esophagitis.

- Most effective treatment for chronic reflux esophagitis and symptomatic hiatal hernias is use of **gravity.** Place 4-inch blocks under the bedposts at head of patient's bed.
- Heal esophagus by using **deglycyrrhizinated licorice.**
- **Enteric-coated peppermint oil** is very helpful for nonulcer dyspepsia and reflux esophagitis.

Hypochlorhydria (Insufficient Gastric Acid)

For chronic indigestion, rather than focusing on blocking digestive process with antacids, focus on aiding digestion. More-common cause of indigestion is lack of gastric acid secretion, based on symptoms and signs. A number of specific diseases are linked to insufficient gastric acid. See boxes "Common Signs and Symptoms of Low Gastric Acidity" and "Diseases Associated with Low Gastric Acidity."

- Ability to secrete gastric acid decreases with age.
- Best method of diagnosing gastric acid is Heidelberg gastric analysis (*Textbook*, "Heidelberg pH Capsule Gastric Analysis"). Response to bicarbonate challenge during Heidelberg gastric analysis, not simply resting pH, is true test of functional ability of stomach to secrete acid. Heidelberg gastric acid analysis is not widely available; clinical trial of hydrochloric acid (HCl) supplements can be used as described in *Textbook* Appendix 7.

Common Signs and Symptoms of Low Gastric Acidity

- Bloating, belching, burning, and flatulence immediately after meals
- A sense of "fullness" after eating
- Indigestion, diarrhea, or constipation
- Multiple food allergies
- Nausea after taking supplements
- Itching around the rectum
- Weak, peeling, and cracked fingernails
- Dilated blood vessels in the cheeks and nose
- Acne
- Iron deficiency
- Chronic intestinal parasites or abnormal flora

- Undigested food in stool
- Chronic *Candida* infections
- Upper digestive tract gassiness

Diseases Associated with Low Gastric Acidity

- Addison's disease
- Asthma
- Celiac disease
- Chronic autoimmune disorders
- Dermatitis herpetiformis
- Diabetes mellitus
- Eczema
- Gallbladder disease
- Graves' disease
- Hepatitis
- Hives (chronic)
- Hyperthyroidism or hypothyroidism
- Myasthenia gravis
- Osteoporosis
- Pernicious anemia
- Psoriasis
- Rheumatoid arthritis
- Rosacea
- Sjögren's syndrome
- Systemic lupus erythematosus
- Thyrotoxicosis
- Vitiligo

Etiology

- Like peptic ulcer disease, achlorhydria and hypochlorhydria are linked to overgrowth of bacterium *H. pylori:* 90% to 100% of patients with duodenal ulcers, 70% with gastric ulcers, and 50% of people older than 50 years test positive for *H. pylori.*
- Presence of *H. pylori* is determined by measuring level of antibodies to *H. pylori* in blood or saliva or by culturing material collected during an endoscopy and measuring breath for urea. A breath test is also available for assessment of current *H. pylori* activity.
- Low gastric output predisposes to *H. pylori* colonization; and *H. pylori* colonization increases gastric pH, setting up positive feedback scenario and increasing likelihood of colonization of stomach and duodenum by other organisms.
- HCl antisecretory drugs (H_2 receptor antagonists and proton pump inhibitors) may actually promote *H. pylori* overgrowth. Patients with *H. pylori* experience exaggerated response in

elevations of pH with antisecretory therapy. Eradication of *H. pylori* restores normal gastric acidity and pepsinogen ratio.

- Research focus on attacking the microbe leaves little information on protective factors against infectivity. Proposed protective factors: maintaining low pH and ensuring adequate antioxidant defense mechanisms.
- Low levels of vitamins C and E and other antioxidants in gastric juice lead to progression of *H. pylori* colonization and contribute to ulcer formation, because mechanism by which *H. pylori* damages stomach and intestinal mucosa is oxidative.
- Antioxidant status and gastric acid output explain observation that most people infected with *H. pylori* do not experience peptic ulcers or gastric cancer; for more information on natural approaches for eradicating *H. pylori,* (*Textbook* "Peptic Ulcer-Duodenal and Gastric").
- Bovine lactoferrin is useful against *H. pylori.* Lactoferrin exerts broad-spectrum antimicrobial action because it inhibits growth of disease-causing protozoa, yeasts, bacteria, and viruses. It can actually kill organisms and prevents attachment of microbes to cells that line the mouth and entire gastrointestinal tract. Lactoferrin boosts health-promoting bacteria—*Bifidobacterium* and *Lactobacillus* species. Lactoferrin assists in development of proper intestinal flora.
- Standard medical treatment of *H. pylori* is a 1- or 2-week course of triple therapy—two antibiotics to kill bacteria and acid suppressor drug.
- Lactoferrin alone or in combination with triple therapy may become treatment of choice. Effective dose of lactoferrin in this application: 300 mg/day.

Pancreatic Insufficiency

- Most severe exocrine pancreatic insufficiency (EPI) is seen in cystic fibrosis. Next in severity is EPI of late stages of pancreatitis. These severe causes of EPI are most often easily recognized; but causes of mild EPI are more insidious and difficult to diagnose.
- Patients with diabetes also have decreased pancreatic exocrine function, especially those with type 1 diabetes.
- Both physical symptoms and laboratory tests can help assess pancreatic function when mild EPI is suspected.
- Common symptoms of EPI: abdominal bloating and discomfort, gas, indigestion, and passing undigested food in stool.

- Laboratory diagnosis: comprehensive stool and digestive analysis (*Textbook*, "Biomarkers for Stool Analysis"); measurement of fecal elastase-1 concentrations using an enzyme-linked immunosorbent assay is indirect test of exocrine pancreatic function. It shows higher sensitivity and specificity for EPI than fecal chymotrypsin determination and is comparable to oral pancreatic function tests—pancreolauryl test.

Pancreatic Enzyme Supplements

- Effective treatment for EPI; widely used.
- Commercial preparations are prepared from fresh hog pancreas (i.e., pancreatin) (*Textbook*, "Pancreatic Enzymes").
- Dose of pancreatic enzymes is based on level of enzyme activity as defined by United States Pharmacopoeia (USP).
- A 1× pancreatic enzyme (pancreatin) product has in each milligram no less than 25 USP units of amylase activity, no less than 2.0 USP units of lipase activity, and no less than 25 USP units of protease activity.
- Pancreatin of higher potency is given a whole-number multiple indicating its strength. Example: full-strength undiluted pancreatic extract that is 10 times stronger than USP standard is termed 10× USP.
- Full-strength products are preferred; lower-potency products are diluted with salt, lactose, or galactose to achieve desired strength (e.g., 4× or 1×).
- Dose for 10× USP pancreatic enzyme product: 350 to 1000 mg t.i.d. immediately before meals when used as digestive aid and 10 to 20 minutes before meals or on empty stomach when anti-inflammatory effects are desired.
- Enzyme products are often enteric coated to protect fragile porcine lipase. Non–enteric-coated enzymes actually outperform enteric-coated products if given before a meal (for digestive purposes) or on empty stomach (for anti-inflammatory effects).
- Alternatives to porcine pancreatin: plant enzymes (e.g., bromelain, papain) and enzymes extracted from microbes or yeast (e.g., *Aspergillus oryzae*). These enzymes are more resistant to digestive secretions and have a broader range of activity, including pH range (*Textbook*, "Bromelain" and "Microbial Enzyme Preparations"). In clinical trials, fungal enzyme preparations produced similar benefits at three fourths the dose of enteric-coated pancreatic enzyme and one fifth the dose of non–enteric-coated pancreatic enzyme preparations.

Menopause

DIAGNOSTIC SUMMARY

- Last spontaneous menstrual period 12 months prior.
- Average age of onset is 51 years.
- Symptoms can, but do not necessarily, include hot flashes, night sweats, palpitations, headache, insomnia, mood swings, anxiety, vaginal dryness, urinary incontinence, rheumatism, fatigue, hair thinning, skin dryness, acne, facial hair, low libido, bladder infections, vaginal infections, nausea, and mild cognitive changes (irregular bleeding with perimenopause).
- Physical examination: vaginal thinning, hair thinning and facial hair, height, weight, abdominal fat, general physical examination.
- Laboratory analysis: increase in follicle-stimulating hormone (FSH).
- Laboratory analysis and imaging may be used to assess risks for osteoporosis and cardiovascular disease.

Baseline Evaluation of Menopausal Woman

- Detailed personal medical history, chief complaint, review of systems, medical history, past and present medications, family history, dietary history, exercise history, social history, occupational hazards.
- General physical examination.
- Breast examination.
- Pelvic examination.
- Laboratory tests: consider complete blood count, blood chemistry, lipid panel with subfractions, thyroid function panel, FSH, homocysteine, C-reactive protein, estrogen metabolites.
- Screening mammography.
- Bone density testing.
- Cervical cytology (Pap smear or liquid-based technologies).
- Electrocardiogram.
- Colonoscopy.

Indications and frequency for these and other tests are based on history, disease risks, current health problems, and family history.

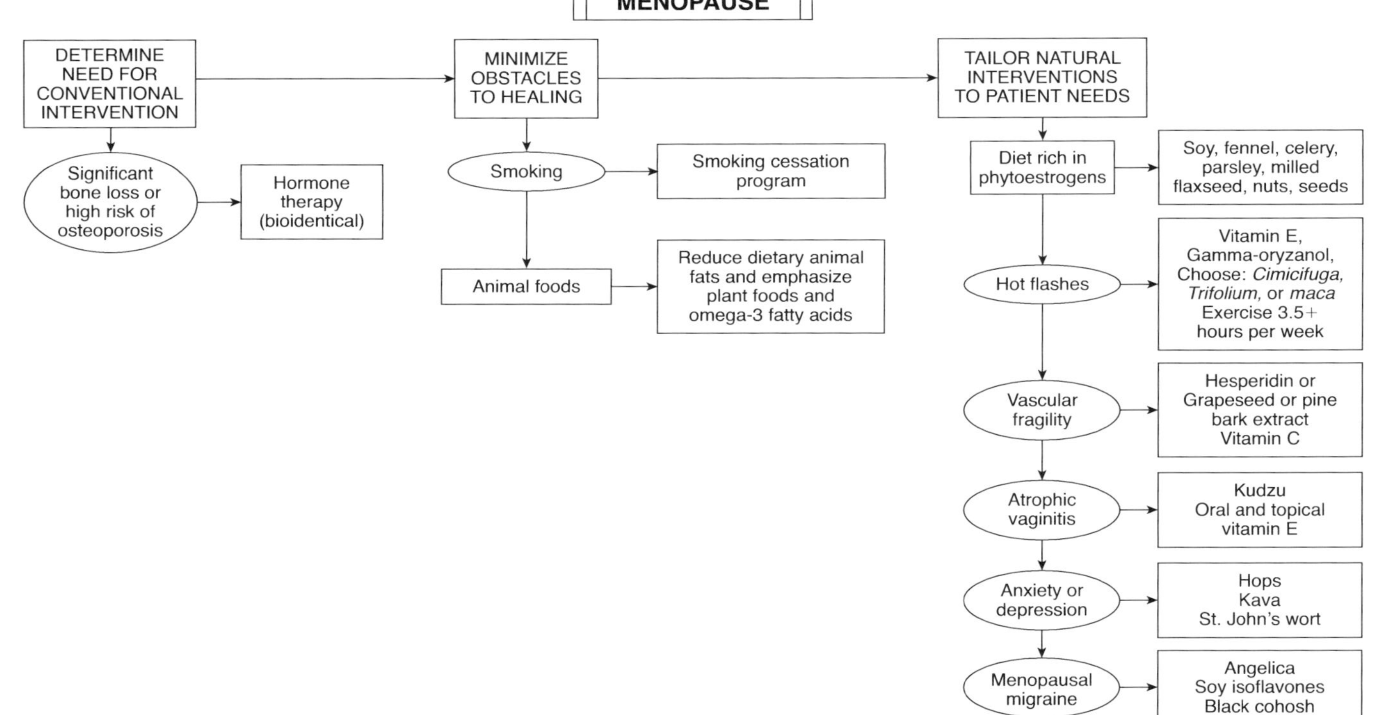

MENOPAUSE
DETERMINE NEED FOR CONVENTIONAL INTERVENTION
Significant bone loss or high risk of osteoporosis
Hormone therapy (bioidentical)
MINIMIZE OBSTACLES TO HEALING
Smoking
Smoking cessation program
Animal foods
Reduce dietary animal fats and emphasize plant foods and omega-3 fatty acids
TAILOR NATURAL INTERVENTIONS TO PATIENT NEEDS
Diet rich in phytoestrogens
Soy, fennel, celery, parsley, milled flaxseed, nuts, seeds
Hot flashes
Vitamin E, Gamma-oryzanol, Choose: Cimicifuga, Trifolium, or maca Exercise 3.5+ hours per week
Vascular fragility
Hesperidin or Grapeseed or pine bark extract Vitamin C
Atrophic vaginitis
Kudzu Oral and topical vitamin E
Anxiety or depression
Hops Kava St. John's wort
Menopausal migraine
Angelica Soy isoflavones Black cohosh

GENERAL CONSIDERATIONS

Goals of integrative approach to menopause: (1) provide relief from symptoms; (2) prevent and/or treat osteoporosis, cardiovascular disease, and other diseases of aging and minimize risks of breast cancer, coronary heart disease (CHD), venous thromboembolism (VTE), strokes, and gallbladder disease.

Cessation of menstruation usually occurs at approximately 51 years. Perimenopause is the period before menopause. Postmenopause is the period after menopause. During the perimenopausal period, many women ovulate irregularly, indicating changes in menstrual cycle, with or without other symptoms.

- **Causes of menopause:** thought to occur when no eggs are left in the ovaries. At birth a female has approximately 1 million eggs (ova), a number that drops to 300,000 to 400,000 at puberty. Only 400 actually mature during the reproductive years. The absence of active follicles reduces estrogen and progesterone, causing the pituitary to increase production of FSH in large and continuous quantities. Luteinizing hormone (LH) and FSH cause ovaries and adrenals to secrete androgens, which can be converted to estrogens by fat cells of the hips and thighs. Converted androgens are the source of most circulating estrogen in postmenopausal women. Total estrogen is still far below reproductive levels.
- **Menopause as social construct:** social and cultural factors contribute greatly to how women react to menopause. Modern society values allure of everlasting youth, culturally devaluing of older women. The cultural view of menopause is directly related to symptoms of menopause. If the cultural view is negative, symptoms are common; if menopause is viewed in a positive light, symptoms are less frequent. In a study of rural Mayan Indians, no women had hot flashes or any other symptoms, and no women showed evidence of osteoporosis despite hormonal patterns identical to postmenopausal women in the United States. Mayan women saw menopause as a positive event, providing acceptance as a respected elder as well as relief from childbearing.
- **Options for managing menopause:** diet, exercise, stress management, nutrition, botanicals, natural hormones, conventional hormones, additional pharmaceuticals.

Estrogen Replacement Therapy

The key question: "Is hormone replacement therapy necessary?" Estrogen replacement therapy (ERT) without appropriate progestogen increases the risk of endometrial cancer. Hormone replacement therapy (HRT) combines estrogen with a progestogen (either progestin or oral micronized progesterone [OMP]) to reduce the risk of endometrial cancer such that it is lower than a natural perimenopause transition without HRT. Current conventional medical treatment involves short-term HRT (1 to 5 years) for menopausal symptoms. North American Menopause Society (NAMS) comprehensive position statement: although there are many benefits (vasomotor symptoms, urogenital atrophy, urinary health, osteoporosis, reduced type 2 diabetes), there are also slight statistical risks (breast cancer, stroke, VTE, ovarian cancer). A still-unfolding picture focuses on cardiovascular disease, cognitive decline, and dementia. Women and their physicians must make the best decisions based on what we know, what we do not know, and what is uncertain.

Benefits and Risks of Conventional Hormone Replacement Therapy and Natural Hormone Replacement Therapy

- **Reasons to discontinue conventional HRT (cHRT):** uterine bleeding, mood changes, breast tenderness, bloating and weight gain, fear of breast cancer, misunderstanding or disbelief in need for long-term use, lack of patient education.
- **Benefits of continuing cHRT:** symptomatic relief from hot flashes, night sweats, vaginal dryness, insomnia, mood swings, depression, incontinence, infections. ERT controls vasomotor symptoms and genitourinary symptoms. Vaginal estrogen is as efficacious as oral or transdermal estrogen for genitourinary symptoms and is advantageous because of local delivery and effect. Sex steroids affect sleep, libido, cognitive function, motor coordination, and pain sensitivity. In perimenopause or early menopause, depression and mood disorders are more common than in reproductive years. HRT benefits many women.
- **Osteoporosis:** inhibits age-related bone loss, reduces risk of vertebral and hip fracture, decreases bone resorption, prevents osteoporosis, and reduces fractures. However, ERT is no longer approved by the Food and Drug Administration (FDA) for treating osteoporosis in deference to drugs such as bisphosphonates (risedronate and alendronate). Continuous combined estrogen-progestogen therapy reduced relative risk for hip, vertebral, other osteoporotic, and total fractures. Estrogen agents approved for prevention of osteoporosis are as follows:
  — Oral micronized estradiol: 1.0 mg
  — Conjugated equine estrogens (CEE): 0.625 mg
  — Ethinyl estradiol: 5 mcg

— Transdermal estradiol: 50 mcg
— Esterified estrogen: 0.3 mg

Dual-energy x-ray absorptiometry (DXA) scans provide the most reliable objective information on the status of bone mineral density and efficacy of dosing.

Risks

- **Colorectal cancer:** ERT reduces risk of colorectal cancer and risk of dying from colon cancer.
- **Endometrial cancer:** unopposed ERT is linked to increased risk of endometrial cancer by a factor of 8 to 10 over more than 10 years. Risk decreases after discontinuation of ERT but remains elevated after more than 10 years. Proven dose and delivery of progestogen (progestins or progesterone), opposing estrogen, minimizes risk and helps prevent endometrial hyperplasia and cancer. OMP and cyclic OMP (200 mg q.d. for 12 days per month) protect endometrium. OMP is equally appropriate as medroxyprogesterone acetate (MPA) to protect endometrium. Compounded OMP and Prometrium are indicated products.
- **VTE:** deep vein thromboembolism is expected complication of HRT. For women at risk for thromboembolism or those who are older, absolute risks of HRT are higher.

Coronary Heart Disease.

ERT reduces plasma low-density–lipoprotein cholesterol (LDL-C) and increases plasma high-density–lipoprotein cholesterol (HDL-C). ERT reduces lipoprotein A, inhibits oxidation of low-density lipoprotein (LDL), improves endothelial vascular function, reduces fibrinogen, and reduces thickening in arterial walls. However, ERT may increase triglycerides, clotting, and C-reactive protein, thereby overriding the beneficial effects. HRT does not reduce overall rate of CHD, but actually increases it.

Consider cardioprotective effects of nutrition, exercise, stress management, and selected nutrients (vitamin B_3, red yeast rice, magnesium, fish oils, pantethine, vitamin C, vitamin E, folic acid, vitamin B_{12}, vitamin B_6, garlic, soy, hawthorne, gugulipid, and policosanols).

Problem with HRT and CAD: HRT (CEE [Premarin] and MPA [Provera]) for women with established CHD is linked to similar rates of myocardial infarction (MI) death and nonfatal MI as placebo, with 50% increase in risk of CHD events (thromboembolism) and early risk of blood clots in legs and lungs, MIs, and stroke.

A subgroup of women could be predisposed to hyperinsulinemia, hypertension, hyperhomocysteinemia, increased C-reactive protein and lipoprotein A, obesity, and elevated LDL-C. Rate of CHD and thromboembolic events after 1 year is much lower in users of HRT plus statins than in those who did not use statins.

Neither estrogen alone nor estrogen plus progestin affects progression of coronary atherosclerosis. In women with coronary artery disease (CAD), MPA does not cancel out beneficial effects of ERT. HRT does not affect the progression of atherosclerosis in women with established heart disease. HRT (transdermal natural estradiol alone or with progestin norethindrone) may slightly increase rates of cardiovascular events during the first 2 years.

Unopposed natural (human) estradiol halts or mildly regresses thickening of arteries. Concurrent lipid-lowering drugs made no difference in rate of progression with either estrogen or placebo.

HRT does not appear to reduce risk of cardiovascular events in postmenopausal women who already have CAD.

Most common HRT in the United States (0.625 mg Premarin plus 2.5 mg Provera [Prempro]) increases the risk of CHD combined with increased risk of breast cancer. Estrogen plus progestin does not confer a benefit for preventing CHD among women with a uterus.

Stroke.

No excess risk of stroke occurred with an estrogen plus progestin group in the first year, but the risk does rise in the second year and persists. The mechanism is not related to increased blood pressure. Estrogen plus progestin increases risk of strokes in women determined to be healthy. Do different kinds of estrogens have different effects? CEE, but not esterified estrogens, are associated with venous thrombotic risk.

Gallstones.

The risk of gallstones or cholecystectomy is increased in postmenopausal women taking ERT.

Areas of Uncertainty

- **Breast cancer:** no data clearly and consistently demonstrate an increased risk of breast cancer associated with HRT. An analysis showed that 90% of postmenopausal women who had ever used HRT had a small but statistically significant increase in risk compared with those who had never used HRT. Among current users or recent users, relative risk increased by factor of 1.02 to 1.04 for each year of use. After not using HRT for 5 years, no significant excess risk remains. Breast cancers diagnosed in HRT users tend to be less advanced and more localized. No studies found an increased risk of breast cancer with short-term use of HRT. If long-term use increases risk, it is a small increase.

- **Cognitive function:** HRT may prevent or delay Alzheimer's disease (AD). In women symptomatic from menopause, ERT improves verbal memory, vigilance, reasoning, and motor speed, but no consistent effects were seen on visual recall, working memory, complex attention, mental tracking, mental status, or verbal functions. ERT does not enhance asymptomatic women's performance. HRT may decrease the risk of dementia. Efficacy of preparations or doses, progestin use, and duration of treatment have not been assessed because of insufficient data. Prior use of HRT reduces risk of AD, but duration of use specifically affects benefit. No apparent benefit is found with currently using HRT unless use exceeds 10 years.
- **Ovarian cancer:** a weak possible positive association exists between HRT and ovarian cancer risk. Women currently using HRT may have higher death rates from ovarian cancer than those who have never used HRT. Given the low incidence of ovarian cancer, even if relative risk increases significantly, it may not affect absolute risk. Ovarian cancer mortality rate in postmenopausal women is extremely low, and more than 7 years of oral contraceptive use during the reproductive age lowers the incidence of ovarian cancer. A twofold increased risk exists among long-term users of HRT and ERT. Users of ERT for longer than 10 years have a much increased risk of ovarian cancer, with a relative risk of 1.8. Users of ERT for longer than 20 years have a relative risk of 3.2. Users of short-term combination HRT are not at increased risk.

Key Clinically Relevant Issues from Women's Health Initiative Estrogen Replacement Study

- CHD is reduced by half youngest age group (most common age group to initiate ERT).
- Stroke risk increases only slightly for youngest women.
- Risk of VTE increases in all age groups, but degree of risk increases with age of initiation of ERT.
- Risk of invasive breast cancer declines in all age groups.

- Risk of colorectal cancer decreases in younger patients, especially age 50 to 59; it increases at age 70 and older.
- Overall reduction in fracture risk is most evident in younger women.
- ERT is associated with lower death rate in those youngest at initiation of therapy.

ERT with CEE is safe for most menopausal women without a uterus. ERT reduces risk of CHD in women who start ERT near the age of menopause. It decreases risk of fractures; it did not increase risk of breast cancer. Risk of colorectal cancer increases in women who start therapy at age 70 or older. ERT is associated with a slight increase in risk of stroke and VTE, but there is no increase in death rates. ERT alone for women without a uterus appears safer than use of estrogen plus a progestin.

Natural Hormones

The natural compounded estrogens are estriol, estrone, and estradiol. Estriol is unique; it has one quarter the potency of estradiol and estrone. Natural compounded estrogens are used in lower doses because of the combined effect of weaker estriol plus estradiol and/or estrone. Natural estrogens may be metabolized differently by the body, have a shorter half-life, are customizable for dosage and potency, and can be adjusted to be stronger or weaker in small units to taper someone off or onto hormones. Bioidentical and nonbioidentical hormones may have different metabolic consequences: cytotoxicity to estrogen-sensitive tissues, alteration of binding of other hormones to receptors, or the alteration of liver metabolism of carcinogens.

Natural progesterone has fewer adverse effects on the cardiovascular system than synthetic progestins (e.g., MPA). It lowers HDL less than MPA, is less atherogenic, and does not cause coronary artery spasm as MPA does.

Natural estradiol is used in a half-strength dose (0.5 mg total q.d.) because it is combined with weaker estriol. Estriol acts as an antiestrogen in the breast, with little impact on the cardiovascular system.

Holistic approach includes hormones plus other strategies to reduce risk of breast cancer and heart disease: soy, flaxseed, cabbage family foods, and supplements to promote metabolism of estrogens to anticarcinogenic metabolites. Use breast cancer and heart disease prevention diets with nutrients and botanicals: vitamins E and C, carotenes, soy, coenzyme Q10, green tea, garlic.

Women using CEE and MPA should consider natural regimens or nonharmonic approaches. Women using natural estrogens and progesterone should reevaluate their regimen to find the lowest dose to achieve benefits and minimize risks. Reconsider yearly continuation of use on an individual basis. Women without a uterus need only estrogen.

Black cohosh, red clover, soy, bioflavonoids, kava, and the proprietary formula Women's Phase II have proven scientific efficacy for menopausal symptoms. Many women need only nonhormonal supplements for symptom relief and never need HRT. Others may be able to lower the dose of cHRT or natural hormones by using them in combination with herbal and nutritional supplements.

Major Symptoms of Perimenopause and Menopause

- Irregular bleeding (perimenopause)
- Hot flashes (or night sweats)
- Vulvovaginal thinning, dryness, dyspareunia, burning (known as atrophic changes)
- Bladder frequency, urgency, leakage
- Mood changes
- Cognitive changes
- Body aches
- Sleep disturbances
- Others: fatigue, sexual dysfunction, hair thinning, facial hair, headache, dry skin, voice impairment, joint pains, bladder infections, urinary incontinence

THERAPEUTIC CONSIDERATIONS

Treatment Overview

Goal of holistic integrative approach: to recognize that there are many options for symptom management, disease prevention, and disease treatment.

Levels of intervention are as follows:

1. Diet, exercise, stress management
2. Nutritional supplementation
3. Botanical medicines
4. Compounded bioidentical hormone therapy (cbHT)
5. Bioidentical hormone therapy (bHT) (FDA-approved prescription items)
6. Nonbioidentical hormone therapy (HT) (FDA-approved prescription items)

7. Condition-specific nonestrogen pharmaceuticals (for symptom relief or disease prevention and/or treatment)

Diet, exercise, lifestyle, and/or nutritional supplements and botanical therapies will be effective for managing menopausal symptoms in the majority of women. When these are not adequate, apply HT or other medicine.

Nutrition

- Diet rich in whole "natural" and unprocessed foods; emphasis on vegetables, whole grains, beans, seeds, nuts, fruits, lean low-fat proteins, and healthful fats. Minimize saturated fats and fried foods, simple carbohydrates, alcohol, sugar, and salt.
- **Soy foods:** moderate hot flashes, slow bone loss, improve lipid profile and blood pressure, and lower risk for CAD. Results of studies of isoflavones (from soy and red clover *[Trifolium pratense]*) are somewhat positive but inconsistent. NAMS reports many diverse effects of soy. Isoflavones appear to relieve menopausal symptoms. Supplements with higher genistein or increased *S*-equol may be more beneficial. Soy food consumption is linked to lower risk of breast and endometrial cancer. Efficacy of soy on bone health has yet to be adequately proved. Cardiovascular benefits are evolving. Soy may lessen arterial stiffness, yet evidence is mixed on lipid effects in postmenopausal women. Younger postmenopausal women derive more cognitive benefit, within the first few years of menopause, compared with older women. Another study has shed some light on why the research on soy isoflavones and vasomotor symptoms is so contradictory. Studies involving a higher percentage of women who are equol producers might have been the determining factor in the effectiveness of soy isoflavones. A woman's ability to produce equol determines her response to soy isoflavones. Daidzein and genistein are the key phytoestrogens in soy. Daidzein is converted to equol, a metabolite of daidzein, by colon bacterial flora. For clinicians, consider testing for equol production before treatment and/or improve colon microflora to enhance transformation of soy isoflavones to equol. In traditional Asian diets, the average adult daily intake of soy isoflavones is 50 to 150 mg. The isoflavone content of soy foods varies with the form.
- **Flaxseed (Linum usitatissimum):** another dietary source of phytoestrogens. Flaxseed lignans matairesinol and secoisolariciresinol have estrogenic activity. Lignans are converted by colon

bacteria into estrogenic mammalian lignans and absorbed in the circulation to exert both estrogenic and antiestrogenic effects. Women who consume 2 tbsp of flaxseed b.i.d. may cut in half the number of hot flashes within 6 weeks and reduce the intensity of hot flashes by 57%.
- **Disease prevention diet:** high in fruits, vegetables, whole grains, vegetarian proteins, nuts, seeds, legumes; low in saturated fats, *trans* fats, simple carbohydrates, fast foods.

Exercise

Benefits of exercise for perimenopausal and postmenopausal women are as follows:
- Relief from hot flashes
- Decreased bone loss
- Improved heart function
- Improved circulation
- Reduced blood pressure
- Decreased blood cholesterol levels
- Improved ability to deal with stress
- Improved oxygen and nutrient use in all tissues
- Increased self-esteem, mood, and frame of mind
- Increased endurance and energy level

Stress Management

- Depression, as defined by the *Diagnostic and Statistical Manual of Mental Disorders* (DSM-V), is no more common during menopause than at any other time of life.
- Perimenopausal transition is associated with depressive symptoms.
- Women experience mood changes but fail to meet DSM-V criteria for the diagnosis of depression.
- A woman's ability to manage stress can be enhanced with self-care tools (e.g., meditation, yoga, breathing exercises, being out in nature, and regular exercise).

Nutritional Supplements

Basic recommendations: multivitamin providing 70% to 100% of recommended daily allowances of vitamins and minerals. Supplements for specific symptoms: melatonin, L-tryptophan, and 5-hydroxytryptophan (5-HTP) for insomnia; vitamins B_6 and B_{12}, folic acid, and L-tyrosine for depression; gamma-aminobutyric acid (GABA) and L-theanine for anxiety.

- **Hesperidin, vitamin C, and procyanidolic oligomers (PCOs):** hesperidin improves vascular integrity and relieves capillary permeability. Combined with vitamin C, hesperidin and other citrus flavonoids may relieve hot flashes. Dose: 900 mg hesperidin, 300 mg hesperidin methyl chalcone (citrus flavonoid), and 1200 mg vitamin C q.d. Side effect: slightly offensive body odor and perspiration-discoloring clothing. In women aged 45 to 55 years given 100 mg of PCOs (as pycnogenol) b.i.d. for 6 months, HDL-C increases and LDL-C decreases significantly from baseline. Perimenopausal symptoms of depression, vasomotor symptoms, memory, anxiety, sexual function, and sleep all improve in both severity and frequency as soon as 1 month after starting treatment.
- **Gamma-oryzanol (ferulic acid):** growth-promoting substance in grains and isolated from rice bran oil. It enhances pituitary function and endorphin release by the hypothalamus. It is effective even in surgically induced menopause. It also lowers cholesterol and triglycerides. It is an extremely safe natural substance with no significant side effects. Dose: 300 mg q.d.
- **Fish oils:** In women aged 40 to 55 years, ethyl-eicosapentaenoic acid (E-EPA) plus omega-3 fatty acid given as a 500-mg capsule taken t.i.d. for 8 weeks, with each capsule containing 350 mg of eicosapentaenoic acid (EPA) and 50 mg of docosahexaenoic acid (DHA), reduced hot flash frequency (2.8 daily at baseline) by a mean of 1.58 daily. EPA induced a 55% reduction in frequency of hot flashes. Responders to fish oil have lower pretreatment DHA levels than nonresponders.
- **Vitamin E:** Studies done in the 1940s found vitamin E to be effective in relieving hot flashes and menopausal vaginal complaints. Unfortunately, there have been no further clinical trials. Vitamin E improved not only symptoms but also blood supply to the vaginal wall. Vitamin E (400 international units [IU] q.d) was effective in 50% of postmenopausal women with atrophic vaginitis. Vitamin E oil, creams, ointments, or suppositories used topically can provide symptomatic relief from atrophic vaginitis. Vitamin E may relieve dryness and irritation of atrophic vaginitis and other forms of vaginitis.

Botanical Medicines

Plants that tone the female glandular system are termed *uterine tonics.* Phytoestrogens improve blood flow to female organs and nourish and tone female glands and organ system. Plants for specific symptoms: valerian (sedative) for insomnia, and chaste tree (increases LH with indirect progesterone-like effect) for dysfunctional uterine bleeding. Herbal phytoestrogens have no side effects and inhibit mammary tumors.

Phytoestrogens in medicinal herbs, compared with estrogen, are at most only 2% as strong. Modulating effect: if estrogens are low, they increase estrogen effect; if estrogens are high, binding of phytoestrogens to receptors decreases estrogens' effects.

- **Black cohosh *(Cimicifuga racemosa):*** most studied herbal alternative to HRT for menopause. Collective findings and long-term clinical anecdotal evidence: *Cimicifuga* is most effective for daytime or nighttime hot flashes, mood swings, sleep disorders, and body aches. Complete disappearance of symptoms has occurred in 50% of study participants. Black cohosh combined with St. John's wort (264-mg tablet containing 0.364 mL of extract from black cohosh, equivalent to 1 mg terpene glycosides, and 84 mg of St. John's wort extract with 0.25 mg hypericin) has induced an average decrease in the Kupperman Index score of test subjects by 20 points. Vaginal dryness and low libido did not improve, but hot flash frequency improved. A combination of black cohosh, red clover, soy, chaste tree, valerian, and vitamin E lowered Kupperman Index scores after 6 months. It contained 72 mg of total isoflavones with 60 mg of soy isoflavones, 12 mg of red cover isoflavones, 40 mg of black cohosh extract, 30 mg of chaste tree extract, 250 mg of valerian extract, and 121 mg of vitamin E. Black cohosh does not appear to affect thrombotic biomarkers, as does oral estrogen therapy (OET), nor does it increase triglycerides, as seen with OET.
- **Hops *(Humulus lupulus):*** positively affect mood (e.g., anxiety and restlessness) for sleep disruptions. Dose of 120 mg to 300 mg of standardized hop extract (providing 100 mcg to 250 mcg of 8-prenylnaringenin) induces rapid decreases in menopausal symptoms. The higher dose is not any better than the lower one. Hops therapy leads to significant improvement in Kupperman Index and visual analog scale (VAS) scores.
- **Maca *(Lepidium peruvianum):*** unlike HT and phytoestrogenic botanicals, maca root can increase the body's production of estrogen and lower levels of cortisol and adrenocorticotropic hormone. Maca does not contain phytoestrogens. Maca's therapeutic actions may rely on plant sterols stimulating the hypothalamus, pituitary, adrenal, and ovarian glands, thereby also affecting the thyroid and pineal glands. Consequently, maca can

improve sleep, mood, fertility, energy, and hot flashes. Maca tends to treat menopausal symptoms as a whole rather than only one specific symptom. At a dose of 2 500-mg capsules of proprietary Maca-GO b.i.d. for a total of 2 g/day for 2 months, this maca product stimulated estradiol production and suppressed FSH, triiodothyronine (T_3), adrenocorticotropic hormone, and cortisol. It also mildly increased bone density and alleviated numerous menopausal symptoms—hot flashes, insomnia, depression, nervousness, and diminished concentration. After administration of 3.5 g of powdered maca *(Lepidium peruvianum)*, the Greene Climacteric Scale revealed a significant reduction in psychological symptoms—anxiety, depression, and sexual dysfunction. These findings were independent of androgenic or alpha-estrogenic activity present in the maca.

- **Siberian rhubarb *(Rheum rhaponticum)*:** a special extract, ERr 731, from roots of rhapontic rhubarb has been used in Germany specifically for menopausal symptoms. Medicinal species of rhubarb are not garden rhubarb used for food. Other rhubarb species—*Rheum officinale, Rheum palmatum, Rheum polygonatum* —are traditional laxatives because of anthraquinone glycosides (e.g., emodin and aloe-emodin). *R. rhaponticum* of clinical studies and extract ERr 731 do not contain emodin or aloe-emodin; thus they have no laxative effects. Standardized extract ERr 731 from roots of *R. rhaponticum* (Siberian rhubarb), given at 1 tablet (250 mg) containing 4 mg of dried extract, induced decreases in the Menopause Rating Scale II (MRS II). The overall menopause quality-of-life score also improved. *R. rhaponticum* dried extract also improved the Hamilton Anxiety Scale total score and anxiety score. The MRS revealed the most significant improvement in hot flashes, irritability, sleep problems, depressive mood, and physical and mental exhaustion.
- **St. John's wort (*Hypericum perforatum*):** research has focused on mild to moderate depression. St. John's wort was compared to a placebo in women with perimenopausal and menopausal hot flashes. St. John's wort, administered at 20 drops t.i.d. of an extract (Hypiran) containing hypericin 0.2 mg/mL, reduced frequency of hot flashes within 2 months, as measured by the Blagg-Kupperman Index. St. John's wort extract (900 mg t.i.d.), after 3 months, can reduce hot flash frequency and severity. At 900 mg of St. John's wort for 12 weeks, about three quarters of women may experience improvement in psychological and psychosomatic symptoms as well as a feeling of sexual well-being.

- **Chaste tree** ***(Vitex agnus-castus):*** no monoingredient studies on this plant have documented its effects on menopausal symptoms. *Vitex* helps when combined with black cohosh. In combination with St. John's wort, it has shown no significant difference from placebo.
- ***T. pratense*** **(red clover):** constituents include flavonoid glycosides, coumestans, volatile oils, L-dopa caffeic acid conjugates, polysaccharides, resins, fatty acids, hydrocarbons, alcohols, chlorophylls, minerals, and vitamins. A 40-mg standardized extract reduces hot flashes. Other effects: no endometrial thickening; increased HDL-C; no abnormalities in liver function test results, complete blood count, or estradiol; reduced coronary vascular disease by increasing arterial elasticity.
- **Kava** ***(Piper methysticum):*** associated with analgesic, sedative, anxiolytic, muscle relaxant, and anticonvulsant effects, but overlooked for menopause. However, anxiety, irritability, tension, nervousness, and sleep disruption are common perimenopausal and menopausal symptoms. Kava reduces anxiety and depression.
- ***Panax*** **ginseng (Korean or Chinese ginseng):** contains 13 triterpenoid saponins (ginsenosides); reduces mental and physical fatigue, enhances ability to cope with physical and mental stressors by supporting adrenal glands, treats atrophic vaginal changes from estrogen loss.
- **Kudzu** ***(Pueraria mirifica):*** studied for its effect on vaginal symptoms, vaginal health index, vaginal pH, and vaginal cytology in postmenopausal women. At 20, 30, or 50 mg of *P. mirifica* daily, kudzu improved vaginal symptoms and maintained vaginal health throughout treatment. Kudzu lessened frequency of dyspareunia. Changes in the Vaginal Health Index (scoring vaginal appearance with regard to moisture, fluid volume, elasticity, epithelial integrity, and pH on a scale of 1 [poorest] to 5 [best]) score were improved. Vaginal pH lowered from alkaline (pH of approximately 8) to acidic (pH of approximately 5). The maturation value and maturation index score also rose in value. In essence, kudzu improved the parabasal, intermediate, and superficial cells, as occurs when vaginal estrogen is used. No notable changes in endometrial thickness occurred.
- **Dong quai** ***(Angelica sinensis):*** menopausal symptoms are the most popular reason for use of *Angelica* species. Traditional use of *Angelica* has been in combination with other plants. A combination of *A. sinensis, Paeonia lactiflora, Ligusticum monnieri,*

Atractylodes chinensis, sclerotium poriae, and *Alisma orientale* was effective in 70% of women with menopausal symptoms. The combination of 100 mg *Angelica*, 60 mg soy isoflavones, and 50 mg black cohosh extract reduced menstrual migraines. On human bone, an aqueous extract of *A. sinensis* directly stimulated proliferation, alkaline phosphatase activity, protein secretion, and type I collagen synthesis in a dose-dependent manner. Thus *A. sinensis* may help prevent age-related bone loss.

- **Valerian:** for sleep quality in postmenopausal women experiencing insomnia. With use of the Pittsburgh Sleep Quality Index (PSQI), administration of 530 mg concentrated valerian extract b.i.d. improved sleep quality in 30% of women taking valerian, compared with 4% taking placebo.

Hormone Therapy

Use any HT—bioidentical or nonbioidentical—in lowest dose for shortest duration and in safest way possible. Each type of estrogen and progestogen, route of administration, timing of initiation, and duration of use have distinct benefits and adverse effects.

North American Menopause Society Recommended Terminology for Describing Hormone Therapy for Menopause

- EPT: combined estrogen-progestogen therapy (form of estrogen and progestogen is not specific)
- ET: estrogen therapy (form of estrogen is not specific)
- HT: hormone therapy (encompassing ET and EPT; the form of estrogen and progestogen is not specific)
- Local therapy: vaginal ET administration that does not result in clinically significant systemic absorption (form of estrogen is not specific)
- Progestogen: encompassing both progesterone and progestin
- Systemic therapy: HT administration with absorption in blood high enough to provide clinically significant effects
- Timing of HT initiation: length of time after menopause occurs when HT is initiated

Additional Terms (Not North American Menopause Society) Distinguishing Hormone Regimens

- cHT: conventional HT (FDA-approved prescription items)
- cET: conventional estrogen therapy (FDA-approved prescription items)

- bHT: bioidentical HT (FDA-approved prescription items)
- bET: bioidentical estrogen therapy (FDA-approved prescription items)
- cbHT: compounded bioidentical HT (from a compounding pharmacy)
- cbET: compounded bioidentical estrogen therapy (from a compounding pharmacy)

Bioidentical or Natural Hormones

- Bioidentical estrogens require prescription and are available at regular pharmacies or as nonpatented forms prepared by compounding pharmacies. Advantages of conventional pharmaceuticals: years of study and standardization. Insurance pays for pharmaceuticals, but not always for compounded hormones. Pharmaceuticals are limited in dosage forms and combinations; they contain harmful additives.
- Advantages of compounded hormones: greater array of doses, hormone combinations, and delivery options. Forms of compounded hormones: capsules, sublingual lozenges or pellets, creams, gels, vaginal creams or gels or tablets, nasal sprays, injections, and subcutaneous implanted pellets. Any combination can be formulated.

Bioidentical Estrogens

- Bioidenticals have superior safety profile over nonbioidenticals; it cannot be stated with science-based facts that an equivalent dose of bioidentical estradiol is innately safer or better than the synthetic. There are however, better safety profiles with bioidentical progesterone versus progestins. cbHT provides endless customization for flexible dosage and delivery. The combination of estriol with estradiol and bioidentical progesterone and testosterone with estrogens provides potential maximum benefit and individualized approach.
- Estriol: symptoms of menopause (e.g., hot flashes); better safety profile than estradiol and estrone. Estriol is one fourth as potent as estradiol. Forms: capsules, tablets, vaginal cream and suppositories.
- Vaginal estriol: vaginal dryness (dominance of estriol receptors in vagina and vulva); restores normal vaginal cytology and decreases incidence of bladder infections; restores vaginal flora; improves vaginal and bladder health; increases lubrication, elasticity, and thickness of vaginal epithelium. Dose: 1 mg estriol per

gram of cream inserted vaginally daily for 2 weeks and then twice a week for maintenance.

- Combinations: compounded bioidentical estriol with small doses of estradiol and estrone. Typical formula: 80% estriol, 10% estradiol, 10% estrone. Add progesterone at a minimum of 100 mg/day to protect the uterus from estrogenic thickening of endometrium. Estrogen only, without adequate progesterone, in women with uterus might increase risk for endometrial hyperplasia or cancer.
- Biestrogen formula: estriol plus estradiol; popular because estrone might be more linked to carcinogenic estrogen metabolites and breast cancer.

Progesterone

- Prescription forms: oral capsules, sublingual drops, sublingual pellets, lozenges, transvaginal or rectal suppositories, injection.
- Over the counter: cream.
- Progesterone is added to compounded biestrogen and triestrogen formulas at minimum of 100 mg/day to prevent endometrial hyperplasia and uterine cancer in women with a uterus.
- Progesterone is a natural hormone. The term *progestin* applies to synthetic derivatives. Progestins in cHT and birth control pills often account for the side effects (e.g., irritability, depression, bloating, mood swings). Progestins can cause water retention, can affect brain chemistry, and alter other steroid pathways. The term *progestogen* applies to any substance possessing progesterone properties—progesterone or progestin.
- Advantages of bioidentical progesterone over progestins; better validated advantages of estrogens; minimizes side effects of progestogens; more-favorable effect on lipid profiles and cardiovascular function.
- In some women, insomnia, fatigue, anxiety, and mood swings may be more responsive to progesterone than estrogen.

Progesterone Cream

- Bioidentical progesterone by itself can help perimenopause issues—regulation of menstrual cycle, hot flashes, night sweats, mood swings, sleep disruption, and premenstrual symptoms.
- Transdermal progesterone cream can improve hot flashes in a significant percentage of patients. Finding the right dose for each patient is a key to success.

Testosterone

- The majority of women treated with estrogen replacement have resolution of their menopausal symptoms. For those who do not, especially with loss of libido, try estrogen with testosterone, which helps restore sexual desire.
- Administration of 1.25 mg of esterified estrogen and 2.5 mg of methyltestosterone daily for 2 years after surgical menopause reduced intensity of hot flashes and vaginal dryness. Postmenopausal women with hypoactive sexual desire given 300-g testosterone patches, without estrogen or progesterone, experienced increased frequency of satisfying sexual episodes. Formulations of CEE and methyltestosterone combined either 0.625 or 1.25 mg of CEE with 5 mg of methyltestosterone. Others are available as either 1.25 or 0.625 esterified estrogens combined with 2.5 or 1.25 mg of methyltestosterone, respectively.
- Bioidentical testosterone is prepared by compounding pharmacists; 4 to 6 mg of bioidentical testosterone is formulated alone or with biestrogen or triestrogen. Testosterone cream applied to genital region is an alternative delivery method. Common prescriptions: 1 to 10 mg/g of cream. Apply to external genitalia just before sexual activity to enhance sensitivity to touch and orgasm.
- Frequency: no more than twice weekly to avert local testosterone side effects (e.g., clitoral enlargement). Rule out other causes of low libido. Conduct laboratory testing of testosterone levels to monitor before and during therapy.
- Testosterone therapy is contraindicated in women with breast or uterine cancer or cardiovascular or liver disease. Give testosterone at lowest dose for shortest duration that meets treatment objectives.

Dehydroepiandrosterone (DHEA)

- Dehydroepiandrosterone (DHEA) is a bioidentical androgenic hormone that is the most abundant circulating steroid in humans. It is a "precursor hormone" used to make other steroids.
- Many claims are made about DHEA's effects, but exact effect DHEA has on body cells is unclear. DAWN trial: DHEA given at 50 mg/day did not improve well-being or cognitive performance in healthy older adults.
- At 10 mg/day, DHEA alone or with HT in postmenopausal women can restore androgenic milieu and positively affect estrogenic tone. DHEA may have an insulin-sensitizing effect,

reducing abdominal visceral fat, lowering elevated insulin level, and increasing insulin sensitivity.

- DHEA also helps vaginal atrophy and/or sexual dysfunction. Oral DHEA induces beneficial change in vaginal epithelial cells, pH, and bothersome symptoms in 2 weeks, with no effect on endometrial histology and minimal effects on serum estrogens and androgens and their metabolites.
- Intravaginal DHEA was studied for effects on sexual dysfunction parameters of libido, arousal, orgasm, and dyspareunia in postmenopausal women who had vaginal atrophy. At 12 weeks, the 13-mg ovule had improved abbreviated sexual function arousal or sensation, arousal or lubrication in orgasm, dryness during intercourse, and menopause-specific quality of life.

Nonbioidentical Hormones

- Examples: manufactured pharmaceutical estrogens that are not identical in chemical structure to endogenous hormones. CEE derived from urine of pregnant mares. Esterified estrogens are part estrone sulfate and part equilin sulfates. Progestins are synthetic.
- Oral capsules containing 1 mg of bioidentical hormones are equivalent to 0.625 mg of CEE. Estrogen patches that contain 0.05 mg of bioidentical estradiol are considered equivalent to 0.625 mg CEE (Premarin) or 0.625 mg of esterified estrogens and equivalent to 1 mg of oral bioidentical estradiol. Products are available through NAMS.
- Recommended dose ratios for triestrogen and biestrogen with progesterone:
  - — A triestrogen is considered comparable with 0.625 mg Premarin/2.5 mg Provera = estriol 1 mg/estradiol 0.125 mg/estrone 0.125 mg/Prog 50 mg 1 cap b.i.d.
  - — Or estriol 2 mg/estradiol 0.25 mg/estrone 0.25 mg/Prog 100 mg 1 cap/day
- A biestrogen is considered comparable with the following:
  - — 0.625 mg Premarin/2.5 mg Provera = estriol 1 mg/estradiol 0.250 mg/Prog 50 mg 1 cap twice a day; or estriol 2 mg/estradiol 0.50 mg/Prog 100 mg 1 cap/day
  - — Vaginal estriol: estriol cream 1 mg/g insert 1 g nightly for 2 weeks then a maintenance dose of twice a week

Additional Medications

For hot flashes: clonidine 0.1 to 0.2 mg q.d. at bedtime; neuroleptic Gabapentin 300 mg t.i.d.; venlafaxine and paroxetine 37.5 to 75 mg and 10 to 20 mg q.d., respectively. However, selective serotonin reuptake inhibitors and selective norepinephrine reuptake inhibitors can cause vasomotor symptoms. Bellergal, an old ergot and belladonna combination, is now available only from compounding pharmacies. There are no studies, and empiric reports show mixed results.

Perimenopause-Menopause Evaluation

- Comprehensive medical history and complete physical examination.
- Assess risk factors for stroke; CHD; VTE; osteoporosis; diabetes; and breast, ovarian, and uterine cancer.
- DXA testing, lipid profiles, fasting glucose, and mammography according to national guidelines, age, and medical judgment.
- Other tests depend on age, symptoms, and other medical problems. There is no one test for menopause.
- Ovarian function tests are not routinely done; diagnosis is made based on medical history. Hormone testing can differentiate menopause from thyroid problems, abnormal causes of cessation of menses (elevated prolactin or premature ovarian failure [premature menopause]).
- FSH testing is not accurate in perimenopause. FSH can fluctuate during perimenopause. In woman having irregular or random menses, FSH fluctuates unpredictably. FSH tests are frequently normal in perimenopause. Two scenarios to consider for ordering FSH testing: (1) Woman's clinical presentation is perimenopausal or menopausal, and she is using contraception: FSH can determine if she still needs contraception. If FSH is above 30 mIU/mL and when test is repeated 1 month later FSH is also above 30 mIU/mL, diagnosis of menopause is justified. Continue contraception during that 1-month period until this is determined. (2) Woman reporting irregular menses, irritability, fatigue, insomnia; FSH and thyroid-stimulating hormone (TSH) tests help sort out her problems.
- Can saliva, serum, or urinary hormone testing determine hormone management? There is little value in these tests in a perimenopausal woman for diagnosing hormone levels. A momentary snapshot of variable hormone levels is not diagnostic of perimenopause. There is no scientific evidence to support claims of increased efficacy, enhanced safety, or need for testing to determine dose of hormonal prescriptions. Numerous problems affect

saliva testing for estrogen and progesterone. Salivary testing of cortisol and DHEA is promising; these do not fluctuate so much and have higher levels in saliva.

- Serum testing of estrogen, progesterone, and testosterone is more accurate with standardized procedures. However, even these are unnecessary in perimenopausal and menopausal women. Even if accurate, neither salivary nor serum hormone testing is necessary or helpful for perimenopausal women because it is difficult to draw conclusions from tests on fluctuating hormones. For women taking HT, there is no mathematical equation connecting hormone levels in the blood or saliva to dose of corresponding hormones. It is not known exactly what dose to give to keep a patient within a reference range. Women absorb and metabolize hormones differently. The form and delivery method also differ.
- Urinary testing of estrogen metabolites can be considered in evaluating risk of health problems linked to certain estrogen metabolites. Such data are limited, yet the use of estrogen metabolism testing to assess risk of or to prevent recurrence of cervical and breast cancer is warranted. The primary value of these tests is that they give valuable feedback in the use of nutrients, botanicals, and lifestyle to facilitate optimal metabolism of hormones.
- It is rarely necessary to test estrogen levels of a postmenopausal woman on HT for prescription management; but testing may help to assess absorption or delivery and dosage issues involving lack of response or adverse response. For difficult cases, consider testing of neurotransmitters, amino acids, and nutrients while ensuring diligent history taking, physical examination, and conventional testing.

Lifestyle Factors

- **Exercise:** hypothesis is that impaired endorphin activity in hypothalamus may provoke hot flashes. Regular physical exercise decreases frequency and severity of hot flashes. Exercise may obviate need for HRT. Women with no hot flashes spent 3.5 hr/wk exercising. Exercise also elevates mood. Benefits are derived for women both on and off HRT.
- **Cigarette smoking:** increases risk of early menopause and doubles the risk of menopause between ages of 44 and 55 years. Former smokers have lower risk, indicating a partial reversal of effect.

THERAPEUTIC APPROACH

Menopause is normal and natural, but premature, surgical, or medication-induced menopause is not normal and must be managed with tailored therapy.

Natural measures can help alleviate most common symptoms. In most cases, HRT either is not necessary or is needed for only 1 to 4 years. HRT may be indicated in women at high risk for osteoporosis who already had significant bone loss and menopausal symptoms or who do not tolerate osteoporosis medicines. For women with intolerable menopausal symptoms, try natural HRT (nHRT) with periodic attempts at reducing or discontinuing hormones.

Diet

- Whole-foods diet that addresses prevention or management of cardiovascular disease, diabetes, and osteoporosis. Increase soy foods, legumes, milled flaxseeds, fennel, celery, parsley.

Supplements

- **Vitamin E (mixed tocopherols):** 800 IU q.d. until symptoms have improved, then 400 IU q.d. thereafter
- **Hesperidin:** 900 mg q.d. or PCOs from grapeseed or pine bark: 200 mg q.d.
- **Vitamin C:** 1200 mg q.d.
- **Gamma-oryzanol:** 300 mg q.d.

Botanical Medicines

- Choose one or more of the following for general symptom relief:
  - *C. racemosa* **(black cohosh):** standardized extract based on content of 27-deoxyactein, 40 mg to 80 mg q.d.
  - **Gelatinized maca extract:** 1000 mg b.i.d. or dose equivalent to 3500 mg dried powdered maca root a day
  - *T. pratense* **(red clover) isoflavones extract:** 40 to 80 mg q.d.
- Choose one of the following if symptoms of anxiety or depression are significant (can be used with previous list):
  - **Hops extract** standardized for 8-prenylnaringenin: 120 to 300 mg q.d.
  - **Kava extract:** 45 to 80 mg of kavalactones t.i.d.
  - **St. John's wort extract** standardized to 0.3% hypericin, 900 to 1800 mg q.d.

- Choose the following if symptoms of vaginal atrophy do not respond after 2 months of treatment with other botanical(s):
  - **Kudzu:** dried powdered root, 20 to 50 mg q.d.
- Choose the following if symptoms of menopausal migraine are significant:
  - 100 mg *A. sinensis* extract, 60 mg soy isoflavones, and 50 mg of black cohosh extract q.d.
  - If symptoms do not sufficiently improve consider HT.

Lifestyle

- **Regular exercise program:** at least 30 minutes four times a week

Menorrhagia

DIAGNOSTIC SUMMARY

- Excessive menstrual bleeding (blood loss of more than 80 mL) occurring at regular cyclic intervals (cycles are usually, but not necessarily, of normal length).
- May be caused by dysfunctional uterine bleeding (DUB; no organic cause) or local lesions (e.g., uterine myomas [fibroids], endometrial polyps, endometrial hyperplasia, endometrial cancer, adenomyosis, and endometritis). Other causes include bleeding disorders and hypothyroidism.

Key to diagnosis begins with history and physical examination. The following tests and procedures are performed for diagnosis and management on an as-needed basis: pelvic examination, pelvic ultrasound, and/or pelvic sonohysterogram; cervical cytology; thyroid function studies; pregnancy test; complete blood count (CBC); ferritin; liver function or coagulation studies; follicle-stimulating hormone (FSH) and luteinizing hormone (LH) levels; serum progesterone; testosterone; dehydroepiandrosterone sulfate; sexually transmitted disease testing; hysteroscopy; endometrial biopsies or dilation and curettage (D&C)—used for diagnosis and management as needed.

GENERAL CONSIDERATIONS

Other patterns of abnormal bleeding are oligomenorrhea (interval longer than 35 days), polymenorrhea (interval shorter than 21 days), metrorrhagia (irregular or frequent intervals with excessive flow and duration), menometrorrhagia (prolonged heavy bleeding at irregular intervals), and intermenstrual bleeding (variable amounts occurring between regular menses).

Normal menstrual cycle: length of 28 days (±7 days), duration of 4 days (±4 days), blood loss of 40 mL (±20 mL).

Menorrhagia is largely subjective; an objective measure of blood loss is rarely done. Measured blood loss correlates poorly with

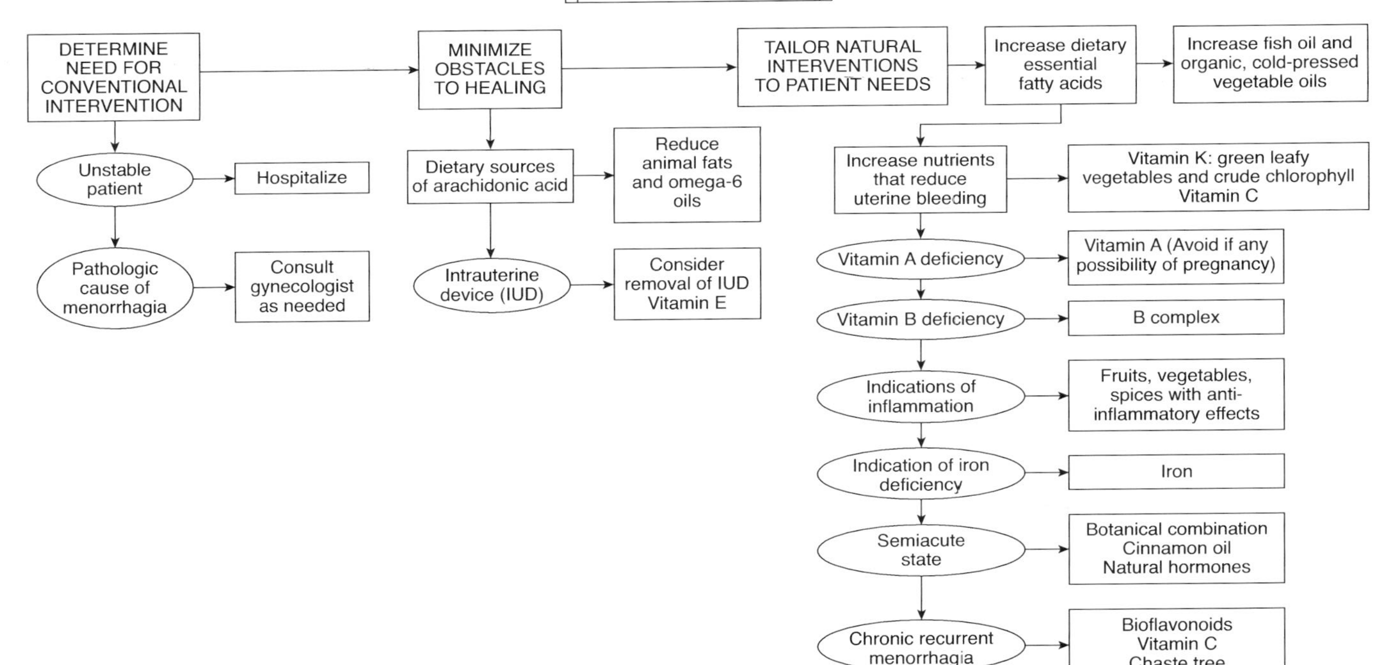
MENORRHAGIA
DETERMINE NEED FOR CONVENTIONAL INTERVENTION
Unstable patient
Hospitalize
Pathologic cause of menorrhagia
Consult gynecologist as needed
MINIMIZE OBSTACLES TO HEALING
Dietary sources of arachidonic acid
Reduce animal fats and omega-6 oils
Intrauterine device (IUD)
Consider removal of IUD
Vitamin E
TAILOR NATURAL INTERVENTIONS TO PATIENT NEEDS
Increase dietary essential fatty acids
Increase fish oil and organic, cold-pressed vegetable oils
Increase nutrients that reduce uterine bleeding
Vitamin K: green leafy vegetables and crude chlorophyll
Vitamin C
Vitamin A deficiency
Vitamin A (Avoid if any possibility of pregnancy)
Vitamin B deficiency
B complex
Indications of inflammation
Fruits, vegetables, spices with anti-inflammatory effects
Indication of iron deficiency
Iron
Semiacute state
Botanical combination
Cinnamon oil
Natural hormones
Chronic recurrent menorrhagia
Bioflavonoids
Vitamin C
Chaste tree

patient assessment of bleeding. Patients with menorrhagia have increased menstrual blood flow during first 3 days (up to 92% of total menses lost at this time), indicating that mechanisms responsible for ceasing menses are as effective in women with menorrhagia as in normal women, despite high blood loss.

Etiology

Consult gynecology textbook to rule out pathologic causes. Realize scope of causes and do not assume DUB.

- **DUB definition:** abnormal uterine bleeding without demonstrable organic cause. DUB includes menorrhagia, oligomenorrhea, polymenorrhea, metrorrhagia, menometrorrhagia, and intermenstrual bleeding.
- **Abnormal bleeding categories:** hormonal, mechanical, and clotting abnormalities. Not all cause menorrhagia, but rather other abnormal bleeding patterns.
- **Hormonal causes:** anovulation and luteal phase defects and stress (DUB), exogenous hormones, hypothyroidism, ovarian cysts.
- **Mechanical causes:** uterine polyps, uterine fibroids, uterine cancer, intrauterine devices, ectopic pregnancy, pregnancy, endometriosis, endometritis.
- **Clotting abnormalities:** vitamin K deficiency, drug-induced hemorrhage (heparin, warfarin, aspirin), dysproteinemias, disseminated intravascular coagulation, severe hepatic disease, primary fibrinolysis, circulating inhibitors of coagulation.
- **Abnormalities in prostaglandin metabolism:** menorrhagic endometrium excessively incorporates arachidonic acid (AA) into neutral lipids and inadequately incorporates it into phospholipids. Increased AA release during menses increases production of series 2 prostaglandins—a major factor in excess menstrual bleeding and dysmenorrhea. Excessive bleeding during first 3 days is caused by vasodilation by prostaglandin E_2 (PGE_2) and PGI_2 and antiaggregating activity of PGI_2; pain of dysmenorrhea is caused by excess PGF_{2alpha}.
- **Thyroid abnormalities:** overt hypothyroidism and hyperthyroidism are linked to menstrual disturbances. Minimal, subclinical insufficiency (thyroid stimulation test) may cause menorrhagia and other menstrual disturbances. Minimal hypothyroid patients with menorrhagia may respond dramatically to thyroxine. Consider thyroid-stimulating hormone testing for patients with longstanding menstrual dysfunction (with no obvious uterine pathosis). This is preferred to empiric use of thyroid hormone.

Estimating Menstrual Blood Loss

- Assessing blood loss by asking for an estimate of number of pads or tampons used during each period and duration of period is inaccurate. Forty percent of women losing more than 80 mL considered their periods only moderately heavy or scanty; 14% with loss of less than 20 mL judged their periods to be heavy.
- Serum ferritin is best indicator of blood loss but may be impractical for immediate information. Attempt to understand blood loss. Be concerned about excess bleeding for longer than 7 straight days, more frequently than every 21 days, new pad or tampon every hour for more than half a day. Changing pad or tampon every half hour or more frequently requires urgent attention; it may be an emergency. Symptoms of light-headedness, dizziness, and fainting are cause for immediate concern. Any bleeding in postmenopausal women is abnormal.

Pathologic Causes of Menorrhagia

Bleeding disorders

Cause	Possible Etiology
Anovulation	Excessive estrogen Failure of midcycle surge of luteinizing hormone Hypothyroidism Hyperprolactinemia Polycystic ovary disease
Intrauterine structural defects	Fibroids Polyps Cancer Ectopic pregnancy Intrauterine devices

Acquired Generalized Hemorrhagic Disorders

Factor	Possible Cause
Deficiency of vitamin K	Low intake, impaired absorption, antimicrobial inhibition of gut flora that synthesize vitamin K
Drug-induced hemorrhage	Heparin, warfarin
Dysproteinemias	Myeloma, macroglobulinemia
Disseminated intravascular coagulation	
Severe hepatic disease	
Circulating inhibitors of coagulation	
Primary fibrinolysis	

- **Abnormalities of prostaglandin metabolism:** menorrhagic endometrium incorporates AA into neutral lipids to much greater extent than normal, and incorporation into phospholipids is decreased; increased AA release during menses increases production of series 2 prostaglandins, a major factor in excess bleeding and dysmenorrhea; excess bleeding during first 3 days from the vasodilatory properties of PGE_2 and PGI_2 and antiaggregating activity of PGI_2; pain of dysmenorrhea is a result of overproducing PGF_{2alpha}.
- **Other contributing factors:** iron (Fe) deficiency, hypothyroidism, vitamin A deficiency, intrauterine devices, local factors (uterine myomas, endometrial polyps, adenomyosis, endometrial hyperplasia, salpingitis, endometritis).

THERAPEUTIC CONSIDERATIONS

Needless hysterectomies have been performed because of inadequate management of heavy menses. Factors to consider for hysterectomy: inability to manage menorrhagia, patient safety and health, lack of clear diagnosis, stress and fatigue wearing on patient. Hysterectomy is needed in selected circumstances, but most cases of menorrhagia can be treated without surgery with botanicals, nutraceuticals, hormones, and pharmaceuticals. Less-permanent surgical procedures may spare the uterus—D&C, hysteroscopic resections and ablations, and uterine artery embolization.

- **Psychological stress:** directly affects bleeding patterns by influencing the hypothalamic-pituitary-ovarian axis. This causes anovulation and subsequent lack of progesterone. Endometrium is in estrogen-dominant state with plump thickening without opposing, stabilizing progesterone, causing heavy bleeding at next menses. Adolescents account for many of these cases; remainder are perimenopausal women.
- **Fe deficiency:** blood loss of greater than 60 mL per period causes negative Fe balance. Chronic Fe deficiency can cause menorrhagia.
  - Many patients without organic pathosis respond well to Fe supplements alone.
  - High rate of organic pathosis (fibroids, polyps, adenomyosis) in patients unresponsive to Fe supplements.
  - Serum Fe levels rise in many patients given Fe supplements.
  - Fe therapy is less effective when initial serum Fe is high.
  - Menorrhagia correlates with depleted tissue Fe stores (bone marrow) irrespective of serum Fe level.

— Seventy-five percent of patients on Fe supplements improve compared with 32.5% on placebo.

Hematologic screening and serum ferritin (first indicator of decreased Fe stores, whereas hemoglobin concentration, mean corpuscular volume, and mean corpuscular hemoglobin may be normal) are essential. Fe supplementation dose: 100 mg elemental Fe q.d. as prophylactic therapy to prevent menorrhagia and depletion of Fe-containing enzymes before hematologic changes are observed. Decreased serum ferritin is a good indicator of need for Fe supplementation.

- **Vitamin A:** serum retinol is significantly lower in women with menorrhagia than healthy control subjects. A dose of 60,000 international units (IU) vitamin A for 35 days can reduce or normalize blood loss in such patients. Although potentially effective, do not use this therapy in women with any possibility of pregnancy. The research is clear that high dose vitamin A is potentially teratogenic. This may be a result of not the vitamin A but rather the concomitant vitamin D deficiency. Nonetheless, contraindicated at this time.
- **Vitamin C and bioflavonoids:** capillary fragility is believed to play a role in many cases of menorrhagia. Ascorbate and bioflavonoids strengthen capillary walls. Bioflavonoids may also reduce heavy bleeding because of their anti-inflammatory effect, as with anti-inflammatory drugs. Vitamin C (200 mg t.i.d.) and bioflavonoids can reduce menorrhagia. Natural anti-inflammatories (e.g., bioflavonoids) may reduce heavy bleeding, just as conventional medicine uses nonsteroidal anti-inflammatories. Vitamin C increases Fe absorption; the therapeutic effect also may be from enhanced Fe absorption.
- **Vitamin E:** free radicals may play a causative role in endometrial bleeding, particularly with an intrauterine device. Vitamin E (100 IU every 2 days) has improved patients within 10 weeks. Vitamin E may work by antioxidant activity or prostaglandin metabolism.
- **Vitamin K and chlorophyll:** although bleeding time and prothrombin levels usually are normal in patients with menorrhagia, vitamin K (crude preparations of chlorophyll) has clinical and limited research support. Also, some women may have inherited or acquired bleeding disorders.
- **Essential fatty acids:** menorrhagia is associated with increased omega-6 AA in uterine tissues. The majority of tissue AA is derived from the diet. Reducing dietary animal products and

ordinary omega-6 vegetable oils and increasing fish oil, flax oil, borage oil, and evening primrose oil may curtail blood loss by decreasing AA. Increasing fish, nuts, and seeds in the diet may also alter production of AA.

- **Vitamin B complex:** menorrhagia may correlate with B-vitamin deficiency. The liver loses its ability to inactivate estrogen in B-complex deficiency. Some cases of menorrhagia are caused by an excessive estrogen effect on endometrium. Supplementing B vitamins may normalize estrogen metabolism. B-complex vitamins can give prompt improvement in menorrhagia and metrorrhagia. Preparations used: thiamin 3 to 9 mg, riboflavin 4.5 to 9 mg, and up to 60 mg niacin.

Botanicals

- ***Zingiber officinale*** **(ginger):** inhibits prostaglandin synthesis, linked to altered PG_2 ratio associated with excessive menstrual loss. Inhibition of prostaglandin and leukotriene formation explains traditional use of ginger as an anti-inflammatory.
- ***Vitex agnus-castus*** **(chaste tree):** best-known herb in Europe for hormonal imbalances and abnormal bleeding in women; most important herb to normalize menstrual flow, but not a fast-acting herb. Results may not be achieved for 3 to 4 months. Seeds are the part used. It acts on the hypothalamic-pituitary axis to increase LH and mildly inhibit release of FSH. Result: shift in ratio of estrogen and progesterone, causing progesterone-like action. It improves amenorrhea, polymenorrhea, oligomenorrhea, and menorrhagia. In polymenorrhea, time between periods lengthened from 20.1 days to 26.3 days; the number of heavy bleeding days was shortened. Dose: 15 drops chaste tree liquid extract.
- **Traditional astringent herbs:** reduce blood loss from reproductive tract, gastrointestinal tract, respiratory tract, and skin. Astringents for uterine blood loss are high in tannins (not the only helpful constituents). Major astringent and hemostatic herbs used in chronic and acute menorrhagia (used in combination formulations for weeks and months to bring about results) are as follows:
  - — Yarrow *(Achillea millefolium)*
  - — Ladies' mantle *(Alchemilla vulgaris)*
  - — Cranesbill *(Geranium maculatum)*
  - — Beth root *(Trillium erectum)*
  - — Greater periwinkle *(Vinca major)*

— Horsetail *(Equisetum arvense)*
— Goldenseal *(Hydrastis canadensis)*
— Shepherd's purse *(Capsella bursa-pastoris)*: was traditionally used to manage obstetric and gynecologic hemorrhage. Intravenous and intramuscular injections have been effective in menorrhagia because of functional abnormalities and fibroids. Its hemostatic action may arise from high levels of oxalic and dicarboxylic acids.

- **Traditional uterine tonics:** used to ease menstrual flow. Traditionally and empirically, if the uterus is hypotonic, heavy bleeding may be occurring. Improving uterine tone may normalize or regulate menstrual bleeding. Uterine tonics and/or amphoterics that regulate tone and potentially reduce bleeding include the following:
  — Blue cohosh *(Caulophyllum thalictroides)*
  — Helonia *(Chamaelirium luteum)*
  — Squaw vine *(Mitchella repens)*
  — Raspberry leaves *(Rubus idaeus)*
  — Life root *(Senecio aureus)*
- **Astringent and uterine tonic herbs:** can be used in formulations for weeks to several months as tea, liquid extract, or powdered capsule.
- **Traditional herbs for semiacute or acute blood loss in a stable patient:** some of these herbs have dose-specific toxicities; use only after consulting botanical reference text to ensure proper dose. Cinnamon essential oil dose: 1 to 5 drops every 3 to 4 hours. Other herbs: do not exceed 20 drops every 2 hours or 1 capsule every 4 hours.
  — Cinnamon essential oil *(Cinnamomum verum)*
  — Life root *(S. aureus)*
  — Canadian fleabane *(Erigeron canadensis)*
  — Greater periwinkle *(V. major)*
  — Shepherd's purse *(C. bursa-pastoris)*
  — Yarrow *(A. millefolium)*
  — Savin *(Sabina officinalis)*
  — Beth root *(T. erectum)*

Use these botanicals only in women who are stable. In unstable patients, use them as adjuncts to intravenous estrogens, other pharmaceuticals, or surgical interventions. They can be used for patients with chronic menorrhagia who are stable and for semiacute blood loss or acute blood loss if patient shows no signs of instability and improves within 12 to 24 hours.

Bioidentical Hormones

Natural estradiol and progesterone can effectively manage menorrhagia, just as conjugated equine estrogens (CEE) or synthetic estrogens and progestins are used in conventional medicine. To control an acute bleeding episode, natural estradiol should be just as effective as CEE. These hormones are prescription items administered by qualified practitioners. Cyclic natural progesterone can correct recurring menorrhagia; a short course of natural progesterone can be used in acute menorrhagia. Natural progesterone creams are not as effective as higher-dose pills or oral micronized natural progesterone.

THERAPEUTIC APPROACH

- Unstable patients (hypotensive, dizzy, loss of consciousness, chills or fever, or passage of large amounts of tissue) require transfer to hospital for intravenous estrogens, D&C, hysterectomy, or uterine ablation.
- First step in treating menorrhagia is to control the cause: correct prothrombin time, hematologic status, or thyroid function. Mechanical causes, such as endometrial polyp or uterine fibroid, may be managed without removing cause; but if no improvement occurs, consider conventional treatment, including surgery. Endometrial hyperplasia requires definitive, proven progesterone and progestin with biopsy-proven improvement. Endometrial cancer requires hysterectomy. Uterine infections need appropriate treatment. Ectopic pregnancy with or without bleeding requires immediate conventional intervention. In chronic menorrhagia or effectively managed episodic acute blood loss, CBC and serum ferritin can be used to monitor anemia status.
- Diet: low in sources of AA (animal fats) and high in fish oils, linolenic and linoleic acids (vegetable oils), green leafy vegetables, and other sources of vitamin K. Fruits, vegetables, and spices with anti-inflammatory effects: garlic, onions, cumin, pineapple, citrus.
- Supplements:
  - — High-potency multiple vitamin-mineral formula
  - — Vitamin C: 1 g t.i.d. with meals
  - — Bioflavonoids (mixed from citrus): 1000 mg q.d.
  - — Chlorophyll: 25 mg/day (use a crude form) or 1 mg vitamin K_1

If low serum ferritin is confirmed:

— Fe: 30 mg, bound to pyrophosphate, succinate, glycinate, or fumarate, b.i.d. between meals. (If this recommendation causes abdominal discomfort, try 30 mg with meals t.i.d.)

Botanical Medicines

Chronic Recurring Menorrhagia

- ***V. agnus-castus* (chasteberry):** chasteberry extract (often standardized to contain 0.5 % agnuside) in tablet or capsule: 175 to 225 mg q.d. If using liquid extract: 2 to 4 mL (½ to 1 tsp) q.d.

  Semiacute:
- **Botanical combination tincture** of equal parts of each herb (20 to 30 drops every 2 to 3 hours): yarrow, greater periwinkle, shepherd's purse, life root
- **Cinnamon oil:** 1 to 5 drops every 3 to 4 hours

Bioidentical Hormones

- **Oral micronized progesterone:** 100 mg b.i.d. during luteal phase for 12 days per month for recurring menorrhagia. A dose of 200 to 400 mg q.d. for 7 to 12 days may be used for semiacute blood loss, followed by a cyclic hormone product for 21 days on and 7 days off.
- **Progesterone cream** (containing at least 400 mg of progesterone per ounce): ¼ to ½ tsp b.i.d. for 12 days per month during luteal phase for mild recurring menorrhagia. Use a product containing at least 400 mg progesterone per ounce.
- **Bioidentical estradiol:** high-dose regimen for acute bleeding—4 mg estradiol every 4 hours for 24 hours then single daily dose of 1 mg for 7 to 10 days, followed by oral micronized progesterone at 200 mg before bed for 7 to 12 days.

Migraine Headache

DIAGNOSTIC SUMMARY

- Recurrent, paroxysmal attacks of headache.
- Headache typically is pounding and unilateral but may become generalized.
- Attacks often preceded by psychological or visual disturbances (auras) accompanied by anorexia, nausea, and gastrointestinal upset and followed by drowsiness.
- Physical examination typically reveals no focal neurologic deficit.

GENERAL CONSIDERATIONS

Lifetime prevalence of migraine headache is 18%. Women are more frequently affected than men. More than half of patients have a family history of migraine. Prevalence is highest in North America and lowest in Africa and Asia.

- Auras: migraines can come without warning but often have symptoms (auras) a few minutes before onset of pain: blurring or bright spots of vision, anxiety, fatigue, disturbed thinking, unilateral peripheral numbness or tingling.
- Migraine headaches are caused by excessive dilation of blood vessels in the head; they affect 15% to 20% of men and 25% to 30% of women.
- Vascular headache pain (e.g., migraine): throbbing or pounding sharp pain. Nonvascular headache (tension headache) pain: steady, constant, dull pain starting at base of skull or in forehead and spreading over entire head, giving sensation of pressure or vise grip applied to skull. Pain of headache comes from outside the brain because brain tissue is insensate. Pain arises from meninges and scalp, large cranial vessels, proximal intracranial vessels, and scalp vasculature and muscles when stretched or tensed.
- Most common nonvascular headache is the tension headache, caused by tightened muscles of the face, neck, or scalp, resulting

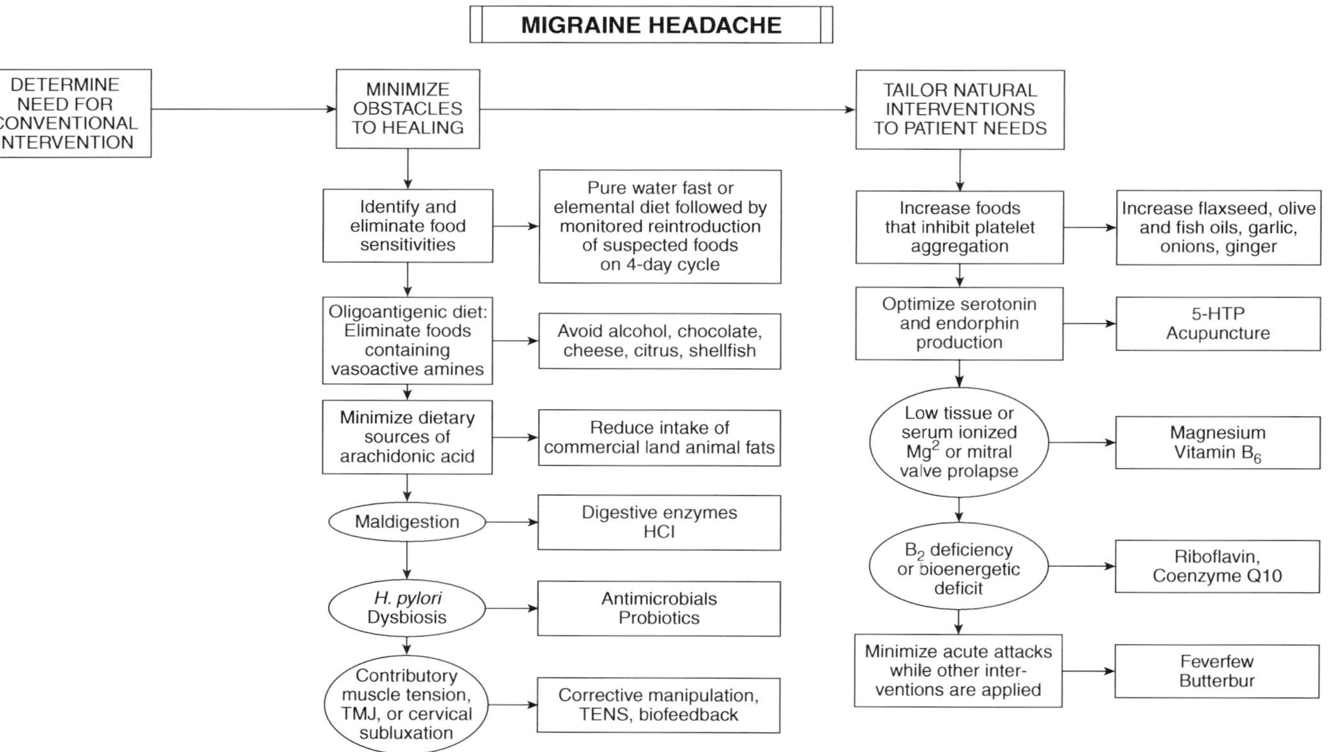
MIGRAINE HEADACHE
DETERMINE NEED FOR CONVENTIONAL INTERVENTION
MINIMIZE OBSTACLES TO HEALING
TAILOR NATURAL INTERVENTIONS TO PATIENT NEEDS
Identify and eliminate food sensitivities
Pure water fast or elemental diet followed by monitored reintroduction of suspected foods on 4-day cycle
Oligoantigenic diet: Eliminate foods containing vasoactive amines
Avoid alcohol, chocolate, cheese, citrus, shellfish
Minimize dietary sources of arachidonic acid
Reduce intake of commercial land animal fats
Maldigestion
Digestive enzymes HCl
H. pylori Dysbiosis
Antimicrobials Probiotics
Contributory muscle tension, TMJ, or cervical subluxation
Corrective manipulation, TENS, biofeedback
Increase foods that inhibit platelet aggregation
Increase flaxseed, olive and fish oils, garlic, onions, ginger
Optimize serotonin and endorphin production
5-HTP Acupuncture
Low tissue or serum ionized Mg^2 or mitral valve prolapse
Magnesium Vitamin B_6
B_2 deficiency or bioenergetic deficit
Riboflavin, Coenzyme Q10
Minimize acute attacks while other interventions are applied
Feverfew Butterbur

from stress or poor posture. Tightened muscles pinch nerves or their blood supply, causing pain and pressure. Relaxation of muscle usually brings immediate relief.

Classification and Diagnosis

Migraine Classification

	Common	Classic	Complicated
Incidence	80%	10%	10%
Pain	Frontal, unilateral or bilateral	Unilateral	Unpredictable, may be absent
Aura	Unusual	Half-hour before striking	Neurologic aura, vertigo, syncope, diplopia, hemiparesis
Duration of headache	1-3 days	2-6 hours	Unpredictable
Physical examination	Unhappiness	Pallor, vomiting	Mild neurotic signs, speech disorder, hemiparesis, unsteadiness, cranial nerve III palsy

- **Cluster headache** was once considered a migraine-type headache because vasodilation is a key component. It is now separately classified. It is also called *histamine cephalgia, Horton's headache,* or *atypical facial neuralgia.* It is much less common than migraine.
- **Chronic daily headache** (CDH) (also called *chronic tension headache, migraine with interparoxysmal headache, transformed migraine, evolutive migraine, mixed headache syndrome, tension-vascular headache*): affects 40% of patients in headache clinics.

Types of Chronic Daily Headache

- Transformed migraine
  - — Drug-induced
  - — Non–drug-induced
- Chronic tension-type headache
- New daily persistent headache
- Posttraumatic headache

Pathophysiology

The sequence of events producing migraine is unclear, but migraine is no longer considered a primary vascular event. Vasomotor changes are considered epiphenomena. A singular pathophysiologic mechanism has not been identified, and many key factors involved relate to prevention and treatment.

- **Vasomotor instability theory:** migraineurs have heightened central nervous system (CNS) activity, mediated by the trigeminovascular system. Stimulation of the trigeminal ganglion releases vasoactive neuropeptides—substance P, calcitonin gene–related peptide (CGRP), and neurokinin A. These neuropeptides induce neurogenic inflammation. Components of this inflammatory response are vasodilation and plasma protein extravasation. Superficial temporal vessels are visibly dilated. Local compression of these vessels or carotid artery temporarily relieves pain. Other types of extracranial vasodilation (heat or exercise induced) are not problematic. Patients are pale during headache despite extracranial vasodilation, and lower skin temperature of the affected side suggests constriction of small vessels. Focal or diffuse cerebral or brainstem dysfunction is attributed to intracranial vasoconstriction. Blood flow is greatly reduced during the prodromal stage, followed by a stage of increased blood flow persisting for longer than 48 hours. Aura may be caused by cortical spreading depression (CSD), a process producing transient depression of spontaneous and evoked neuronal activity. During this time, the brain fails to maintain normal ionic homeostasis and efflux of excitatory amino acids from neurons. CSD may be linked to decreased cerebral blood flow during aura. CSD may play a role in migraine and overall cerebral hyperexcitability. Triggering CSD can require activation of the *N*-methyl-D-aspartate (NMDA) receptor, which augments depolarization. CSD is prevented by ifenprodil, a selective NMDA receptor antagonist, offering a novel therapeutic approach. The anticonvulsant topiramate is a conventional first-line treatment for migraine as a gamma-aminobutyric acid (GABA) agonist and glutamate antagonist. This supports the concept of excessive cerebral excitability related to NMDA receptor activation. CGRP, a potent vasodilator, is elevated after migraine. CGRP antagonists relieve migraine pain without causing vasoconstriction and are being tested for efficacy and safety. This stage may be followed by a phase of increased blood flow that can persist for longer than 48 hours. Migraine patients may have functional abnormality of vasomotor control, suggested by orthostatic symptoms and abnormal sensitivity to vasodilatory effects of physical and chemical agents. Migraineurs experience heightened CNS activity, which appears to be mediated by the trigeminovascular system.

Migraine also has complex relations with disorders of the cerebrovasculature, the cardiovascular system, and the heart. Right-to-left shunt, patent foramen ovale, and mitral valve prolapse are all linked with a higher incidence of migraine. Migraine is also linked to cardiovascular risk factors (total cholesterol/high-density–lipoprotein cholesterol ratio greater than 5; hypertension; and history of early-onset coronary heart disease or stroke). Risk for stroke is highest among young women experiencing migraine with aura, particularly if they smoke or use oral contraceptives; however, male and female migraineurs are at increased risk for ischemic stroke regardless of age. Migraine and epilepsy are co-morbid disorders sharing common physiologic mechanisms and treatments.

- **Platelets and serotonin:** serotonin is normally stored in platelets and released by platelet aggregation and in response to stimuli (e.g., catecholamines). There is no difference in total serotonin content between normal platelets and platelets of migraine patients. However, the quantity of serotonin released by platelets of a migraine patient in response to serotonin stimulation, although normal (or even subnormal) immediately after an attack, becomes progressively higher as the next attack approaches. The rise of plasma serotonin may not cause migraine, but it could be a self-defense mechanism. Platelet activation occurs during migraine, which may be an epiphenomenon of neurogenic inflammation. On the other hand, platelet-deactivating agents (e.g., aspirin, feverfew, and essential fatty acids [EFAs]) help prevent migraine. Serotonin is a stress-response system that involves increased turnover during both acute and longer-term stress. Serotonin metabolite 5-hydroxyindoleacetic acid (5-HIAA) increases in urine during migraine, as a result of increased breakdown of serotonin from increased activity of monoamine oxidase. Individuals with migraine have low tissue serotonin (low serotonin syndrome). Low serotonin may cause a decreased pain threshold. Positive clinical results are seen with serotonin precursor 5-hydroxytryptophan (5-HTP) (*Textbook*, "5-Hydroxytryptophan"). Link between low serotonin and headache is the basis of many migraine prescription drugs. Monoamine oxidase inhibitors (which increase serotonin) prevent headaches. Increasing serotonin relieves chronic migraines. Effects of 5-HTP and drugs on the serotonin system are complex because of the multiple types of serotonin receptors. Binding to 5-hydroxytryptamine (5-HT_{1C}) receptors triggers migraines;

inhibiting 5-HT_{1C} prevents migraines. Binding receptor 5-HT_{1D} may prevent and stop migraines. 5-HT_{1C} receptors are desensitized —that is, they lose affinity for serotonin—when serotonin exposure is increased by use of 5-HTP. Serotonin binds instead to 5-HT_{1D} receptor, decreasing headaches. Evidence for theory: 5-HTP is more effective over time (after 60 days of use rather than after 30). Antimigraine triptan drugs are 5-HT_{1B} and 5-HT_{1D} receptor agonists that constrict blood vessels and block neurogenic inflammation and neural peptide release. They may also inhibit neuronal activity within the trigeminovascular system. Safety issue: triptans activate serotonin receptors on cerebral vessels and coronary arteries; avoid in patients with ischemic heart disease, uncontrolled hypertension, or cerebrovascular disease. Avoid using triptans, ergotamine-based drugs, and selective serotonin reuptake inhibitors (SSRIs) concurrently, although risk of serotonin syndrome is low. Some practitioners use 5-HTP successfully with SSRIs, but caution is advised. Although SSRIs are used for migraine prophylaxis, their biochemical effect is unknown, quality of evidence is poor, and clinical impact is low. Low-serotonin state facilitates activation of the trigeminovascular nociceptive pathway, as induced by CSD.

- **Neuronal disorder:** trigeminovascular neurons, which innervate pial arteries, release CGRP and the peptide substance P, either directly from cellular signals or secondarily to CNS activation. Substance P is a pain mediator, and its release into the arteries induces vasodilation, mast cell degranulation, and increased vascular permeability. Arterial endothelial cells may respond to substance P and CGRP by releasing vasoactive substances (e.g., arachidonic acid metabolites, purine compounds, or molecules containing carbonyl groups). Theory: functional changes within the noradrenergic system constitute the threshold for migraine activation. Modulation of sympathetic activity allows potentiators to exert their effects. Chronic stress is a potentiator in this model.
- **Unified hypothesis:** migraine has a three-stage process: initiation, prodrome, and headache. Initiation depends on accumulation over time of several stressors that ultimately affect serotonin metabolism. At a critical point of susceptibility (or threshold), a cascade event is initiated. Susceptibility is a combination of decreased tissue serotonin, platelet changes, altered responsiveness of key cerebrovascular end organs, increased sensitivity of intrinsic noradrenergic system of the brain, and buildup of

histamine, arachidonic acid metabolites, or other mediators of inflammation. Platelet changes: increased adhesiveness, enhanced tendency to release serotonin, and increased membrane arachidonic acid. When platelets are stimulated to secrete serotonin, platelet aggregation, vasospasm, and inflammatory processes cause local cerebral ischemia. This is followed by rebound vasodilation and release of peptide substance P and other mediators of pain.

THERAPEUTIC CONSIDERATIONS

Pharmaceuticals tend to be inadequate because they fail to address underlying cause. Pharmaceutical prophylaxis (e.g., propranolol, valproic acid, and topiramate) can be effective; but they do not treat the causes, and some preventive drugs can exacerbate other conditions. Avoid using flunarizine (unavailable in the United States), valproate, and amitriptyline in obese patients; these drugs cause weight gain. Amitriptyline and pizotifen can worsen glaucoma and urinary retention. Beta-blockers can exacerbate asthma and diabetes. Topiramate can enhance risk of renal calculi. European countries incorporate nondrug treatments, including behavioral and psychological techniques. Medicines are considered effective if they reduce migraine frequency by 50% or more. The first step in treating migraine is identifying precipitating factors. Food intolerance or allergy is the most important, but many other factors are primary causes or contributors. Assess role headache medicines play, especially in chronic headaches.

Drug Reactions

Medication-overuse headache (MOH) (*analgesic rebound headache, drug-induced headache,* or *medication-misuse headache*) frequently precludes successful treatment of underlying primary headache disorder or migraine or tension headache. MOH may be associated with development or maintenance of CDH syndrome. After successful MOH treatment, preventive medicines for underlying primary headache disorder have a greater chance of success. Patients able to discontinue daily symptom-modifying drugs experience improvement in chronic headaches in addition to greater efficacy of prophylactic medicines. All drugs used regularly for symptomatic relief can produce MOH, but the mechanism of action is unknown. Central sensitization, changes in trigeminal pain processing, receptor downregulation, and biobehavioral factors are proposed mechanisms. Drugs with the highest potential for causing MOH: opioids, butalbital-containing analgesics, and aspirin/acetaminophen/caffeine combinations. Triptans have intermediate to high potential for causing MOH when used frequently, and nonsteroidal anti-inflammatory drugs (NSAIDs) carry the lowest risk. Regular ergotamine use can cause MOH and other symptoms. Regular use of ergotamine in migraine can result in dependency cycle in which headaches escalate in severity on cessation of medication. Ergotamine withdrawal predictably causes debilitating headaches, often accompanied by nausea and vomiting, generally resulting in an improved status by 72 hours. Ginger preparations can be helpful during ergotamine withdrawal.

Diet

Food allergy or intolerance: plays role in many cases. Detection and removal of allergens or foods to which patient is intolerant eliminate or greatly reduce symptoms in the majority of patients (success ranges from 30% to 93%). Incidences of food allergy are similar for the three major types of migraine. Few studies have been performed since the 1980s, when the groundwork relating food intolerance to migraine was laid. Mechanism is unknown, but several theories have been proposed.

- Idiopathic response to a pharmacologically active substance, such as tyramine
- Monoamine oxidase deficiency
- Platelet phenolsulfotransferase deficiency; immunologically mediated food allergy
- Platelet abnormalities
- **Egger theory:** chronic alteration of nonspecific responsiveness of cerebral vascular end organ from long-term antigenic stimulation (analogous to asthmatic response of bronchioles to exercise or cold after antigen contact). Food allergies cause platelet degranulation and serotonin release. Common migraine triggers in children: cheese, chocolate, citrus fruits, hot dogs, monosodium glutamate (MSG), aspartame, fatty foods, ice cream, caffeine withdrawal, and alcoholic drinks, especially red wine and beer. Tyramine, phenylethylamine, histamine, nitrites, and sulfites are involved in food intolerance headache; but immunoglobulin E (IgE)–mediated food allergy is an infrequent cause. Laboratory detection of food allergies is most convenient for patient. A major drawback of food intolerance testing with IgG antibodies can

be a lack of reproducible findings with split blood samples among various laboratories. However, when migraineurs remove foods to which they have mounted IgG responses, they experience robust improvement and even complete remission after 1 month of specific food elimination. Challenge testing is most reliable but has a delayed response, requiring several days of repeated challenge. Ingestion of large amounts of several foods is needed to detect the marginally reactive.

- **Dietary amines:** chocolate, cheese, beer, and wine precipitate migraines because they contain histamine and/or other vasoactive compounds, triggering migraines in sensitive individuals by causing blood vessels to expand. Tyramine, a component of these foods, is considered a migraine trigger; but controlled studies have yielded conflicting findings.
- **Red wine** is more problematic than white wine because it has 20 to 200 times the amount of histamine, and it stimulates release of vasoactive compounds by platelets. Being much higher in flavonoids, it inhibits enzyme (phenolsulfotransferase), which breaks down serotonin and other vasoactive amines in platelets. Migraine sufferers have much lower levels of this enzyme. High vasoactive amine foods (cheese, chocolate) worsen the problem.
- Standard treatment of histamine-induced headache is a histamine-free diet plus vitamin B_6.
- Enzyme diamine oxidase, which breaks down histamine in small intestine mucosa before absorption into circulation, influences whether a person reacts to dietary histamine. Persons sensitive to dietary histamine have less of this enzyme than control subjects. Diamine oxidase is vitamin B_6 dependent. Compounds inhibiting B_6 (that also inhibit diamine oxidase): food coloring agents (hydrazine dyes: FD&C yellow No. 5), drugs (isoniazid, hydralazine, dopamine, penicillamine), birth control pills, alcohol, and excessive protein intake. Yellow dye No. 5 (tartrazine) is consumed in greater quantities (15 mg q.d.) than the recommended daily allowance for vitamin B_6 (2.0 mg for males and 1.6 mg for females).
- **Vitamin B_6** (1 mg/kg body weight) improves histamine tolerance, presumably by increasing diamine oxidase activity. Women have lower diamine oxidase. This may explain the higher incidence of histamine-induced headaches among women. Women are more frequently intolerant of red wine. Level of diamine oxidase in women increases by more than 500 times during

pregnancy; women with histamine-induced headaches commonly have complete remission during pregnancy.

- **Diet-related triggers:** hypoglycemia can trigger migraine and is correctable by dietary manipulation. Hypoglycemia may arise from refined carbohydrate intake, especially when insulin becomes elevated. Excessive sodium intake may increase angiotensin in response to sodium ingestion. For lactose intolerance, avoiding dairy may afford improvement. Aspartame, a common sweetener, may increase migraine incidence. Sucralose, another commonly used artificial sweetener, might be a migraine trigger. MSG is a well-recognized migraine trigger that can directly activate the NMDA receptor.
- **Dysbiosis and detoxification:** migraine is not just food intolerance; digestive and detoxification aberrations complicate matters. Metabolic waste of pathogenic organisms may produce headache. Correct intestinal dysbiosis is identified clinically or by stool culture, organic acids analysis, or intestinal permeability assessment. *Helicobacter pylori* was detected in 40% of migraine patients; eradication of the bacterium improved headache intensity, duration, and frequency in 100% of patients treated. Toxic overload or suboptimal function of detoxification enzymes may trigger headache. Susceptibility to toxicity is produced by excessive environmental exposures, genetic polymorphisms in detoxification enzyme production, and depletion of nutrient cofactors catalyzing phase I and/or phase II detoxification reactions.
- ***H. pylori:*** migraine headaches improve dramatically in 100% of patients for whom *H. pylori* was identified and treated with standard measures. *H. pylori* infection prevalence is significantly higher in migraineurs without aura compared with controls, indicating that *H. pylori* infection is an independent environmental risk factor for migraine without aura, especially in patients not genetically or hormonally susceptible. Incidental *H. pylori* positivity is more relevant in migraineurs compared with controls, because a high percentage experienced relief from migraines when the infection was eradicated.

Nutritional Supplements

- **5-HTP:** 5-HTP, the molecular intermediate between L-tryptophan and serotonin, is readily absorbed when taken orally and easily crosses the blood-brain barrier. It augments serotonin (see earlier). It also increases endorphins and is at least as effective as pharmaceuticals used to prevent migraine but much safer and better tolerated. Doge: 200 to 600 mg q.d.

- **Essential fatty acids (EFAs) and arachidonic acid:** have received little research attention for migraine. Platelet aggregation and arachidonic acid metabolites play a major role mediating events causing prodromal cerebral ischemia. Manipulating dietary EFAs may be very useful. Reducing animal fats and increasing fish significantly change platelet and membrane EFA ratios and decrease platelet aggregation. Sixty percent of the brain is composed of lipids. Omega-3 fatty acids can reduce headache frequency and intensity. Fish oil and olive oil improve migraine frequency, duration, and severity. Proposed mechanisms of action of omega-3s: reduced platelet serotonin release, modulation of prostaglandin synthesis, and diminution of cerebral vasospasm. Elevated blood lipids and free fatty acids are associated with increased platelet aggregability, decreased 5-HT, and increased prostaglandin levels. Biologic states that produce increased free fatty acids and lipids: high fat intake, obesity, insulin resistance, vigorous exercise, hunger, intake of alcohol and caffeine, oral contraceptives, tobacco abuse, and stress.
- **Riboflavin (vitamin B_2):** Another hypothesis states that migraines are caused by reduced energy production within mitochondria of cerebral blood vessels. B_2 is the precursor of flavin mononucleotide and flavin adenine dinucleotide, which are required for activity of flavoenzymes of electron transport chain. Riboflavin can increase mitochondrial complex I and II activity in mitochondrial energy metabolism without changing neuronal excitability—allowing excellent tolerance and lack of CNS adverse effects. Dose for prophylaxis: 400 mg q.d. for more than 3 months. It improved patients 68.2% as determined by migraine severity score used by researchers. Diarrhea and polyuria may be associated with administration of high-dose B_2. Advantages: well tolerated, inexpensive, reduces brain oxidative toxicity. Riboflavin prophylaxis at 200 mg/day for pediatric and adolescent migraine was an adequate dose, but it takes 4 months to achieve optimal results. Other prophylactic B vitamins: folic acid.
- **Coenzyme Q10 (CoQ10):** a critical component of the electron transport chain that also functions as an antioxidant. CoQ10 reduces frequency of migraines by 61%. After 3 months at 150 mg daily at breakfast, the average number of headache days decreased from 7 to 3 per month. Water-soluble CoQ10 at 100 mg t.i.d. induced similar results. CoQ10 deficiency may be common

in children and adolescents; it deserves therapeutic consideration in these age groups. Like riboflavin, CoQ10 is well tolerated (but expensive), with little risk of toxicity. It is ideal for women of childbearing age and for children. Liquid gel formulations are favored for their high bioavailability. Use CoQ10 with caution in patients taking warfarin, because CoQ10 may antagonize anticoagulation effects of warfarin. Many drugs can interfere with CoQ10 activity—statins, beta-blockers, and certain antidepressants and antipsychotics.

- **Magnesium (Mg):** low Mg is linked to migraine and tension headache. Low brain and tissue Mg levels are found in patients with migraines. Key Mg functions are to maintain tone of the blood vessels and prevent overexcitability of nerve cells. Mg supplements may be effective only in patients with low tissue or low ionized levels of Mg. Cerebrospinal fluid Mg tends to be low in migraine. Low Mg can predispose to many physiologic dysfunctions prominent in migraine—for example, induction of cerebral vasospasm; potentiation of contractile response of blood vessels to vasoactive compounds (e.g., serotonin); enhanced sensitivity of NMDA receptors to glutamate; and increased platelet aggregation, leading to serotonin release. Mg deficiency facilitates pathogenesis of migraine by promoting CSD. In migraineurs without aura, 600 mg of Mg citrate daily improves cortical blood flow. Low tissue Mg is common in migraine patients but is unnoticed because serum Mg is normal. Serum Mg, however, is an unreliable indicator because most body Mg stores are intracellular. Low serum Mg is an end-stage deficiency. Use red blood cell (erythrocyte) Mg and ionized Mg^{2+} (most biologically active form) in serum. Patients with acute migraine and low serum ionized Mg^{2+} (below 0.54 mmol/L) are more likely to respond to intravenous magnesium sulfate ($MgSO_4$) than patients with higher serum ionized Mg^{2+}. Pain relief lasts at least 24 hours in patients with serum ionized Mg^{2+} below 0.54 mmol/L. Average ionized Mg^{2+} in patients most relieved by intravenous Mg is significantly lower than in less-responsive patients. Intravenous Mg is extremely effective in some cases of acute migraine, tension, and cluster headaches. Dose of 1 to 3 g intravenous Mg (over 10-minute period) has 90% success rate in patients with low ionized Mg^{2+}. $MgSO_4$ completely eliminates migraine-associated symptoms of nausea and photosensitivity. Adverse effects include a brief flushed feeling. Mg improves mitral valve prolapse, which can damage platelets, causing release of histamine, platelet-activating factor, and serotonin. Eighty-five percent of patients with mitral valve prolapse have chronic Mg deficiency. Mg bound to citrate, malate, aspartate, or other Krebs cycle compound is better absorbed and tolerated than inorganic forms with laxative effect. (Be advised concerning possible neuroexcitatory effect of aspartate.) Typical Mg dosage ranges from 200 to 800 mg/day, depending on bowel tolerance. Use 50 mg vitamin B_6 q.d. to increase intracellular Mg.

Botanical Medicines

- *Tanacetum parthenium* **(feverfew):** most popular antimigraine botanical. Seventy percent of surveyed migraine sufferers eating feverfew leaves q.d. for prolonged periods claimed decreased frequency and/or intensity of attacks (many of these patients were unresponsive to orthodox medicines). Carbon dioxide–based feverfew extract MIG-99 has been effective in migraine prophylaxis involving only 6.25 mg t.i.d. for up to 4 months. It has been claimed to inhibit serotonin release, inhibit prostaglandin synthesis and platelet aggregation, inhibit polymorphonuclear leukocyte degranulation and phagocytosis of neutrophils, inhibit mast cell release of histamine, promote cytotoxic activity against human tumor cells, and possess both antimicrobial activity and antithrombotic potential. Studies indicate feverfew treats and prevents migraine by inhibiting release of serotonin from platelets. Constituents: sesquiterpene lactone (e.g., parthenolide). Avoid or use with caution in patients on anticoagulants because of platelet inhibition. Side effects: well tolerated; oral ulceration (from chewing feverfew leaves) and gastrointestinal symptoms are the most common adverse events, but these effects are mild and reversible with discontinuation. It is in same family as ragweed and chamomile; avoid in allergic persons.
- *Zingiber officinale* **(ginger):** ginger root has significant effects against inflammation and platelet aggregation. Much anecdotal information on migraine exists, but little experimental evidence. Most active anti-inflammatory components are found in fresh preparations and ginger oil.
- **Butterbur** *(Petasites hybridus):* vascular wall antispasmodic, especially for cerebral vessels. In medieval times, it was used to treat fever and bubonic plague; in the seventeenth century, it was an oral remedy for cough and asthma and a topical for

skin wounds. It inhibits leukotriene synthesis and lipoxygenase activity. Active principles petasine and isopetasine also produce vasodilation. This plant can decrease migraine frequency by 60% (and improve dysmenorrhea). Use prophylactically as daily supplement for 4 to 6 months; taper until migraine incidence begins to increase. It is well tolerated. Side effects: diarrhea in some patients. No drug interactions have been identified, but it is not known to be safe during pregnancy or lactation. Pyrrolizidine alkaloids are hepatotoxic and carcinogenic; use only extracts from which these have been removed. Adult dose: 50 to 100 mg b.i.d. with meals. Butterbur has diverse properties. It can be especially helpful for migraineurs with dysmenorrhea and/or allergic rhinitis. No allergic reactions have been reported, but patients hypersensitive to the Asteraceae family (e.g., ragweed, marigolds, daisies, chrysanthemums) should exercise caution because of risk of cross-reactivity.

Hormones

- **Melatonin:** downstream metabolite of dietary tryptophan. Ninety percent of serotonin is produced in the walls of the gastrointestinal tract, stored in platelets, and distributed to the rest of the body except the CNS (serotonin cannot cross the blood-brain barrier). Tryptophan and 5-HTP cross the blood-brain barrier to be converted into serotonin in the pineal gland, which contains 90% of CNS serotonin and most of the melatonin. The pineal gland is the interface between the environment and CNS and is involved in triggering external and internal factors—certain foods, toxins or odors, flickering lights, sleep deprivation, travel through time zones, menses. Migraine patients have decreased plasma and urinary melatonin. Melatonin deficit excessively stimulates the trigeminovascular system. Melatonin therapy helps migraineurs with delayed sleep phase syndrome and may resynchronize circadian rhythms to lifestyle, relieving triggers and symptoms. Melatonin produces headache in susceptible persons. Regular sleep, regular meals, exercise, avoidance of excessive stimulation and relaxation, and evasion of dietary triggers help reduce activation. Melatonin at 3-mg dose can reduce migraine frequency by over 50%; some patients get complete relief. The mechanism of action is not understood, but melatonin is anti-inflammatory in the brain, prevents translocation of nuclear factor kappa B to the nucleus, scavenges free radicals, inhibits CGRP-induced vasodilatation, increases inhibitory neurotransmitter activity, exerts direct analgesic effects, inhibits adhesion molecules, inhibits nitric oxide synthase, and has hypnotic effects from GABAergic upregulation.

- **Sex steroid hormones:** onset of migraine rises with menarche. Migraines are linked to menstruation in 60% of female migraineurs (menstrual migraine) and improve with pregnancy (sustained estrogens). Many women report that menstrual migraines are more disabling, longer-lasting, and less responsive to traditional treatment. Oral contraceptives can induce, improve, or exacerbate migraine. Incidence tends to decrease with advancing age but either regress or worsen during menopause. Headaches occur during and after simultaneous decline of both estrogen and progesterone. Falling estrogen levels are linked to menstrual migraine. Estrogens given premenstrually can delay migraine but not menstruation; progesterone given premenstrually delays menstruation but not migraine. Percutaneous estradiol gel perimenstrually reduces headaches. Estrogens increase number of progesterone, muscarinic, and serotonin ($5\text{-}HT_2$) receptors and decrease number of $5\text{-}HT_1$ and beta adrenergic receptors. Estrogens increase trigeminal mechanoreceptor receptive fields, increasing receptive input from trigeminal system. Progesterone blocks estrogen-induced increase in $5\text{-}HT_2$ receptors. Transdermal progesterone therapy can prevent migraine for some patients. Hysterectomy or oophorectomy has not been helpful. Although estrogen therapy can be effective for menstrual migraine, migraineurs (especially with aura) are at higher risk for ischemic strokes. Estrogen replacement, particularly with factors that promote coagulation, could be risky. Medicines or supplements used daily for a portion of the luteal phase have also prevented menstrual migraine (e.g., naproxen, Mg, and triptans).

Manual Medicine

- Modalities include spinal manipulation, massage, myofascial release, and craniosacral therapy. Practitioners identify loss of mobility in the cervical and thoracic spine in migraineurs.
- Many forms of physical medicine may shorten the duration and intensity of an episode, but literature support is sparse on prevention. Chiropractic spinal manipulation has demonstrated improvement in migraine frequency, duration, disability.
- Spinal manipulation has performed as favorably as amitriptyline for migraine prophylaxis.

- Tension headache may also respond favorably to these techniques, because of the structural component of muscular tension. The incidence of migraine in patients with temporomandibular joint (TMJ) dysfunction is similar to that in the general population, whereas the incidence of tension headache in patients with TMJ dysfunction is much higher than in the general population.
- Physical therapy is most effective when combined with other treatments (e.g., thermal biofeedback, relaxation training, and exercise).

Acupuncture

- Relieves migraine pain.
- Mechanism of relief is not endorphin mediated. Acupuncture increases endorphins in controls, but low levels of serum endorphins in migraine patients do not increase with treatment. Mechanism may be by normalization of serotonin levels.
- It is effective in relieving pain when it normalizes serotonin levels, but ineffective in relieving pain and raising serotonin in patients with very low serotonin. It offers some success reducing frequency of migraine attacks; 40% of patients experienced a 50% to 100% reduction in severity and frequency in one study; five treatments (over a period of 1 month) decreased recurrence in 45% of patients over a period of 6 months.

Biofeedback

- Ask patients about their emotional stressors to enhance your therapeutic relationship by sending a message of caring and validating effects of stress rather than dismissing symptoms as "just stress."
- Teach patients that stress management is a critical component of daily maintenance. Ask patients why they think they are experiencing their condition.
- Traditional peripheral biofeedback can effectively treat migraines. Thermal biofeedback uses hand temperature to learn that inducing relaxation response will raise hand temperature and facilitate other positive physiologic changes. Acquiring active control over the body may reduce headache frequency and severity. These techniques can be as effective as beta-blockers for prevention but without adverse effects.
- Biofeedback is costly and no more effective than simpler relaxation techniques in migraine and tension headache.

- Consider also cognitive behavioral therapy, neurolinguistic programming, hypnotherapy, transcutaneous electrical nerve stimulation (TENS), electromyographic biofeedback, massage, and laser therapy. Consider especially relaxation training, thermal biofeedback combined with relaxation training, electromyographic biofeedback, and cognitive behavioral therapy for prophylaxis. Neurofeedback, using electroencephalographic feedback to teach alteration of brainwave activity, has demonstrated efficacy sustained for 14.5 months after discontinuation of treatment.
- Exercise for 30 minutes three times a week can improve headache parameters. Pre-exercise beta-endorphin levels are inversely proportional to degree of improvement in postexercise headache parameters.
- Patient education is paramount to high-quality care. Patients experience greater reduction in headache frequency when provided educational materials—general migraine information, headache diary, instructions on range-of-motion stretching, and biofeedback tapes. Subjects who worry about impending migraines benefit from higher self-efficacy and coping skills.

THERAPEUTIC APPROACH

Migraine is a multifaceted disorder that may be a symptom rather than a disease. Determine which factors are responsible for each patient's migraine process. Identifying and avoiding precipitating factors reduce frequency and cumulative effect of initiators.

- **Identify problematic foods:** high incidence (80% to 90%) of food allergy or intolerance in migraine warrants 1 week of careful avoidance of all foods to which patient may be allergic or intolerant; follow a pure water fast or elemental diet. (Oligoantigenic diet may be used but is less desirable because allergens may be inadvertently included.) Avoid all other possible allergens (vitamin preparations, unnecessary drugs, herbs). Food-sensitive patients will exhibit strong exacerbation of symptoms early in the week, followed by almost total relief by the end of fast or modified diet. This sequence is caused by the addictive characteristics of reactive foods. When patient is symptom free, one new food is reintroduced (and eaten several times) daily, with symptoms carefully recorded. Some recommend reintroduction on 4-day cycle. Suspected foods (symptom onset ranges from

20 minutes to 2 weeks) are eliminated, and apparently safe foods are rotated through the 4-day cycle (*Textbook,* "Food Allergy Testing"). When symptom-free period of at least 6 months is established, 4-day rotation diet is no longer necessary.

- **Oligoantigenic diet:** effective in some patients, but a longer trial (4 to 8 weeks) is necessary, depending on frequency of episodes. Eliminate dairy, gluten, eggs, corn, chocolate, peanuts, coffee, black tea, soft drinks, alcohol, and processed foods. Food allergy immunoglobulin testing gives mixed results.
- **Optimize digestive function,** as needed.
- **Correct intestinal dysbiosis,** including *H. pylori.*
- **Reduce toxic overload** and support detoxification enzymes.
- **Diet:** eliminate food allergens. Use 4-day rotation diet until patient is symptom free for 6 months. Eliminate foods containing vasoactive amines and reintroduce carefully after symptoms are controlled. Eliminate alcohol, cheese, chocolate, citrus fruits, and shellfish. Reduce sources of arachidonic acid (land animal fats). Increase foods inhibiting platelet aggregation (olive and flaxseed oils, fish oils, garlic, onion).
- **Supplements:**
  — Mg: 250 to 800 mg q.d. in divided doses; titrate to symptoms and bowel tolerance
  — Vitamin B_6: 50 to 75 mg q.d., as a separate supplement, balanced with vitamin B complex
  — 5-HTP: 100 to 200 mg q.d. to b.i.d.
  — Vitamin B_2 (riboflavin): 400 mg q.d., balanced with vitamin B complex
  — CoQ10: 150 mg q.d.

Hormonal Therapies

- Trial of melatonin: 0.3 to 3 mg at bedtime
- Trial of estradiol, carefully individualized to clinical picture

Botanical Medicines

- *T. parthenium* (feverfew): 0.25 to 0.5 mg parthenolide b.i.d.
- *Z. officinale* (ginger): fresh ginger, approximately 10 g q.d. (6-mm slice); dried ginger, 500 mg q.i.d.; extract standardized to contain 20% of gingerol and shogaol, 100 to 200 mg t.i.d. for prevention and 200 mg every 2 hours (up to six times daily) in the treatment of an acute migraine
- *P. hybridus* (butterbur): 50 to 100 mg b.i.d. with meals.

Physical Medicine

- TENS to control secondary muscle spasm
- Acupuncture to balance meridians
- Biofeedback
- Guided imagery

Primary Classifications of Headache

Vascular Headache	Cluster Headache
• Migraine headache • Classic migraine • Common migraine • Complicated migraine • Variant migraine	• Episodic cluster • Chronic cluster • Chronic paroxysmal hemicrania

Miscellaneous Vascular Headaches

- Carotidynia
- Hypertension
- Exertional
- Hangover
- Toxins and drugs
- Occlusive vascular disease
- Nonvascular
- Tension headache
- Common tension headache
- Temporomandibular joint (TMJ) dysfunction
- Increased or decreased intracranial pressure
- Brain tumors
- Sinus infections
- Dental infections
- Inner or middle ear infections

Factors that Trigger Migraine Headaches

- Low serotonin levels
- Genetics
- Shunting of tryptophan into other pathways
- Foods
- Food allergies
- Histamine-releasing foods
- Histamine-containing foods
- Alcohol, especially red wine
- Chemicals
- Nitrates
- Monosodium glutamate (MSG)
- Nitroglycerin
- Withdrawal from caffeine or other drugs that constrict blood vessels
- Stress
- Emotional intensity: letdown, anger
- Hormones: menstruation, ovulation, birth control pills
- Too little or too much sleep
- Exhaustion
- Poor posture
- Muscle tension
- Weather: barometric pressure, sun exposure
- Glare or eyestrain

Foods that Most Commonly Induce Migraine Headaches

- Cow's milk
- wheat
- chocolate
- egg
- orange
- benzoic acid
- cheese
- tomato
- tartrazine
- rye
- rice
- fish
- grapes
- onion
- soy
- pork
- peanuts
- alcohol
- MSG
- walnuts
- beef
- tea
- coffee
- nuts
- goat's milk
- corn
- oats
- cane
- sugar
- yeast
- apple
- peach
- potato
- chicken
- banana
- strawberry
- melon
- carrot

Factors Involved with Histamine-Induced Headaches

Histamine Levels Increased By	Histamine Breakdown Inhibited By
• Histamine in alcoholic beverages (red wine)	• Vitamin B_6 antagonists
• Histamine in food	• Alcohol
• Histamine-releasing foods	• Drugs
• Food allergy	• Food additives (e.g., yellow dye No. 5, monosodium glutamate)
• Vitamin B_6 deficiency	• Vitamin C deficiency

Histamine Release Prevented By	Histamine Breakdown Promoted By
• Disodium cromoglycate	• Vitamin B_6
• Quercetin	• Vitamin C
• Antioxidants (e.g., vitamin C, vitamin E, selenium)	

Multiple Sclerosis

DIAGNOSTIC SUMMARY

- Episodic neurologic symptoms depending on the parts of the central nervous system (CNS) affected
- Typically occurs between 20 and 55 years of age
- Symptoms not consistent with a single neurologic lesion

GENERAL CONSIDERATIONS

- Multiple sclerosis (MS) is a CNS disease characterized by relapses and remissions, a variety of symptoms (depending on parts of the CNS are affected), and permanent disability. MS is the most common disabling neurologic disease of young and middle-aged adults in North America and Europe.
- MS is an inflammatory disorder of multifocal destruction of myelin sheaths (demyelination) and axons within the brain, spinal cord, and optic nerves. Areas of demyelination are termed *plaques.* Destruction of the myelin sheath around axons occurs with relative sparing of the axons, but axon damage also occurs. Macrophages and lymphocytes are present in active demyelination within plaques.
- Neurologic problems depend on location and severity of plaques.
- In 85% of cases, relapsing MS begins with a remitting course—relapses or attacks of a new problem, return of an old problem that had resolved, or worsening of preexisting symptoms. Relapses develop over a few days or weeks; improvement and stability then ensue, with an average of one relapse every 2 years. Between relapses the patient is clinically stable, but the effects of previous relapses are permanent. Relapses causing symptoms are the tip of the iceberg of disease activity. Asymptomatic new lesions appear within the brain five to 10 times more commonly than symptomatic lesions. Asymptomatic relapses cause permanent damage.
- Fifty percent of patients with relapsing-remitting MS enter a progressive phase (secondary progressive MS) 5 to 15 years after onset, characterized by steady worsening with or without

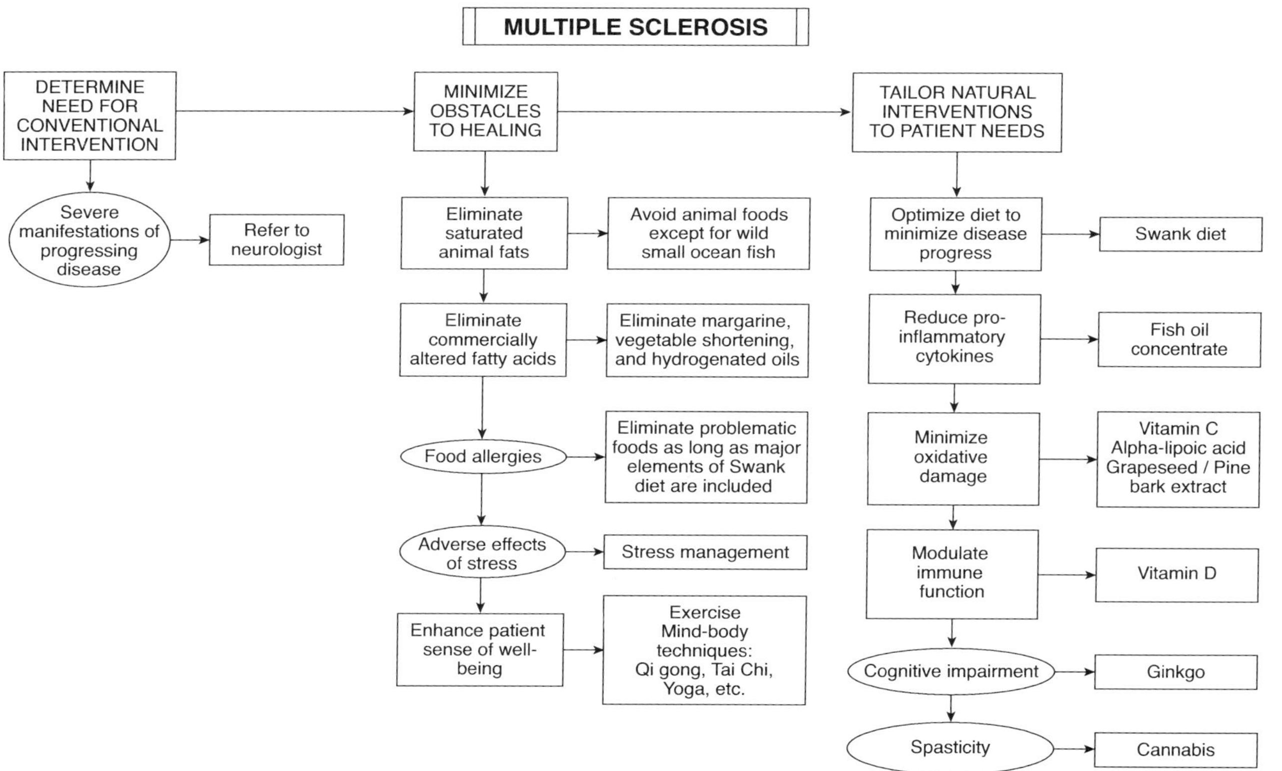
MULTIPLE SCLEROSIS
DETERMINE NEED FOR CONVENTIONAL INTERVENTION
Severe manifestations of progressing disease
Refer to neurologist
MINIMIZE OBSTACLES TO HEALING
Eliminate saturated animal fats
Avoid animal foods except for wild small ocean fish
Eliminate commercially altered fatty acids
Eliminate margarine, vegetable shortening, and hydrogenated oils
Food allergies
Eliminate problematic foods as long as major elements of Swank diet are included
Adverse effects of stress
Stress management
Enhance patient sense of well-being
Exercise
Mind-body techniques:
Qi gong, Tai Chi, Yoga, etc.
TAILOR NATURAL INTERVENTIONS TO PATIENT NEEDS
Optimize diet to minimize disease progress
Swank diet
Reduce pro-inflammatory cytokines
Fish oil concentrate
Minimize oxidative damage
Vitamin C
Alpha-lipoic acid
Grapeseed / Pine bark extract
Modulate immune function
Vitamin D
Cognitive impairment
Ginkgo
Spasticity
Cannabis

relapses. Fifteen percent of patients have progressive worsening from disease onset (primary progressive MS).
- MS is rarely fatal but is disabling; one third of patients lose the ability to walk 15 to 20 years after onset.
- Benign forms (up to 15% of patients) never develop complete disability from MS but develop varying degrees of permanent disability.

Symptoms of Multiple Sclerosis and Their Neurologic Causes

Symptoms	Causes
Weakness, numbness, and tingling in legs and arms; stiffness in legs	Spinal cord lesions
Urinary urgency, retention, and incontinence and recurrent infections	Spinal cord lesions
Constipation	Spinal cord lesions; diet
Sexual dysfunction	Spinal cord lesions
Blurred vision and blindness	Optic nerve lesions
Double vision	Brainstem lesions
Imbalance	Spinal cord and cerebellar lesions
Tremor of arms	Cerebellar lesions
Impaired memory and concentration	Cerebral lesions
Fatigue	Effects of inflammatory cytokines on neuronal function; nerve fiber fatigability resulting from demyelination
Heat sensitivity	Sensitivity of demyelinations to elevations in body temperature
Depression and other mood changes	Cerebral lesions and changes; disorders in neurotransmitters

Epidemiology

- Incidence: one person per 1000 in the United States, Canada, and Northern Europe.
- Begins typically between ages 20 and 55 years but may occur at any age.
- Women are more commonly affected than men; 60% of cases are in women.
- Racial influence: most common among whites of Northern European descent; rare among Asians and black Africans;

relatively common among African Americans. Genetic predisposition is linked to risk of MS.
- Geographic distribution: highest prevalence in higher latitudes of northern and southern hemispheres in persons who lived their first two decades of life there. Environmental exposure in first two decades of life influences risk.

Pathogenesis

- Pathologic features: demyelination of axons and, to a lesser extent, loss of axons.
- T lymphocytes, macrophages, and plasma cells cause destruction during development of acute plaques.
- Subset of T lymphocytes initiates acute lesions, recognizes antigens within CNS, becomes activated, and initiates inflammatory cascade that injures myelin and axons.
- Mediators of tissue damage: macrophages releasing soluble inflammatory mediators, cytokines, and free radicals or stripping myelin from axon sheath. Activated T cells can release cytokines. Antimyelin antibodies can damage myelin by initiating complement cascade or facilitating macrophage phagocytosis of myelin.
- Disease process is "turned off" by apoptosis of initiating T cells and by recruitment of regulatory T cells into the CNS.

Role of Free Radicals

- Oxygen and nitrogen free radicals are implicated in myelin and axon damage and upregulation of proinflammatory tumor necrosis factor-alpha (TNF-α), inducible nitric oxide, and nuclear transcription factor kappa B.
- They are also implicated in activating matrix metalloproteinase (MMP), a mediator of T-lymphocyte trafficking into CNS.
- Metabolites of oxidative and nitrosative stress are elevated in the cerebrospinal fluid (CSF) of patients with MS, who also have decreased glutathione and increased oxidized glutathione in the CSF. A specific genotype for glutathione *S*-transferase is linked to an increased number of active lesions and impaired ability to detoxify oxidized lipids and DNA.

ETIOLOGY

- Why people develop MS remains uncertain. Genes and the environment influence risk.

Genes

- Having a first-order relative (parent or sibling) increases risk fivefold to tenfold.
- Twins in which one has MS: for nonidentical twins, chances of the second twin having MS are 1% to 2% (similar to nontwin siblings). For identical twins, the chance of the second twin having MS is 25%.
- Ten to 15 different genes affect risk, including human leukocyte antigen (HLA)-*DR2* among northern Europeans.

Viruses

- Viruses and microbial agents might be linked to increased risk of MS.
- Evidence for viral involvement: inflammatory nature of MS and environmental effect on MS, suggesting the possibility of an infectious cause.
- There is no convincing evidence linking any infectious agent to MS. However, the lack of evidence does not exclude infectious causality.

Environment: Geographic and Seasonal Influences

- **Latitude:** mixed results, and assessment is confounded by migration, lifestyle, biologic influences, and social factors. However, MS is more prevalent in latitudes far from the Equator (high risk) and less prevalent in the Tropics (low risk). People who move from low-risk to high-risk areas before age 15 acquire higher risk. Those who make the same move after adolescence retain a lower risk. Early sunlight exposure, correlated to serum vitamin D, may influence risk.
- **Season of birth:** lower risk for births occurring after summer, and higher risk for births occurring after winter. Suggestion: maternal vitamin D during the third trimester of pregnancy may influence MS risk—lower risk when maternal vitamin D is high (summer), and higher when vitamin D is low (winter).
- **Sunlight:** Sun exposure and vitamin D levels at a young age may influence MS risk.

Diet

- One review study found risk of MS to be correlated with consumption of animal fat, animal protein, and meat from nonmarine mammals.

- Another study found that intake of plant omega-3 alpha-linolenic acid (ALA), but not fish oil omega-3s (e.g., docosahexaenoic acid [DHA]), was associated with a lower risk for MS.
- No relation between intake of fruits and vegetables and risk of MS has been found.
- A protective effect of cereals and breads, vegetable protein, dietary fiber, vitamin C, thiamin, riboflavin, calcium, and potassium for all cases and fish in cases in women only has been identified.

DIAGNOSTIC CONSIDERATIONS

- Only neurologists have sufficient training and experience to make an accurate diagnosis.
- Diagnosis of MS rests on objective demonstration of two or more areas of demyelination in CNS occurring at more than one time point. It is not solely based on patient's symptoms.
- Evidence: neurologic examination, magnetic resonance imaging (MRI) of brain and spinal cord as well as electrophysiologic tests, called *evoked potentials,* that assess visual, auditory, and somatosensory pathways.
- CSF examination for plasma cells producing immunoglobulins—qualitative (oligoclonal bands) and quantitative (total immunoglobulin G [IgG], IgG index, and IgG synthesis rate) changes.
- Rule out other disorders: unusual causes of cerebrovascular disease; vitamin B_{12} deficiency; spinal cord compression from tumors, herniated disks, or spinal canal stenosis; vascular malformations of spinal cord; Lyme disease.
- MRI allows diagnosis at early stages and helps exclude other diseases.

THERAPEUTIC CONSIDERATIONS

Conventional Treatments

- Medicines that help decrease disease activity in relapsing-remitting MS: human recombinant interferon-beta (Avonex, Betaseron, and Rebif) and glatiramer acetate (Copaxone), a random polymer of four amino acids that stimulates protective T cells; a monoclonal antibody against alpha-4-integrin (Tysabri); fingolimod (Gilenya), the only oral agent that prevents activated lymphocytes from entering the CNS by sequestration in lymph

nodes; and a chemotherapy agent (Novantrone). These agents decrease relapse rate by one third, decrease new lesion formation in the brain, and decrease risk of permanent neurologic disability. Corticosteroids, such as methylprednisolone, in high doses can decrease duration of relapses but do not affect degree of eventual recovery from relapses.
- Immunosuppressant (chemotherapy agent) mitoxantrone (Novantrone) decreases MS activity in rapidly progressing forms of MS.
- Monoclonal antibody (Tysabri) that prevents inflammatory cells from entering the CNS decreases rate of MS exacerbations and reduces disease activity (MRI lesions).
- Fingolimod (Gilenya) reduces CNS inflammation and axonal damage by retaining lymphocytes in lymph nodes to inhibit entry into CNS. Fingolimod reduces relapse rates by 50%, decreases disease progression, and decreases disease activity (MRI lesions). Conventional medicines can reduce disease activity in relapsing-remitting MS, but they have limitations: only modest effect on prolonging time to disability, high monetary cost, and side effects (e.g., injection site reactions, neutralizing antibodies for interferon-beta; bradycardia, arrhythmia for fingolimod).

Natural Medicine

Interventions used in combination with appropriate allopathic therapies:
- Dietary therapy
- Nutritional supplements
- Exercise
- Stress management

Diet Therapy

Dr. Roy Swank Low-Saturated-Fat Diet

- Diet low in saturated fats over a long period can retard disease process, reduce number of attacks, and decrease mortality rate. A low-fat diet supplemented with cod liver oil decreased the incidence of MS in populations eating diets low in animal fats and high in cold-water fish.
  - Saturated fat intake: below 15 g q.d.
  - Unsaturated fat intake: 20 to 50 g q.d.
  - No red meat for first year (including dark meat of turkey and chicken); only 3 oz of red meat per week thereafter.

— White meat poultry, fish, and shellfish in any amounts if low in saturated fats
— Eliminate dairy containing 1% butterfat or more
— 1 tsp or 4 capsules nonconcentrated cod liver oil; one multiple vitamin-mineral

- Benefits: anti-inflammatory and neuron membrane–stabilizing effects of omega-3 fatty acids eicosapentaenoic acid (EPA) and DHA.
- Recent uncontrolled open-label study diet for newly diagnosed relapsing-remitting MS: low in saturated fats; increased intake of fish plus fish oil, vitamin B complex, and vitamin C; reduced intake of sugar, coffee, tea, and alcohol; no smoking. Over a 2-year period, plasma omega-3 increased and plasma omega-6 decreased, with a reduction in both relapse rates and disability.
- A diet low in saturated fats with fish oil and olive oil supplementation might promote better physical and mental health for people with MS.

Nutritional Supplements

Omega-3 Fatty Acids

- "Marine lipids" EPA and DHA: MS patients have increased proinflammatory cytokines, TNF-α, interferon-gamma (IFN-γ), and interleukin-2 (IL-2), mediators of immunopathogenesis of MS linked to disease activity in peripheral blood, CSF, and brain lesions.
- MMPs are also implicated. These proteases aid in remodeling extracellular matrix, basement membrane, and other tissues by digesting collagen components. MMPs play a role in transmigration of inflammatory cells into the CNS by disrupting the blood-brain barrier. MS patients have elevated serum levels of MMP-9. Fish oil induces reduction in MMP-9 secreted from unstimulated immune cells. Dose: 8 g/day (providing 2.9 g EPA and 1.9 g DHA).
- Omega-3s decrease mRNA and protein levels of cytokines: TNF-α, IFN-γ, IL-1, IL-2, and vascular cell adhesion molecule 1. Fish oil supplements decrease proinflammatory cytokines participating in pathogenesis of MS in patients and healthy control subjects. Fish oil decreases gene expression and protein levels of proinflammatory cytokines and MMPs.
- Omega-3s help treat depression in MS. Inflammatory cytokines are correlated with depression in MS. Gene expression levels of

TNF-α and IFN-γ positively correlate with scores on depression inventory (high score indicating greater depression) in MS patients during relapses. Depression is common in MS. Ethyl-EPA significantly improves primary depression in non-MS patients. Dose: 1 to 4 g q.d. Omega-3 supplementation might help in conjunction with counseling and, when indicated, antidepressant drugs.

Omega-6 Fatty Acids

- Supplementing omega-6 increased transforming growth factor beta 1 (TGF-β1) in peripheral blood mononuclear cells of healthy subjects. TGF-β1 is an anti-inflammatory cytokine that might be beneficial for MS. Animal study models of MS report that supplementing linoleic acid decreases severity of disease and reduces inflammation in the CNS.
- MS patients supplemented with linoleic acid had a smaller increase in disability and reduced severity and duration of relapses compared with patients supplemented with olive oil. Dose: sunflower seed oil emulsion at sufficient dose to provide daily 17.2 g linoleic acid.
- Evening primrose oil (EPO) contains omega-6 gamma-linoleic acid (GLA). GLA might be more effective than linoleic acid because of easier incorporation into brain lipids and greater effect on immune function. However, EPO contains low levels of GLA and is expensive; EPO also showed no benefit in a clinical trial. EPO is not recommended for MS.

Vitamin D

- Low vitamin D intake and low serum vitamin D may increase risk of MS. Among MS patients, 84% are vitamin D deficient. Vitamin D decreases immune cell–mediated inflammation and prevents disease. Vitamin D may affect the ability of inflammatory cells to enter the CNS. Oral calcitriol at a target dose of 2.5 mcg/dL is safe and tolerable for up to a year of supplementation.
- Higher circulating levels of vitamin D in women are correlated with lower MS-related disability. In relapsing-remitting MS patients, there is a positive correlation between serum vitamin D levels and levels of anti-inflammatory cytokine IL-4.
- Vitamin D may benefit MS patients, but 30% to 50% of the general population may be deficient in vitamin D. Assess serum levels of vitamin D and treat deficiency in MS.

Antioxidants

- **Alpha-lipoic acid:** alpha-lipoic acid and its reduced form, dihydrolipoic acid (DHLA), are potent antioxidants with multiple modes of action. Alpha-lipoic acid or DHLA regenerates other antioxidants (glutathione peroxidase [GSH-Px], vitamins C and E), scavenges reactive oxygen species, repairs oxidative damage, and chelates oxidizing metallic ions. DHLA restores reduced GSH. Alpha-lipoic acid is absorbed in the diet and synthesized de novo, is converted intracellularly to DHLA, and crosses the blood-brain barrier. Both alpha-lipoic acid and DHLA are present in extracellular and intracellular environments. At doses of 10 to 100 mg/kg/day, alpha-lipoic acid suppressed an animal model of MS by inhibiting T-lymphocyte trafficking into the spinal cord.
- Alpha-lipoic acid given at 600 mg b.i.d. to relapsing-remitting MS patients was barely measurable in serum; but alpha-lipoic acid given at 1200 mg once daily showed much higher serum levels. Higher alpha-lipoic acid serum levels was associated with lower MMP-9 levels and lower soluble intercellular adhesion molecule 1 (ICAM-1) levels. Thus alpha-lipoic acid is linked to increased immunomodulatory activity that may benefit MS patients.

Botanical Medicines

- ***Ginkgo biloba* (GB):** cognitive impairment affects 40% to 50% of MS patients, and currently there are no effective conventional therapies. GB has a modest effect in slowing progressive cognitive dysfunction in MS, but benefits for improving cognitive impairment and dementia are not predictable. MS patients receiving GB have significantly improved performance on the Stroop test (a measure of attention and executive function) and improved subjective cognitive complaint deficits. GB extract is safe and well tolerated in MS patients. GB in people with dementia displays mixed results.
- **Cannabis:** the major psychoactive constituent is delta-9-tetrahydrocannabinol (THC). THC binds to cannabinoid receptors (CBs) in the CNS and acts as a partial agonist to both CB_1 and CB_2 receptors. Cannabidiol (CBD) is a nonpsychoactive constituent and the major constituent in cannabis. It is thought to decrease the clearance of THC by affecting liver metabolism. It binds to both CB_1 and CB_2 receptors in the CNS, with a higher affinity to the CB_2 receptor. A combination of THC and CBD (Marinol), given for spasticity in MS, is well tolerated and improves patient self-reports of spasticity, although objective measures for spasticity

(e.g., Ashworth score) do not show significant improvement. Side effects are mild. Researchers conclude that there is significant improvement in patient-reported spasticity with the combination of THC and CBD. Unlike dietary supplements discussed, Marinol is a controlled substance and requires a prescription in the United States.

OTHER CONSIDERATIONS

- **Exercise:** in the past, MS patients were advised not to exercise because increased body temperature and nerve fiber fatigue were thought to induce transient symptomatic worsening without long-term benefit. Research shows that regular exercise benefits MS patients. Exercise improved patients' reports of fatigue, quality of life, well-being, and walking ability.
- **Stress:** worsens MS symptoms and triggers exacerbation. Increased conflicts and disruptions in routine are followed by increased risk of developing new brain lesions 8 weeks later. However, stress at a point in time does not reliably predict clinical exacerbations in individual patients. Distraction moderates effect of stress on new lesions. Emotional preoccupation is linked to increased relation between stress and new lesions. Coping can moderate effect of stress on MS disease activity. Stress management training decreases anxiety and somatization. Patients are less preoccupied with physical symptoms after undergoing stress management training. Approaches to stress management include exercise, yoga, tai chi, prayer, meditation, massage therapy. Meditation lowers stress and improves symptoms in patients with chronic illnesses. Experienced meditators have enhanced biochemical and physiologic functioning compared with those who do not meditate.
- **Food allergy:** although no convincing evidence exists that gluten-free or allergy elimination diets are beneficial in MS, food allergens should be eliminated as long as other dietary measures are also included (e.g., low-fat diet, Swank diet).
- **Mind-body interventions:** few scientific studies have evaluated mind-body interventions (e.g., yoga, meditation, and prayer) in MS. Mind-body techniques to reduce stress in cancer patients are effective in decreasing stress, improving quality of life, and improving sleep. Training in principles of "mindfulness of movement" from tai chi and qi gong in MS patients has improved self-reported measures of MS-related symptoms. Tai chi

training twice weekly has improved walking speed, hamstring flexibility, and subjective reports of well-being and quality of life. Yoga has improved quality of life and physical measures. Mind-body interventions can reduce stress, improve fatigue, and improve quality of life in MS.

THERAPEUTIC APPROACH

Diet, nutritional supplementation, exercise, and stress reduction comprise the natural medicine approach to MS. This approach also can be used in conjunction with allopathic therapies.

Diet

Swank's dietary protocol is recommended:

- 15 g or less of saturated fat intake per day
- A daily unsaturated fat intake between 20 and 50 g
- No red meat consumption for the first year (including the dark meat of turkey and chicken); after the first year, only 3 oz of red meat per week
- White-meat poultry, fish, and shellfish are permissible in any amounts as long as they contain low levels of saturated fats
- Elimination of dairy products containing 1% butterfat or more

Although the Swank diet calls for 1 to 4 capsules of nonconcentrated cod liver oil, substitute fish oil concentrate (see section on nutritional supplements). Emphasize fresh whole plant foods; reduce or avoid animal foods (except small wild cold-water fish).

Nutritional Supplements

- **Multiple vitamin-mineral supplement**
- **Fish oil concentrate:** 3000 mg EPA plus DHA q.d.
- **Vitamin E (mixed tocopherols):** 800 international units (IU) q.d.
- **Vitamin C:** 500 to 1000 mg q.d.
- **Vitamin D_3:** 2000 to 8000 IU q.d. with the goal of achieving an ideal range of 50 to 80 ng/mL of serum 25-(OH)D_3
- **Alpha-lipoic acid:** 600 to 1200 mg once daily with meal.

Choose one of the following:

- **Grapeseed extract** (more than 95% procyanidolic oligomers): 150 to 300 mg q.d.
- **Pine bark extract** (more than 90% procyanidolic oligomers): 150 to 300 mg q.d.
- **Proteolytic enzymes** (e.g., mixed enzyme preparations or pancreatin (8× to 10× USP), 350 to 750 mg between meals t.i.d.; or

bromelain, 250 to 750 mg (1800 to 2000 MCU) between meals t.i.d.

Botanical Medicine

- **GB extract** (24% *Ginkgo* flavon glycosides, 6% terpenoids): 120 to 160 mg t.i.d. for patients with cognitive impairment

Exercise and Stress Management

- **Exercise:** type and amount tailored for patient. Mild to moderate exercise for at least 30 minutes, three times per week. Types: walking, stretching, bicycling, low-impact aerobics, stationary bicycle, swimming or water aerobics, yoga, tai chi.
- **Stress management:** tailored for patient. Stress reduction therapies recommended for MS: exercise, meditation, deep breathing or breath exercises, prayer.

Obesity

DIAGNOSTIC SUMMARY

- Body mass index (BMI) above 30
- Body fat percentage above 30% for women and above 25% for men

GENERAL CONSIDERATIONS

- Obesity is a major contributor to mortality risk and morbidity, having surpassed smoking as the number one cause of premature death. Definition: excessive body fat distinguished from being overweight (excess body weight relative to height). A muscular athlete may be overweight but have a low body fat percentage. Body weight alone is not an index of obesity. BMI is the standard for classifying body composition. BMI correlates well to total body fat.

BMI calculation: BMI = (pounds × 703)/square inches (height)

Metric: BMI = kilograms/square meters (height)

Morbidity Associated with Increased Risk from Obesity

- **Cardiovascular system:** angina, atherosclerosis, congestive heart failure, deep vein thrombosis, heart attack, hypertension, high cholesterol, pulmonary embolism, stroke
- **Dermatology:** cellulitis, hirsutism, intertrigo, lymphedema, stretch marks
- **Endocrinology and reproduction:** complications during pregnancy, diabetes mellitus (DM), infertility, menstrual disorders, intrauterine fetal death, polycystic ovary syndrome
- **Gastrointestinal (GI) system:** gastroesophageal reflux disease, cholelithiasis, fatty liver disease
- **Neurology:** carpal tunnel syndrome, dementia, idiopathic conditions, intracranial hypertension, migraine headaches, multiple sclerosis

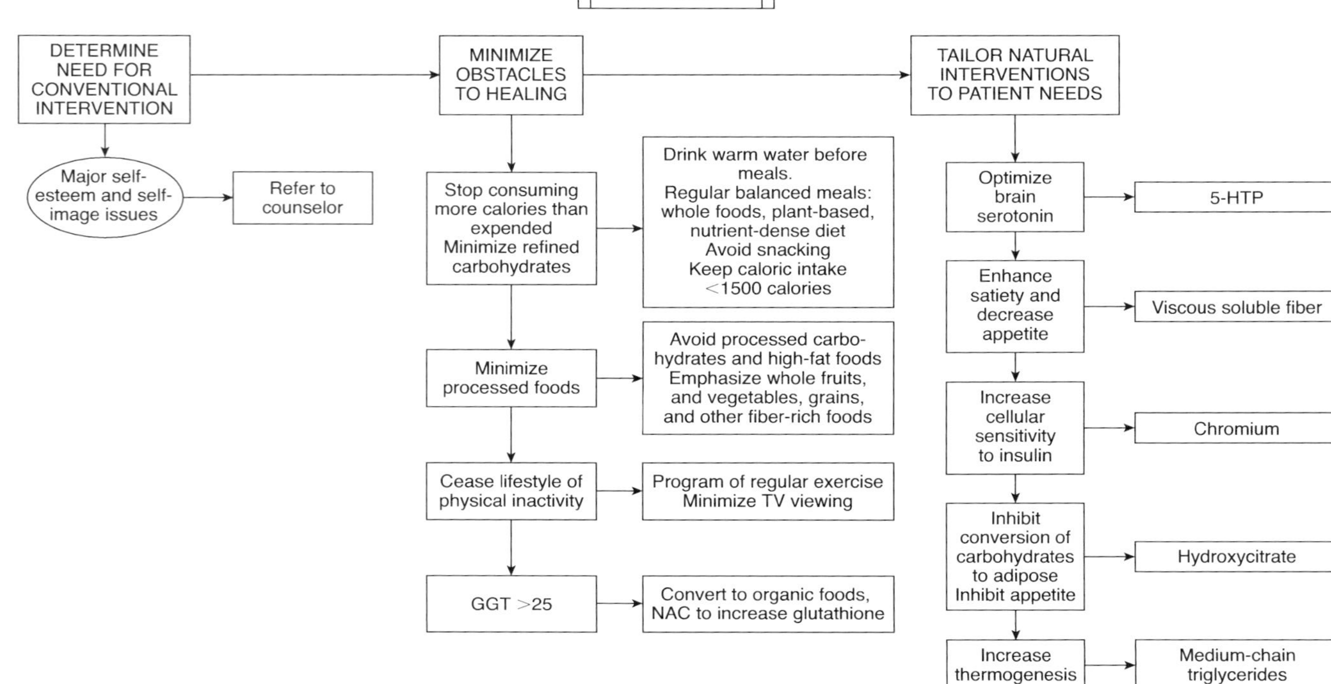
OBESITY
DETERMINE NEED FOR CONVENTIONAL INTERVENTION
Major self-esteem and self-image issues
Refer to counselor
MINIMIZE OBSTACLES TO HEALING
Stop consuming more calories than expended
Minimize refined carbohydrates
Drink warm water before meals.
Regular balanced meals: whole foods, plant-based, nutrient-dense diet
Avoid snacking
Keep caloric intake <1500 calories
Minimize processed foods
Avoid processed carbohydrates and high-fat foods
Emphasize whole fruits, and vegetables, grains, and other fiber-rich foods
Cease lifestyle of physical inactivity
Program of regular exercise
Minimize TV viewing
GGT >25
Convert to organic foods, NAC to increase glutathione
TAILOR NATURAL INTERVENTIONS TO PATIENT NEEDS
Optimize brain serotonin
5-HTP
Enhance satiety and decrease appetite
Viscous soluble fiber
Increase cellular sensitivity to insulin
Chromium
Inhibit conversion of carbohydrates to adipose
Inhibit appetite
Hydroxycitrate
Increase thermogenesis
Medium-chain triglycerides

- **Oncology:** cancer
- **Psychiatry:** depression, social stigmatization
- **Respiratory:** asthma, obstructive sleep apnea
- **Rheumatology and orthopedics:** chronic low back pain, gout, osteoarthritis
- **Urology and nephrology:** chronic renal failure, erectile dysfunction, hypogonadism, urinary incontinence

Classification of Body Mass Index

Underweight	<18.5
Normal	18.5-24.9
Overweight	24.9-29.9
Obesity	30.0-39.9
Extreme obesity	>40.0

Height and weight indexes are still used to determine obesity; tables of desirable weights for height provided by the Metropolitan Life Insurance Company are criticized for three shortcomings, as follows:

- Stated weight ranges merely reflect weights of those with lowest mortality rate of insured persons, which may not reflect U.S. population.
- Weight ranges for lowest mortality rate do not necessarily reflect optimal healthy weight for height.
- Standard values make assessing degree of obesity difficult; a person within proper weight range may have excess fat and lower than optimal lean body mass (LBM), and a person with increased musculature may be "overweight" despite low body fat percentage.

Prevalence

- Obese persons have a 5- to 7-year shorter life expectancy, with greater relative risk for mortality associated with greater degree of obesity. Most of the risk is from cardiovascular causes: type 2 diabetes mellitus (T2DM), elevated cholesterol, hypertension, and atherosclerosis.
- Determination of body composition: obesity is defined as body fat percentage above 30% for women and above 25% for men. Indirect methods of measurement must be used.

- Visual observation: qualitative analysis of obesity. Classifying by body types (somatotyping) is the physical anthropologic classification of physique based on body size and proportion.
  - **Endomorph:** relatively large body, short arms and legs
  - **Mesomorph:** large muscular chest that dominates abdomen, prominent bony joints
  - **Ectomorph:** relatively small frame (slender, delicate bone structure), long arms and legs

Endomorphs are at greatest risk for obesity; mesomorphs are at moderate risk, and ectomorphs are extremely unlikely to develop obesity.

- Distribution of body fat: gynecoid (female) and android (male). See the section on the types of obesity.
- Skinfold or fat fold thickness: measuring thickness of subcutaneous fat (skinfold or fat fold thickness) with skinfold calipers at several sites to improve accuracy—triceps, biceps, subscapular, suprailiac skinfolds. Limitations: inability to control intersubject and intrasubject variation in skinfold compressibility; inability to palpate fat-muscle interface; impossibility of obtaining interpretable measurements on very obese persons; interobserver variability; errors from use of different types of calipers. Skinfold measurements give easiest and least expensive method for estimating fat percentage. More precise tools: bioelectrical impedance, ultrasound, total body electrical conductivity, hydrostatic weighing.

Measurement of Body Density

- Quantitative measure of body fat determined from specific gravity by measuring different weights of body in and out of water. Weigh patient under water and out of water, taking into account residual volume of lungs. Factual basis: fat is lighter than water; other tissues are heavier than water. This is the gold standard of body composition determination. Limitation of hydrostatic weighing: requires subject cooperation to exhale completely and then submerge completely underwater up to 10 times—impossible for elderly, ill, or hospitalized patients.
- Sophisticated body composition analysis has replaced hydrostatic weighing procedure, but many experts still consider it to be the gold standard. However, dual-energy x-ray absorptiometry (DXA) is becoming the new gold standard: it provides greater precision with only one measurement and shows exactly where fat is distributed. DXA divides the body into total body mineral, fat-free soft (lean) mass, and fat tissue mass. DXA uses

a whole-body scanner with two low-dose x-ray beams from different sources reading bone and soft tissue mass simultaneously.

- Bioelectrical impedance: measures conduction of applied electrical current through body tissues. In biologic structures, constant low-level alternating current (AC) results in impedance to flow of current that is frequency dependent, according to type of tissue. Fluids act as electrical conductors; cell membranes act as electrical condensers. At low frequencies (1 kHz), current mainly passes through extracellular fluids; at higher frequencies (500 to 800 kHz), it penetrates intracellular and extracellular fluids. Fat-free mass has greater conductivity than fat does, explaining the strong relation between conductance and LBM. This method is safe, noninvasive, and rapid. Home scales with bioelectrical impedance are available for $50 to $200.

Types of Obesity

Categories are based on size and number of fat cells and how fat is distributed in the body (e.g., abdomen versus hips).

- **Hyperplastic obesity:** increased number of fat cells throughout body; dependent on the diet of the mother during pregnancy and on early infant nutrition. Excess calories during early stages of development increase number of fat cells for life. Hyperplastic obesity begins in childhood and is linked to fewer serious health effects.
- **Hypertrophic obesity:** increased size of fat cells; linked to DM, heart disease, hypertension. Fat distribution is around waist, considered male patterned or android. Android obesity is a waist larger than hips. In female-patterned or gynecoid obesity, the hips are larger. Waist/hip ratio: measure waist circumference (WC) one half inch above navel; measure hip circumference (HC) at the greatest protrusion of buttocks. Divide WC by HC. Ratio greater than 1.0 for men and greater than 0.8 for women is linked to metabolic syndrome (syndrome X) and increases risk of T2DM, hypertension, coronary heart disease, stroke, and gout.
- **Hyperplastic-hypertrophic obesity:** increase in number and size of fat cells.

CAUSES OF OBESITY

- Tendency to be overweight is inherited. However, even high-risk persons can avoid obesity; dietary and lifestyle factors (physical inactivity) are responsible.

- Psychological factors: insensitivity to internal signals for hunger and satiety plus extreme sensitivity to external stimuli (sight, smell, taste), increasing appetite. Watching television: linked to onset of obesity with dose-related effect; linked to obesity in children and smoking and hypercholesterolemia in adolescence and adulthood. Time spent watching television is positively linked to risk of obesity and T2DM. Each 2-hour increment in television watching daily is linked to a 23% increase in obesity and 14% increase in risk of DM. Each 2-hour increment in sitting at work daily is linked to a 5% increase in obesity and 7% increase in DM. Physiologic effects of watching television: reducing physical activity and lowering resting (basal) metabolic rate to a level during trance states.

Physiologic Factors

- **Theory:** obese persons are extremely sensitive to specific internal cues for dysfunctional appetite control because of genetic, dietary, and lifestyle factors. Central issue: insulin resistance as a conditioned reaction to a high-glycemic diet. Vicious positive feedback cycle of obesity: insulin resistance, central adiposity, alterations in adipokine secretion by adipocytes and gut-derived hormones, impaired diet-induced thermogenesis, and low brain serotonin. Obesity is an adaptive physiologic response.
- **"Set point":** weight that a body tries to maintain by regulating food and calories consumed. Each person has programmed set point weight. Fat cells may control set point: when enlarged fat cells in obese persons become smaller, either they send messages to brain to eat or they block action of appetite-suppressing compounds (leptin). Signals are too strong to ignore indefinitely, causing rebound overeating and set point at a higher level, increasing difficulty for weight loss—known as a *ratchet effect* or *yo-yo dieting.* Key to overcoming fat cells' set point: increase sensitivity of fat cells to insulin by exercise, specially designed diet, and key nutritional supplements. Diet that does not improve insulin sensitivity will fail to provide long-term results.
- **Fat cell engorgement:** when fat cells (especially in the abdomen) become full of fat, they secrete resistin, leptin, tumor necrosis factor, and free fatty acids that dampen the effect of insulin, impair glucose use in skeletal muscle, and promote liver gluconeogenesis. Increased number and size of fat cells induce reduced secretion of compounds that promote insulin action—adiponectin (novel protein produced by fat cells). Adiponectin improves

insulin sensitivity, is anti-inflammatory, lowers triglycerides, and blocks development of atherosclerosis. Fat cells severely stress blood sugar control and promote a complication of DM—atherosclerosis. Adipose tissue is now considered part of the endocrine system.

- **Adiponectin and gut-derived hormone alterations:** obese persons are more sensitive to internal signals to eat. Appetite, for human survival during famine, is extremely biased toward weight gain. People who survived famines were more adept at storing fat with a built-in tendency to overeat. Normal physiologic processes that curb appetite must be advanced. The hypothalamus controls appetite and eating. Adipokines (e.g., leptin, triggering appetite control) originate in the GI tract. GI nerve signals feed back to the central nervous system; gut-derived hormones and peptides (neuropeptide Y, ghrelin, cholecystokinin [CCK]). Peptide YY (PYY) 3-36 dramatically reduce appetite in obese and normal persons. Stomach-derived hormone ghrelin increases appetite, with highest levels when the stomach is empty and during calorie restriction. Obese persons have elevated ghrelin, which rises during dieting. Gastroplasty may succeed because of reduced ghrelin production.
- **Human compensatory actions:** may negate the effect of appetite regulators. A perfect agent should increase insulin sensitivity, reduce factors that increase appetite, and increase factors that decrease appetite. Highly viscous dietary fiber blends may be useful.
- **Gut-derived appetite regulators:** main hormones inhibiting food intake are CCK, glucagon-like peptide 1 (GLP-1), oxyntomodulin (OXM), and PYY. Hormonal stimulators of appetite are ghrelin and orexin A. Enteroendocrine cell function is regulated by the presence or absence of viscous dietary fiber; the main target for these neurotransmitters is vagal afferent neurons, and the appetite-inhibiting effects of CCK are enhanced by the mechanical effects of dietary fiber (gastric distention). Gut-derived appetite regulators include the following:
  - **CCK:** controls gastric emptying and delivery of enzymes from the pancreas. It inhibits appetite, and its effect is enhanced with moderate gastric distention triggering gastric mechanoreceptors. Viscous dietary fiber increases CCK secretion.
  - **GLP-1:** distal intestinal peptide GLP (7-36)-1 is derived from different regions of glucagon precursor. It inhibits food intake, decreases sensations of hunger, and inhibits plasma

ghrelin. Secretion of GLP-1 is influenced by food intake, but specifics are unknown.

— **OXM:** released from gut postprandially in proportion to food volume and energy content. OXM is elevated during anorexia and suppresses ghrelin. Elevated OXM is linked to GI disorders and may contribute to anorexia.

— **PYY:** secreted by enteroendocrine cells of the ileum and colon; the related compound pancreatic polypeptide is secreted by the pancreas. Plasma PYY in obese subjects, basal and postprandial, is subnormal. PYY inhibits food intake, with long-term action. Viscous dietary fiber raises PYY.

— **Ghrelin:** peptide from X cells in stomach lining. It makes the stomach "rumble" and is a powerful appetite stimulator. Plasma ghrelin is depressed in anorexia nervosa and elevated in obesity. Ghrelin levels decline on feeding, especially fiber. Effect is mediated by insulin; insulin resistance is associated with higher ghrelin levels.

— **Orexin A:** peptide in hypothalamus, enteric neurons, and gut endocrine cells (enterochromaffin cells). It stimulates appetite and inhibits CCK-stimulated excitation of vagal afferent fibers (negating appetite-suppressing effect of CCK). Plasma orexin A increases with fasting. It may contribute to overeating during or immediately after a meal by suppressing satiety signaling by CCK.

Diet-Induced Thermogenesis

- In lean persons, a meal stimulates up to a 40% increase in diet-induced thermogenesis; overweight persons display up to a 10% increase. In the obese, food energy is stored, not converted to heat.
- Insulin insensitivity contributes to decreased thermogenesis. Enhancing insulin sensitivity may restore thermogenesis and normal set point. Even after weight loss, obesity-prone persons still have decreased diet-induced thermogenesis.
- Brown fat cells: contain multiple fat storage compartments localizing triglycerides into smaller droplets surrounding numerous mitochondria. Blood vessel network and density of mitochondria give the brown color and increased capacity to metabolize fats. Brown fat does not metabolize fatty acids to adenosine triphosphate efficiently, causing increased heat production. Lean people may have a higher ratio of brown fat to white fat than overweight people have. The amount of brown fat in human

beings is extremely small (0.5% to 5% of body weight). It has a profound effect on thermogenesis; just 1 oz of brown fat (0.1% of body weight) makes the difference between having a stable body weight or adding an extra 10 pounds per year.

- For overfed lean persons to increase and maintain excess weight, caloric intake must increase by 50% over previous intake. To maintain a reduced weight, formerly obese persons must restrict intake to 25% less than a lean person of similar weight and body size.
- Decreased diet-induced thermogenesis worsens weight gain in obese individuals on a high-fat diet compared with lean people; it increases intake of fat and decreases exercise tendency.

Low Serotonin Theory

- Diets deficient in tryptophan induce increased appetite, causing binge eating of carbohydrates. Tryptophan deficit causes low brain serotonin and brain sense of starvation that stimulates appetite control centers, with a preference for carbohydrates. Carbohydrate foods increase tryptophan delivery to the brain, elevating serotonin synthesis.
- Carbohydrate craving may play a major role in obesity.
- Blood tryptophan and brain serotonin levels plummet with dieting. Brain starvation signals cannot be ignored; this is why most diets fail.
- Upper end of spectrum of carbohydrate addiction is bulimia, a serious eating disorder of binge eating and purging by forced vomiting or laxatives. Medical consequences of bulimia: rupture of stomach, erosion of dental enamel, and heart disturbances from the loss of potassium.

Environmental Toxin Theory

Recent research has shown that both individual persistent organic pollutants (POPs) and total chemical toxin load increase the risk of obesity. The primary mechanism of action appears to be the blocking of insulin receptor sites. Of particular concern, research is now showing that elevated levels of POPs in pregnant women significantly increase the risk of obesity in their children. In fact, researchers are now referring to POPs as "obesogens." An indirect measure of total POP load is the liver enzyme gamma-glutamyltransferase (GGT). Within the normal range, GGT increases in proportion to POP load and has a strong correlation with obesity. This reflects the increased regeneration of glutathione, which is critical to the detoxification and excretion of POPs.

THERAPEUTIC CONSIDERATIONS

- Only 5% of obese persons attain and maintain "normal" body weight for a year or more; 66% of those a few pounds overweight do.
- Basic foundations: positive mental attitude, healthy lifestyle (regular exercise), health-promoting diet, supplements.
- For an individual to lose weight, energy intake must be less than energy expenditure; decrease caloric intake and increase metabolizing of calories.
- To lose 1 pound, a person must consume 3500 fewer calories than expended. Loss of 1 lb/wk requires a negative caloric balance of 500 calories/day—achievable by decreasing calories and/or increasing exercise.
- Reducing intake by 500 calories/day or increasing metabolism by 500 calories/day by exercise (45-minute jog, playing tennis for 1 hour, or brisk walk for 1.25 hours) is a challenge. Sensible approach: both diet and exercise.
- Weight loss begins at a caloric intake below 1500 calories/day with exercise for 15 to 20 minutes three to four times per week.
- Starvation and crash diets: rapid weight loss (muscle and water) with rebound weight gain.
- Most successful approach: gradual weight reduction (0.5 to 1 lb/wk) through long-term dietary and lifestyle habits.
- Exercise maintains muscle mass and bone mineral density. It prevents accumulation of visceral fat during active weight loss and after weight loss has been achieved.
- Even modest weight reductions help: 5% to 10% reduction in weight improves cholesterol, blood pressure, blood glucose.

Behavioral Therapy

- Despite behavioral approaches, lost weight is generally regained; most patients return to pretreatment weight within 3 years.
- Main behavioral characteristics have been identified of persons who avoid weight regain:
  — High level of physical activity (1 hour daily)
  — Eating a low-calorie, low-fat, low-glycemic diet
- Eating breakfast regularly.
  — Active self-monitoring of body weight
- Maintaining consistent eating pattern across weekdays and weekends

- Healing depression
- Boost to self-esteem and self-confidence plus improving appearance, feeling more attractive, and being able to wear more fashionable clothing give motivation for continued weight loss until goals or effective maintenance of weight loss is achieved.
- Majority of people want to lose weight for changes in physical appearance, not health benefits. Key to success: identify primary goals of weight loss.

Dietary Strategies

Stress adequate protein intake. Recommendation: 2.0 g of protein per 2 pounds (kg) body weight unless there are signs of renal or liver failure.

Water

- Water consumption can acutely reduce mealtime caloric intake, especially among middle-aged and older adults.
- Drinking 500 mL water before each daily meal leads to 44% greater weight loss long term than diet alone. When combined with a hypocaloric diet, consuming water before each main meal induces greater weight loss than a hypocaloric diet alone in middle-aged and older adults.

Atkins Diet

- High-protein, high-fat, low-carbohydrate diet: unlimited amounts of all meats, poultry, fish, eggs, most cheeses.
- Four phases:
  - — Induction phase (first 14 days): carbohydrates limited to less than 20 g/day. No fruit, bread, grains, starchy vegetables, or dairy, except cheese, cream, and butter.
  - — Ongoing weight loss phase: dieters experiment with levels of carbohydrate intake to find most liberal level of carbohydrate intake that allows continued weight loss. Dieters maintain this level until weight loss goals are met.
  - — Premaintenance and maintenance phases: dieters determine level of carbohydrate intake that allows stable weight. Dieters must stick to this level of intake for life.
- Diets high in sugar and refined carbohydrates cause weight gain and obesity. Atkins dieters are spared feelings of hunger and deprivation of other regimens, but this diet is not conducive to long-term health.

- In the long term, Atkins dieters gain back all the weight lost plus more. Findings from clinical trials indicate that although strict adherence to the Atkins diet (dramatically reducing carbohydrates and allowing high-fat, high-protein foods) can lead to more weight loss in the first 6 months, a healthier diet is equally effective long term with fewer risks. High protein level in the Atkins diet stresses liver and kidneys.

Natural Weight Loss Aids

- **Meal replacement (MR) formulas:** are a popular strategy; effectiveness confirmed in several clinical trials; improve dietary compliance and convenience. Formulations should contain high-quality nutrition low in glycemic load and high in viscous, soluble fiber. Protein target: 2.2 g protein/kg LBM daily produces greater fat loss than 1.1 g protein/kg LBM daily. Medifast is a popular physician-supervised weight-loss program that relies heavily on MR formulas. It has been compared with a self-selected isocaloric food-based (FB) meal plan. Medifast plan: 5 MRs (90 to 110 kcal each), 5 to 7 ounces lean protein, 1½ cups nonstarchy vegetables, and up to two fat servings daily (providing daily 800 to 1000 kcal). MRs are low fat, low glycemic index, and low sugar, with a balanced ratio of carbohydrates to proteins. MRs are based on soy and/or whey protein. FB plans include 3 ounces of grains, 1 cup of vegetables, 1 cup of fruit, 2 cups of milk, 5 to 7 ounces of lean protein, and 3 tsp of fat daily (1000 kcal/day). Weight loss at 16 weeks is significantly better with Medifast versus the FB approach.
- **Fiber supplements:** dietary fiber promotes weight loss. Best supplements for weight loss: glucomannan, gum karaya, psyllium, chitin, guar gum, pectin—rich in water-soluble fibers. Taken with water, they form a gelatinous mass, inducing satiety. Benefits: enhanced glycemic control, decreased insulin levels, reduced calories absorbed. They can reduce number of calories absorbed by 30 to 180 calories/day, inducing a 3- to 18-pound weight loss in a year.
  - — Avoid products that contain a lot of sugar or sweeteners to camouflage taste.
  - — Drink adequate amounts of water with fiber supplement, especially in pill form.

PGX (PolyGlycopleX) is made of three natural fiber compounds (glucomannan, alginate, and xanthan gum) that coalesce into an entirely new matrix that is the most viscous fiber known to date.

PGX benefits: reduces appetite, promotes weight loss, increases compounds that block appetite and promote satiety, decreases compounds that stimulate overeating, reduces postprandial (after-meal) and delayed (second meal) blood glucose when added to or taken with foods, reduces glycemic index of any food or beverage by 15% to 70%, increases insulin sensitivity and decreases blood insulin levels, stabilizes glycemic control in overweight and obese patients, and lowers blood cholesterol and triglycerides. To avoid minor side effects (e.g., flatulence, bloating, loose stools, or constipation), start with small amounts and gradually increase dose over a few days to a week.

- **Chromium:** essential to glycemic control and insulin sensitivity. No recommended dietary allowance exists, but optimal health requires 200 mcg/day. Chromium levels are depleted by refined sugars and flour and lack of exercise. Chromium decreases fasting glucose, improves glucose tolerance, lowers insulin, decreases total cholesterol and triglycerides, increases high-density lipoprotein. It is effective in DM and hypoglycemia, improving glucose tolerance and number of insulin receptors on red blood cells. Chromium supplements lower body weight yet increase LBM by increasing insulin sensitivity. Results are most striking in elderly and in men. Dose: in picolinate form, 400 mcg is more effective than 200 mcg q.d. Greater muscle mass means greater fat-burning potential. Women in an exercise program did not show significant changes in body composition. Effects of chromium arise from increased insulin sensitivity. Forms: chromium picolinate, chromium polynicotinate, chromium chloride, and chromium-enriched yeast.
- **Medium-chain triglycerides (MCTs):** saturated fats (from coconut oil) in six to 12 carbon chains. The body uses MCTs differently than long-chain triglycerides (LCTs) in common fats found in nature. LCTs are storage fats in human beings and plants, with 18 to 24 carbons. MCTs promote weight loss rather than weight gain by increasing thermogenesis and energy expenditure. LCTs are stored in fat deposits; their energy is conserved. A diet high in LCTs decreases metabolic rate. Excess energy of MCTs is not efficiently stored as fat, but wasted as heat. MCT oil given over a 6-day period can increase diet-induced thermogenesis by 50%. LCTs elevate blood fats by 68%; MCTs have no effect on blood fat level. To benefit from MCTs, keep diet low in LCTs. Use MCTs as oil for salad dressing, as bread spread, or as supplement. Dose: 1 to 2 tbsp/day.

Closely monitor diabetics and persons with liver disease when using MCTs; they may develop ketoacidosis. Compared with LCTs, when used as the exclusive cooking oil, MCTs induce much greater decreases in body weight, BMI, body fat, WC, WC/HC ratio, total fat area, and subcutaneous fat area in the abdomen, as well as blood triglycerides and low-density–lipoprotein cholesterol.

- **Hydroxycitric acid (HCA):** natural substance isolated from fruit of Malabar tamarind *(Garcinia cambogia),* a yellowish fruit the size of an orange, with thin skin and deep furrows similar to acorn squash. It is native to southern India, where it is dried and used in curries. Dried fruit has 30% HCA. HCA is powerful lipogenic inhibitor in animals, reducing food intake and weight gain in rats. It also suppresses appetite. Still maintain a low-fat diet; it only inhibits conversion of carbohydrates into fat. By itself, HCA may offer a safe, natural aid for weight loss when taken at a dose of 1500 mg t.i.d. HCA helps reduce low-density lipoprotein (LDL) and triglycerides and increases high-density lipoprotein (HDL). HCA decreases serum leptin and increases serotonin and urinary excretion of fat metabolites.
- **5-Hydroxytryptophan (5-HTP):** genetically decreased activity of tryptophan hydroxylase (which converts tryptophan to 5-HTP, itself subsequently converted to serotonin) is linked to overeating and obesity in animals. Many human beings are genetically predisposed to obesity. Preformed 5-HTP can bypass this genetic defect to increase serotonin synthesis (*Textbook,* "5-Hydroxytryptophan"). 5-HTP reduces calorie intake and promotes weight loss in women despite no conscious effort to lose weight. Weight loss during 5-week period of 5-HTP support: 3 pounds. 5-HTP helps overweight people adhere to dietary recommendations. It promotes early satiety. Dose: 300 mg t.i.d. Side effects: mild nausea during first 6 weeks of therapy; never severe enough to stop therapy.

THERAPEUTIC APPROACH

- Implement four cornerstones of good health.
  - — Proper diet: whole-food, plant-based, nutrient-dense diet.
  - — Adequate protein: 2 g daily per kilogram of body weight.
  - — Drink 2 cups of warm water or herbal tea before each meal.
  - — Adequate exercise is critical (*Textbook,* "The Exercise Prescription").

- Psychological support: consider referral for counseling to heal assaults on self-esteem and self-image; maintain positive mental attitude.
- Support body through natural measures.

Supplements

- **Viscous, soluble fiber** (e.g., PGX, milled flaxseed, chia seed): 2.5 to 5 g, thoroughly hydrated, before meals.
- **5-HTP:** begin at 50 to 100 mg 20 minutes before meals for 2 weeks; then double dose (to maximum of 300 mg) if weight loss is less than 1 lb/wk. Higher doses of 5-HTP (e.g., 300 mg) are associated with nausea, but this symptom disappears after 6 weeks of use.
- **Chromium:** 200 to 400 mcg q.d.
- **MCTs:** incorporate 1 to 2 tbsp daily into diet.
- ***N*-acetylcysteine (NAC):** 500 mg bid to increase glutathione production if elevated POPs.

Botanical Medicines

- **HCA** *(G. cambogia):* 1500 mg t.i.d.

Indirect Methods of Analyzing Body Fat Composition

- Visual observation (somatotypes)
- Anthropometric measurements
- Height and weight
- Circumferences and diameters
- Skinfold thickness
- Isotope or chemical dilution
- Body water
- Body potassium
- Body fat
- Body density and body volume
- Conductivity
- Total body electrical conductivity
- Bioelectric impedance
- Neutron activation
- Imaging techniques
- Ultrasound
- Computed tomography
- Nuclear magnetic resonance imaging
- Nuclear magnetic spectroscopy

Osteoarthritis

DIAGNOSTIC SUMMARY

- **Symptoms:** mild early morning stiffness, stiffness after periods of rest, pain that worsens with joint use, and loss of joint function
- **Signs:** local tenderness, soft tissue swelling, joint crepitus, bony swelling, restricted mobility, swelling of Heberden's nodes (proximal interphalangeal joints) and/or less commonly Bouchard's nodes (distal interphalangeal joints), and other signs of degenerative loss of articular cartilage
- **Radiographic findings:** narrowed joint space, osteophytes, increased density of subchondral bone, subchondral sclerosis, bony cysts, soft tissue swelling, and periarticular swelling

GENERAL CONSIDERATIONS

Osteoarthritis (OA) characteristics include joint degeneration, loss of cartilage, and alterations of subchondral bone. It is the most common form of arthritis, with the highest morbidity rate of any illness. It primarily affects the elderly, but 35% of its incidence in the knee starts as early as age 30 years (often diagnosed as chondromalacia patellae). The incidence dramatically increases with age. More than 40 million Americans have OA, including 80% of persons older than 50 years. OA is responsible for 25% of all office visits to primary care physicians. Men and women are equally affected, but symptoms occur earlier and appear to be more severe in women.

- Diseases thought to be OA of specific joints: hands (Heberden's and Bouchard's nodes), hips (malum coxae senilis), temporomandibular joint (Costen's syndrome), knees (chondromalacia patellae), and spine (ankylosing hyperostosis, interstitial skeletal hyperostosis).
- Weight-bearing joints and peripheral and axial articulations are principally affected. Hyaline cartilage destruction is followed by hardening and formation of large bone spurs (calcified

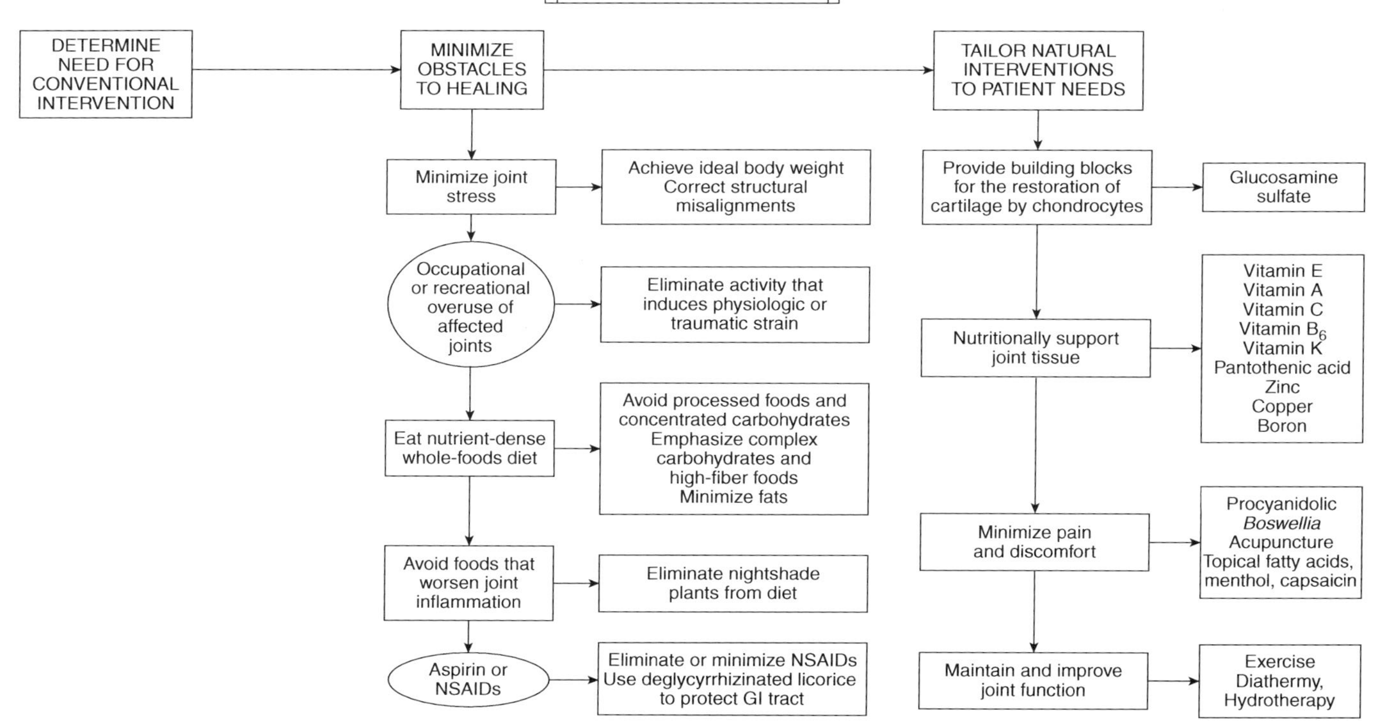
OSTEOARTHRITIS
DETERMINE NEED FOR CONVENTIONAL INTERVENTION
MINIMIZE OBSTACLES TO HEALING
TAILOR NATURAL INTERVENTIONS TO PATIENT NEEDS
Minimize joint stress
Achieve ideal body weight
Correct structural misalignments
Occupational or recreational overuse of affected joints
Eliminate activity that induces physiologic or traumatic strain
Eat nutrient-dense whole-foods diet
Avoid processed foods and concentrated carbohydrates
Emphasize complex carbohydrates and high-fiber foods
Minimize fats
Avoid foods that worsen joint inflammation
Eliminate nightshade plants from diet
Aspirin or NSAIDs
Eliminate or minimize NSAIDs
Use deglycyrrhizinated licorice to protect GI tract
Provide building blocks for the restoration of cartilage by chondrocytes
Glucosamine sulfate
Nutritionally support joint tissue
Vitamin E
Vitamin A
Vitamin C
Vitamin B_6
Vitamin K
Pantothenic acid
Zinc
Copper
Boron
Minimize pain and discomfort
Procyanidolic
Boswellia
Acupuncture
Topical fatty acids, menthol, capsaicin
Maintain and improve joint function
Exercise
Diathermy,
Hydrotherapy

osteophytes) in joint margins, causing pain, deformity, and limited joint motion. Inflammation usually is minimal.
- Two categories of OA: (1) primary OA arises from wear and tear after the fifth and sixth decades, with no predisposing abnormalities. The cumulative effects of decades of use stress collagen matrix. Damage releases enzymes that destroy collagen components. With aging, the ability to synthesize restorative collagen decreases. (2) Secondary OA entails predisposing factors for degeneration. Factors include congenital abnormalities in joint structure or function (e.g., hypermobility and abnormally shaped joint surfaces), trauma (obesity, fractures along joint surfaces, surgery), crystal deposition, presence of abnormal cartilage, previous inflammatory disease of joint (rheumatoid arthritis [RA], gout, septic arthritis).
- OA severity, as determined by radiography, does not correlate with degree of pain. Normal-looking joints, with little joint-space narrowing, can be excruciatingly painful. Conversely, joints with tremendous deformity may have little pain. In fact, 40% of patients with the worst x-ray classification for OA are pain free. The cause of pain is ill defined, but there are numerous potential causes. Depression and anxiety increase the experience of OA pain.

DIAGNOSIS

Onset is subtle; morning joint stiffness is the first symptom, then pain on joint motion worsened by prolonged activity and relieved by rest. No signs of inflammation are present. Clinical picture varies with joint(s) involved. Disease of the hands causes pain and limitation of use; knee involvement causes pain, swelling, and instability; hip OA causes local pain and limping; spinal OA (very common) involves compression of nerves and blood vessels, causing pain and vascular insufficiency. RA is associated with much more inflammation of surrounding soft tissues. After a complete medical history, the best diagnostic tool is a radiograph of the suspected joint, which should reveal joint-space narrowing, loss of cartilage, and presence of bone spurs (osteophytes).

Causes of Misdiagnosis of Osteoarthritis

- Source of pain is not OA, but the following:
  - Arthritis of other origin
  - Pathologic changes of adjacent bone (tumor, osteomyelitis, metabolic bone disease)

- — Mechanical injuries
- — Pathologic fractures
- — Referred pain of neuritis, neuropathy, or radiculopathy
- — Other neurologic disorders causing stiffness of joints

- Source of pain is OA, but not at joint suspected:
  - — OA of hip, pain localized to knee
  - — OA of cervical spine, causing pain in shoulder
  - — OA of lumbar spine, causing pain in hip, knee, or ankle
  - — OA of shoulder, causing pain in elbow
- Source of pain is secondary soft tissue alterations of OA:
  - — Tendonitis or ligamentitis (especially of knee)
  - — Enthesopathy, tendinopathy from joint contracture
  - — Bursitis
- Misinterpretation of deformity:
  - — Pseudohypertrophic osteoarthropathy
  - — Psoriatic arthritis
  - — Flexion contracture of joints
  - — Mucopolysaccharidoses
  - — Neurogenic arthropathies
  - — Calcium pyrophosphate dihydrate crystal deposition disease
  - — Genu varum and valgum
- Misinterpretation of x-ray films:
  - — Arthritis with previous OA changes
  - — Initial stage of OA, may have normal radiograph
  - — Flexion contracture can cause virtual loss of joint-space width
  - — Neurogenic and metabolic arthropathies
  - — Pain: severity of OA (by radiograph) does not correlate with degree of pain. Forty percent of patients with the worst radiographic classification for OA are pain free. The cause of pain in OA is still not well defined. Depression and anxiety increase OA pain.

THERAPEUTIC CONSIDERATIONS

Cellular and tissue response is purposeful and aimed at repair of anatomic defects. Disease process is arrestable and sometimes reversible. Therapeutic goal: enhance collagen matrix repair and regeneration by chondrocytes. Studies to determine natural course of OA show marked clinical improvement and radiologic recovery of joint space in almost 50% of patients with no therapy. Medical intervention may promote disease progression.

Conventional Pharmacologic Treatment

- Nonsteroidal anti-inflammatory drugs (NSAIDs) are the main conventional treatment for OA. NSAIDs provide short-term symptomatic relief, but they may accelerate degeneration of joint cartilage.
- Aspirin and other NSAIDs inhibit collagen matrix synthesis and accelerate destruction of cartilage. NSAID use is associated with accelerated OA and increased joint destruction. NSAIDs suppress symptoms but accelerate progression of OA.
- A patient is unlikely to die of OA, but NSAIDs are linked to higher risk for mortality. With older NSAIDs, the risk involves gastrointestinal (GI) bleeding; newer cyclooxygenase-2 (COX-2) inhibitors celecoxib (Celebrex) and rofecoxib (Vioxx) are linked to more-frequent cardiovascular events.

Physical Therapy

- **Simple but only recently documented concept:** skewed musculoskeletal dynamics increase stress on involved joints.
- Decline is greater for patients with more-extensive misalignments.
- Consider musculoskeletal dynamics in evaluating any OA patient. Those with misalignments may need manual manipulation therapies, orthotics, and extremity adjustments, along with regular massage therapy, to relax hypertonic muscles.
- From a prevention standpoint, assessing and treating younger patients may decrease risk of OA later in life.
- Various physical therapy modalities (e.g., exercise, heat, cold, diathermy, ultrasound) often improve joint mobility and reduce pain in OA, especially when administered regularly.
- Much of the benefit of physical therapy results from achieving proper hydration within joint capsules.
- Short wave diathermy may offer the greatest benefit. Combining short wave diathermy with periodic ice massage, rest, and appropriate exercises might be the most effective approach.
- Ultrasound and laser therapy may also help.
- The best exercises are isometrics and swimming because they increase circulation to joints and strengthen surrounding muscles without placing excess strain on joints.
- Increasing quadriceps strength improves clinical features and reduces pain in knee OA. Walking improves functional status and relieves pain of knee OA.
- Patient-specific physical therapies may also be useful.

Dietary and Exercise Considerations

- Achieve normal body weight to minimize stress on weight-bearing joints affected by OA.
- Obesity is a major risk factor for OA of the knee. OA is linked to metabolic syndrome because of the negative effects of insulin resistance, inflammatory adipokines, and metabolic syndrome on inflammation and joint structures. Insulin stimulates chondrocytes to generate proteoglycans. The most prominent early change in articular cartilage in OA is diminished proteoglycan content and aggregation; thus, insulin insensitivity or deficiency predisposes to OA.
- Lack of exercise decreases hydration of joint cartilages and retards diffusion of nutrients into the affected area. OA pain causes reduced activity, decreasing muscle strength. Muscle weakness increases joint wear; inactivity causes weight gain, exacerbating OA and the cycle of degeneration. Diabetics and cardiovascular patients increase risks as their exercise diminishes. Weight loss, dieting, and exercise independently decrease causative factors of OA.
- Healthy diet rich in complex carbohydrates and dietary fiber (*Textbook,* "Role of Dietary Fiber in Health and Disease").
- Regimens combining diet and exercise are superior to protocols using only one, not both.
- **Nightshade vegetables:** Childers' theory is that genetically susceptible individuals might develop arthritis from long-term, low-level consumption of the *Solanum* alkaloids found in Solanaceae (nightshade) plants: tomatoes, potatoes, eggplant, peppers, and tobacco. Alkaloids may inhibit normal collagen repair. This theory is as yet unproven, but diet is beneficial to some patients.
- **Mediterranean diet:** consists of abundant plant foods (fruits, vegetables, whole-grain cereals, beans, nuts, seeds); minimally processed, seasonally fresh, and locally grown foods; fish and poultry; olive oil as the main source of lipids; controlled intake of dairy, red meat, and wine. This diet is rich in omega-3 polyunsaturated fatty acids and oleic acid (omega-9 monounsaturated), antioxidants, and plant fiber.

Nutritional Supplements

Americans spend more on natural remedies for OA than for any other medical condition.

- **Glucosamine sulfate (GS):** stimulates manufacture of glycosaminoglycans (GAGs) by chondrocytes and promotes incorporation of sulfur into cartilage. With age comes a reduced ability to synthesize sufficient glucosamine; cartilage loses its gel-like nature and ability to absorb shock. Inability to manufacture glucosamine may be the major factor leading to OA. GS was significantly more effective than placebo in improving pain and movement after 4 weeks (1500 mg q.d.) in a double-blind crossover study. Longer GS use gives greater therapeutic benefit. Rate and severity of GS side effects are not different from placebo. Head-to-head studies: GS gives better long-term results than NSAIDs in relieving OA pain and inflammation despite little direct anti-inflammatory or analgesic effect from GS. NSAIDs offer only symptomatic relief and may promote disease process. GS treats root cause (cartilage synthesis), improving symptoms and helping the body repair damage. Higher doses may be required for heavy or obese patients. Patients with peptic ulcers should take GS with food. Individuals taking diuretics may need an increased dose to compensate for reduced efficacy. Improvement with GS lasts 6 to 12 weeks after end of treatment. GS should be taken for long periods or in repeated short-term courses. GS has high safety and excellent tolerability and is suitable for long-term use (*Textbook,* "Glucosamine"). Glucosamine hydrochloride at 2000 mg q.d. for 5 months provided significant pain relief and improved function after 8 weeks. With respect to concerns about effects on blood sugar in diabetics, 1500 mg of glucosamine (and 1200 mg of chondroitin) given daily to diabetics, most on antiglycemic medicines, had no effect on hemoglobin A_{1c} after a 90-day trial.

- **Chondroitin sulfate (CS), shark cartilage, bovine cartilage extracts, sea cucumber:** contain a mixture of intact or partially hydrolyzed GAGs of molecular weights 14,000 to 30,000. CS is composed of repeating units of derivatives of GS. Absorption rate of GS is 90% to 98%; absorption of intact CS is 13%. CS is 50 to 300 times larger than GS. Key reason why GS is effective is its small molecular size, allowing diffusion through joint cartilage to chondrocyte. CS levels typically are elevated in synovial tissues of OA patients; CS is less effective than GS. Any benefit from CS is likely from the absorption of sulfur or smaller GAG molecules broken down by the digestive tract. No evidence exists that shows using both GS and CS together is more effective than either alone. GS gives more-impressive results; it is faster acting and has greater overall benefit. Evidence of modification of joint-space pathology makes CS a reasonable addition to GS regimen for OA. Also, in OA patients, levels of CS in synovial tissues are typically elevated. These absorption problems suggest that any direct effect of these compounds in OA is unlikely. However, conflicting evidence supports the notion that exogenous CS is indeed absorbed as a high-molecular-weight polysaccharide together with derivatives originating from a partial depolymerization, desulfation, or both.

- **Hyaluronic acid (HA):** important GAG in joints, providing a structural framework and supporting ability of cartilage to hold water. HA is the matrix network that holds the body together. By age 70, body HA content has dropped by 80% from the level at age 40, predisposing loss of connective tissue integrity (e.g., skin and joints). Weekly injections of HA (e.g., Synvisc, Hyalgan, Supartz) into OA-affected joints (viscosupplementation) is an effective treatment, improving pain, function, and patient global assessment. Best results occur at the 5- to 13-week postinjection period. Oral HA supplementation can increase body HA stores. HA supplements feature HA derived from rooster combs or cow eyes or from bacterial fermentation. Clinical trial dose: 80 to 100 mg HA q.d. for 8 weeks. Significant reductions in pain scores and total symptom scores are seen with the 200-mg dose.
- **Niacinamide:** Kaufman and Hoffer treatment of RA and OA with high-dose niacinamide (900 to 4000 mg q.d. in divided doses) improves joint function, range of motion, muscle strength and endurance, and sedimentation rate. Benefits are noted within 1 to 3 months of use; peak benefits occur after 1 to 3 years of continuous use. Use of 3000 mg q.d. in six divided doses resulted in a 29% improvement in global arthritis impact versus 10% worsening with placebo. Pain levels did not change, but niacinamide patients reduced NSAID use. It reduced erythrocyte sedimentation rate by 22% and increased joint mobility by 4.5 degrees over control subjects (8 vs. 3.5 degrees). No other changes in blood chemistry were noted. Side effects were mild GI complaints, managed by taking with food or fluids. High doses can result in significant side effects (e.g., glucose intolerance and liver damage); strict supervision is required.
- **S-adenosylmethionine (SAM):** is formed in the body by converting the essential amino acid methionine to adenosyl-triphosphate. SAM deficiency in joint tissue causes loss of gel-like nature and shock-absorbing qualities of cartilage. SAM is important in the synthesis of cartilage components. Supplemental SAM increases cartilage formation (determined by magnetic

resonance imaging) in OA of the hands. It shows mild analgesic and anti-inflammatory effects in animal studies. SAM induces reductions in pain scores and clinical symptoms similar to reductions with NSAIDs. SAM administered orally at dose of 1200 mg q.d. is significantly more effective than NSAIDs (physicians' and patients' judgments). It is better tolerated than placebo. Its efficacy has been described as very good or good in 71% of cases, moderate in 21%, and poor in 9%. Tolerance was assessed as very good or good in 87%, moderate in 8%, and poor in 5% of patients. SAM offers significant advantages over NSAIDs. Side effects: occasional GI disturbances, mainly diarrhea.

- **Vitamin C:** high intake of antioxidants, especially vitamin C, may markedly and dose-dependently reduce risk of cartilage loss and OA progression. Recommend foods rich in plant-based antioxidants. Deficient intake is common in the elderly, causing altered collagen synthesis and compromised connective tissue repair. In vitro, vitamin C has anabolic effect on cartilage. Excess of ascorbic acid is needed in human chondrocyte protein synthesis. In vivo study of experimental OA in guinea pigs found cartilage erosion is much less, and overall histologic and biochemical changes in and around OA joint are much milder, in animals on high doses of vitamin C. Patient self-reported vitamin C supplementation indicated halting progression of OA. Vitamins C and E have synergistic effects that enhance stability of sulfated proteoglycans in cartilage.
- **Vitamin D:** low intake and low serum levels of vitamin D are both linked to increased risk for progression of OA of knee, especially in people younger than 60. Low serum vitamin D predicts loss of cartilage, indicated by joint space and osteophyte growth. Vitamin D deficiency lowers likelihood of excellent outcomes from total hip replacement. Sunlight and sufficient intake in childhood and young adulthood may decrease risk of OA. Whether increasing vitamin D intake helps decrease or reverse already established OA is not known.
- **Pantothenic acid:** acute deficiency in rats causes pronounced failure of cartilage growth and lesions similar to OA. Pantothenic acid clinically improves OA symptoms at a dose of 12.5 mg. Results often do not manifest for 7 to 14 days. A larger, double-blind study of RA patients found no significant benefit at dose of 500 mg q.d.
- **Vitamins A and E, pyridoxine, zinc, copper, and boron:** required for synthesis of collagen and maintenance of normal

cartilage. Deficiency of any one of these allows accelerated joint degeneration. Supplements at appropriate potencies may promote cartilage repair. Boron has been used to treat OA in Germany since the mid-1970s. At a dose of 6 mg boron q.d. (sodium tetraborate decahydrate), 71% of patients improved compared with 10% on placebo. Open trial: boron at 6 to 9 mg q.d. gave effective relief in 90% of arthritis patients, including OA, juvenile arthritis, and RA. Boron is of value in arthritis; many OA patients experience complete resolution.

- **Vitamin K:** low vitamin K status is associated with OA. Of dietary factors studied in OA, only vitamin K intake is inversely associated with preventing radiographic knee OA. Knee joint-space narrowing is also inversely associated with vitamin K intake. Vitamin K may protect against knee OA and might lead to a disease-modifying treatment. Study protocol: 500 mcg of phylloquinone (part of a single daily effervescent multivitamin), as well as separate elemental calcium (600 mg/day) and vitamin D (400 international units [IU]/day). Although vitamin K did not affect radiographic OA outcomes, patients with insufficient vitamin K at baseline who attained sufficient levels at follow-up had 47% less joint-space narrowing. Vitamin K food sources: green tea, kale, turnip greens, spinach, and other green leafy vegetables.

Physical Therapy

- Skewed musculoskeletal dynamics play a role in abnormally stressing involved joints. Patients with varus alignment have a fourfold increased risk of medial OA progression; those with valgus alignment have five times the risk of lateral OA progression. Decline is greater for those with more-extensive misalignments. Consider musculoskeletal dynamics when evaluating any patient with OA. Misalignments may need manual manipulation, orthotics, and extremity adjustments plus massage to relax hypertonic muscles. Assessing and treating younger persons may reduce risk of OA later on in life.
- Exercise, heat, cold, diathermy, and ultrasound often improve joint mobility and reduce pain in OA, especially when administered regularly. Benefit of physical therapy is achieving proper hydration within the joint capsule.
- Short wave diathermy may be of greatest benefit. Combining short wave diathermy with periodic ice massage, rest, and appropriate exercises may be the most effective approach. Ultrasound and laser therapy also are helpful.

- Best exercises are isometrics and swimming; they increase circulation to joints and strengthen surrounding muscles without excess strain on joints. Increasing quadriceps strength improves clinical features and reduces pain in knee OA. Walking helps improve functional status and relieve pain in knee OA.

Magnetic Therapies

- Used to treat a wide variety of chronic pain syndromes. Magnetic fields may stimulate chondrocyte proliferation and synthesis of proteoglycans. Studies support use in knee OA.
- Low-frequency and low-amplitude pulsed fields improve pain, functionality, and physician global evaluation of patients' condition.
- High-strength magnetic knee sleeve treatment for 4 hours in a monitored setting and self-treatment 6 hours daily for 6 weeks decreased pain scores.

Relaxation

- Relaxation techniques, such as meditation, deep breathing, and guided imagery, are applied to many types of pain.
- Daily listening to music of Mozart for 20 minutes over a 14-day period caused patients to have less pain compared with those who sat quietly for 20 minutes and did not listen to music. Pain decreased incrementally over a 14-day study period.

Botanical Medicines

When inflammation is present, botanicals and nutritional factors possessing anti-inflammatory activity are indicated, such as bromelain, curcumin, and ginger.

- ***Boswellia serrata:*** large branching tree native to India, yielding an exudative gum resin (salai guggul). Newer preparations concentrated for active components (boswellic acids) have antiarthritic effects. *Boswellia* inhibits inflammatory mediators, prevents decreased GAG synthesis, and improves blood supply to joint tissues. Clinical studies show good results in knee OA—decreased pain and swelling and increased knee flexion and walking distance. Corroborating improvements in pain and joint function were reductions in synovial fluid matrix metalloproteinase-3, indicating improved stability of collagen matrix. Standard dose for boswellic acids in arthritis is 400 mg t.i.d. No side effects have been reported.

- **Procyanidolic oligomers:** pycnogenol (100 mg daily for 3 months) induced a 56% reduction in the score of the global Western Ontario and McMaster Universities Osteoarthritis Index (WOMAC) questionnaire for OA. Pycnogenol increases treadmill walking distance. Pharmaceutical use is decreased. Moreover, foot edema is decreased.
- **Limbrel (Flavocoxid):** a proprietary mixture of flavonoid molecules baicalin and catechin. It is promoted for balanced inhibition of COX-1 and COX-2 and 5-lipoxygenase without cardiovascular, renal, or GI side effects of NSAIDs. Clinical results are comparable with those of naproxen in relieving OA pain scores. Dose: 500 mg b.i.d. Flavocoxid does not increase bleeding time, inhibit platelet aggregation, or inhibit or potentiate anticoagulant effect of warfarin.
- ***Zingiber officinale*** **(ginger):** ginger extract had moderate effect on symptoms of knee OA, reducing need for acetaminophen and reducing knee pain on standing and after walking. Side effect: mild GI upset. Dose: 170 mg of ginger extract t.i.d. Other studies have indicated no benefit. More research is needed. Note that ginger inhibits CYP2D6. Because this liver enzyme detoxifies approximately 25% of prescribed drugs, check to see if any drug a patient is taking is detoxified by this route to prevent induction of an adverse drug reaction (ADR).
- ***Harpagophytum procumbens*** **(devil's claw):** South African plant in regions bordering the Kalahari. Secondary tuberous roots yield powders or extracts standardized for active compound harpagoside. Dose of 60 mg of harpagoside q.d. shows moderate efficacy for spine, hip, and knee OA. In experimental animal models of inflammation, devil's claw has an anti-inflammatory and analgesic effect comparable to that of phenylbutazone. Dose: 670 mg powder t.i.d. Adverse events occur at a rate of 3% and do not exceed the rate experienced with placebo. Long-term use appears to be safe and without toxicity.
- ***Yucca:*** double-blind trial found saponin extract of *Yucca* has positive therapeutic effect. Results are gradual with no direct joint effects. Improvement is caused by indirect effects on GI flora. Bacterial lipopolysaccharides (endotoxins) depress the biosynthesis of proteoglycans. *Yucca* may decrease bacterial endotoxin absorption, reducing inhibition of proteoglycan synthesis. Other saponin-containing herbs and other ways of reducing endotoxin load may be useful.

Additional Therapeutic Considerations

Topical Analgesics

Mainstay natural topical preparations for OA contain menthol-related compounds (e.g., camphor 4%, menthol 10%, and methyl salicylate 30%) and/or capsaicin (creams containing 0.075%). They can provide significant relief; yet each has compliance issues. Alternative products contain Celadrin—a mixture of cetylated fatty acids (Celadrin) with cetyl myristoleate, cetyl myristate, cetyl palmitoleate, cetyl laureate, cetyl palmitate, and cetyl oleate. Celadrin affects several factors that contribute to inflammation. Celadrin enhances integrity of cell membranes, halting production of inflammatory prostaglandins. It also reduces negative immune factors (e.g., interleukin [IL-6]). Studies have assessed both the oral and topical use of Celadrin. Oral Celadrin for knee OA improves knee range of motion and overall joint function compared with placebo. Celadrin cream was studied in OA of the knees. It improved stair-climbing ability and Timed Up and Go test results 30 minutes after first administration and after 1 month of use. Range of motion of the knees increased with Celadrin both 30 minutes after the initial application and after 1 month's use. Celadrin also improves static postural stability (ability to stand comfortably in one place for a period of time). Unlike many other natural approaches, Celadrin produces almost immediate results.

Proteolytic Enzymes

Proteolytic enzymes (e.g., pancreatic proteases chymotrypsin and trypsin, bromelain, and fungal proteases) are useful in OA. A combination of bromelain 90 mg, trypsin 48 mg, and rutin 100 mg (Phlogenzym) at a dose of 2 tablets t.i.d. or 3 tablets b.i.d. on an empty stomach reduces OA pain scores on par with the drug diclofenac (100 mg q.d.). However, bromelain alone (800 mg q.d.) produced no significant effects in OA.

Acupuncture

- **Traditional Chinese medicine** (TCM) views OA as a "bi" or pain syndrome, with pathogenic causes stemming from coldness, dampness, heat, and wind. Each one of these types has a separate clinical picture and requires manipulation of specific acupuncture points. Acupuncture reduces pain from OA. As many as 75% of patients may have a reduction in pain of 45% or more with acupuncture. These benefits can be maintained during the 1 month after a course of acupuncture. TCM considers a cause of pain to be "stuck qi." In this case, the addition of electrical energy to the area can reestablish qi flow, thus alleviating pain.

- **Electroacupuncture** and a Western electrical treatment called **transcutaneous electrical nerve stimulation (TENS)** have been used to alleviate OA-induced knee pain. Electroacupuncture protocol: low-frequency (2 Hz) treatment at two local acupuncture points (ST-35, Dubi and Neixiyan) of the painful knee for 20 minutes. TENS protocol: low-frequency treatment of 2 Hz and pulse width of 200 micro ohms at the same acupuncture points for 20 minutes. Course of treatment for both modalities involves a total of eight sessions in 2 weeks. Both electrical modalities can significantly reduce knee pain, with prolonged analgesic effect at 2-week follow-up. Electroacupuncture also lowers scores for the Timed Up and Go test, which TENS does not achieve. Electroacupuncture, tested head to head against the NSAID diclofenac in knee patients, proved superior to the drug and placebo. When acupuncture is being considered, it may be most effective when employed early in the treatment plan. To avoid a rebound effect, administer treatments with a tapering, methodical decrease in frequency once acute treatment is completed. Because the density of peripheral nerve endings in the skin or muscles is much greater at acupuncture points compared with areas beyond these points, it is possible that an abrupt lack of stimulation in these areas may untowardly affect neurotransmitter release to contribute to a rebound effect.

THERAPEUTIC APPROACH

Clinical study of comprehensive, integrated program for OA has yet to be conducted. Therapeutic approach: reduce joint stress, promote collagen repair, and eliminate foods and other factors that inhibit collagen repair. Control all diseases or predisposing factors. Avoid NSAIDs as much as possible. If aspirin is used, deglycyrrhizinated *Glycyrrhiza glabra* (licorice) (DGL) may protect GI tract from damaging effects, and aspirin should be discontinued as soon as possible.

- **Diet:** the achievement of ideal body weight is the primary dietary goal. Avoid simple, processed, and concentrated carbohydrates. Emphasize complex-carbohydrate, high-fiber foods. Minimize fats. Eliminate Solanaceae foods (tomatoes, potatoes, eggplant, peppers, and tobacco). Liberally consume flavonoid-rich berries or extracts.

- **Supplements**:
  - GS: 1500 mg q.d.
  - Niacinamide: 500 mg six times a day (under strict supervision; monitor liver enzymes)
  - Vitamin E: 600 IU q.d. (mixed tocopherols)
  - Vitamin A: 5000 IU q.d.
  - Vitamin C: 1000 to 3000 mg q.d.
  - Vitamin B_6: 50 mg q.d.
  - Vitamin K: 0.5 mg/day
  - Pantothenic acid: 12.5 mg q.d.
  - SAM: 400 mg t.i.d.
  - Zinc: 45 mg q.d.
  - Copper: 1 mg q.d.
  - Boron: 6 mg q.d.
- **Botanical medicines:**
  - *B. serrata:* equivalent to 400 mg boswellic acids t.i.d.
  - Procyanidolic oligomers from either pine bark (Pycnogenol) or grapeseed extract: 100 to 300 mg q.d.
  - Limbrel (Flavocoxid): 500 mg twice a day
  - *H. procumbens:* dose that provides a minimum of 60 mg harpagoside q.d.
    - Dried root powder (tablet or capsule): 2000 mg t.i.d.
    - Fluid extract (1:1): 2 mL t.i.d.
    - Dried powdered extract (standardized to contain 2.5% harpagoside): 750 to 1000 mg t.i.d.
  - *Yucca* leaves: 2 to 4 g t.i.d.
- **Topical applications:**

Choose one of the following:
  - Cetylated fatty acid cream (Celadrin): applied to affected area b.i.d.
  - Menthol preparations: applied to affected areas b.i.d.
  - Capsaicin preparations can be applied to affected areas b.i.d.
- **Physical therapy and exercise:** avoid physical activity that induces physiologic or traumatic strain (occupational or recreational overuse). Normalize posture; orthopedically correct structural abnormalities to limit joint strain. Prescribe monitored daily nontraumatic exercise (isometrics and swimming). Use short wave diathermy, hydrotherapy, and other physical therapy modalities that improve joint perfusion.
- **Acupuncture:** administer two to four times weekly until acute symptoms resolve. Then frequency should be gradually decreased. Maintenance treatments every 2 weeks to monthly may help prevent recurrence.

Osteoporosis

DIAGNOSTIC SUMMARY

- Usually asymptomatic until severe backache
- Common in postmenopausal (PM) women and men who are older than 70 or taking aromatase inhibitors, corticosteroids
- No trauma fractures of the hip and vertebra
- Decrease in height
- Defined as a T-score at or below a bone mineral density (BMD) of −2.5 standard deviations below that of a young normal adult

GENERAL CONSIDERATIONS

- Osteoporosis (OP) is the most common bone disease in human beings and is a serious health threat for PM women. Features include low bone mass, deterioration of microarchitecture of bone tissue, fragility of bones, diminished bone strength, and increased risk of fracture.
- Approximately 1.5 million OP fractures occur each year in the United States, of which 250,000 are hip fractures.
- After an osteoporotic hip fracture, a woman's risk of dying doubles; a man's risk of dying triples.
- Of those who sustain an osteoporotic hip fracture, 10% to 20% die in the subsequent 6 months, 50% of those who survive will be unable to walk without assistance, and 25% will require long-term home care.
- Although African Americans are the ethnic group at the lowest risk, OP is projected to occur in 53% of African American women and 24% of African American men. This translates to more than half of all African American women and one quarter of all African American men developing osteopenia or OP.
- Among Caucasians, risk for low bone mass and OP is even higher; it is currently projected to develop in three out of four (77%) women and close to one of every two (43%) men.
- Hispanic Americans, however, fare the worst: 86% of Hispanic American women and 53% of Hispanic American men will lose

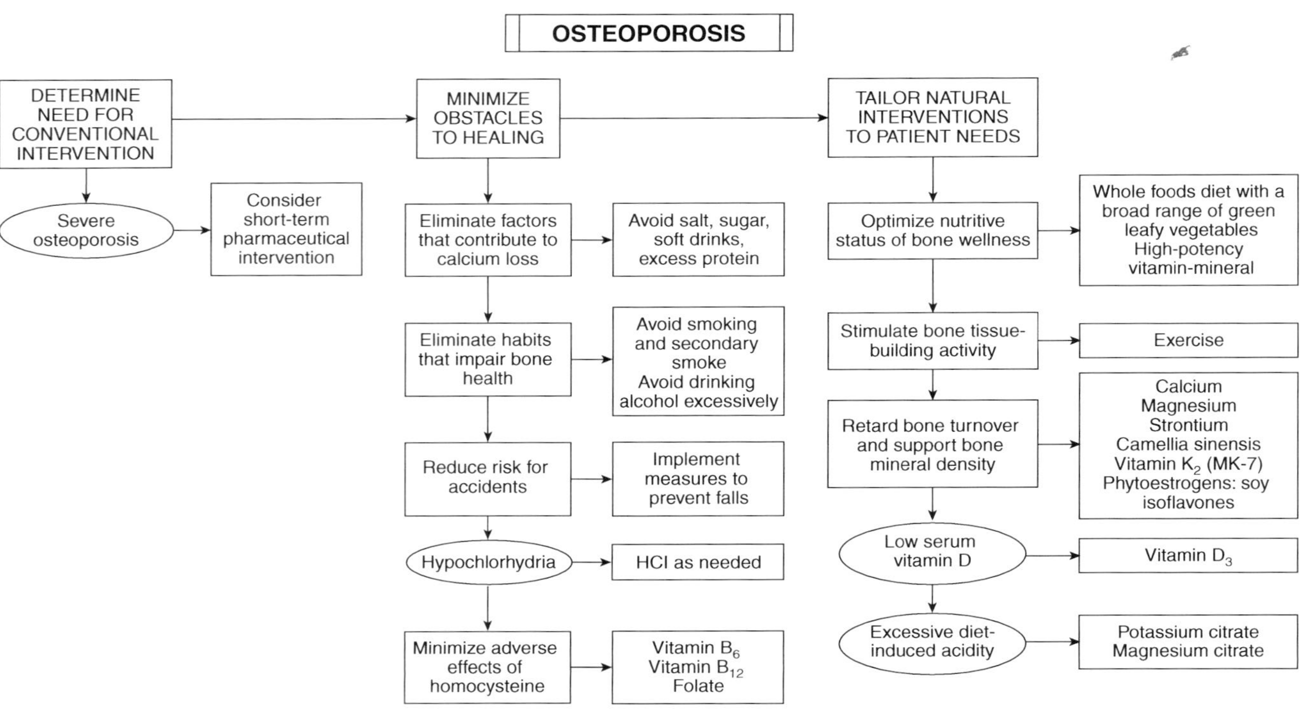
OSTEOPOROSIS
DETERMINE NEED FOR CONVENTIONAL INTERVENTION
Severe osteoporosis
Consider short-term pharmaceutical intervention
MINIMIZE OBSTACLES TO HEALING
Eliminate factors that contribute to calcium loss
Avoid salt, sugar, soft drinks, excess protein
Eliminate habits that impair bone health
Avoid smoking and secondary smoke
Avoid drinking alcohol excessively
Reduce risk for accidents
Implement measures to prevent falls
Hypochlorhydria
HCl as needed
Minimize adverse effects of homocysteine
Vitamin B_6
Vitamin B_{12}
Folate
TAILOR NATURAL INTERVENTIONS TO PATIENT NEEDS
Optimize nutritive status of bone wellness
Whole foods diet with a broad range of green leafy vegetables
High-potency vitamin-mineral
Stimulate bone tissue-building activity
Exercise
Retard bone turnover and support bone mineral density
Calcium
Magnesium
Strontium
Camellia sinensis
Vitamin K_2 (MK-7)
Phytoestrogens: soy isoflavones
Low serum vitamin D
Vitamin D_3
Excessive diet-induced acidity
Potassium citrate
Magnesium citrate

so much bone that they will be at greatly increased risk of osteoporotic fractures. From 2005 to 2025, a 175% increase in incidence of osteoporotic fractures is projected to occur in Hispanic Americans. More than half of fragility fractures occur in women with osteopenia, and women with osteopenia who have experienced a fragility fracture have the same fracture risk as women with OP.

- Vertebral fractures of the thoracic and/or lumbar region cause pain, height loss, and exaggerated kyphosis or deformity of thoracic spine, with restricted range of motion, changes in posture, restricted lung function, and digestive problems. A vertebral fracture means at least a fivefold to sevenfold increase in risk of subsequent vertebral fractures.
- Depression, anxiety, low self-esteem, and tooth loss are also caused by OP.

Pathophysiology

- Bone remodeling is process of bone resorption (breakdown) and bone formation. Osteoclasts induce enzymatic dissolution of minerals and protein for bone resorption. Osteoblasts create protein matrix of collagen for remineralization and bone formation. Bone remodeling is normally a balance of resorption and formation. Imbalance between removal and replacement causes bone loss and risk of fracture.
- Bone mass rapidly increases in childhood; this increase slows in the late teens but continues during the 20s. In women, the building process is complete by age 17 years. Peak bone mass is at 28 years, then bone mass is slowly lost at a rate of 0.4% per year in the femoral neck. After menopause, the loss accelerates to 2% per year during the first 5 to 10 years. Loss continues in women older than 70 years at much slower rate.

Risk Factors

- **Genetic factors:** level of peak bone mass is attributable to genetic factors. History of fracture in a first-degree relative increases fracture risk. Young daughters of women with OP fractures and first-degree relatives of women with OP have subnormal bone mass. Black women have greater bone mass compared with white women. Genomic testing is now available to assess the genetic predisposition to a defect in the vitamin D receptor sites (VDRs). Women with the VDR defect require substantially greater levels of vitamin D, preferable as D_3. New key genetic factor: polymorphisms of VDR site, some of which may increase need for vitamin D.

- **Vitamin D deficiency:** Vitamin D's role in bone health is underappreciated. Bone density correlates directly with serum 25-hydroxycholecalciferol (25(OH)D_3) and inversely with fractures of all types.
- **Vitamin K_2 deficiency:** osteocalcin, which pulls calcium (Ca) into bone, and matrix Gla protein, which prevents calcium deposition in arteries, are vitamin K–dependent proteins.
- **Lifestyle:** lifestyle, hormonal factors, Ca, vitamins D and K_2 intake, exercise, age of menarche, menstrual regularity, and alcohol and tobacco use have a greater impact than genetics, which accounts for only 30% of OP risk. Several lifestyle factors affect OP risk after menopause: physical activity; animal protein intake; acid-base homeostasis; Ca, vitamin D, vitamin K, and magnesium (Mg) intake; heavy smoking; and alcohol intake. Requirements for peak bone mass: balanced diet, adequate calories, protein and Ca throughout life. Ca, Mg, vitamin K_2, and vitamin D_3 are critical in older women. Ca requirements change with age; menopause increases Ca needs. After age 65 years, women absorb 50% less Ca than do young women. Renal enzymatic activity that produces active vitamin D decreases.
- **Dietary protein:** high intake of animal protein, but not plant protein, is linked to increased risk of forearm fracture. Red meat is acid producing, inducing release of salts from bone to balance acid and maintain acid-base homeostasis. Diets high in fruits and vegetables and plant proteins are alkaline forming.
- **Smoking:** cigarettes are loaded with cadmium and nicotine, both of which cause bone loss. Women smokers lose bone more rapidly, have lower bone mass, and have higher fracture rates. Smokers reach menopause up to 2 years earlier. Smoking increases hepatic clearance of estrogen.
- **Alcohol:** consuming 7 oz of alcohol daily (heavy intake) increases the risk of falls and hip fractures. Moderate alcohol intake lowers risk of hip fractures in older women; it inhibits bone resorption by increasing estradiol levels and calcitonin excretion.
- **Physical activity:** highly active persons have higher bone mass; prolonged bed rest or confinement to a wheelchair causes rapid, dramatic bone loss. Exercise reduces OP risk by stimulating osteoblasts.

Hormonal Factors

- Menopause: all women lose bone, but this loss is accelerated in the first 5 years of menopause. Estrogen decline increases rate of bone resorption. The earlier that occurs before the average age of menopause (51 years), the sooner the bones lose the protective effect of endogenous estrogen. Premature menopause (before 40 years), late onset of menarche in adolescence, periods of amenorrhea because of low estrogen in reproductive years (e.g., hypothalamic amenorrhea), or infrequent menses increase risk of OP. Women who missed up to half of their expected menstrual periods have 12% less vertebral bone mass; those who missed more than half had 31% less bone mass than healthy controls.
- Ca blood concentration is strictly held within narrow limits. Ca decline triggers increased secretion of parathyroid hormone (PTH) and decreased secretion of calcitonin from the thyroid and parathyroids. Ca excess triggers decreased secretion of PTH and increased secretion of calcitonin.
- PTH increases serum Ca by increasing osteoclast catabolism of bone, decreases excretion of Ca by kidneys, increases absorption of Ca in intestines, and increases kidney conversion of 25-(OH) D_3 to 1,25-$(OH)_2D_3$.

Additional Factors

The more risk factors present, the greater the potential for lower bone mass and risk of fracture. Risk factors alone do not adequately assess low bone mass but can guide clinical assessment risks that contribute to optimal preventive strategies. The individual woman's risk is the most relevant parameter for her future bone health. Diseases and medicines can interrupt normal bone metabolism.

- Secondary causes of bone loss:
  - — Medicines: aromatase inhibitors, cytotoxic agents, excessive thyroid therapy, gonadotropin-releasing hormone agonists or analogues, some long-term anticonvulsants (e.g., phenytoin), glucocorticoid use for more than 3 months
  - — Genetic disorders: hemochromatosis, hypophosphatasia, osteogenesis imperfecta, thalassemia, Ca balance disorders, urinary Ca excretion
  - — Endocrinopathies: cortisol excess, Cushing's disease, hyperthyroidism, primary syndrome, gonadal insufficiency, hyperthyroidism, primary hyperparathyroidism, hypercalciuria, vitamin D deficiency, gallbladder disease, primary type 1

diabetes mellitus, hypothalamic amenorrhea, premature ovarian failure

— Gastrointestinal diseases: primary biliary cirrhosis, fat malabsorption, hypochlorhydria, lactose intolerance, celiac disease, Crohn's disease, total gastrectomy, gastric bypass

— Other conditions: ankylosing spondylitis, chronic renal disease, lymphoma and leukemia, multiple myeloma, anorexia nervosa, bulimia, rheumatoid arthritis

DIAGNOSTIC CONSIDERATIONS

- Assess all PM women for risk factors of OP—history, physical examination, diagnostic tests. Goals of evaluation: identify women at risk for OP or fracture; diagnose OP and/or determine severity of OP; rule out secondary causes of bone loss; identify risk factors for falls or injuries.
- **World Health Organization (WHO) Fracture Risk Assessment (FRAX) risk factors:** patient history (personal history of fracture after age 40, history of hip fracture in a parent, current cigarette smoking, alcohol abuse, glucocorticoid use, rheumatoid arthritis or other secondary causes of OP), bone density testing, and the FRAX risk calculator are tools for ascertaining fracture risk. Use FRAX risk calculator for PM women who have low bone density but not OP. It determines 10-year probability of OP fracture and 10-year probability of hip fracture. FRAX risk calculator is available online.
- Focus history and physical examination on identifying risk factors. Physical signs of OP: loss of height of more than 1½ inches (measure height annually), excess kyphosis of thoracic spine, dowager's hump, dental caries, tooth loss, receding gums, back pain.
- Radiologic tests of BMD: BMD testing is optimal to diagnose OP. Gold standard is dual energy x-ray absorptiometry (DXA). Other methods include computed tomography (CT) scans, ultrasound of heel, radiographs; none of these tests is optimal for diagnosis and follow-up.
- Record weight to identify women with low BMI and therefore increased risk for low bone density. Inquire and examine patient for acute or chronic back pain, signs of percussion tenderness, and bone density testing. Assess for risk of falls, which increases with medication that affects balance and coordination; muscle weakness; impaired vision; a history of falls, fainting, or loss of

consciousness; difficulty standing or walking; arthritis and/or neuropathy of lower extremities.

Bone Mineral Density Testing

- BMD testing is the optimal method to confirm diagnosis of OP. There are several techniques to measure BMD, but the gold standard is DXA.
- DXA test requires less radiation exposure than radiographs or CT scans. It can measure both hip and lumbar densities. Hip is the preferred site for BMD testing, especially in patients older than 60 years, because spinal measurements are unreliable because of extraosseous ossification. The spine is useful in early PM women; rates of bone loss are greater because of lower estrogen. Peripheral DXA sites are accurate but less useful; they may not correlate with fracture risk and BMD at hip and spine.
- North American Menopause Society guidelines for indications for BMD testing are as follows:
  - — PM women with secondary causes of bone loss (e.g., steroid use, hyperparathyroidism)
  - — Radiologic evidence of osteopenia
  - — All women age 65 years and older
  - — PM women age 50 and older with additional risk factors (fracture after menopause, body weight below 127 pounds, personal history of hip fracture, current smoker, rheumatoid arthritis, alcohol intake of more than two units daily [one unit = 12 oz of beer, 4 oz of wine, or 1 oz of liquor])
  - — PM women, regardless of age, with fragility fractures since menopause, low body weight, or family history of spine or hip fracture
- Reporting of results of BMD tests: standard deviations of either a Z-score or a T-score. Z-score is based on standard deviation from the mean BMD of women in the same age group. T-score is based on mean peak BMD of normal, young adult women. WHO criteria for diagnosing OP use T-scores.

Laboratory Tests of Bone Metabolism

- Biochemical markers of bone turnover
  - — Urine test for breakdown products of bone: cross-linked N-telopeptide of type I collagen or deoxypyridium.
  - — Measure bone turnover correlated with rate of bone loss; not intended to be used for diagnosis of OP or monitoring bone loss.

- — Use to monitor success (or failure) of therapy; provide quicker feedback compared with DXA, which can take up to 2 years to detect therapeutic response.
- — Use DXA to measure bone density; use urinary bone resorption assessments to measure rate of turnover.
- — Reducing urinary markers of breakdown over a 2-year period has produced increases in bone density measurements, but value of markers in clinical practice has yet to be confirmed.
- Additional tests for secondary causes of bone loss: serum Ca, 24-hour urinary Ca, PTH, thyroid-stimulating hormone, free thyroxine, serum albumin, serum alkaline phosphatase, erythrocyte sedimentation rate, complete blood count, and vitamin D levels. Indirect tests of Ca absorption: gastric acid levels, vitamin D levels.

THERAPEUTIC CONSIDERATIONS

Goals for treating and preventing OP are as follows:

- Preserve adequate bone mass
- Preserve bone strength
- Prevent skeletal fragility
- Prevent deterioration of microarchitecture
- Prevent or reduce the risk of fractures

OP is largely preventable, but not by using the pharmaceuticals currently available. The number needed to treat (NNT) to prevent one hip fracture in women aged 55 to 64 years is 4406 for the bisphosphonates (BPs). For denosumab, 334 women must be treated for 3 years for one hip fracture to be prevented. Despite these facts, the North American Menopause Society guidelines recommend pharmaceutical therapy for the following:

- All PM women with previous OP vertebral or hip fracture.
- All PM women who have BMD values of −2.5 or lower at lumbar spine, femoral neck, or total hip region.
- All PM women with T-scores from −1.0 to −2.5 and a 10-year risk, based on FRAX calculator results, of major OP fracture (spine, hip, shoulder, or wrist) of at least 20% for hip fracture and at least 3% at high risk.

Pharmacologic therapies: numerous for OP treatment (e.g., BPs, selective estrogen receptor modulators [SERMs], raloxifene, PTH, estrogens, and calcitonin). These therapies, except estrogen, have been studied for effect on fracture only in patients with either a clinical or BMD diagnosis of OP. Absolute reduction in fracture risk is greatest in women at high risk for fracture.

Drug Therapy

- **Hormone replacement therapy (HRT):** both estrogen replacement therapy (ERT) and HRT reduce rate of bone turnover and resorption. ERT can lower resorption rates to those of premenopausal women. ERT and HRT reduce risk by 54%. ERT and HRT are more effective at reducing fracture risk if begun within 5 years of menopause. If used more than 10 years, they produce even greater risk reduction—75% for wrist fractures and 73% for hip fractures. Systemic oral or transdermal estrogen and estrogen-progestogen at standard doses increase BMD at all sites in PM women. The average difference in BMD after 2 years of treatment is 6.8% at lumbar spine and 4.1% at femoral neck. Daily doses of 0.625 mg conjugated equine estrogens with or without progestogen (either medroxyprogesterone acetate or oral micronized progesterone) for 3 years can increase spinal BMD by 3.5% to 5.0%, with a 1.7% increase in hip BMD. HRT can reduce risk of hip fractures (34%), vertebral fractures (34%), and total body fractures (24%). Even doses lower than standard for estrogen can increase spine and hip BMD 1% to 3%, as has systemic estrogen via vaginal ring (Femring). Standard doses of estrogen or estrogen-progestogen can reduce fracture risk in PM women by 27%. Despite these studies, estrogen-only or estrogen-plus-progestogen products are approved for prevention but not treatment of PM OP. Risks of breast cancer, blood clots, strokes, nonfatal myocardial infarction, cholelithiasis, breast tenderness, fluid retention, uterine bleeding, and headache are increased. Individualize treatment; identify risk/benefit ratio. ERT and HRT work best during first 5 to 10 years after menopause. The optimal duration and maximal duration have not yet been determined. ERT and HRT are not to be seen as primary long-term treatment except in those who do not tolerate BPs or who have menopausal symptoms that are not responding to other therapies.
- **BPs:** inhibit osteoclasts, reducing bone resorption. Increase BMD at spine and hip in PM women regardless of age. Although BPs are claimed to reduce risk of vertebral fractures in OP women by 40% to 70% and reduce incidence of hip and other fractures by half of this, these number are very misleading, as shown earlier in

discussion of NNT. Most BPs in the United States (alendronate, ibandronate, and risedronate) are intended for use in daily or intermittent oral doses. Zoledronic acid is given intravenously (IV). BMD responses show similar results for weekly oral administration of alendronate and risedronate, monthly oral administration of ibandronate and risedronate, and intravenous administration of ibandronate every 3 months. Use BPs only with caution, weighing potential benefit versus potential serious risk. Unresolved questions about BPs exist regarding the quality of bone; possibly increased fractures long term in some patients; and potential oversuppression of bone turnover long term, causing brittle bone. Problematic case reports: unusual, poorly healing fractures; atypical femur fractures. Clinicians' responses to these concerns: "drug holidays," the frequency and duration of which are under study. Other BP problems: OP of the jaw (osteonecrosis of the jaw [ONJ]) in patients on high-dose intravenous BPs and those treated with radiation for head and neck cancers. Characteristics of ONJ: delay in healing of oral lesions after surgery or extraction for more than 6 to 8 weeks. Incidence of ONJ with intravenous BPs in those without neck radiation: 12%. Oral incidence: 0.03% to 0.06%. However, oral surgery increases incidence sevenfold. Controversy: whether to discontinue BPs before dental extraction. Many practitioners suspend BPs until oral lesion heals. Uncommon long-term BP complication: insufficiency fractures of femoral shaft, which manifests with prodromal thigh pain and may be bilateral. Accordingly, BP use is now limited to a maximum of 5 years to allow bone remodeling. Monitor BMD closely to ensure stable or minimal bone loss after discontinuation. BP use for 5 years may provide long-term protection as effectively as BP therapy for more than 5 years. Side effects of oral BPs: upper gastrointestinal disorders (e.g., dysphagia, esophagitis, and esophageal and gastric ulcers). Precautions: hypocalcemia and renal impairment; uncommon transient flulike illness with large oral or intravenous doses. Follow administration directions carefully. Major benefits: life-altering relief of pain and suffering; save lives (hip fractures). Use FRAX tool for determining fracture risk in those with low BMD but not OP. With proper care and monitoring for adverse events and loss of bone remodeling, use BPs when truly indicated and only if natural interventions described herein fail to produce satisfactory results.

- **SERMs:** nonsteroidal estrogen agonists and/or antagonists. Raloxifene, at 60 mg q.d., is approved for prevention and treatment of OP and is the only SERM currently approved to treat OP. Raloxifene can significantly improve lumbar BMD by 1.6% to 2.6% and femoral neck BMD by 1.2% to 2.1%.

- **PTH:** anabolic agent, given by subcutaneous injection q.d., that stimulates osteoblastic bone formation and increases trabecular bone density in OP women. Teriparatide (Forteo) is approved to treat OP in PM women. At 20 mcg per injection q.d., teriparatide increased spine BMD by 8.6% and femoral neck BMD by 3.5% compared with placebo. It also reduced incidence of new vertebral fractures by 65% and nonvertebral fractures by 53%. Unfortunately, even chronic intermittent elevation of PTH by the standard dose of teriparatide (20 mcg/day) has been found to cause a number of undesirable side effects, including not only nausea, leg cramps, and dizziness, but hypercalcemia, hypercalciuria, and hyperuricemia plus hypomagnesemia. Also, because osteogenic sarcoma (a very aggressive bone cancer) occurred in almost half the animals in the rat studies, teriparatide comes with an FDA "black-box" warning about this potential long-term side effect. Lastly, chronic elevations in PTH promote cognitive decline.
- **Calcitonin:** approved for PM OP treatment but not prevention; available as nasal spray and subcutaneous injection. Intranasal spray delivering 200 international units (IU) q.d. for 5 years in PM women with OP reduced risk of new vertebral fractures by 33% compared with placebo. No effect was seen on hip or nonvertebral fractures. Calcitonin spray may also reduce bone pain from vertebral compression fractures.
- **New therapies being researched:** some of them are not currently available in the United States (e.g., tibolone and oral strontium ranelate [Protelos]). Denosumab (Prolia), a human monoclonal antibody to receptor activator of nuclear factor kappa B ligand, is approved and indicated to treat PM women with OP who are at high risk for fracture, who have a history of OP fracture, or who are intolerant of other OP therapies or in whom these therapies have failed. Other developing drugs: SERMs and full-length PTH.

Lifestyle Factors

Lifestyle approaches alone are insufficient to prevent bone loss or fractures; however, they do provide foundation for natural therapies to prevent and manage OP. Smoking accelerates bone loss and reduces bone mass. Smokers experience menopause 2 years earlier than nonsmokers. PM smokers have higher fracture rates. Hip fracture risk may be increased in current smokers, especially among women older than 60. A history of smoking increases risk for future fracture independent of BMD. Moderate alcohol intake is associated with increased BMD in PM women, but alcohol consumption greater than seven units a week is linked to increased risk of falls. Drinking more than two units a day of alcohol increases risk of OP fracture (one unit = 12 oz of beer, 4 oz of wine, or 1 oz of liquor).

- **Exercise:** physical fitness is the major determinant of bone density. One hour of moderate activity three times per week prevents bone loss and increases bone mass in PM women. Both weight bearing and strength training benefit bone development, function, and maintenance. Women who exercise can increase spine BMD by 2%. In surgically menopausal women who have used estrogen, adding strength training enhances BMD. Although a particular exercise may not increase BMD, it can reduce risk of fractures from falling. Muscle-strengthening and balancing exercises reduce risk of falls and related injuries by 75% in women age 75 and older. Immobilization doubles the rate of urinary and fecal Ca excretion, causing negative Ca balance. The most effective practice for strengthening bones is physical activity. Simple weight-bearing exercises: walking or tai chi. Simple strength-training exercises: home barbells or resistance bands. Consult resources that give guidance about effective exercises, safe activities, and exercises to be avoided.

General Dietary Factors

Dietary factors suggested as causes of OP include the following:

- **Low Ca, low vitamin K_2**, low Mg, high phosphorus intake
- **High-protein diet**
- **High acid-ash diet**
- **High salt intake** (half of diet-induced acidosis—much of which is neutralized by extracting Ca from bone—is caused by excessive consumption of salt, which apparently impairs renal excretion of acid)
- **Trace mineral deficiencies**
- **Vegetarian diet** (both lacto-ovo and vegan): lowers risk of OP. Bone mass in vegetarians does not differ from omnivores in third, fourth, and fifth decades but does in later decades. Decreased incidence of OP in vegetarians is caused by decreased

bone loss in later years. High-protein and high-phosphate diets increase excretion of Ca in urine. Raising daily protein from 47 to 142 g doubles urine Ca excretion. Opposing point of view: high-protein diets increase urinary Ca excretion and acid production, causing negative Ca balance only if daily Ca intake is inadequate. Rather than reduce protein, increase intake of Ca plus fruits and vegetables for alkalinizing effect. Reasonable compromise: ensure at least 20 g q.d. of protein, especially in the elderly older than 80, with an upper limit of 60 g. The key issue here is systemic pH effects of foods. Diet-induced acidosis, typical of high-protein and high-salt eating, causes the body to normalize pH by buffering with Ca taken from bones. Although Ca supplements can prevent bone loss in excess doses, they can increase Ca kidney stones in those susceptible. Possible strategy to reduce this risk of kidney stones: use Ca citrate.

- **Gastric acid:** Ca must be ionized in the stomach acid to be absorbed. Poor ionization of Ca is a major problem with Ca carbonate. Decreased gastric acidity occurs in 40% of PM women, but the effects of increased gastric pH appear only when poorly soluble Ca salts such as Ca carbonate are taken after an overnight fast. Fasting patients with insufficient stomach acid only absorb 4% of oral Ca as Ca carbonate, whereas normal stomach acid allows absorption of 22%. Preionized Ca is preferred: Ca citrate, lactate, or gluconate. Forty-five percent of Ca is absorbed from citrate with reduced stomach acid. However, if calcium is taken with meals, little difference in Ca absorption is found, even in elderly subjects with atrophic gastritis or those taking H_2-receptor antagonists.
- **Sugar:** after refined sugar intake, urinary excretion of Ca increases. The average American consumes 125 g of sucrose, 50 g of corn syrup plus other simple sugars, a glass of carbonated beverage loaded with phosphates, and a high amount of protein every day.
- **Soft drinks:** are high in phosphates but not Ca. Per capita intake in the United States: 15 oz/day. Soft drink intake in children is a major risk factor for impaired calcification of growing bones. Serum Ca levels are inversely correlated with number of bottles of soft drinks consumed each week.
- **Green leafy vegetables:** eating green leafy vegetables (e.g., kale, collard greens, parsley, lettuce) protects against OP. They are rich sources of broad range of vitamins and minerals that maintain healthy bones (Ca, vitamin K_1, boron).

- **Soy isoflavones:** the potential for soy protein or soy isoflavones to alter bone metabolism and bone resorption is contradictory and inconclusive. Soybeans contain phytoestrogens—genistein, daidzein, and glycitein—molecularly similar to 17-beta-estradiol. Binding of isoflavones to estrogen receptors is preferential for estrogen receptor beta, indicating that isoflavones act as selective estrogen receptor modulators. Daidzein is molecularly similar to the drug ipriflavone, used in Europe to treat OP. Ipriflavone is a nutritional supplement in the United States. BMD is the gold standard parameter for determining nontraumatic fracture risk, and bone turnover is an independent predictor. Soy may play a role in slowing bone turnover and increasing BMD in women because of estrogenic effect on bone. Variations in dose, duration, soy formulation used, and different study populations are possible reasons for inconsistent results regarding effects of isoflavones on bone turnover and BMD. However, how isoflavones are metabolized in the gut is also a factor. Significant effects on urinary peptides occur in Asian women but not white women, perhaps because of conversion of daidzein into its active metabolite equol by intestinal flora and the fact that only one third of white women can metabolize isoflavones into equol, whereas more than half of Asian women can do so. Soy isoflavones may also have more effect in PM women than premenopausal or perimenopausal women. An overlooked nutritional influence of soy foods may be the amount of Ca in some soy foods or in diets containing soy foods. Some soy foods offer as much Ca as dairy foods. Prudent clinical advice: increase soy foods as prevention for premenopausal, perimenopausal, and PM women. For all women with significant risk for OP, add soy supplements so that total daily isoflavone intake would be 90 mg q.d. Use isoflavones to treat perimenopausal and PM women with OP , as part of a larger protocol.

Nutritional Supplements

Bone needs a constant supply of many nutrients. Deficiency of any one adversely affects bone health. In addition to vitamin K and boron, bone needs the following:

- **Ca:** adequate Ca intake is essential in very young women and the elderly. However, Ca is only modestly effective in slowing loss of BMD in perimenopausal and early PM women. Supplementation may improve efficacy of pharmaceutical agents intended to treat bone loss. Higher Ca intake and supplementation

(500 to 2000 mg q.d.) are not associated with lower incidence of hip fractures. Ca at 1000 mg/day plus 400 IU of vitamin D per day decreases hip fractures by 29% compared with placebo. In PM women, Ca supplements decrease bone loss by 50% at non-vertebral sites. Effects are greatest in women whose baseline Ca intake was low, in older women, and in women with established OP. Vertebral bone loss has been reduced with 1000 to 2000 mg of Ca per day for 1 year. Dietary Ca is essential throughout a woman's life; requirements increase with advancing age because of less absorption and less renal Ca conservation. However, Ca supplementation alone does not prevent accelerated bone loss occurring soon after menopause. Ten years after menopause, Ca supplementation again helps reduce age-related bone loss. Adequate Ca is important but can be given at excessive doses. Ca is only one of many nutritional and lifestyle factors that affect bone health.

- **Vitamin D:** supports Ca balance by enhancing intestinal Ca absorption. Increased Ca absorption reduces PTH-mediated bone resorption. Fortified dairy foods are main sources in the United States. Intake declines with age. Vitamin D doses must be adequate to raise serum $25(OH)D_3$ levels into the effective range. Nonetheless, in elderly PM women, even inadequate dose of 700 to 800 IU/day is associated with reduced risk of hip and nonvertebral fractures. Especially in older women, vitamin D, combined with Ca supplements, reduces rate of PM bone loss. Vitamin D also improves muscle strength and balance, thereby reducing the risk of falling.
- **Mg:** may be as important as Ca supplementation to prevent and treat OP. Women with OP have lower bone Mg than those without OP. Human Mg deficiency is linked to diminished serum levels of most active vitamin D ($1,25\text{-}[OH]_2D_3$), also seen in OP. Mechanism: either enzyme responsible for converting $25\text{-}(OH)D_3$ to $1,25\text{-}(OH)_2D_3$ is Mg dependent or Mg mediates PTH and calcitonin secretion. Supplementing at 250 to 750 mg (as Mg hydroxide) for 1 year slightly improved BMD. Cofactor for alkaline phosphatase, involved in bone mineralization. Low Mg status is common in women with OP, and Mg deficiency is associated with abnormal bone mineral crystals. Some women with reduced BMD do not have an increased fracture rate, possibly because their bone mineral crystals are of high quality, owing in part to high tissue Mg. In PM women, supplementing Mg at 250 to 750 mg/day for 6 months followed by

250 mg/day for 6 to 18 months increased BMD in 71% of these women without Ca supplementation.

- **Strontium:** nonradioactive earth element physically and chemically similar to C. Strontium ranelate specifically is used for OP in clinical trials but is unavailable in the United States. Strontium in large doses stimulates bone formation and reduces bone resorption. Clinical trials are inconclusive. Clinical study: among PM women with history of vertebral fractures, the incidence of new vertebral deformities was lowest (38.8%) with lowest dose of strontium. Strontium chloride is the most common form in in the United States, but it has not been researched. Owing to potential adverse effects of higher doses, including rickets, bone mineralization defects, and interference with vitamin D metabolism, it is prudent to use low doses until more research is conducted.
- **Zinc (Zn):** essential for the formation of osteoblasts and osteoclasts. Zn enhances biochemical action of vitamin D and supports synthesis of bone proteins. Zn deficits are found in the serum and bone of the elderly with OP.
- **Copper (Cu):** deficiency produces abnormal bone development in growing children and contributes to OP. Cu supplementation inhibits bone resorption—3 mg/day for 2 years significantly decreased bone loss in PM women.
- **Manganese (Mn):** Mn deficiency is an esoteric but important factor in OP. Mn deficiency causes a reduction in Ca deposition in bone. Mn stimulates mucopolysaccharide production, providing a framework for calcification.
- **Zn, Cu, and Mn:** this combination with Ca might be more effective than Ca alone for preventing bone loss in PM women.
- **Boron:** supplementation reduces urinary excretion of Ca and Mg and increases serum 17-beta-estradiol and testosterone in PM women. Boron supplementation might help to prevent bone loss.
- **Silicon:** during bone growth and early calcification, silicon supports cross-links between collagen and proteoglycans. Silicon-deficient diets produce abnormal skull development and growth retardation in animals; supplemental silicon may partially prevent trabecular bone loss.
- **Folate and vitamin B_{12}:** high homocysteine (Hcys) may contribute to PM bone loss. A breakdown product of methionine, Hcys can promote OP if it is not eliminated. Women with high

Hcys have twice the risk of nonvertebral OP fractures as do women with low Hcys. However, there is no association between Hcys levels and femoral neck or lumbar BMD. This suggests that fracture risk is a result of poorer bone quality. Folate promotes remethylation of Hcys to methionine; supplementing PM women reduces Hcys levels. B_{12} also reduces Hcys. Research dosage: 5 mg of folate plus 1500 mcg of B_{12} for 2 years reduced hip fracture incidence by 78% compared with placebo.

- **Vitamin B_6:** also helps control Hcys. In people with genetic disorder homocystinuria, B_6 supplementation reverses elevated Hcys. B_6 deficiency can prolong fracture healing time, impair cartilage growth, cause defective bone formation, and promote OP. B_6 may influence progesterone production and exert a synergistic effect on estrogen-sensitive tissue. B_6 deficits are common, even among healthy persons.
- **Vitamin C:** promotes formation and cross-linking of some structural proteins in bone. Ascorbate deficiency can cause OP. Scurvy, caused by vitamin C deficiency, is also associated with bone abnormalities.
- **Vitamin K_1 and K_2** (menaquinone): K_1's anti-inflammatory actions help prevent excessive osteoclast activation. K_2 is required for the activation of the two proteins essential to Ca regulation: osteocalcin, which draws Ca ions to bone tissue, enabling Ca crystal formation, and matrix Gla protein, which prevents Ca deposition in the vasculature. Vitamin K_2 is required for bone formation, remodeling, and repair because osteocalcin is a vitamin K–dependent protein. Low intake of vitamin K increases risk of OP hip fractures in women. Forms of vitamin K: vitamin K_1 (phylloquinone), MK-4 (a form of vitamin K_2) and MK-7 (a longer-chain form of vitamin K_2). Low intake of vitamin K is linked to increased bone loss in the elderly. Meta-analysis of randomized controlled trials of K_1 or MK-4 supplements at the high dose of 45 mg q.d. (15 mg every 6 to 8 hours) for more than 6 months reported reduction in bone loss with supplemental vitamin K. The recommended intake is 90 to 120 mcg/day; however, the optimal protective dose and form of vitamin K are unknown. Most studies used MK-4 at doses 400-fold higher than recommendations for K_1, and they involved exclusively Japanese PM women, thereby skewing results toward Japanese diets and genetics. MK-7 is found in natto (highest concentration in

fermented soybeans) and cheese and in lower concentrations in meat and other dairy. Small amounts may be produced by health-promoting gut bacteria from dietary vitamin K_1 if the body's supply of K_1 exceeds needs for the production of clotting factors. MK-7 is more potent and bioavailable with a much longer half-life than MK-4. As a daily supplement (0.22 μmol/day), MK-7 is more effective than MK-4 in carboxylating osteocalcin. MK-7 has longer residence time and higher serum levels during prolonged intake. Longer-chain menaquinones (MK-7) are more hydrophobic, increasing half-life. In Japanese PM women, natto consumption is inversely linked to incidence of hip fractures. A likely reason for inconsistent clinical results is the confounding effect of vitamin D status. Vitamin D deficiency affects the results.

- **Ipriflavone:** semisynthetic isoflavonoid similar to soy isoflavonoids and approved in Japan, Hungary, and Italy for treatment and prevention of OP. It has been impressive in clinical studies. Ipriflavone (200 mg t.i.d.) increased BMD measurements by 2% and 5.8% after 6 and 12 months, respectively, in women with OP. Ipriflavone (600 mg/day) produced 6% increase in BMD after 12 months, whereas BMD of controls declined by 0.3%. Naturally occurring isoflavonoids such as genistein and diadzein in soy may exert similar benefits. Given benefits of soy isoflavonoids against breast cancer, soy foods are encouraged. Mechanism of action: enhanced calcitonin effects (see earlier) on Ca metabolism; ipriflavone exerts no estrogen-like effects. Most recent and extensive study has not shown positive results. Ipriflavone may not have an important role in treating OP. It may be more appropriate for women with osteopenia or for prevention of OP and not OP treatment. Because of the incidence of decreased lymphocytes and lack of effect, the risk/benefit ratio of ipriflavone must be considered. Ipriflavone may be considered for women for whom other OP treatments are unacceptable, not tolerated, or contraindicated. Monitor BMD to confirm benefit; monitor lymphocyte levels to detect adverse effects.

Botanical Medicine

***Camellia sinensis* (green tea):** Green tea consumption may protect against OP. Green tea is rich in polyphenols and is a major source of vitamin K_1. Dose: 3 to 5 cups daily, providing 250 mg daily of polyphenols (catechins), *or* a green tea extract providing the same quantity of polyphenols. Green tea polyphenols impaired bone resorption and stimulated osteoblast activity in laboratory experiments.

THERAPEUTIC APPROACH

The most effective approach to OP is prevention. Optimize peak bone mass during younger years, and minimize subsequent bone loss in elderly women. To maximize peak bone mass (even with hereditary and other nonmodifiable risk factors), prescribe bone-supportive lifestyle, whole-foods nutrition, and moderate weight-bearing exercise during childhood and adolescence. Add avoidance of smoking and excessive alcohol intake thereafter. Lifestyle improvements and supplements may reduce risk in many women but not all. For women already diagnosed, nutritional and lifestyle factors serve as adjuncts to conventional therapies. Primary goals: prevent bone loss and reduce fracture risk. In cases of actual OP (vs. osteopenia), use the following recommendations in conjunction with appropriate conventional care, including prescription drugs.

- **Exercise:** weight-bearing exercise four times per week plus strength training and/or weight training twice per week.
- **Habits:**
  - — Drink less than seven units of alcohol per week
  - — Avoid smoking and secondhand smoke
  - — Implement measures to prevent falls
- **Diet:** balanced diet with focus on adequate protein, daily soy isoflavones, green leafy vegetables, adequate Ca and vitamin D, vitamin K, and Mg. Avoid factors that promote Ca excretion (e.g., salt, sugar, excessive protein, and soft drinks).

Supplements

- High-potency multiple vitamin-mineral formula
- Key individual nutrients:
  - — Ca: 1000 to 1200 mg q.d.
  - — Mg: 350 to 500 mg q.d.
  - — Vitamin D_3: 2000 to 5000 IU q.d. (measure blood levels and adjust dose accordingly)
  - — Vitamin B_6: 25 to 50 mg q.d.
  - — Folate, optimally 5-MTHF: 800 mcg q.d.

— Vitamin B_{12}: 800 mcg q.d.
— Vitamin K_2 (MK-7): 100 mcg q.d.
— Fish oils: 1000 mg eicosapentaenoic acid (EPA) plus docosahexaenoic acid (DHA) q.d.
— Soy isoflavones: 90 mg q.d; or ipriflavone: 600 mg q.d.
— Strontium: 170 to 680 mg q.d. (see earlier discussion)

Botanical Medicine

- **Green tea:** either 3 to 5 cups q.d. or a green tea extract providing 250 to 300 mg polyphenols (catechins) q.d.

Otitis Media

DIAGNOSTIC SUMMARY

Acute Otitis Media

- Earache or irritability
- History of recent upper respiratory tract infection or allergy
- Red, opaque, bulging eardrum with loss of the normal features
- Fever and chills

Chronic or Serous Otitis Media

- Painless hearing loss
- Dull, immobile tympanic membrane

GENERAL CONSIDERATIONS

Otitis media (OM) is inflammation, swelling, or infection of the middle ear. Two types of OM are diagnosed.

- **Acute OM:** usually preceded by upper respiratory tract infection or allergy. Common microorganisms are *Streptococcus pneumoniae* (40% to 50%), *Haemophilus influenzae* (30% to 40%), and *Moraxella catarrhalis* (10% to 15%).
- **Chronic OM** (also known as *serous, secretory,* or *nonsuppurative OM; chronic OM with effusion;* or *glue ear*): constant swelling of middle ear. Acute OM affects two thirds of American children by age 2 years; chronic OM affects two thirds of children younger than 6 years. OM is the most common diagnosis in children and accounts for more than 50% of all visits to pediatricians. Eight billion dollars are spent annually on medical and surgical treatment.

Standard Medical Treatment

- Interventions: antibiotics, analgesics (e.g., acetaminophen), and/or antihistamines. If longstanding infection is unresponsive to drugs, surgery is performed that involves placing a tiny plastic myringotomy tube through the eardrum to drain fluid into the throat by the eustachian tube (ET).

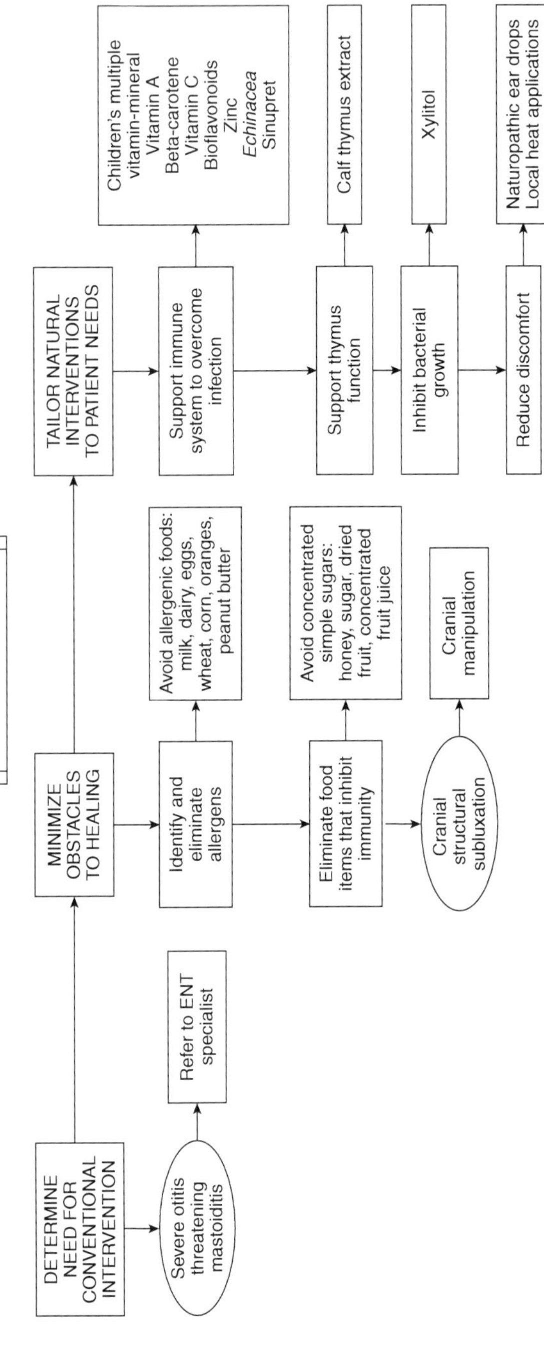
OTITIS MEDIA
DETERMINE NEED FOR CONVENTIONAL INTERVENTION
Severe otitis threatening mastoiditis
Refer to ENT specialist
MINIMIZE OBSTACLES TO HEALING
Identify and eliminate allergens
Avoid allergenic foods: milk, dairy, eggs, wheat, corn, oranges, peanut butter
Eliminate food items that inhibit immunity
Avoid concentrated simple sugars: honey, sugar, dried fruit, concentrated fruit juice
Cranial structural subluxation
Cranial manipulation
TAILOR NATURAL INTERVENTIONS TO PATIENT NEEDS
Support immune system to overcome infection
Children's multiple vitamin-mineral
Vitamin A
Beta-carotene
Vitamin C
Bioflavonoids
Zinc
Echinacea
Sinupret
Support thymus function
Calf thymus extract
Inhibit bacterial growth
Xylitol
Reduce discomfort
Naturopathic ear drops
Local heat applications

- Children with tubes in their ears are more likely to have further problems with OM. Surgery is unnecessary for most children. Only 42% of these surgeries are judged appropriate. No significant differences in clinical course of acute OM have been found between conventional treatments and placebo. No differences have been found among nonantibiotic treatment, ear tubes, ear tubes with antibiotics, and antibiotics alone. Children not receiving antibiotics may have fewer recurrences than those receiving antibiotics because of immune suppression and disturbance of respiratory microflora by antibiotics.
- Because most children with acute OM (70% to 90%) have spontaneous resolution within 7 to 14 days, antibiotics should not initially be routinely prescribed for all children.
- Results of extensive international review: antibiotics are not recommended for OM in most children. Conventional alternative: analgesics (e.g., acetaminophen) and close observation by parent; 80% of children with acute OM respond to placebo within 48 hours. A natural alternative to avoid analgesic toxicity is botanical ear drops (see later).
- Risks of antibiotics: allergic reactions, gastric upset, accelerated bacterial resistance, unfavorable changes in nasopharyngeal bacterial flora. Antibiotics fail to eradicate microbe, may induce middle ear superinfection, and increase return office visits. Concurrent antibiotic and steroid treatment yields poor results.
- Antibiotics induce chronic candidiasis and "superbugs" resistant to antibiotics. They should be used only for underlying systemic infection.
- OM is normally self-limiting. Eighty percent of children's cases spontaneously remit within 2 to 14 days; children younger than 2 years have a lower spontaneous resolution of 30% after a few days.
- Evaluate each child individually. Follow-up: devise physician-family communication before making a decision not to use conventional medicine.
- Special circumstances to prevent hearing loss–induced developmental delays suggest use of ear tubes.
- Pneumococcal and viral vaccines have little benefit because of the multifactorial nature of OM. With risks and complications, vaccinations are warranted at this time for the prevention of OM.

Causes

- Primary risk factors for OM: day care attendance, wood-burning stoves, parental smoking or exposure to other secondhand smoke, food allergies, not being breastfed, pacifier use, previous antibiotic use, winter season, underlying rhinitis, cleft palate, Down's syndrome.

- Common mechanism is abnormal ET function, the underlying cause in virtually all cases of OM.
- ET regulates gas pressure in the middle ear, protects the middle ear from nose and throat secretions and bacteria, and clears fluids from the middle ear. Swallowing opens the ET by action of surrounding muscles. Infants and small children are susceptible to ET problems because of a smaller diameter and more-horizontal orientation.
- ET obstruction allows fluid buildup and bacterial infection if immunity is impaired and pathogenic microbes are present. Obstruction results from collapse of tube (weak tissues and/or abnormal opening mechanism), blockage by allergy-induced mucus, mucosal edema, or infection.
- Genetic factors: monozygotic twins have a higher concordance rate in OM history than do dizygotic twins. No genetic influence has been identified in studies of immunoglobulin markers and human leukocyte antigens.
- Blood type: children with blood type A have 50% higher rate of infection and are susceptible to more-severe and repeated bouts of OM. Children whose mothers have blood type A and who have OM before age 1 year have greater risk of having recurrent ear infections by an astounding 2677%.

THERAPEUTIC CONSIDERATIONS

Treatment goals: ensure ET patency and drainage by identifying and addressing causative factors; support immune system (*Textbook,* "Immune Support"). Bottle feeding: recurrent ear infection is linked to early bottle feeding. Breastfeeding (minimum 3 to 4 months) is protective, possibly because of cow's milk allergy and protective effect of human milk against infection. Bottle feeding while the child is lying on his or her back (bottle propping) leads to regurgitation of bottle contents into the middle ear. Human milk is protective because of its high antibody content, inhibiting microbes. Breastfed infants have thymus glands 20 times larger than formula-fed infants.

- **Food allergy:** the role of allergy as the major cause of chronic OM has been firmly established in research literature. The middle and inner ear are immunologically responsive, including responsiveness to food hypersensitivities. From 85% to 93% of children with OM have allergies: 16% to inhalants only, 14% to food only, 70% to both. Prolonged breastfeeding may prevent OM by avoiding food allergens, particularly if mother avoids sensitizing foods (those to which she is allergic) during pregnancy and lactation. Excluding or limiting foods to which children are commonly allergic (wheat, egg, fowl, dairy), particularly during the first 9 months, also is of value. The child's digestive tract is permeable to antigens, especially during the first 3 months. Control eating patterns (infrequent repetition of any food, avoid common allergenic foods, and introduce foods in controlled manner—one food at a time, carefully watching for reaction).

- **Allergic reaction:** causes blockage of ET—inflammatory edema of ET mucosa and nasal edema causing Toynbee phenomenon (swallowing with both mouth and nose closed, forcing air and secretions into the middle ear).
- **Chronic OM:** always consider allergy. A total of 93.3% of children tested were allergic to foods, inhalants, or both. Ninety-two percent of children with OM improve when treated with serial dilution titration therapy for inhalants and elimination diet for food allergens. A statistically significant association exists between food allergy and recurrent OM in 78% of patients. Elimination diet ameliorates chronic OM in 86% of patients. Challenge diet with suspected offending food(s) provokes recurrence of serous OM in 94% of patients.
- **Most common food allergens** (in order of frequency): cow's milk, wheat, egg white, peanut, soy, corn, tomato, chicken, apple.
- **Reflux:** there might be a link between gastroesophageal reflux disease in infants and young children with OM. Disease burden from OM and hearing loss decreases with acid-blocking pharmaceuticals. Dose: 15-mg dose of lansoprazole in the morning and, depending on age, ranitidine (4 mg/kg q.d.) or nizatidine (5 mg/kg q.d.) at bedtime. The Pediatric Reflux Finding Score, which assesses extraesophageal reflux via fiberoptic laryngoscopy, showed improvements. However, there was a high dropout rate, perhaps because of side effects. From the naturopathic perspective, the role of digestive function is important for OM and health in general. Drugs mentioned earlier are not recommended because they will impair digestive function and increase risk of food allergies as well as unhealthy gut flora.

Use food allergen avoidance, a focus on healthful foods, and measures to support digestive health.

- **Thymus gland extract:** the thymus secretes hormones acting on white blood cells to ensure proper development and function. Oral calf thymus extracts given to children improve immune function, decrease food allergies, and improve resistance to chronic respiratory infections. They may be of particular benefit in chronic OM (*Textbook,* "Food Allergy Testing").
- **Naturopathic herbal ear drops:** otalgia (ear pain) can persist during period of improvement, motivating anxious parents to request unnecessary antibiotics. Naturopathic botanical eardrops are as effective as either antibiotic or anesthetic drops, with much less toxicity. Herbal ear drop combination: *Calendula officinalis* flowers (marigold, 28%), *Hypericum perforatum* complete herb (St. John's wort, 30%), and *Verbascum thapsus* flowers (mullein, 25%) in olive oil with essential oils *Allium sativum* (garlic) 0.05% in olive oil (10%), *Lavandula officinalis* (lavender, 5%), and tocopherol acetate oil (vitamin E, 2%). Dose: 5 drops t.i.d.
- ***Echinacea:*** effective for upper respiratory infection and stimulates components of cytokine cascade. As monotherapy, the efficacy of *Echinacea* is unclear. Given its long history of benefit, *Echinacea* might be helpful in combination with other natural treatments.
- **Xylitol:** a commonly used sweetener with anticariogenic properties. It is a sugar alcohol derived from birch and other hardwood trees. It inhibits *S. pneumoniae.* Xylitol reduces acute OM incidence by 40%. It can be given as xylitol (8.4 g/day) chewing gum or lozenge to reduce incidence of OM in day care centers and schools. Xylitol administration needs to be four or five times per day, which may decrease compliance and overall efficacy. Side effect is diarrhea.
- **Sinupret:** herbal combination originating in Germany, consisting of sorrel (aerial) *(Rumex acetosa),* 36 mg; European elder (flower) *(Sambucus nigra),* 36 mg; cowslip (flower with calyx) *(Primula veris),* 36 mg; European vervain (aerial) *(Verbena officinalis),* 36 mg; and gentian (root) *(Gentiana lutea),* 12 mg. Sinupret works with antibiotics and may have more-effective antibiotic properties than amoxicillin for OM. It may also reduce the frequency of complications. Sinupret may be a reasonable choice for children already started on antibiotics.
- **Vitamin A:** helps prevent oxidative tissue damage, support immune function, and maintain mucous membrane integrity.

Although not studied in children, pretreatment with vitamin A in animals before *S. pneumoniae* inoculation conferred protection by increasing antioxidant enzyme activity and reducing formation of malondialdehyde and nitric oxide.

- **Humidifiers:** are popular treatments for OM and upper respiratory infections in children. Significantly more effusions (fluid in ETs) are observed in laboratory animals kept in low-humidity environments compared with those kept in more-moderate environments. Low humidity may induce nasal swelling and reduce ventilation of ET or may dry ET lining, causing inability to clear fluid and increased secretions. Mast cells of ET mucosa may release histamine and produce edema. Increasing humidity with a humidifier may be an important modality to treat OM with effusion.
- **Osteopathic manipulation:** may decrease frequency of recurrent OM in children. Osteopathy acknowledges abnormal structural dynamics, which can contribute to change in function. These dynamics may be modulated with cranial manipulative. In young patients with structural dysfunction, this may be beneficial in conjunction with other therapies.

THERAPEUTIC APPROACH

Goals: recognize and eliminate allergies, particularly food allergies; support immune system and digestive function.

- **Diet:** determining the exact allergen during an acute attack typically is not possible. Eliminate most common allergenic foods: milk and dairy, eggs, wheat, corn, oranges, peanut butter, chocolate. Eliminate concentrated simple carbohydrates (sugar, honey, dried fruit, concentrated fruit juice) that inhibit the immune system.
- **Nutritional supplements:**
  - — Children's multiple vitamin-mineral formula
  - — Vitamin A: 50,000 international units (IU) q.d. for 2 days in children younger than 6 years, and 4 days in children older than 6 years
  - — Beta-carotene (natural mixed carotenoids): age in years × 20,000 IU q.d. (up to 200,000 IU q.d.)
  - — Vitamin C: age in years × 50 mg every 2 hours
  - — Bioflavonoids: age in years × 50 mg every 2 hours
  - — Zinc: age in years × 2.5 mg q.d. (up to 30 mg) for maximum of 2 weeks

- — Thymus extract: equivalent of 120 mg pure polypeptides with molecular weights below 10,000 daltons or 500 mg of crude polypeptide fractions daily
- **Botanical medicines:**
  - — *Echinacea* species: half of adult dose for children younger than 6 years; full adult dose for children older than 6 years (*Echinacea* is safe for children); all doses can be given up to three times daily. Dried root (or as tea), 0.5 to 1 g; freeze-dried plant, 325 to 650 mg juice of aerial portion of *Echinacea purpurea* stabilized in 22% ethanol, 2 to 3 mL; tincture (1:5), 2 to 4 mL; fluid extract (1:1), 2 to 4 mL; solid (dried powdered) extract (6.5:1 or 3.5% echinacoside), 150 to 300 mg.
  - — Xylitol: 8 g/day as either chewing gum chewed throughout day or 10 g of syrup per day in divided doses.
  - — Naturopathic ear drop formula: 5 drops in affected ear t.i.d.
  - — Sinupret: as adjunctive treatment when antibiotics are employed.
- Consider cranial manipulation.
- **Physical medicine:** local application of heat is often helpful in reducing discomfort; apply as hot pack with warm oil (mullein oil) or by blowing hot air into ear with straw and hair dryer. These tactics help reduce pressure in the middle ear and promote fluid drainage.

Parkinson's Disease

DIAGNOSTIC SUMMARY

- **Motor symptoms are considered cardinal in Parkinson's disease (PD).**
  - — Tremor: most common feature—resting tremor, maximal when limb is at rest and diminishing with voluntary movement and sleep. Tremor affects the most distal part of the extremity; typically unilateral at onset, progressing to bilateral. Thirty percent of PD patients do not have tremor at onset, yet most progress into it.
  - — Combination of joint stiffness, increased muscle tone, and resting tremor produce "ratchety" cogwheel rigidity during passive motion.
  - — Slow movement (bradykinesia) or inability to move (akinesia): difficulties not only with executing movement but also with planning and initiating movement. Performance of sequential and simultaneous movements is hindered. Most disabling feature in early stages: bradykinesia.
- **Other common motor symptoms:**
  - — Postural instability in late stages, causing impaired balance and frequent falls, but often absent in initial stages, especially in younger patients.
  - — Pill-rolling motion of thumb and forefinger.
  - — Stooped posture, progressively shortened and accelerated steps that get progressively faster and may lead to falling *(festinating gait).*
  - — Reduced or fixed facial expressions ("masked face"), low-volume and/or monotone voice, or both.
  - — Small handwriting (micrographia) that decreases in size toward end of a writing sample.
  - — Gastrointestinal symptoms: constipation can be an early symptom. Difficulty swallowing (dysphagia) may arise later.

Neuropsychiatry

- Cognitive disturbances: may occur early, but progress to dementia in 80% of cases by the tenth year. Most common cognitive

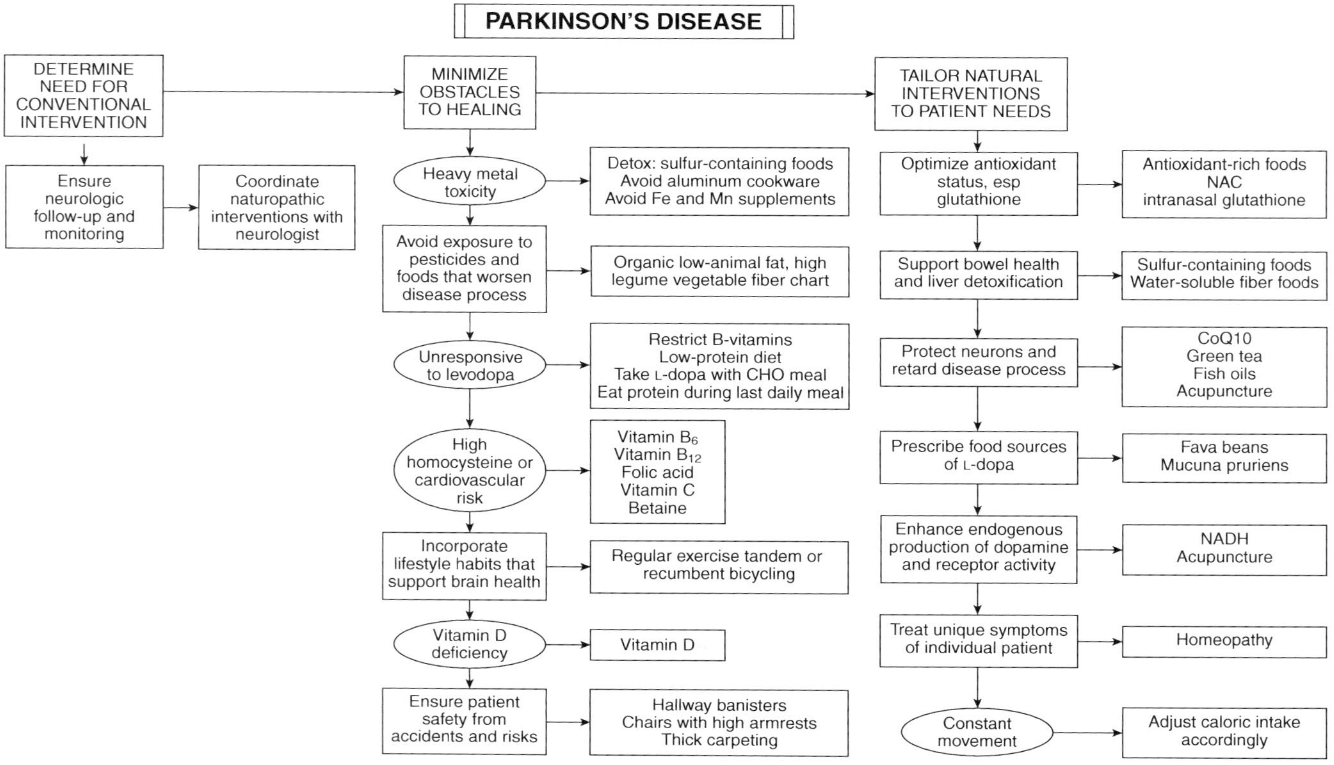
PARKINSON'S DISEASE
DETERMINE NEED FOR CONVENTIONAL INTERVENTION
Ensure neurologic follow-up and monitoring
Coordinate naturopathic interventions with neurologist
MINIMIZE OBSTACLES TO HEALING
Heavy metal toxicity
Detox: sulfur-containing foods
Avoid aluminum cookware
Avoid Fe and Mn supplements
Avoid exposure to pesticides and foods that worsen disease process
Organic low-animal fat, high legume vegetable fiber chart
Unresponsive to levodopa
Restrict B-vitamins
Low-protein diet
Take L-dopa with CHO meal
Eat protein during last daily meal
High homocysteine or cardiovascular risk
Vitamin B_6
Vitamin B_{12}
Folic acid
Vitamin C
Betaine
Incorporate lifestyle habits that support brain health
Regular exercise tandem or recumbent bicycling
Vitamin D deficiency
Vitamin D
Ensure patient safety from accidents and risks
Hallway banisters
Chairs with high armrests
Thick carpeting
TAILOR NATURAL INTERVENTIONS TO PATIENT NEEDS
Optimize antioxidant status, esp glutathione
Antioxidant-rich foods
NAC
intranasal glutathione
Support bowel health and liver detoxification
Sulfur-containing foods
Water-soluble fiber foods
Protect neurons and retard disease process
CoQ10
Green tea
Fish oils
Acupuncture
Prescribe food sources of L-dopa
Fava beans
Mucuna pruriens
Enhance endogenous production of dopamine and receptor activity
NADH
Acupuncture
Treat unique symptoms of individual patient
Homeopathy
Constant movement
Adjust caloric intake accordingly

deficits: decision making, adapting to new environments, problem solving, attention span, cognitive speed, and memory—specifically recalling learned information, with improvement when given cues.
- Alterations in behavior and mood: depression, apathy, anxiety. Poor impulse control can lead to "punding," binge eating, craving, hypersexuality, or pathologic gambling. These are linked to dopamine dysregulation syndrome associated with pharmaceuticals for PD.
- Psychotic symptoms: hallucinations or delusions are common in later stages.

GENERAL CONSIDERATIONS

Epidemiology

- Occurs in 0.3 % of the general population and 1% of the population older than 55 to 60 years. It affects 500,000 people in the United States.
- Progressive neurologic disorder caused by the deterioration of neurons in the brain region that controls muscle movements, causing shortage of neurotransmitter dopamine and leading to movement impairments.
- Features: trembling, muscle rigidity, difficulty walking, problems with balance and coordination.
- Prevalence and incidence rise with age; average age of onset is 60 years; rates are very low in those younger than 40 years and rise in the 70s and 80s.
- Found in many regions of world. True ethnic and/or geographic differences are unclear.

Pathophysiology

- Primary contributors to cell death: oxidative and nitric oxide stress, inflammation, and mitochondrial dysfunction. Decreased glutathione (GSH), the brain's primary antioxidant, is an early biochemical event in the substantia nigra.
- Mitochondrial dysfunction: several PD-associated genes interface with pathways regulating mitochondrial function, morphology, and dynamics.
- Primary pathology of PD: degeneration of neurons in the brain substantia nigra pars compacta. These neurons produce dopamine, a critical signaling molecule. Dopamine loss induces profound, multifaceted disruption of information flow through the basal ganglia.

- Lewy bodies: hallmark of classic PD; found in substantia nigra; abnormal accumulations of alpha-synuclein, a normal cellular protein, marked for degradation by ubiquitin complex, but escaping normal degradation process. Presence of Lewy bodies is not a diagnostic criterion because they are found only at autopsy. Autopsies reveal Lewy bodies in surprising numbers of the elderly without diagnosed PD. Symptoms do not occur until nervous system "reserve" is exhausted and significant damage has already been done. More than 50% of substantia nigra has been lost by time of PD diagnosis.
- Several neurodegenerative disorders have excessive protein deposition as pathophysiologic mechanism; the primary differences are the location of deposition and/or the protein(s) that accumulate.

Substantia Nigra Cell Death

- Loss of brain neurons is a pathologic feature of Parkinson's, Alzheimer's, and Huntington's diseases as well as amyotrophic lateral sclerosis (Lou Gehrig's disease).
- Elevated apoptosis arises from deficits in nerve growth factor and free radical damage.
- Long-term delivery of nerve growth factors can protect against programmed cell death.
- Some natural therapeutics may decrease programmed cell death (e.g., melatonin).

Oxidative Stress and Glutathione Deficiency

- Biochemical changes—increased neurotoxic metals, inhibition of mitochondrial complex I activity, and depleted GSH in substantia nigra—suggest that oxidative stress is involved in PD.
- Compared with healthy controls, PD patients have 40% reduced GSH levels; oxidized GSH is insignificantly elevated. Brain GSH depletion may be an early component of pathogenesis: suboptimal levels occur in presymptomatic PD, also termed *incidental Lewy body disease.*
- GSH deficiency may be a common denominator in all PD conditions associated with nigral damage (as well as all neurodegeneration).
- GSH has several functions in the brain, acting as antioxidant and redox regulator. GSH depletion affects mitochondrial function, probably via selective inhibition of mitochondrial complex I activity. Oxidative damage due to GSH depletion may also

encourage aggregation of defective proteins, leading to cell death of nigral-striatal dopaminergic neurons.

- GSH depletion may enhance susceptibility of substantia nigra to destruction by endogenous or exogenous toxins.

Environmental Exposures

- There is an association between PD and many environmental risk factors: rural residence, farming, well-water drinking, exposure to pesticides (e.g., organochlorines, carbamates, paraquat, maneb, rotenone, diethyldithiocarbamate), long-term occupational exposure to copper, iron, lead, and manganese.
- Pesticides and metals may act synergistically with other exposures to increase risk.
- Iatrogenic parkinsonism is caused by exposure to central dopamine antagonists.
- MPTP: 1-methyl-4-phenyl-1,2,3,6-tetrahydropyridine (MPTP) is a neurotoxic product of pesticide production and contaminant in synthetic heroin. MPTP freely crosses the blood–brain barrier, is selectively taken up by dopaminergic cells, and inhibits mitochondrial complex 1 in the respiratory chain, a factor in PD pathogenesis. MPTP is the only environmental agent directly linked to P.D.
- **Rotenone:** mimicking MPTP, chronic, systemic inhibition of mitochondrial complex I by lipophilic pesticide rotenone can cause highly selective nigrostriatal dopaminergic degeneration, linked behaviorally with hypokinesia and rigidity. Nigral neurons in rotenone-treated rats accumulate fibrillar cytoplasmic inclusions that contain ubiquitin and alpha-synuclein—major constituents of intracellular protein inclusions forming Lewy bodies and Lewy neuritis in dopaminergic neurons of substantia nigra. Long-term rotenone exposure can increase nitric oxide and lipid peroxidation products in the brain cortex and striatum and mimic PD symptoms (akinesia and rigidity) in rats. Interestingly, rotenone is a natural pesticide and until recently was used in organic produce.
- **Pesticides:** occupational pesticide exposure has the most consistent causative association with PD. Specific pesticides: 2,4-dichlorophenoxyacetic acid, paraquat, permethrin. All affect dopaminergic neurons. Maneb and paraquat are associated with PD. Exposure of children, teenagers, and young adults induces younger-onset PD (diagnosed before age 60). People are four to six times more likely to develop PD if exposed to both pesticides.

- **Trauma:** repeated traumatic loss of consciousness is associated with increased risk.
- **Solvents:** sustained cumulative exposure is key. No evidence has been found of increased risk for those exposed for shorter periods. Pathogenesis may be worsened by older solvents: trichloroethylene, 1,1,1-trichloroethane, carbon tetrachloride, kerosene, white spirit, and acetone.
- **Heavy metals:** risk increases with occupational exposure to specific metals—manganese, copper, lead, iron, mercury, zinc, and aluminum. Elevated levels of these metals are present in the substantia nigra of patients with PD. Several divalent and trivalent cations accelerate alpha-synuclein fibril formation: aluminum, copper (II), iron (III), cobalt (III), and manganese (II). Long-term mercury inhalation is tied to cortical and cerebellar atrophy, dementia, PD syndrome, and ataxia of lower limbs.
- **Manganese:** induces damage in the substantia nigra, globus pallidus, and caudate nucleus, with depletion of dopamine and serotonin. It also is linked to psychiatric changes followed by impaired motor activity with muscle rigidity and tremors. Although this phenomenon is poorly understood, welders, commonly exposed to manganese, do not have higher incidence of PD, but PD manifests 11 years earlier than in other PD patients. Other sources of manganese: well water and industrial waste.
- **Iron buildup:** linked to neurologic disorders such as Alzheimer's disease, PD, and type I neurodegeneration with brain iron accumulation. Elevated iron, lipid peroxidation, and decreased GSH and superoxide dismutase (SOD) are present in substantia nigra of patients with PD. Iron may trigger dopaminergic neurodegeneration of PD.

Detoxification Dysfunction

- Xenobiotic metabolizing enzymes (XMEs): defects in both phase I and phase II reactions may be involved with PD and motor neuron disease (MND). PD and MND can be associated with problems in xenobiotic metabolism.
- Dysfunction of detoxification may underlie chronic neurologic diseases, such as a defective ability to metabolize sulfur-containing xenobiotics. Altered detoxification may render susceptible persons at higher risk for neurotoxicity when exposed to sulfur-containing compounds.
- This issue may underlie various chronic neurologic diseases, even Alzheimer's.

- Genetics is one contributing factor; nutritional and environmental factors also play a role.

DIAGNOSTIC CONSIDERATIONS

- No diagnostic test can clearly identify PD. PD is diagnosed by a neurologist evaluating symptoms and severity and applying clinical judgment. A therapeutic trial of dopamine with positive response is suggestive.
- Diagnosis entails thorough neurologic examination. Brain imaging with blood and urine tests can help distinguish true PD from vascular parkinsonism.
- From 25% to 40% of patients with PD develop dementia, making differentiation of PD with Lewy bodies and Alzheimer's disease with parkinsonian characteristics difficult. Patients with PD may not exhibit classic resting tremor, but an essential tremor, characterized by unilateral postural tremor, mostly in the upper extremities. Key sign of PD: accompanying bradykinesia and rigidity.
- Lewy bodies in the substantia nigra are a pathologic hallmark of classic PD. They are acidophilic inclusions of cytoplasm with a dense core and peripheral halo associated with diffuse neuronal loss in substantia nigra linked to deficient dopamine production in nigrostriatal pathway. Lewy bodies cannot be a diagnostic criterion; they are seen only during autopsy. But they also are found in people without PD: 8% of people older than 50 years, 13% of people older than 70 years, and 16% of those older than 80 years.
- Unified Parkinson's Disease Rating Scale (UPDRS) grades patients on a number of criteria: behavior, activities, motor function, complications, staging by symptoms, and scale of daily living. Neuroimaging tests aid diagnosis (positron emission tomographic scan with 18-fluorodopa, beta-carboxymethyoxy-3-beta-(4-iodophenyl) tropane (CIT) single-photon emission computed tomography). But UPDRS and neurologic examination are sensitive enough for a diagnosis to be made.
- Differential diagnosis: normal aging, essential tremor, drug-induced parkinsonism, Parkinson-plus syndromes, vascular parkinsonism, normal pressure hydrocephalus, dopa-responsive dystonia, juvenile-onset Huntington's disease, and pallidopontonigral degeneration.
- Related diagnoses include the following:
  - **Parkinsonism-plus syndrome:** parkinsonism with other abnormal neurologic symptoms. An example is progressive

supranuclear palsy—early symptoms of PD, then later abnormal eye movements, neck dystonia, dysphagia, decreased response to levodopa.
— **Shy-Drager syndrome (multisystem atrophy):** parkinsonism with autonomic nervous system abnormalities, cranial nerve abnormalities, peripheral polyneuropathy, spasticity, and/or anterior horn cell dysfunction.
— **Drug-induced parkinsonism:** phenothiazines, butyrophenones, reserpine and related hypertensives, manganese poisoning, carbon monoxide poisoning.

THERAPEUTIC CONSIDERATIONS

Naturopathic philosophy prioritizes disease prevention, especially difficult where slow, insidious degenerative process begins a decade before symptoms are diagnosed. There is little conventional effort to identify susceptible persons, because there are no conventional neuroprotective agents and an identified high-risk person must wait until symptoms appear. Naturopathically, lifestyle modifications and neuroprotective nutraceuticals can be employed. Immediate family members are at increased risk; symptoms (e.g., restless legs, loss of smell, and constipation) may precede onset of tremor by several years.

Conventional Medicine

- No conventional therapy can modify the pathologic progression of the PD neurologic degeneration. But PD is somewhat treatable.
- Levodopa (L-dopa) is a mainstay, synthesized by the enzyme tyrosine hydroxylase from food-derived aromatic amino acid tyrosine. Modern treatment combines levodopa with a peripheral decarboxylase enzyme inhibitor to minimize conversion of levodopa to dopamine outside the nervous system. L-Dopa provides only symptomatic relief without altering disease progression, and it loses efficacy with time. L-Dopa side effects: motor complications (fluctuations and dyskinesias), nausea and vomiting, orthostatic hypotension, sedation, hallucinations, delusions, propensity to gamble, and accelerated growth of malignant melanoma. L-Dopa contributes to decreased slow-wave peristaltic activity and impaired digestion. Concomitant naturopathic care can drastically reduce side effects of L-dopa. In spite of side effects, L-dopa is excellent for controlling symptoms and must be considered as part of overall treatment.

However, be clear that L-dopa may increase rate of neuronal oxidative damage.

- Deep brain stimulation (DBS): involves implanting a brain stimulator in certain areas of the brain. Desired effect is to decrease overactivity of excitatory glutamatergic subthalamo-internal pallidum pathway caused by loss of dopaminergic neurons within the substantia nigra. Stimulation may modulate neuronal activity and thus prevent disease-related abnormal neuronal discharges. Candidates for DBS are selected with strict criteria. DBS may control symptoms so drugs can be reduced.

NUTRITIONAL CONSIDERATIONS

Diet

- Detoxification of heavy metals: high sulfur-containing foods such as garlic and onions and water-soluble fibers such as guar gum, oat bran, pectin, psyllium seed.
- Antioxidants: vegetables and fruits.
- PD patients consume fewer raw vegetables, more carbohydrates, less alcohol and coffee, more meat and equivalent protein and fat compared with control subjects. PD patients may have a higher intake of animal fats.
- Recommendation: higher intake of vegetables, low intake of fat.

Food Sources of Levodopa

- **Broad beans:** give PD patients improved symptom control. Response to *Vicia faba* (fava beans) may be even greater than to levodopa medication. Fava beans contain levodopa: 100-g serving of *V. faba* pods contains 250 mg levodopa, equal to levodopa in one drug formulation. However, unsupervised replacement or coadministration of L-dopa with fava beans is not recommended.
- ***Mucuna pruriens* (kapikacchu seed; velvet bean):** L-dopa-containing seed powder of this legume is used in Ayurvedic medicine for PD. Dose: 30 g seed powder q.d. *Mucuna* may be superior to pharmaceutical L-dopa because of rapid onset of longer action without side effects (increased dyskinesias).

Calorie Restriction

- Overeating is a major modifiable risk factor for several age-related diseases, including PD. Calorie restriction (CR): 10% to 25% fewer calories than average Western diet. The luxury of large populations to overeat is new in human history.

- In a primate model of PD, CR diet (30% reduced) decreased PD progression, supported brain dopamine levels, and supported glial cell line–derived neurotrophic factor (GDNF), a protein that promotes survival of neurons. GDNF supports survival of dopaminergic and motoneurons.
- CR extends life span and increases resistance of the brain to insults involving metabolic compromise and excitotoxicity. Exogenous antioxidants have been largely unsuccessful, but a proposed mechanism of CR is enhanced production of antioxidants via intrinsic pathways.

Low-Protein Diet

- May be useful for patients taking levodopa.
- A diet of 50 g protein per day for men and 40 g protein per day for women, compared with a high-protein diet of 80 g/day for men and 70 g/day for women, improved performance scores, tremor, hand agility, and mobility.
- Levodopa absorption is delayed or diminished by dietary amino acids. Eating a majority of protein in the evening also improved symptoms. Recommendation: take levodopa with a high-carbohydrate meal and delay protein intake until final meal of the day to optimize efficacy of the drug.

Nutritional Supplements

Antioxidants

- Excessive free radical burden contributes to PD; antioxidant augmentation might be therapeutic. However, PD-antioxidant research has been disappointing.
- Antioxidants prevent damage from oxidation and may reduce risk of PD. They slow progression of PD in patients not yet taking drugs. High doses are required; increasing antioxidant levels in brain tissue is more difficult.
- Pilot study: 3000 mg of vitamin C per day and 3200 international units (IU) of vitamin E per day over a 7-year period delayed the need for medication for up to 2 to 3 years longer than in patients not taking antioxidants.
- Prospective study: health care professionals—76,890 women during 14 years and 47,331 men during 12 years—completed dietary and supplement surveys every 2 to 4 years. Results: vitamin C and carotenoids did not lower PD risk; vitamin E supplements also were not helpful. However, vitamin E–rich foods in the diet were protective.

Glutathione

- Combined intravenous and oral liposomal GSH replacement is safe and well tolerated and provides ongoing benefit.
- Precursors *N*-acetylcysteine and antioxidant alpha-lipoic acid may also be of use.
- GSH is a systemic antioxidant; repletion may help ameliorate PD-related damage in the heart, liver, muscles.
- Other antioxidants work synergistically with GSH. High-dose vitamin C provides antioxidant-reducing equivalents that conserve GSH.
- Intranasal GSH has anecdotal support.

Vitamin D

- This fat-soluble prohormone is linked to maintaining physiologic function and preventing bone, cardiovascular, autoimmune, and neurologic disorders. Endogenous synthesis in skin exposed to ultraviolet-B radiation from sunlight.
- Dietary sources—fortified foods and certain fish—can provide minor amounts.
- Deficiency causes: inadequate sun exposure, metabolic or absorption disorders, and other genetic factors.
- Patients with chronic neurodegenerative disease are at increased risk for vitamin D insufficiency from advanced age, obesity, and decreased sun exposure. Vitamin D regulates multiple cellular processes abnormal in PD—cellular differentiation, proliferation, and apoptosis.
- Check PD patients regularly for low 25-hydroxyvitamin D to minimize PD complications.

Coenzyme Q10

- Ubiquinone (coenzyme Q10 [CoQ10]) is a cofactor in the electron-transport chain of redox reactions that synthesize adenosine triphosphate (ATP). Used in cardiovascular diseases, acquired immunodeficiency syndrome (AIDS), and cancer, it may also be helpful in neurodegenerative conditions.
- High-dose CoQ10 may slow symptom progression in early PD. At doses of 300, 600, and 1200 mg/day over a 6-month period, patients on CoQ10 faired significantly better than did a placebo group, with 1200 mg showing greatest results. At 360 mg for 4 weeks, CoQ10, in treated and stable PD patients, gave mild symptomatic benefit and much better improvement of visual defects compared with placebo.

- High doses (1200, 1800, 2400, and 3000 mg/day) of CoQ10 are safe in the short term (2 weeks). Ubiquinone reaches a blood plateau at a dose of 2400 mg/day. Although serum levels of CoQ10 are not necessarily lower in PD patients versus healthy controls, doses up to 2400 mg may have an added benefit for symptomatic patients. Because of the expense of CoQ10, start at 1200-mg dose and ramp it up if benefits are not seen in the first few months.

Melatonin

- Hormone manufactured from serotonin and secreted by the pineal gland.
- Powerful antioxidant and treatment option for jet lag, sleep problems, and cancer.
- May be protector of neuronal cells by supporting mitochondrial function and preventing apoptosis.
- Directly scavenges oxidants produced during the normal metabolism and indirectly promotes activity of antioxidant enzymes SOD and catalase.
- Increases activities and expression of electron transport chain complexes. Melatonin increases ATP production and promotes GSH homeostasis. It may interact with the mitochondrial genome to enhance production of proteins. Melatonin may help prevent neuronal apoptosis.
- Theoretically, melatonin may actually exacerbate symptoms because of its putative interference with dopamine release. However, most studies agree that PD is caused by multiple issues of compromised mitochondrial activity in substantia nigra and loss of GSH, oxidative damage, and increased apoptosis. Clinical studies are needed to evaluate efficacy in PD. If melatonin is used, start with low dose (1 to 5 mg); gradually increase, and carefully monitor symptoms.

Reduced Nicotinamide Adenine Dinucleotide

- Coenzyme reduced nicotinamide adenine dinucleotide (NADH) enhances endogenous dopamine production by supplying reducing equivalents to rate-limiting, tyrosine hydroxylase–catalyzed step of dopamine synthesis.
- Both intravenous and intramuscular NADH gave a moderate to very good improvement of disability. Effect of NADH depends on dose and severity of the case. Optimal dose: 25 to 50 mg/day.
- Intravenous administration seems to work better than intramuscular administration.

- Homovanillic acid in urine increases; this metabolite indicates stimulation of endogenous L-dopamine biosynthesis.
- One 10-mg treatment over a 30-minute period every day for 7 days in patients also taking levodopa improved UPDRS scores and significantly increased plasma levodopa.
- More rigorous studies are needed to confirm benefit and elucidate any side effects.

Creatine

- Body-building supplement that acts as a temporal and spatial buffer for cytosolic or mitochondrial pools of cellular energy currency ATP and its regulator, adenosine diphosphate.
- Creatine may have neuroprotective potential to combat cellular energy impairment in neurodegenerative disease.

Botanical Medicines

Camellia Sinensis (Green Tea)

- Drinking green and black tea protects against developing PD.
- Polyphenols penetrate the blood-brain barrier with antioxidant actions, free radical scavenging, iron-chelating properties, (3)H-dopamine and (3)H-methyl-4-phenylpyridine uptake inhibition, catechol-*O*-methyltransferase activity reduction, protein kinase C or extracellular signal-regulated kinase signal pathway activation, and cell survival or cell cycle gene modulation.
- Green tea polyphenols such as (−)-epigallocatechin-3-gallate (EGCG) are being considered as therapeutic agents to alter brain aging processes and serve as neuroprotective agents.
- Clinical data are limited, but several recent studies suggest green tea polyphenols may protect against PD and other neurodegenerative diseases.
- In animal models of PD, both green tea and oral EGCG prevented loss of tyrosine hydroxylase–positive cells in the substantia nigra and tyrosine hydroxylase activity in striatum and prevented neurotoxin-induced elevations in antioxidant enzymes SOD and catalase. These treatments also retained striatal levels of dopamine and its metabolite homovanillic acid and inhibited nitric oxide synthetase in the substantia nigra.

Ginkgo Biloba

- *Ginkgo biloba* extract (GBE) effects: stabilizes membranes, is an antioxidant, scavenges free radicals, enhances use of oxygen and

glucose, is an extremely effective inhibitor of lipid peroxidation of cellular membranes.
- No clinical studies in PD exist, but it is proven beneficial in Alzheimer's disease and useful in animal models of PD, where it is protective in vivo and in vitro.
- Mechanism of action: antioxidation and antiapoptosis.

Mucuna Pruriens

- In Ayurveda, PD ("kampavata") is seen as an imbalance of vata dosha.
- *M. pruriens:* a legume; rich source of antioxidant vitamin E.
- Clinical trial: powdered preparation of this legume is called HP-200; a 7.5-g sachet mixed with water and given orally three to six times per day was given to 26 patients taking synthetic levodopa-carbidopa before treatment and to 34 not using medications. Results: statistically significant reductions in Hoehn and Yahr stage and UPDRS scores from baseline to end of 12-week treatment. Adverse effects: mild gastrointestinal upset.
- Randomized study: single doses of 200/50 mg L-dopa/carbidopa (LD/CD) versus 15 and 30 g of velvet bean preparation at weekly intervals. Compared with standard LD/CD, 30 g velvet bean preparation led to much faster onset of effect (34.6 vs. 68.5 minutes), reflected in shorter times to peak L-dopa blood levels, with fewer, milder side effects of mainly gastrointestinal nature.
- For patients taking medicines such as Sinemet and L-dopa, velvet bean may overelevate L-dopa levels.

Piper Methysticum (Kava Kava)

- No side effects reported with standardized kava extracts at recommended levels in clinical studies.
- **Caution:** isolated reports of kava causing onset of parkinsonian symptoms; case reports that kava may interfere with dopamine and worsen PD. Avoid kava in PD patients or those genetically susceptible.

OTHER THERAPEUTIC CONSIDERATIONS

Smoking

- Smoking is linked to lower incidence and delayed onset of PD.
- Postulated mechanism: nicotine may enhance striatal stimulation of dopaminergic neurons selectively damaged in PD.

- Risk/benefit ratio is quite high with smoking; smoking is not a reasonable prevention for PD.

Estrogen

- Estrogens may modulate activity of dopamine, act as an anti-apoptotic agent, and affect neuronal pathways affected in PD.
- Animal studies: estrogens influence synthesis, release, and metabolism of dopamine and may modulate dopamine receptor expression and function.
- Clinical studies: conflicting findings regarding whether PD symptoms may worsen after menopause and whether hormone replacement therapy can be protective. Several variables—age, dose and formulation, timing and length of dosage period—may determine effect. Monitor menstrual pattern correlations to symptoms to make best patient-specific choices for hormone replacement therapy.

Homeopathy

No clinical studies available to support homeopathy in PD; however, anecdotal success has occurred. Consider the following:

- *Agaricus muscarius:* crawling sensations; vertigo with impulse to fall backward; symptoms worse in cold weather
- Antimonium crudum: parkinsonian movements associated with gastric symptoms; desire for sour foods that do not sit well in digestive tract; thickly white-coated tongue; stubbornness; anxiousness; general feeling of disgust with symptoms, worsened by heat, wine, or moonlight
- Argentum nitricum: tremulousness

Acupuncture and Tui Na

- In traditional Chinese medicine, "pathogenic wind" is the main agent responsible for PD symptoms.
- Treatment strategy: calm this wind and tranquilize the mind. Acupuncture may increase brain dopamine and augment excitability of dopamine neurons.
- Acupuncture can be neuroprotective of the nigrostriatal system. Acupuncture and tui na (Chinese therapeutic massage) can improve symptoms and signs and possibly delay disease progression.
- Areas of objective improvement: sleep, rest, and auditory-evoked brainstem potential examinations, with no other obvious improvements. However, 85% of patients report subjective

improvement (e.g., in tremor, walking, handwriting, slowness, pain, sleep, depression, and anxiety).

THERAPEUTIC APPROACH

Diagnosis: in addition to standard neurologic rating scales and imaging, serum iron, ferritin, and total iron binding identify iron overload. Rule out blood homocysteine. Careful history and testing for heavy metal and pesticide toxicities.

Dietary Recommendations

- Diet low in animal fats, high in fiber—legumes and vegetables.
- Antioxidant-rich foods: nuts and seeds, green leafy vegetables (e.g., bok choy, chard), beans, spices (turmeric, clove, cinnamon), dark chocolate.
- Avoid pesticides: eat organic foods whenever possible.
- To maintain bowel health and facilitate liver detoxification, recommend high sulfur-containing foods—garlic, onions, eggs—and water-soluble fibers (e.g., milled flaxseed, chia seed, guar gum, oat bran, pectin, psyllium seed).
- Patients taking levodopa: lower protein intake—50 g q.d. for men and 40 g q.d. for women. To optimize medicine's therapeutic efficacy, such patients should take their medicines 30 to 45 minutes before protein-containing meals.
- Because of constant movement, weight loss may be an issue; adjust caloric intake to specific patient needs.

Lifestyle Recommendations

- Avoid cooking in aluminum pots.
- Exercise regularly; tandem and recumbent bikes are especially suitable.
- Banisters along walls and chairs with higher arms ease the ability to walk through halls and sit.
- Thick carpeting may be helpful to avoid falls.

Nutritional Supplementation

- Vitamin D_3: 2000 to 4000 IU q.d. (measure blood levels; adjust dose accordingly).
- Fish oils: 1000 to 3000 mg combined eicosapentaenoic acid (EPA) plus docosahexaenoic acid (DHA) q.d.
- Exogenous GSH: best delivery system is unknown. Intranasal GSH has been anecdotally effective. *N*-acetylcysteine (500 mg b.i.d.) and ketogenic diets can boost brain GSH levels.

- Vitamins B_6 and B_{12} and folic acid: doses sufficient to maintain homocysteine levels below 10. If homocysteine levels do not drop adequately, add betaine to the regimen.
- NADH (tradename: Enada): 10 to 20 mg q.d.
- CoQ10: estimated daily dose to achieve target levels in PD based on available forms; for best results, take in divided doses:
  - — Ubiquinone powder in hard gelatin capsule: 1200 to 2400 mg in divided doses
  - — Ubiquinone suspended in oil in soft gelatin capsule with rice bran oil: 600 to 1200 mg in divided doses
  - — Ubiquinone solubilized (e.g., Q-gel) in soft gelatin capsule: 300 to 400 mg in divided doses
  - — Ubiquinone nanonized in soft or hard gelatin capsule: 250 to 400 mg in divided doses
  - — Ubiquinone emulsified with soy peptide (BioQ10 SA) in soft or hard gelatin capsule: 200 to 400 mg in divided doses
  - — Ubiquinol in soft gel capsule: 200 to 400 mg in divided doses
- Intranasal GSH: 200 mg GSH/mL. One sniff per nostril two or three times a day. Keep refrigerated. Half-life refrigerated less than 1 month.

Botanical Medicines

- **Green tea:** 3 cups q.d. or 3 g of soluble components providing 240 to 320 mg polyphenols. For green tea extract standardized for 80% total polyphenol and 55% EGCG content: 300 to 400 mg q.d.
- ***M. pruriens:*** Dose equivalent to 30 g dried powdered seed q.d.

Acupuncture

- Treatments involving needling and tui na massage according to traditional Chinese medical diagnosis.

Pelvic Inflammatory Disease

DIAGNOSTIC SUMMARY

- Dyspareunia
- Mucopurulent cervical discharge
- Pelvic pain; bilateral adnexal tenderness
- Palpable adnexal mass
- Elevated temperature (above 101°F)
- Cervical motion tenderness
- White blood cell (WBC) count 20,000/μL, with marked leukocytosis, elevated erythrocyte sedimentation rate (ESR), or both
- *Neisseria gonorrhoeae* (gonococcus [GC]) and *Chlamydia trachomatis* (CT) most common, followed by *Ureaplasma urealyticum, Mycoplasma hominis, Streptococcus* species, *Escherichia coli, Haemophilus influenzae, Peptostreptococcus,* and *Peptococcus*
- Transvaginal ultrasound showing thickened, fluid-filled tubes or tubo-ovarian mass
- Acute and chronic endometritis on endometrial biopsy
- Laparoscopy: gold standard

GENERAL CONSIDERATIONS

Pelvic inflammatory disease (PID) is a categoric name for a range of pelvic infections and inflammations. The Centers for Disease Control and Prevention (CDC) defines PID as abdominal and adnexal tenderness and cervical motion tenderness in the absence of another definable cause of symptoms. Diagnosis does not require elevated WBC count, elevated ESR, or fever. Salpingitis is a particular condition under PID (adnexa always involved by definition); noninfectious states (pelvic adhesions and chronic salpingitis) also are included. PID leads to 2.5 million outpatient visits annually in the United States. Twenty-five percent of patients have serious long-term sequelae with risk of recurrence. Risk of ectopic pregnancy increases sixfold after one episode of PID. PID carries a 13% risk of infertility after one infection and a 70% risk after three.

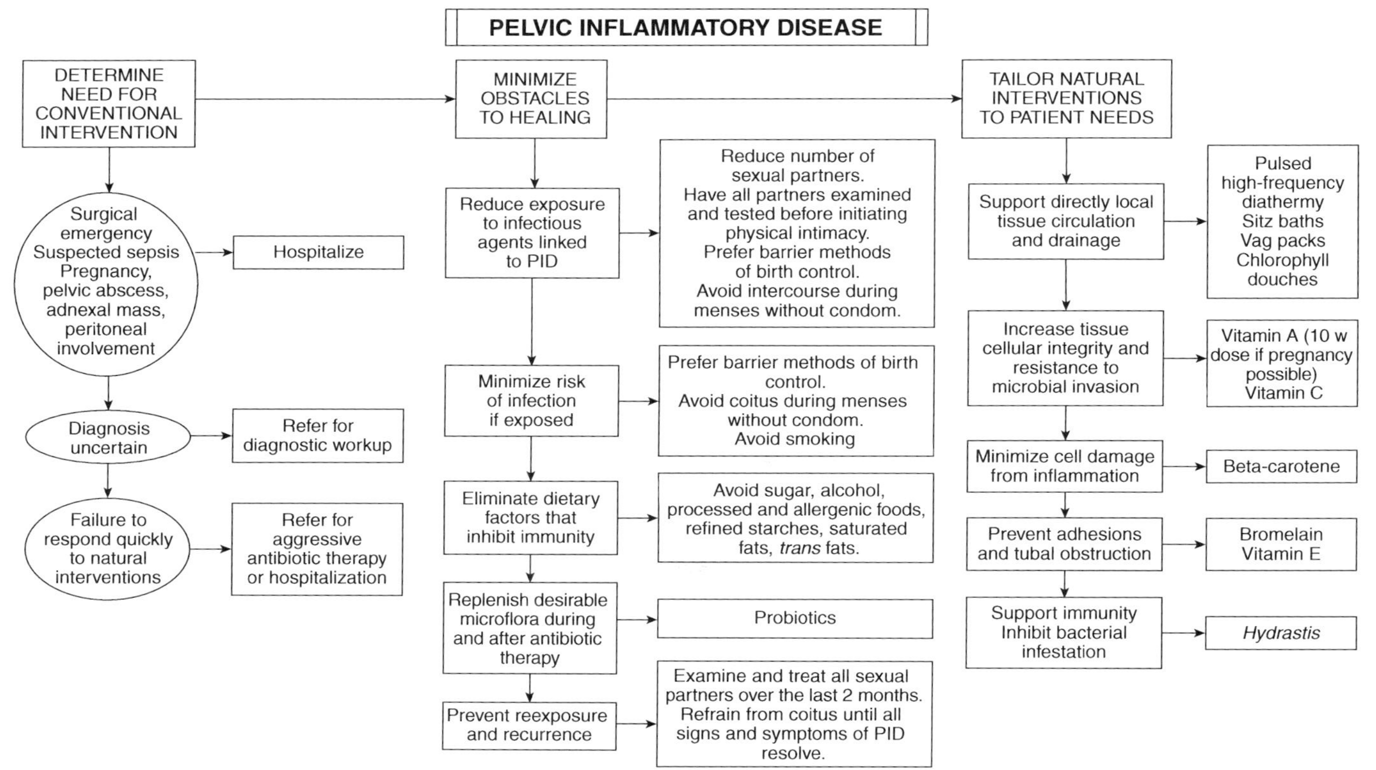
PELVIC INFLAMMATORY DISEASE
DETERMINE NEED FOR CONVENTIONAL INTERVENTION
Surgical emergency
Suspected sepsis
Pregnancy, pelvic abscess, adnexal mass, peritoneal involvement
Hospitalize
Diagnosis uncertain
Refer for diagnostic workup
Failure to respond quickly to natural interventions
Refer for aggressive antibiotic therapy or hospitalization
MINIMIZE OBSTACLES TO HEALING
Reduce exposure to infectious agents linked to PID
Reduce number of sexual partners.
Have all partners examined and tested before initiating physical intimacy.
Prefer barrier methods of birth control.
Avoid intercourse during menses without condom.
Minimize risk of infection if exposed
Prefer barrier methods of birth control.
Avoid coitus during menses without condom.
Avoid smoking
Eliminate dietary factors that inhibit immunity
Avoid sugar, alcohol, processed and allergenic foods, refined starches, saturated fats, trans fats.
Replenish desirable microflora during and after antibiotic therapy
Probiotics
Prevent reexposure and recurrence
Examine and treat all sexual partners over the last 2 months.
Refrain from coitus until all signs and symptoms of PID resolve.
TAILOR NATURAL INTERVENTIONS TO PATIENT NEEDS
Support directly local tissue circulation and drainage
Pulsed high-frequency diathermy
Sitz baths
Vag packs
Chlorophyll douches
Increase tissue cellular integrity and resistance to microbial invasion
Vitamin A (10 w dose if pregnancy possible)
Vitamin C
Minimize cell damage from inflammation
Beta-carotene
Prevent adhesions and tubal obstruction
Bromelain
Vitamin E
Support immunity
Inhibit bacterial infestation
Hydrastis

Etiology

Organisms listed earlier are implicated in the etiology of PID; GC and CT are the most common. Asymptomatic chlamydial infections are a major cause of PID. A higher proportion of PID cases are ascribed to CT than to GC.

- **GC:** incidence 40% to 60%: a delicate and fastidious species with high infectivity, preferring human columnar and transitional epithelia. In less than 1 hour after intercourse, GC can establish itself on the urethral mucosa, resisting the flow of urine. Favored sites in the lower female genital tract are Bartholin's and Skene's glands, urethra, and endocervical canal. Spreading occurs from the endocervix across endometrium to tubal mucosa or by migration through subendothelial vascular and lymphatic channels. The most common method of spreading is via vectors; GC attached to spermatozoa are physically carried to the fallopian tubes. Retrograde menstruation or uterine contractions during intercourse are other modes of dissemination. Acute state: GC and polymorphonuclear leukocytes accumulate in subepithelial connective tissue, causing patchy destruction of overlying mucosa. Consequent mucosal thinning may facilitate GC penetration into deeper tissue; GC survives only a short time in the fallopian tubes. Descent of the microbe beyond surfaces being examined makes it difficult to detect. Concomitant infections occur; the primary role of GC is paving the way for secondary invaders from normal vaginal flora. CT and anaerobic bacteria superinfections are possible.
- **CT:** 20% to 30% of PID cases are caused by CT; acute chlamydial PID may be subclinical or silent in 66% to 75% of cases. Laboratory diagnosis is difficult. It is frequently asymptomatic.
- **Anaerobes:** most commonly isolated from fallopian tubes or cul-de-sacs of PID patients. They are probably not the chief causative agents, but opportunists commonly found in immunocompromised hosts. They typically are of endogenous origin; cervix and vagina of normal healthy women contain anaerobes and aerobes. Anaerobic infections are more common in older patients and women with a history of prior PID.
- **Other organisms:** facultative aerobic organisms in tuboperitoneal fluids from women with salpingitis include coliforms, *H. influenzae*, streptococci, and *M. hominis*. *M. hominis* is a common agent of polymicrobial milieu of PID, present in 81% of female patients with GC and 64% of those without.

Complications

Sequelae of PID are abdominal pain, infertility, ectopic pregnancy, dyspareunia. Dyspareunia often is not investigated but is frequently found in the post-PID patient.

- **Death** from salpingitis is rare and generally from rupture of tubo-ovarian abscess with subsequent peritonitis, with mortality rate of 5.2% to 5.9% for tubo-ovarian abscesses.
- **Fitz-Hugh–Curtis syndrome:** perihepatitis complicating primary PID. It has characteristic violin-string adhesions attaching liver to abdominal wall. Adhesions are from local peritonitis involving the anterior liver surface and adjacent abdominal wall. CT is a more-frequent cause than GC.
- **Infertility:** PID puts women at risk for recurrence. After fallopian tubes are damaged by infection, normal defense mechanisms are impaired. Reinfection is the most important cause of infertility after PID.
- **Ectopic pregnancy:** sevenfold to tenfold increased risk.

Risk Factors

Risk factors include sexual contact, age, use or history of use of intrauterine device (IUD), previous history of PID, earlier sexual debut, especially with multiple sexual partners.

- Risk in sexually active 15-year-olds is 1 in 8; in average 24-year-olds, the risk is 1 in 80. Cervical mucus in younger women may be estrogen dominated, creating an environment more accessible to pathogens.
- Women with multiple partners have a 4.6-fold greater risk than do monogamous women.
- IUDs increase risk. Oral contraceptive (OC) users have less risk of GC but more risk for CT invasion. Barrier methods of birth control decrease PID risk. (Women with vasectomized partners may have less risk.)
- Iatrogenic: the following invasive procedures may introduce pathogens or disturb tract flora and induce PID: cervical dilation, abortion, curettage, tubal insufflation, hysterosalpingography, insertion of IUD. PID may not strictly be a sexually transmitted disease (STD).

Pathogen Access to Upper Female Tract

Menstruation, sperm, and trichomonads help transport pathogens into the salpinx.

- Infections occurring around menses tend to be GC rather than CT. Menstrual regurgitation may carry sloughed endometrium with attached GC or intracellular CT organisms that proliferate in tubal epithelium or on peritoneal surfaces.
- Human sperm: bacteriospermia is a cause of infertility in men; 66% to 75% of men who tested positive for GC were asymptomatic. Sperm are vectors. Cervical mucus is an effective mechanical and immunologic barrier between flora of the vagina and upper tract. Yet organisms attached to sperm can easily traverse mucus column. Sperm migrate through menstrual plasma but not during the luteal phase or through cervical mucus of pregnancy. Sperm is intimately associated with cytomegalovirus, *Toxoplasma, U. urealyticum,* and *Chlamydia.*
- Motile trichomonads are another transporter, ascending from the vagina to the fallopian tubes, carrying additional invaders. Key observation: trichomonads are never isolated from human beings when heavy bacterial contamination is absent.

DIAGNOSIS

Pelvic or lower abdominal pain is the most dependable symptom of PID, but it is not specific. Rebound tenderness is not reliable; cervical motion tenderness and adnexal tenderness are much more common. Clinical picture is misleading; many patients with PID have atypical signs and symptoms. Some have no signs and symptoms at all.

Common Signs and Symptoms in Acute Pelvic Inflammatory Disease

Symptom	Incidence (%)
Lower abdominal pain	90
Adnexal tenderness on palpation	90
Pain on movement of the cervix	90
Vaginal discharge	55
Adnexal mass or swelling	50
Fever or chills	40
Irregular vaginal bleeding	35
Anorexia, nausea, and vomiting	25

- Patients with GC may appear more toxic and febrile with leukocytosis. CT PID may give elevated ESR. Most GC PID occurs at or shortly after menses. GC PID has a more-severe clinical picture, but tissue damage and long-term sequelae can be more severe in CT. Many infections are mixed GC and CT.
- Putrid discharge yields anaerobes; an offensive odor is diagnostic of anaerobic infection and indicative of well-developed PID, with opportunistic anaerobes following primary invaders.

Differential Diagnosis of Pelvic Inflammatory Disease

- Acute appendicitis
- Acute cholecystitis
- Acute pyelonephritis
- Ectopic pregnancy
- Endometriosis
- Hemorrhagic ovarian cysts
- Intrauterine pregnancy
- Mesenteric lymphadenitis
- Ovarian cyst with torsion
- Ovarian tumor
- Pelvic thrombophlebitis
- Septic abortion

Note: **Potentially lethal conditions: ectopic pregnancy, tubo-ovarian abscess, ovarian cyst rupture with hemorrhage, appendicitis.**

- **Fitz-Hugh–Curtis syndrome:** symptoms from upper right quadrant in sexually active women may be an indirect sign of genital infection. Pain has sudden onset, overshadowing underlying PID.
- **Rupture of tubo-ovarian abscess:** sudden severe exacerbation of pain. Pain is referred to side of rupture, followed by generalized peritonitis and collapse. Shoulder pain is possible. Pulse is elevated out of proportion to fever, up to 170 beats per minute. Surgery within 12 hours is required or death is probable.
- **Take careful medical history:** STDs, birth control methods, sexual activity, recent medical procedures, and nature and onset of symptoms. Evaluate source, severity, and characteristics of pelvic and abdominal pain.
- Look for mucopurulent cervicitis.
- Culture cervix for GC and CT.

Empiric Treatment of Pelvic Inflammatory Disease

Initiate in sexually active women at risk for STDs if they experience pelvic or lower abdominal pain, if no other cause can be identified, and if the following minimal criterion is present on pelvic examination:

- Cervical motion tenderness or uterine tenderness or adnexal tenderness

  The following additional criteria may enhance diagnosis of PID:
- Oral temperature below 101°F or 38.3°C.
- Abnormal cervical or vaginal mucopurulent cervicitis. Culture cervix for GC and CT discharge.
- High numbers of WBCs on saline microscopy of vaginal secretions.
- Elevated ESR.
- Elevated C-reactive protein.

THERAPEUTIC CONSIDERATIONS

- Hospitalization criteria:
  - — Surgical emergencies (e.g., appendicitis) cannot be excluded.
  - — Suspected sepsis.
  - — Pregnancy.
  - — Lack of clinical response to oral antimicrobials.
  - — Patient unable to follow or tolerate outpatient oral regimen.
  - — Severe illness, nausea and vomiting, or high fever.
  - — Suspected tubo-ovarian abscess.
  - — Adnexal mass.
  - — Peritoneal involvement.
  - — Refer if diagnosis is uncertain or surgical emergency threatens. Give antibiotic therapy plus supportive therapies if patient's clinical and laboratory status can be reassessed in 48 to 72 hours. Laboratory values and objective patient criteria should direct all acute-phase treatment. **CDC guidelines: "Most experts encourage hospitalization and treatment with intravenous antibiotics."**
- **Antibiotics:** broad-spectrum regimens tailored to clinical severity and laboratory findings, patient compliance, cost, and availability of medicines. CDC outpatient recommendations take into account the limited antibiotic activity of any one regimen.
- **Oral treatment:** viable option for women with mild to moderately severe acute PID, because clinical outcomes are similar

to those of parenteral therapy. Reevaluate women who fail to respond within 72 hours, to confirm diagnosis and apply parenteral therapy.

Recommended Antibiotic Regimen

- Ceftriaxone: 250 mg intramuscularly (IM) in single dose
  plus
- Doxycycline: 100 mg orally b.i.d. for 14 days
  with or without
- Metronidazole: 500 mg orally b.i.d. for 14 days
  or
- Cefoxitin: 2 g IM in single dose, and probenecid 1 g orally, administered concurrently in single dose
  plus
- Doxycycline: 100 mg orally b.i.d. for 14 days
  with or without
- Metronidazole: 500 mg orally b.i.d. for 14 days
  or
- Other parenteral third-generation cephalosporin (e.g., ceftizoxime or cefotaxime)
  plus
- Doxycycline: 100 mg orally b.i.d. for 14 days
  with or without
- Metronidazole: 500 mg orally b.i.d. for 14 days

Parenteral and oral therapy have similar clinical efficacy for women with PID of mild or moderate severity. Let clinical experience and judgment guide decisions regarding transition to oral therapy, which usually can be initiated within 24 hours of clinical improvement.

Recommended Parenteral Regimen A

- Cefotetan: 2 g intravenously every 12 hours
  or
- Cefoxitin: 2 g IV every 6 hours
  plus
- Doxycycline: 100 mg orally or IV every 12 hours

Intravenous infusion of doxycycline is painful; administer orally when possible. Bioavailability of oral and intravenous formulations is similar. Parenteral therapy may be discontinued 24 hours after clinical improvement, but complete 14 days of oral doxycycline (100 mg b.i.d.). For tubo-ovarian abscess, clindamycin or metronidazole with doxycycline provides more-effective anaerobic coverage than doxycycline alone.

Recommended Parenteral Regimen B

- Clindamycin: 900 mg IV every 8 hours
  plus
- Gentamicin loading dose IV or IM (2 mg/kg body weight); followed by maintenance dose (1.5 mg/kg) every 8 hours. Single daily dose (3 to 5 mg/kg) can be substituted.

Parenteral therapy may be discontinued 24 hours after clinical improvement; continue oral doxycycline 100 mg b.i.d., or oral clindamycin 450 mg q.i.d. to complete 14-day therapy. For tubo-ovarian abscess, clindamycin or metronidazole with doxycycline provides more effective anaerobic coverage than doxycycline alone.

Antibiotics are not always curative. Antibiotic resistance is increasing rapidly; 15% of women with PID do not respond to primary antimicrobial treatment, 20% have at least one recurrence, and 15% are rendered infertile. Fundamental approach of combining immune enhancement and nontoxic therapies is more sound. However, no evidence-based therapies exclusively using natural therapies for the treatment of PID are available. Antibiotics, herbal or pharmaceutical, can help in the first phase of treatment but are insufficient intervention for devastating sequelae.

Physical Medicine

- **Diathermy:** pulsed high-frequency diathermy is quite beneficial in PID. Pulsing electrical energy of short duration (65 μs every 1600 ms) at a high intensity achieves desired therapeutic result without hyperpyrexia associated with diathermy. Local recovery is enhanced, reticuloendothelial system is stimulated, and gamma-globulin fractions are increased. There is no modern research on this therapy; be very cautious using it as a substitute for antibiotics.
- **Sitz baths:** contrast sitz bath increases pelvic circulation and drainage, stimulates influx of macrophages, and decongests pelvic inflammatory reaction (*Textbook,* "Hydrotherapy").

Nutritional Supplements

- **Vitamin C:** anti-inflammatory effects help decrease tissue destruction. Vitamin C supports collagen tissue repair, which helps prevent spread of infection (important in GC spread through subepithelial connective tissue, disorganizing collagen matrix). Fibrinolytic activity helps prevent pelvic scarring.

- **Beta-carotene:** the normal ovary has high beta-carotene. Maintain optimal carotene to optimize defense against nearby inflammation. It potentiates beneficial effects of interferon and enhances antibody response and WBC activity. It is an antioxidant, limiting cell damage from inflammation (*Textbook,* "Beta-carotene and Other Carotenoids").
- **Bromelain:** adnexal exudate in PID frequently suppurates to form abscesses. Alleviating tissue irritation during initial stages allows resorption of exudate with fewer adhesions. Adhesions form as exudate lingers because structures are overwhelmed by inflammation. Agglutination of villous fold in lumen of the tube may cause scarring and tubal occlusion. Bromelain activates fibrinolysis, diminishing sequelae of exudates. It has antimicrobial properties and penetrates the salpinx (*Textbook,* "Bromelain").
- **Probiotics:** antibiotics disturb gastrointestinal, vaginal, and bladder microflora, causing diarrhea, candidal vulvovaginitis, and acute cystitis. Probiotics are live microorganisms that benefit the host when administered orally. Many species and strains have adhesive properties and can proliferate in these organs, preventing opportunistic overgrowth and side effects from antibiotics. They also restore normal microflora. No one species or strain can be recommended, but consider combinations that include at least one of the following: *Lactobacillus rhamnosus, Lactobacillus plantarum, Lactobacillus reuteri, Lactobacillus acidophilus, Bifidobacterium bifidum, Bifidobacterium lactis, Bifidobacterium breve,* and *Bifidobacterium longum.*

Botanical Medicines

Many botanicals have antimicrobial and immunostimulating effects. Consider allicin extracts from garlic, goldenseal and Oregon grape root, and *Echinacea* as part of therapeutic regimen and as adjuncts to antibiotics.

- **Vaginal depletion packs:** recommended to promote drainage of exudate from involved tissues. They may also stimulate immune cells within the vagina to provide first line of defense (*Textbook,* "Vaginal Depletion Pack").
- ***Hydrastis canadensis* (goldenseal):** immune potentiating. It has specific antichlamydial properties. The general antibacterial nature of goldenseal justifies its use in PID. It is trophorestorative to mucous membranes; use throughout the rehabilitation period (*Textbook,* "Hydrastis canadensis [Goldenseal] and Other Berberine-Containing Botanicals").

Prevention

Woman with no history of PID need to be concerned about asymptomatic male carriers of STDs. Choice of birth control method is pivotal. Barrier methods of contraception reduce risk of PID.

- **OCs:** inhibit GC. Some researchers suggest OC use after first episode of PID to prevent recurrence. Estrogens create thicker cervical plug, protective against GC. OCs decrease length and volume of menstrual flow, thus decreasing exposure of GC to this culture medium. However, OCs may give higher risk of CT. Progesterone induces hyperplasia and hypersecretion, producing cervical eversion, exposing endocervical columnar epithelium, a target tissue of CT. Estradiol may suppress endocervical antibodies necessary to resolve CT. Estrogen-treated individuals may have higher number of infected cervical cells and longer duration of infection. Because women are not selectively exposed to GC versus CT, OCs are not recommended.
- **IUDs:** are associated with a small increased risk of PID, especially in the first 4 months of use. IUDs are an STD disaster; they allow bacterial colonization on the surface and reduce local immunologic capacity. If a woman with suspected PID has an IUD, it needs to be removed 12 to 24 hours after initiation of antibiotic therapy to prevent spread of infection during its removal. IUDs are not recommended.
- **Barrier methods:** excellent choices to prevent PID. Condom is preferred to cervical protectors; sperm reach the vaginal vault more rarely.
- **Douching:** avoid haphazard douching; it disturbs vaginal flora. All forms of douching increase risk of PID and cause organisms to ascend into the upper genital tract. Use with caution; PID has been correlated to frequency of douching; those who douched 3 or more times per month were 3.6 times more likely to get PID than those who douched less than once per month.
- **Intercourse during menses:** intercourse during menses is not recommended unless a condom is used. GC risk is increased by the loss of the protective cervical mucus plug and the prevalence of blood, a medium of choice for GC. The endometrium also is thought to offer local protection against bacterial invasion, and this layer is being sloughed off during menses.
- **Smoking:** current and former smokers, compared with those who have never smoked, have increased risk of PID. Women

who smoke 10 or more cigarettes daily have a higher risk than those who smoke less.

- **Patient education:** discuss signs and symptoms of PID with all sexually active women. Encourage early intervention if clinical picture of PID appears.

THERAPEUTIC APPROACH

Two phases of treatment: (1) eliminate all pathogens and normalize adnexal microflora, and (2) rehabilitate damaged tissues. Avoid intercourse until all signs and symptoms have resolved and male partners have been examined and treated. All partners during 2 months before illness must be examined and treated. Increase bed rest. These therapies are adjunctive to appropriate antibiotic treatment and immune support. *Caution:* referral for aggressive antibiotic treatment or hospitalization is mandatory if patient does not respond quickly.

- **Diet:** limit all dietary inhibitors of immunity (sugar, refined starches, alcohol, saturated fats, *trans* fats, processed and allergenic foods) during both phases of treatment.
- **Supplements:**
  - — Beta-carotene: 100,000 international units (IU) q.d. for 2 or more months.
  - — Vitamin E (mixed tocopherols): 400 IU q.d. for 3 months.
  - — Vitamin C: 500 mg q.i.d. during first week of treatment, then decrease over a 3-day period to 250 mg t.i.d.
  - — Bromelain: 250 mg (potency 1800 milk clotting units [MCU]) q.i.d. for first week and then t.i.d. for 6 weeks.
  - — Probiotics: minimum 1 billion colony-forming units (CFUs) q.d.; consider up to 24 billion CFUs q.d. during antibiotic treatment and for 2 months thereafter.
- **Botanical medicines:**
  - — *H. canadensis:* 500 mg solid extract (4:1 or 8% to 12% alkaloid content) t.i.d. during acute phase; 250 mg t.i.d. during recovery.
  - — Vaginal packs: daily during acute phase until adequate clinical and laboratory response; after acute phase, vaginal packs three times per week, alternating with chlorophyll douches for 3 weeks.
- **Physical medicine:**
  - — Diathermy: pulsed, high-intensity diathermy for 10 minutes over suprapubic area, 10 minutes over liver, and 10 minutes

in area of left adrenal (the right being presumably stimulated with the liver).

— Sitz baths: one or two times per day throughout acute phase; contrast sitz baths are given in groups of three alterations of hot to cold; two separate tubs are necessary to facilitate this process. The hot should be 105°F to 115°F, the cold 55°F to 85°F, with the temperatures dependent on the strength of the patient. Standard treatment is 3 minutes hot and 30 seconds cold; the water level in the hot tub is set 2.5 cm higher than in the cold. Adequate draping is necessary to prevent chilling. As with all hydrotherapy treatments, always finish with the cold.

Peptic Ulcers

DIAGNOSTIC SUMMARY

- Epigastric distress 45 to 60 minutes after meals or nocturnal pain; both are relieved by food, antacids, or vomiting.
- Epigastric tenderness and guarding.
- Symptoms chronic and periodic.
- Gastric analysis shows acid in all cases, with hypersecretion in approximately half the patients with duodenal ulcers (DUs).
- Ulcer crater or deformity usually occurring at the duodenal bulb (DU) or pylorus (gastric ulcer [GU]) on radiograph or fiberoptic examination.
- Positive test for occult blood in stool.

GENERAL CONSIDERATIONS

Peptic ulcers (PUs) occur in the stomach (gastric) and first portion of the small intestine (duodenal). DUs are more common; the prevalence is 6% to 12% in the United States. Ten percent of the U.S. population has clinical evidence of DU during their lifetimes. PU is four times more common in men than in women and four to five times more common than benign GU.

- Most PUs are associated with abdominal discomfort 45 to 60 minutes after meals or during the night described as gnawing, burning, cramplike, aching, or heartburn. Eating or antacids usually give great relief. In the elderly, presentation may be subtle and atypical compared with younger patients, leading to a delay in diagnosis.
- DU and GU result from similar mechanisms—specifically, some influence that damages protective factors lining the stomach and duodenum.
- Gastric acid is corrosive with a pH of 1 to 3. Lining of the stomach and small intestine is protected by a layer of mucin; constant renewing of intestinal cells and secretion of factors neutralizing acid on contact with the mucosa are also protective.

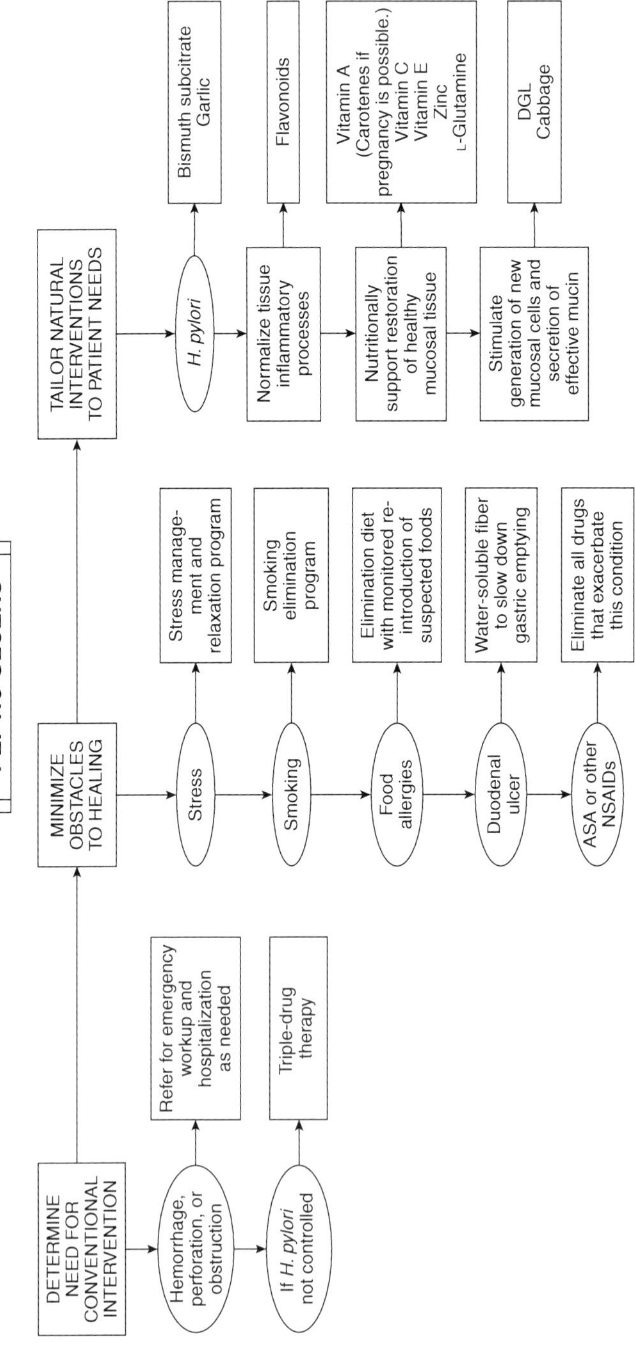
PEPTIC ULCERS
DETERMINE NEED FOR CONVENTIONAL INTERVENTION
Hemorrhage, perforation, or obstruction
Refer for emergency workup and hospitalization as needed
If H. pylori not controlled
Triple-drug therapy
MINIMIZE OBSTACLES TO HEALING
Stress
Stress management and relaxation program
Smoking
Smoking elimination program
Food allergies
Elimination diet with monitored re-introduction of suspected foods
Duodenal ulcer
Water-soluble fiber to slow down gastric emptying
ASA or other NSAIDs
Eliminate all drugs that exacerbate this condition
TAILOR NATURAL INTERVENTIONS TO PATIENT NEEDS
H. pylori
Bismuth subcitrate
Garlic
Normalize tissue inflammatory processes
Flavonoids
Nutritionally support restoration of healthy mucosal tissue
Vitamin A
(Carotenes if pregnancy is possible.)
Vitamin C
Vitamin E
Zinc
L-Glutamine
Stimulate generation of new mucosal cells and secretion of effective mucin
DGL
Cabbage

- GUs are linked to acid output that is normal or reduced; half of patients with DUs have increased gastric acid output. That increase may be attributable to an increased number of parietal cells; patients with DUs have twice as many parietal cells as do normal control subjects. This is problematic only when integrity of protective factors is impaired.

Helicobacter pylori

- Loss of integrity of protective factors can be linked to bacterium *H. pylori,* nonsteroidal anti-inflammatory drugs (NSAIDs), alcohol, nutrient deficiency, stress. *H. pylori* and NSAID use are most significant.
- Chronic diseases associated with increased risk of PUs: Crohn's disease, chronic renal failure, liver cirrhosis, cystic fibrosis, chronic obstructive pulmonary disease, systemic mastocytosis (condition of too many immune mast cells in body), and myeloproliferative disorders (polycythemia vera, chronic myelogenous leukemia, agnogenic myeloid metaplasia, and essential thrombocythemia).
- *H. pylori:* 90% to 100% of patients with DUs, 70% with GUs, and 50% of people older than 50 years test positive for *H. pylori.* However, 80% of *H. pylori*–infected people never develop ulcers. Tests: antibodies to *H. pylori* in blood or saliva, culture of material collected during endoscopy, measure of breath for urea. Low gastric output and low antioxidant content in gastrointestinal (GI) mucosa may predispose to *H. pylori* colonization, which in turn increases gastric pH, setting up positive feedback and increasing the risk for colonization of other organisms.

Aspirin and Other Non-steroidal Anti-inflammatory Drugs

- NSAIDs are linked to significant risk of PU; NSAIDs plus smoking is a harmful combination.
- Increased risk of GI bleeding is present with PU at all doses; 75 mg q.d. aspirin (ASA) is associated with 40% less bleeding than 300 mg q.d. and 30% less bleeding than 150 mg q.d. Thus conventional prophylactic ASA regimen is not free of risk of PU.
- NSAID-induced ulcers have declined with replacement of these drugs with selective cyclooxygenase-2 inhibitors (rofecoxib, celecoxib) for arthritides, but the problem remains an ongoing issue because of the increased use of ASA for cardioprotection.

THERAPEUTIC CONSIDERATIONS

PU complications are hemorrhage, perforation, and obstruction. These are **medical emergencies** requiring immediate hospitalization. Identify causes and eliminate them.

Lifestyle Factors

- **Stress and emotions:** individuals with PUs have distinctly different psychological profiles from those without PUs. The number of stressful life events is not significantly different in patients with PU compared with ulcer-free controls. Patient response to stress is a significant factor. People who perceive more-significant stress in their lives are at increased risk of developing PUs (*Textbook,* "Peptic Ulcer—Duodenal and Gastric"). Psychological factors are important in some patients but not in others. Ulcer patients tend to repress emotions; encourage discovery of enjoyable outlets of self-expression and emotions.
- **Smoking:** increased frequency, decreased response to PU therapy, and increased mortality rate are linked to smoking. Three postulated mechanisms are (1) decreased pancreatic bicarbonate secretion, (2) increased reflux of bile salts into the stomach, and (3) acceleration of gastric emptying into the duodenum. Bile salts are quite irritating to the stomach and first portions of the duodenum. Bile salt reflux induced by smoking is the most likely factor. But psychological aspects of smoking also are important; chronic anxiety and psychological stress linked to smoking worsen ulceration.

Nutritional Factors

- **Food allergy:** this is the prime causative factor. PU lesions are histologically similar to Arthus reaction (local inflammatory response caused by deposition of immune complexes in tissues). Ninety-eight percent of patients with PU had coexisting lower and upper respiratory tract allergic disease. Elimination diet is successful in treating and preventing recurrent ulcers. Food allergy is consistent with high recurrence rate of PUs. Milk should be avoided; the higher the milk consumption, the greater the likelihood of ulcer. Milk significantly increases stomach acid production.
- **Fiber:** a diet rich in fiber is linked to a reduced rate of DUs compared with a low-fiber diet. A high-fiber diet in patients with recently healed DUs reduced recurrence rate by half. Fiber

delays gastric emptying of liquid phase, counteracting rapid movement into duodenum. Supplemental fibers used: pectin, guar gum, psyllium; diet rich in plant foods is best.

- **Cabbage:** raw cabbage juice is effective in treating PUs. Use of 1 L of fresh juice per day in divided doses has induced total ulcer healing in only 10 days. High glutamine content of cabbage juice is a healing factor. A dose of 1.6 g q.d. L-glutamine is more effective than conventional treatment; almost all patients tested showed complete relief and healing within 4 weeks. L-Glutamine is involved in biosynthesis of hexosamine moiety in certain mucoproteins. Cabbage-family isothiocyanates (e.g., sulforaphane [SF]) are active against *H. pylori.* For example, clinically, broccoli sprouts (70 g/day; containing 420 μmol of SF precursor) for 8 weeks decreased levels of urease (urea breath test and *H. pylori* stool antigen, biomarkers of *H. pylori* colonization) and serum pepsinogens I and II (biomarkers of gastric inflammation).
- **Bismuth subcitrate:** bismuth is a naturally occurring mineral antacid and inhibitor of *H. pylori.* Bismuth subsalicylate (Pepto-Bismol) is the most popular form, but bismuth subcitrate produces the best results against *H. pylori* and treating PUs. Bismuth subcitrate is available through compounding pharmacies (International Academy of Compounding Pharmacists, 800-927-4227). The advantage of bismuth over standard antibiotics is the risk of developing bacterial resistance to antibiotics that is unlikely relative to bismuth. Dose for bismuth subcitrate is 240 mg b.i.d. before meals. For bismuth subsalicylate, dose is 500 mg q.i.d. Bismuth preparations are extremely safe at these doses. Bismuth subcitrate may cause temporary and harmless darkening of the tongue and/or stool. Avoid bismuth subsalicylate in children recovering from the flu, chickenpox, or other viral infection because it may mask nausea and vomiting of Reye's syndrome, a rare but serious illness.
- **Flavonoids:** counteract production and secretion of histamine (a factor in ulcer formation). Antiallergy compounds are indicated as a result of probable allergic cause. Catechin inhibits histidine decarboxylase. Catechin displays significant antiulcer activity in various models. A dose of 1000 mg catechin five times per day reduces histamine in gastric tissue of normal patients and those with GUs and DUs and acute gastritis. Several flavonoids inhibit *H. pylori* in a concentration-dependent manner. They augment natural defense factors that prevent ulcer formation. Flavone

(most potent flavonoid studied in this context) has an effect similar to bismuth subcitrate. Sofalcone—a synthetic derivative of the flavonoid sophoradin in Chinese herb *Sophora tonkinensis*—has been effective in healing ulcers after eradication of *H. pylori.*

Miscellaneous

- **Vitamins A and E:** inhibit development of stress ulcers in rats and help maintain integrity of mucosal barrier. High-dose vitamin A may have a useful protective effect on chronic GUs.
- **Zinc:** increases mucin production in vitro and has a protective effect on PUs in animals and curative effect in human beings.
- **Melatonin:** pineal hormone used to treat jet lag and insomnia-like conditions. It also has antioxidant properties. Melatonin mitigates gastric lining breakdown and ulcer formation. Research has focused on hypersecretion situations; therefore melatonin may be most applicable for DUs, entailing acid hypersecretion.

Botanical Medicines

- ***Glycyrrhiza glabra*** **(licorice):** used historically for PUs. The aldosterone-like side effects of glycyrrhizinic acid (GA) are avoided by removal of GA from licorice to form deglycyrrhizinated licorice (DGL).
  — DGL is an antiulcer agent with no known side effects (*Textbook,* "Glycyrrhiza glabra [Licorice]"). DGL stimulates differentiation to glandular cells plus mucus formation and secretion. No significant differences exist in recurrence rates between cimetidine and DGL. It prevents ASA-induced ulceration and gastric bleeding.
  — DGL is composed of several flavonoids that inhibit *H. pylori.*
  — DGL must mix with saliva to be effective; this may promote release of salivary compounds that stimulate growth and regeneration of stomach and intestinal cells. DGL in capsule form has not been shown to be effective
  — Dose: 2 to 4 380-mg chewable DGL tablets between meals or 20 minutes before meals; continue at least 8 to 16 weeks after full therapeutic and symptomatic response.
- Mastic *(Pistacia lentiscus)*
  — Mastic is a resin from the mastic tree *(P. lentiscus),* known in Greece as "tears of Chios," being traditionally produced on the island of Chios. When chewed, the resin becomes a white, opaque gum. The flavor is bitter at first, then refreshing, with a slightly piney or cedar flavor.

- — Mastic gum is traditional Mediterranean medicine for GI ailments and may help heal PUs.
- — In a double-blind clinical trial involving symptomatic and endoscopically proven DU, mastic gum (1 g q.d.) for 2 weeks provided symptomatic relief in 80% of patients versus 50% on placebo, as well as endoscopically proved healing in 70% of patients versus 22% on placebo. Mastic gum has some bactericidal activity against *H. pylori* in vivo but not enough to produce consistent clinical eradication.

- ***Rheum species* (rhubarb):** in cases of active intestinal bleeding, rhubarb is extremely effective. Alcohol-extracted rhubarb tablets (*Rheum officinale* Baill, *Rheum palmatum* L., *Rheum tanguticum* Maxim ex Balf) have been more than 90% effective in clinical trials with bleeding GUs and DUs. Time taken for stool occult blood test to change from positive to negative was 53 to 57 hours. Benefits are from astringent anthraquinones and flavonoids.
- **Plantain banana:** dried extract of unripe plantain banana is antiulcerogenic against a variety of experimentally induced ulcers in rats. The effect is similar to that of DGL—stimulation of mucosal cell growth rather than inhibition of gastric acid secretion.
- ***Zingiber officinale* (ginger root):** used traditionally for GI ailments—indigestion, motion sickness, and nausea associated with pregnancy. A methanol extract of ginger root effectively inhibited 19 strains of *H. pylori*. Given ginger's safety profile and reasonable cost, it is worth trying.
- ***Artemisia douglasiana:*** located on western slopes of the Rocky Mountains, this folk remedy has been used in Argentina to treat GUs and skin lesions for decades. *Artemisia* and its active constituent dehydroleucodine act as antioxidants and, similar to DGL and plantain, confer gastric lining protection by enhancing mucus secretion.
- ***Allium sativum* (garlic):** high intake of garlic and onions reduces the risk of stomach cancer. Garlic inhibits growth of *H. pylori*. Garlic is useful for antibiotic-resistant strains as well. Human clinical trials are needed to verify efficacy.

THERAPEUTIC APPROACH

PU disease refers to a heterogeneous group of disorders with a common final pathway, leading to ulcerative lesions in gastric or duodenal mucosa. Determine which factors are most relevant. A more-general approach may be easier to implement.

- Identify and eliminate or reduce all factors implicated in cause: food allergy, cigarette smoking, stress, drugs (especially ASA and other NSAIDs).
- Inhibit exacerbating factors (e.g., reducing excess acid secretion, if present) and promote tissue resistance.
- Follow proper diet and lifestyle to prevent recurrence.
- **Complications:** hemorrhage, perforation, and obstruction are emergencies requiring immediate hospitalization.
- **Psychological:** stress reduction program to eliminate or control stressors, plus a regular relaxation plan.
- **Diet:** eliminate allergenic foods, emphasize high-fiber foods, encourage cabbage family vegetables.
- **Supplements:**
  — Vitamin A: 20,000 international units (IU) t.i.d. (Avoid these high doses in women with even the slightest possibility of becoming pregnant, because of the teratogenic nature of high dose retinol. Consider the alternative use of mixed carotenes in such patients.) When using high-dose vitamin A, be sure to include vitamins D and K_2 as indicated.
  — Vitamin C: 500 mg b.i.d. (Consider use of buffered ascorbates to minimize aggravation of GU symptoms with ascorbic acid.)
  — Vitamin E (mixed tocopherols): 200 IU b.i.d.
  — Flavonoids: 500 mg b.i.d.
  — Zinc (picolinate or other highly bioavailable form): 20 mg elemental zinc q.d.
  — L-Glutamine: 500 mg t.i.d.
  — Bismuth subcitrate: 240 mg b.i.d. before meals.
- **Botanical medicines:**
  — DGL: 380 to 760 mg dissolved in mouth 20 minutes before meals t.i.d.
  — Mastic gum: 350 to 1000 mg t.i.d.

Periodontal Disease

DIAGNOSTIC SUMMARY

- Gingivitis: inflammation of the gingiva characterized by erythema, contour changes, and bleeding.
- Periodontitis: localized pain, loose teeth, demonstration of dental pockets, erythema, swelling and/or suppuration; radiographs may reveal alveolar bone destruction.

GENERAL CONSIDERATIONS

Periodontal disease (PD) is an inclusive term for the inflammatory condition of gingiva (gingivitis) and/or periodontium (periodontitis). The disease process progresses from gingivitis to periodontitis. It may be a manifestation of a systemic condition (diabetes mellitus, collagen diseases, leukemia or other disorders of leukocyte function, anemia, or vitamin deficiency). It is linked to atherosclerosis by an increased level of serum C-reactive protein, a marker for inflammation and risk factor for coronary artery disease.

- Alveolar bone loss may be noninflammatory; definition of PD excludes processes causing only tooth loss (mainly from osteoporosis or endocrine imbalances). These conditions reflect systemic disease.
- Focus on the underlying condition rather than PD. Noninflammatory alveolar bone loss is a separate entity that involves a different etiology (see the chapter on osteoporosis).
- Focus of this chapter is nutrition and lifestyle improvement as adjuncts to the control and prevention of causes of inflammatory PD.
- Best treated with combined expertise of a dentist or periodontist and nutritionally minded physician. Oral hygiene is paramount but insufficient in many cases; host defense must be normalized; nutritional status determines status of host defense factors.
- Prevalence and epidemiology: prevalence increases directly with age: 15% at age 10 years, 38% at 20 years, 46% at 35 years, and 54% at 50 years. Men have a higher prevalence and severity

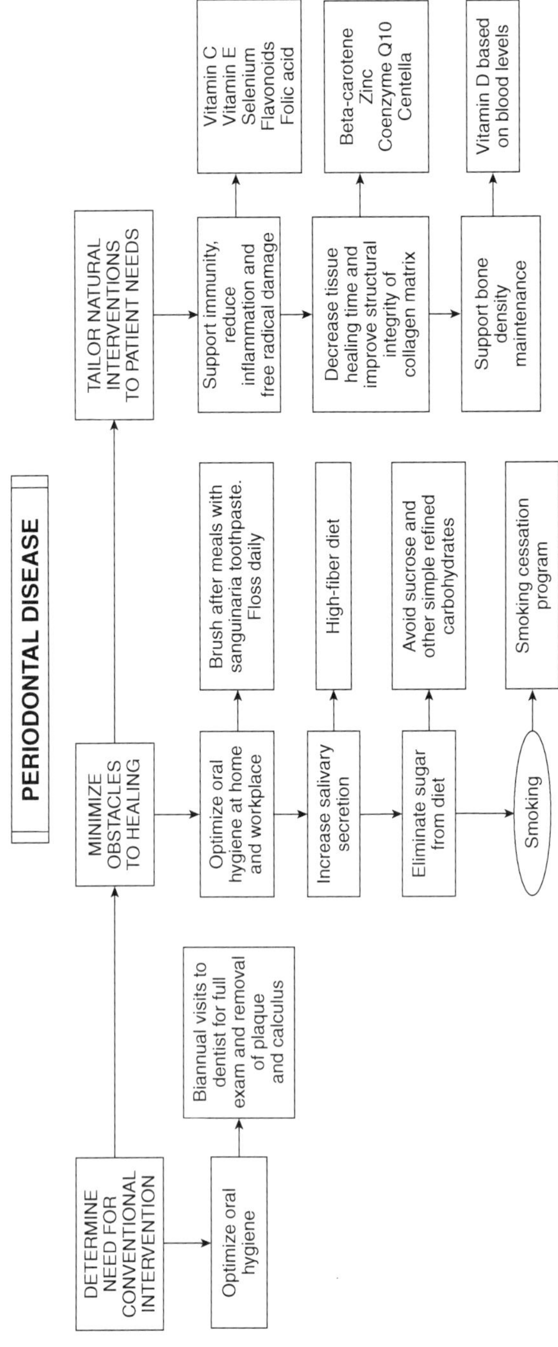
PERIODONTAL DISEASE
DETERMINE NEED FOR CONVENTIONAL INTERVENTION
Optimize oral hygiene
Biannual visits to dentist for full exam and removal of plaque and calculus
MINIMIZE OBSTACLES TO HEALING
Optimize oral hygiene at home and workplace
Brush after meals with sanguinaria toothpaste. Floss daily
Increase salivary secretion
High-fiber diet
Eliminate sugar from diet
Avoid sucrose and other simple refined carbohydrates
Smoking
Smoking cessation program
TAILOR NATURAL INTERVENTIONS TO PATIENT NEEDS
Support immunity, reduce inflammation and free radical damage
Vitamin C
Vitamin E
Selenium
Flavonoids
Folic acid
Decrease tissue healing time and improve structural integrity of collagen matrix
Beta-carotene
Zinc
Coenzyme Q10
Centella
Support bone density maintenance
Vitamin D based on blood levels

than women. Prevalence is inversely related to increasing levels of education and income. Rural inhabitants have higher severity and prevalence than their urban counterparts.

Pathophysiology

Factors involved in host resistance include the following:

- **Gingival sulcus:** V-shaped crevice that surrounds each tooth, bounded by tooth on one side and epithelium lining free margin of gingiva on the other. Sulcus is ideal for bacteria; it is resistant to the cleaning action of saliva. Gingival fluid (sulcular fluid) is a rich nutrient source for microorganisms. Depth of gingival sulcus is a diagnostic parameter. Patients with PD should be monitored biannually by a dentist.
- **Bacterial factors:** bacterial plaque is the causative agent in PD. Bacteria secrete compounds detrimental to host defenses: endotoxins and exotoxins, free radicals and collagen-destroying enzymes, leukotoxins, bacterial antigens, waste products, and toxic compounds.
- **Polymorphonuclear leukocytes (PMNs):** neutrophils (PMNs) are the first line of defense against microbes. PMN functional defects are catastrophic to the periodontium. PMNs are depressed in the elderly and those with diabetes, Crohn's disease, Chédiak-Higashi syndrome, Down's syndrome, and juvenile periodontitis—establishing an extremely high risk for rapidly progressing PD. Transient neutropenia and PMN function defects may cause alternating quiescence and exacerbation in PD. PMNs release numerous free radicals, collagenases, hyaluronidases, inflammatory mediators, and an osteoclast stimulator.
- **Macrophages and monocytes:** increased numbers in PD. They phagocytize bacteria and debris. They are the primary source of prostaglandins in diseased gingiva, and they release abundant enzymes involved in collagen destruction.
- **Lymphocytes:** produce lymphokines. Their role is overshadowed by other immune components. They promote PMN and monocyte chemotaxis, fibroblast destruction, and osteoclast activation.
- **Complement system:** 22 proteins (more than 10% of total serum globulin) whose activation initiates cascade (classic or alternative pathway) triggering immunologic and nonspecific resistance to infection and pathogenesis of tissue injury. Products of

complement activation regulate the release of mediators from mast cells; promotion of smooth muscle contraction; chemotaxis of PMNs, monocytes, and eosinophils; and phagocytosis by immune adherence. Net effect is increased gingival permeability, increased penetration of bacteria and byproducts, and initiation of positive feedback cycle. Other effects include solubilization of immune complexes, cell membrane lysis, neutralization of viruses, and killing of bacteria. In PD, activation of complement by an alternative pathway in the periodontal pocket is a major factor in tissue destruction.

- **Mast cells and immunoglobulin E (IgE):** mast cell degranulation releases inflammatory mediators (histamine, prostaglandins, leukotrienes, kinins, serotonin, heparin, serine proteases). It is initiated by IgE complexes, complement components, mechanical trauma, endotoxins, and free radicals. Increased IgE in gingiva of PD patients suggests allergic factor in progression of PD in some patients.
- **Amalgam restorations:** faulty dental restorations and prostheses are common causes of gingival inflammation and periodontal destruction. Overhanging margins are ideal for plaque and bacteria. Silver amalgam decreases activities of antioxidant enzymes. Mercury accumulation depletes free radical–scavenging enzymes, glutathione peroxidase, superoxide dismutase, and catalase. Proteoglycans and glycosaminoglycans (GAGs) of collagen are sensitive to free radicals.
- **Miscellaneous local factors:** food impaction, unreplaced missing teeth, malocclusion, tongue thrusting, bruxism, toothbrush trauma, mouth breathing, tobacco.
- **Tobacco:** smoking is linked to increased susceptibility to severe PD and tooth loss. The harmful effects are free radical damage to epithelial cells. Smoking greatly reduces ascorbate, potentiating damaging effects. Carotenes and flavonoids greatly reduce toxic effects of smoking.
- **Structure and integrity of collagen matrix:** collagen of periodontal membrane serves as periosteum to alveolar bone. This enables dissipation of tremendous pressure exerted during mastication. Collagen matrix of periodontium (specifically extracellular proteoglycans of gingival epithelium) determines rate of diffusion and permeability of inflammatory mediators, bacteria and byproducts, and destructive enzymes. Because of the high rate of protein turnover in periodontal collagen, integrity of collagen is vulnerable to atrophy when cofactors needed for

collagen synthesis (protein; vitamins C, B_6, and A; zinc [Zn] and copper [Cu]) are absent or deficient. Collagen of periodontium is rich in GAGs: heparin sulfate, dermatan sulfate, and chondroitin-sulfate proteoglycan 4. Stabilizing collagen is the major treatment goal.

THERAPEUTIC CONSIDERATIONS

Therapeutic goals in treating PD from nutritional perspective are as follows:

- Decrease wound healing time
- Improve membrane and collagen integrity
- Decrease inflammation and free radical damage
- Enhance immune status

Vitamin C (ascorbic acid): plays a major role in preventing PD. Classic symptom of gingivitis in scurvy shows ascorbate maintains membrane and collagen integrity and immunocompetence. Deficiency is linked to defective collagen, ground substance, and intercellular cement substance in mesenchymal tissue. Deficiency effects on bone are retardation or cessation of osteoid formation, impaired osteoblastic activity, and osteoporosis. Subclinical deficiency also delays wound healing. Decreased vitamin C is linked to increased permeability of oral mucosa to endotoxin and bacterial byproducts and impaired leukocyte functions (PMNs). It increases chemotaxis and phagocytosis by PMNs; enhances lymphoproliferative response to mitogens; and increases interferon levels, antibody response, immunoglobulin levels, and secretion of thymic hormones. Vitamin C has antioxidant and anti-inflammatory properties and decreases wound healing time.

Vitamin D: low vitamin D is linked to gingivitis; it is a likely cause of both gingivitis and PD. Persons with the highest levels of vitamin D have decreased incidence of gingivitis—across racial and ethnic groups, genders, users and nonusers of vitamin-mineral supplements. Higher vitamin D levels are linked to less periodontal bone loss in both genders. Supplementation reduces bone loss. Vitamin D deficiency correlates with higher incidence of TT VDR (vitamin D receptor) polymorphism and aggressive periodontitis. Vitamin D deficits help link PD and breast cancer in women.

Sucrose: sugar increases plaque accumulation. It decreases PMN chemotaxis and phagocytosis because of osmotic effects and competition with vitamin C. The average American consumes

175 g sucrose q.d. and other refined carbohydrates; this habit increases risk for PD.

Vitamin A: deficiency predisposes to PD. Deficiency is linked to the following:
- Keratinizing metaplasia of gingival epithelium
- Early karyolysis of gingival epithelial cells
- Inflammatory infiltration and degeneration
- Periodontal pocket formation
- Gingival calculus formation
- Increased susceptibility to infection
- Abnormal alveolar bone formation

Vitamin A supports collagen synthesis and wound healing, maintains integrity of epithelial and mucosal surfaces and their secretions, and enhances immune function. Beta-carotene may be better because of its affinity for epithelial tissue and potent antioxidant activity.

Zn and copper (Cu): Zn is synergist with vitamin A. Severity of PD is linked to increased Cu/Zn ratio—consistent with other causes of inflammation—and signifies activation of metallothionein, which increases ceruloplasmin formation and Zn sequestration in response to inflammation. Zn functions in gingiva and periodontium include the following:
- Stabilization of membranes
- Inhibition of calcium influxes
- Antioxidant activity
- Metallocomponent in 40 enzymes, including enzymes for DNA, RNA, and collagen synthesis
- Inhibition of plaque growth
- Inhibition of mast cell degranulation
- Numerous immune activities, including increased PMN chemotaxis and phagocytosis

Zn reduces wound healing time. It is active in calcium- and calmodulin-mediated processes (mast cell degranulation, tissue damage induced by endotoxin, and increased vascular permeability). Twice-daily use of mouthwash with 5% Zn solution inhibits plaque growth.

Vitamin E and selenium (Se): function synergistically in antioxidant mechanisms that deter PD. They potentiate each other's effects. Vitamin E decreases wound healing time. Antioxidant effects of vitamin E are needed for silver amalgam to prevent toxic effects of mercury on antioxidant enzymes. Se and vitamin E prevent free radicals from damaging gingival proteoglycans and

GAGs, deterring PD. Mercury depletes the tissues of the antioxidant enzymes superoxide dismutase, glutathione peroxidase, and catalase. In animal studies, this toxic effect of mercury is prevented by supplementation with vitamin E.

Coenzyme Q10: ubiquinone is a coenzyme in mitochondrial oxidative phosphorylation and an antioxidant; 70% of patients with PD studied responded favorably to supplementation; it was superior to placebo in a double-blind study.

Flavonoids: these are the most important components of an anti-PD program; they reduce inflammation and stabilize collagen by doing the following:

- Decreasing membrane permeability, thereby decreasing load of inflammatory mediators and bacterial products
- Preventing free radical damage by potent antioxidant properties
- Inhibiting enzymatic cleavage by hyaluronidases and collagenases
- Inhibiting mast cell degranulation
- Cross-linking with collagen fibers directly

Supplement biologically active flavonoids: quercetin, catechin, anthocyanidins and proanthocyanidins; rutin has little collagen-stabilizing effect; 3 to 0-methyl-(+)-catechin retards plaque growth and alveolar bone resorption in animal models.

Grapeseed extract is most useful source of flavonoids because its proanthocyanidins possess wide-ranging biologic properties useful against PD. Grapeseed proanthocyanidin extract (GSE) strongly decreases production of reactive oxygen species and protein expression of inducible nitric oxide synthase by murine macrophages stimulated with lipopolysaccharides of periodontopathogens.

Folic acid: most common micronutrient deficiency in the world; given either topically or systemically, it reduces gingival inflammation by reducing color changes, bleeding tendency, exudate flow, and plaque scores. Folate mouthwash (0.1% folic acid) is much more effective than oral supplement at 2 or 5 mg q.d., suggesting a local mechanism; binds plaque-derived endotoxin. Folate mouthwash is particularly indicated for pregnant women and oral contraceptive users and in exaggerated gingival inflammatory response or folate antimetabolites (phenytoin, methotrexate).

- Epithelium of cervix and oral mucosa suffer from end-organ folate deficiency under hormonal influences of pregnancy and oral contraceptives; cervical dysplasia of oral contraception also responds to pharmacologic dose of folate (8 to 30 mg q.d.); sera and leukocytes of pregnant women and oral contraceptive users contain macromolecule that binds folate, a major factor for end-organ folate deficiency.

Botanical Medicines

- *Sanguinaria canadensis* **(bloodroot):** contains benzophenanthridine alkaloids—sanguinarine in commercial toothpastes and mouth rinses. Sanguinarine is antimicrobial and anti-inflammatory; it inhibits bacterial adherence. Bacteria aggregate and become morphologically irregular. It is less effective than chlorhexidine mouthwash but effective in many cases and is a natural compound versus a synthetic.
- *Centella asiatica* **(gotu kola):** triterpenoids demonstrate impressive wound healing; useful in severe PD or if surgery required. It speeds up recovery after laser surgery for severe PD.

THERAPEUTIC APPROACH

Control all relevant factors; general approach is recommended. Smoking greatly decreases the success of any therapy for PD. Because factors that increase risk for osteoporosis (e.g., low calcium and vitamin D, cigarette smoking) also predispose individuals to risk for PD and tooth loss, consult osteoporosis chapter.

- **Hygiene:** periodic visits to the dentist to eliminate plaque and calculus; brush after meals; floss daily; use tiny proxy brushes between teeth as needed.
- **Diet:** high in dietary fiber, which is protective from increased salivary secretion; avoid sucrose and all refined carbohydrates.
- **Supplements:**
  - Vitamin C: 3 to 5 g q.d. in divided doses.
  - Vitamin D: 2000 to 6000 international units (IU) q.d. (monitor dosing effect with blood testing of 25-[OH]D_3).
  - Vitamin E (mixed tocopherols): 400 to 800 IU q.d.
  - Beta-carotenes: 50,000 IU q.d.
  - Se: 400 mcg q.d.
  - Zn: 30 mg q.d. of Zn picolinate; wash mouth with 15 mL of 5% solution b.i.d.
  - Folic acid: 800 mcg q.d.; wash mouth with 15 mL of 0.1% solution b.i.d.

- **Botanical medicines:**
  - — High flavonoid–containing extracts, such as those from bilberry *(Vaccinium myrtillus)*, hawthorn (*Crataegus* species), grapeseed *(Vitis vinifera)*, or green tea *(Camellia sinensis)*. Grapeseed extract and green tea extract (or liberal consumption of green tea) might be most protective. For grapeseed extract with 95% proanthocyanidolic oligomer content or green tea extract with 90% polyphenol content, dose is 150 to 300 mg q.d.
  - — ***S. canadensis:*** use toothpaste containing extract.
  - — ***C. asiatica*** **triterpenoids:** 30 mg b.i.d. of pure triterpenoids.

Porphyrias

DIAGNOSTIC SUMMARY

- Unexplained abdominal pain, possibly including nausea and vomiting
- Acute peripheral or central nervous system dysfunction
- Mental abnormalities ranging from confusion to acute psychosis
- Urinary porphobilinogen (PBG) during attack
- Most carriers are asymptomatic, except when exposed to drugs or chemicals that exacerbate condition

GENERAL CONSIDERATIONS

- Although the condition was once considered rare, the prevalence now may be higher. Allopathic medicine has some therapies, but naturopathy has an array of effective modalities for therapy and prevention.
- Classic triad: abdominal pain, constipation (or diarrhea), and vomiting.
- Acute intermittent porphyria has periods of exacerbation and remission.
- Genetic deficits of porphyria affect all tissues but primarily the hematopoietic tissues of bone marrow and the cytochrome p450 system in the liver because of the greater number of porphyrin precursors required. The liver is the major site where inherited or acquired deficits in heme synthesis manifest.

Classifications of Porphyria

- Hepatic or erythropoietic origin. Both classes are characterized by overproduction of porphyrin or precursors.
- Biosynthesis of heme is controlled differently in the liver and bone marrow. Rate-limiting enzyme in the liver is aminolevulinic acid (ALVA) synthase. In bone marrow, biosynthesis of heme is partly regulated by uptake of iron (Fe).

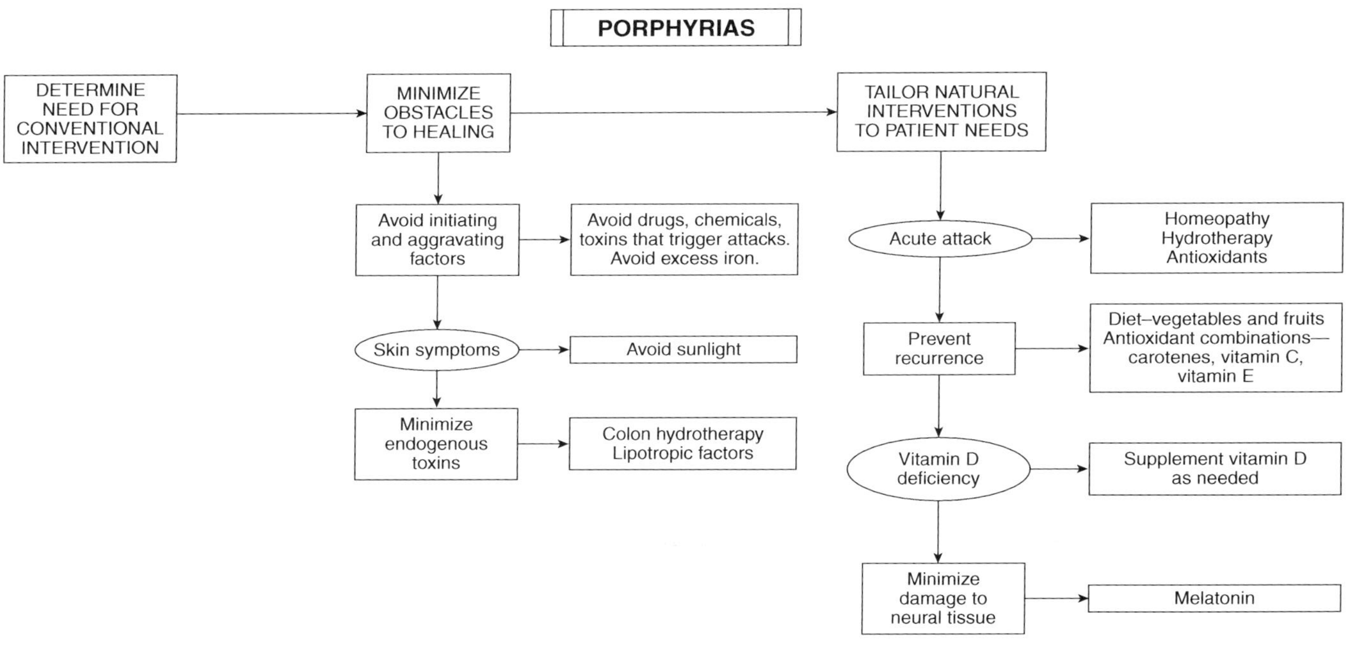
PORPHYRIAS
DETERMINE NEED FOR CONVENTIONAL INTERVENTION
MINIMIZE OBSTACLES TO HEALING
TAILOR NATURAL INTERVENTIONS TO PATIENT NEEDS
Avoid initiating and aggravating factors
Avoid drugs, chemicals, toxins that trigger attacks. Avoid excess iron.
Skin symptoms
Avoid sunlight
Minimize endogenous toxins
Colon hydrotherapy Lipotropic factors
Acute attack
Homeopathy Hydrotherapy Antioxidants
Prevent recurrence
Diet–vegetables and fruits Antioxidant combinations—carotenes, vitamin C, vitamin E
Vitamin D deficiency
Supplement vitamin D as needed
Minimize damage to neural tissue
Melatonin

- Acute hepatic porphyrias: rapid onset of symptoms, largely neurologic; erythropoietic variety manifests primarily in skin as cutaneous photosensitivity.

Primary Porphyrias

Hepatic Porphyrias	Erythropoietic Porphyrias
• Aminolevulinic acid–dehydrase deficiency porphyria	• X-linked sideroblastic anemia
• Acute intermittent porphyria	• Congenital erythropoietic porphyria
• Porphyria cutanea tarda	• Erythrocytic protoporphyria
• Hereditary coproporphyria	
• Variegate porphyria	

Signs and Symptoms of Hepatic Porphyrias

- Acute attacks: wide variety of symptoms ranging from skin lesions to abdominal pain to neurologic symptoms of varying degrees of intensity.
- Abdominal, back, or extremity pains increase over a 24- to 48-hour period (mimics appendicitis or an acute abdomen). Rebound tenderness usually is not present.
- Nausea and vomiting.
- Anxiety and restlessness.
- Constipation that worsens as condition develops.
- Tachycardia, suggesting infectious process or bowel toxicity.
- Severity of symptoms out of proportion to presenting signs. Bowel symptoms are caused by a neurologic disturbance.
- Mental abnormalities: confusion to acute psychosis can be the first presentation.
- Prolonged attacks impair sensory and motor function, causing respiratory paralysis and death.
- Many patients have been misdiagnosed with schizophrenia and confined to mental institutions.
- Majority of carriers are asymptomatic except when exposed to drugs or chemicals that exacerbate the condition.
- Neurologic symptoms and sequelae of acute and/or prolonged attack can take months to clear, but eventual recovery occurs in the majority of cases.

Biochemistry

- Biosynthesis of heme is the main purpose for porphyrogenic pathway. Heme is a member of a group of compounds including cytochromes (oxidation and reduction reactions), chlorophyll (photosynthesis), and vitamin B_{12}. It is formed from succinyl coenzyme A (CoA) and combined with globin chains synthesized on ribosomes in plasma of developing red blood cells (RBCs). In the liver, heme is used to make detoxifying cytochrome p450. Heme synthesis begins and ends in mitochondrion, with part occurring in cytoplasm. All tissues form heme, but primary sites are bone marrow and the liver.

- Rate-limiting enzyme for heme synthesis is ALA synthase, which is the initial enzyme in the cascade. It is regulated by a feedback response to tissue demand for heme. With the formation of uroporphyrinogen, branching generates porphyrin isomers. Isomer III results in the formation of uroporphyrinogen III, modified to be more lipophilic for excretion from the body. The majority of the pathway favors heme production.

Heme Formation

- Regulated by action of ferrochelatase in mitochondria. Reducing substances are required: ascorbic acid, cysteine, or glutathione. Fe must be in ferrous rather than ferric form. Ferrochelatase is inhibited by high levels of heme, which also inhibit ALA synthase.
- Multiple control systems regulate the metabolic pathway.
- RBC incorporation of heme, Fe, and glycine occurs in maturing reticulocytes but is lost as the cell ages. Hypoxia and erythropoietin stimulate ALA synthase in RBCs but not the liver; drugs and chemicals affect the liver but not erythropoietic tissues.

Porphyria Manifestation

- Genetic or acquired deficits limit flow of heme precursors through a cascade that forms hemoglobin. Deficiency manifests from increased demand; certain drugs, chemicals, steroids, estrogens, oral contraceptives, progesterone, or testosterone that burdens cytochrome p450 can precipitate an acute attack.
- This results from partial removal of feedback on ALVA synthase. Depending on enzyme deficit, heme precursors follow different pathways and accumulate in tissues—skin and nervous system—causing signs and symptoms.
- Attacks are more frequent in women than in men, especially premenstrually. Expression of porphyria increases with age from increased exposures to toxins and the aging body's decreasing ability to adapt.

- Skin symptoms: some porphyric precursors absorb light at 400 nm, raising the potential energy of the molecule to an excited state of highly reactive oxygen species. Histamine and proteolytic enzyme release induce oxidative damage. Beta-carotene protects against these injuries.
- Neuropsychiatric changes occur in hepatic porphyrias (ALA-dehydrase deficiency porphyria, acute intermittent porphyria, porphyria cutanea tarda (PCT), hereditary coproporphyria, and variegate porphyria) with excess production of ALA and PBG. Exact mechanism of how porphyrins affect the central nervous system is unknown.
- Familial PCT: occurs at a younger age than spontaneous PCT despite no difference in biochemical features. Reason: either genetic predisposition to sequestering ferritin in the liver or increased sensitivity to alcohol ingestion. Even manifestations among family members vary.

Etiologic Agents

- Prescription medicines, estrogens, some herbal medicines, heavy metals, organophosphates, burdens on cytochrome p450.
- Exogenous estrogens: oral contraceptives, estrogen patches, or estrogen replacement therapy or hormone replacement therapy. Estrogens enhance porphyrin-inducing activities of other agents; women are more vulnerable to environmental exposures than are men.
- Herbicides decrease activity of enzymes of porphyric pathway and increase porphyrins in nerve tissue.
- Theory: unexplained chemical-associated illnesses, such as multiple chemical sensitivity (MCS) syndrome, may be mild chronic porphyria or acquired abnormalities in heme synthesis. Exposures to porphyrogenic substances or severe infection overpower the deficient enzyme system, causing accumulation of specific porphyrins. Symptoms arise from increased porphyrinogen and not accumulation of the toxin itself.
- Expediting the distinction between "real" porphyria and secondary porphyrinopathies: porphyria diagnosis is based on urinary and/or fecal porphyrin excretions twice to 20 times the upper limit of normal. This excludes persons with lesser degrees of porphyrogenic activity, whose conditions may be in remission or not subject to environmental exposures.
- Intensity of symptoms varies widely. Ten percent have acute, severe attacks; 25% have chronic symptoms of varying degrees;

65% have no symptoms but become susceptible under the right circumstances.

- Alternative theory: patients with MCS may, at times, have modest increases in urinary coproporphyrin, commonly found in asymptomatic subjects or those with diverse other conditions (e.g., diabetes mellitus, heavy alcohol use, liver disease, anemias). Secondary coproporphyrinuria does not indicate coproporphyria.
- Modern exposures to offending agents will increase unmasking of underlying deficits.

Laboratory Diagnosis

- Small amounts of porphyrins (coproporphyrin) are excreted in normal human urine. Coproporphyrin also is present in bile and feces. ALA, PBG, and uroporphyrin are excreted in urine; coproporphyrin is preferentially and protoporphyrin exclusively excreted in bile and feces.
- Fecal excretion is affected by diet and bowel flora; arriving at "normal" values is difficult. PBG in urine of healthy persons is less than 1.5 mg q.d. and undetectable by conventional testing. Watson-Schwartz qualitative test for PBG is positive in acute intermittent porphyria in acute attacks and variegate porphyria and hereditary coproporphyria in latent periods. High rate of false negatives is attributable to its subjective nature. A substance present in yeast tablets can induce false-positive Watson-Schwartz test result.
- Cost-effective strategy for acute symptoms:
  - — For neurovisceral features suggesting acute porphyric syndrome, use rapid screening test for urinary PBG.
  - — For solar urticaria and acute photosensitivity (protoporphyria), test for increased RBC porphyrins.
  - — For vesiculobullous formation (PCT, hereditary coproporphyria, or variegate porphyria), test for urinary porphyrins.
  - — Confirm positive screening test results with targeted quantitative testing.
- Enzymatic assays and DNA-based testing usually are not needed for acute disease. They are useful for evaluation and genetic counseling. Isolating specific DNA encoding heme biosynthetic pathway enzymes provides precise heterozygote identification and prenatal diagnosis in families with known defects.
- Cell markers to identify porphyria in the absence of symptoms: white blood cell (WBC) manganese, calcium, Fe, and zinc, plus

RBC calcium differing in concentration among those classified as acute intermittent porphyria gene carriers. Manganese is the most discriminative of all variables. Increased cellular manganese by factor of 4 suggests an increased likelihood of developing acute intermittent porphyria.
- Specific deficit must be determined; successful treatment outcomes depend on correct diagnosis (*Textbook,* "Urinary Porphyrins for the Detection of Heavy Metal and Toxic Chemical Exposure").

THERAPEUTIC CONSIDERATIONS

- Identify patients predisposed or susceptible to porphyric episodes: medical history of periodic psychotic episodes, nervous breakdowns, unexplained abdominal pains, unusual symptoms. Prevention is the first option because porphyric episodes are difficult to control.
- Treatment of acute episodes is demanding because of severity and a changing clinical picture. Presentations differ depending on the degree of toxicity, genetic component, and patient response to therapy.
- Homeopathy has been successful; medicines depend on the clinical picture. Constitutional prescribing does not work as well during the acute state; several prescriptions may be needed to stabilize the patient. Prescriptions may need to be frequently changed as disease stages progress. Frequent follow-up, perhaps daily, is needed to assess clinical state.
- Patient education: helps overcome disbelief and denial. Delineate which symptoms go with each condition. Inform other physicians that patient is seeking to keep prescription drugs to a minimum. Course of therapy to reach state of insusceptibility to toxins is long, with exacerbations and remissions. Help patient understand this.
- Identify and limit offending agents. Take a complete history of environmental and work exposures. Often simply changing work environment eliminates attacks.

Toxins Known to Cause or Exacerbate Porphyria

- Intoxications:
  - **Alcoholism**
  - **Foreign and environmental chemicals** such as hexachlorobenzene, polyhalogenated biphenyls, dioxins, vinyl chloride, carbon tetrachloride, benzene, chloroform

— **Heavy metals,** such as lead, arsenic, mercury
— **Drugs**

Categories of Drugs that Cause Adverse Effects

- Analgesics
- Sedatives
- Hypnotics
- Anesthetics
- Sex hormones
- Sulfa antibiotics

Drugs Known to Cause or Exacerbate Porphyria*

- Aminoglutethimide
- Aminopyrine
- Antipyrine
- Barbiturates
- Captopril
- Carbamazepine
- Carbromal
- Chloral hydrate
- Chloramphenicol
- Chlordiazepoxide
- Chlorpropamide
- Danazol
- Dapsone
- Diazepam
- Diclofenac
- Diltiazem
- Diphenhydramine
- Diphenylhydantoin
- Doxycycline
- Ergot preparations
- Erythromycin
- Estrogen
- Ethanol (acute)
- Ethchlorvynol
- Ethinamate
- Furosemide
- Glutethimide
- Griseofulvin
- Hydralazine
- Hydrochlorothiazide
- Imipramine
- Isopropyl meprobamate
- Lidocaine
- Mephenytoin
- Meprobamate
- Methyldopa
- Methyprylon
- Metoclopramide
- Metronidazole
- *N*-butylscopolammonium bromide
- Nifedipine
- Nitrous oxide
- Novobiocin
- Oral contraceptives
- Orphenadrine
- Oxycodone
- Pentazocine
- Phenobarbital
- Phenylbutazone
- Phenytoin
- Piroxicam
- Pivampicillin
- Primidone
- Progesterone
- Pyrazinamide
- Pyrazolone preparations
- Sodium valproate
- Succinimides
- Sulfonamide antibiotics
- Sulfonethylmethane
- Sulfonmethane
- Synthetic estrogens, progestins
- Terfenadine
- Tetracyclines
- Theophylline
- Tolazamide
- Tolbutamide
- Trimethadione
- Valproic acid
- Verapamil

*This list includes many drugs that can exacerbate porphyria, but it is not complete.

Nutritional Therapies

- **Diet:** during acute intermittent porphyria attacks, increasing complex carbohydrates helps alleviate symptoms. Often the patient is ingesting high amounts of carbohydrates when first seen, and weight gain follows. Intravenous glucose (300 to 400 g/day) can be given. A more-complete parenteral nutritional regimen is preferable. Avoid fasting or rapid weight loss, which can precipitate acute intermittent porphyria. High-fiber fruits and vegetables improve several porphyria measures. In a study of PCT, 500 kcal of fruits and vegetables per day decreased body mass index, serum alanine aminotransferase (ALT) from 122.0 to 75.6 U/L, serum aspartate aminotransferase (AST) from 91.8 to 55.2 U/L, serum Fe from 188.6 to 140.2 mg/dL, and serum ferritin from 574 to 499 ng/mL. Diet also improved skin lesions and decreased urinary coproporphyrin and uroporphyrins.

- **Antioxidants:** along with homeopathy, antioxidants are the mainstay of case management during acute porphyric episodes. Once the condition is stabilized, an ongoing regimen of antioxidants—vitamin C, vitamin E, glutathione (GSH), beta-carotene, *N*-acetylcysteine—should prevent recurrence. Vitamin C is low in patients with PCT.
- **Vitamin C:** (1 g/d) may help reduce erythropoietic protoporphyria photosensitivity.
- **Vitamin E:** high-dose (1 g of alpha-tocopherol per day) in PCT decreases urinary uroporphyrins (50% of C8 carboxyls) with clinical improvement. Effect lasts only as long as vitamin E is supplemented. Vitamin E reduces residual oxidative stress and does not affect increased plasma and whole-blood viscosity present in PCT. Mixed tocopherols may produce better results.
- **Combinations of antioxidants:** for phototoxicity of protoporphyrin IX (PP IX) and uroporphyrin I (UP I).
  - Both beta-carotene with lycopene and combination of beta-carotene, ascorbic acid, and alpha-tocopherol protect cells cultures against PP IX phototoxicity
  - Beta-carotene, ascorbic acid, and alpha-tocopherol combination: for membrane protection against the phototoxicity of both porphyrins, resulting possibly from synergistic processes. PCT and erythropoietic protoporphyria may be treated by combinations of these antioxidants.
- **Vitamin D:** deficits might be worsened by increased oxidative damage from photodermatitis. Vitamin D insufficiency and deficiency are linked directly with total erythrocyte protoporphyrin concentration and inversely with the time in minutes to onset of symptoms after sunlight exposure. In patients with porphyrias involving photodermatitis, consider vitamin D therapy.
- **Melatonin:** as an antioxidant affecting delta-ALA–induced oxidative toxicity in neural tissue and as co-treatment for ALA accumulation. Melatonin (10 mg/kg) may reduce lipid

peroxidation induced by delta-ALA in the cerebellum and hippocampus. Melatonin protects against ALA-related oxidative stress and its oncostatic properties. Because of its low toxicity, consider melatonin as co-treatment for disturbances arising from ALA accumulation.

- **Vitamin B complex:** pantothenic acid (vitamin B_5) facilitates formation of succinyl CoA (by the tricarboxylic acid cycle) and glycine, precursors to ALA; supplementation is helpful. Transformation of succinyl CoA involves vitamin B_{12}–dependent enzyme; check B_{12} and folic acid status. The initial reaction is oxygen dependent; therefore oxygen therapy may be contraindicated in delta-ALA porphyria. ALA formation needs pyridoxal-5-phosphate (P5P); any substance that inhibits enzyme systems is countered in part by P5P. However, P5P may not play an important role.
- **Carotenoids:** all cutaneous porphyrias are alleviated by avoiding sunlight. Treating erythropoietic protoporphyria with large doses of beta-carotene is effective and may improve tolerance to sunlight. Mixed carotenoids (alpha-carotene, beta-carotene, and lycopene) are effective in cell cultures, but single carotenes are ineffective.
- **Fe:** excessive Fe stores and intake aggravate several porphyrias. Avoid Fe unless clearly indicated by low Fe stores.
- **Detoxification:** liver and colon detoxification eliminates toxins that may exacerbate the condition. Methods: colon hydrotherapy, constitutional hydrotherapy, sauna, antioxidants, or oxygen therapy (ozone). Lipotropic factors that enhance the liver cytochrome p450 system are contraindicated during acute attacks but are useful when patient is in a quiet, stable period. Lipotropics and antioxidants help decrease acute attacks. Chelation with ethylenediaminetetraacetic acid (EDTA) and ethanol extracts of botanicals is contraindicated in patients predisposed to porphyria.
- **Constitutional hydrotherapy:** quite effective during acute flare-up, normalizing liver function and neurologic symptoms. Daily sessions may be needed.
- **Ozone therapy:** indicated for deficit of coproporphyrinogen oxidase causing deficit of coproporphyrinogen in hereditary coproporphyria. It is contraindicated in deficit of ALA synthase; oxygen enhances the pathway, resulting in exacerbation of symptoms.

THERAPEUTIC APPROACH

- **Identify condition early:** avoid initiating and aggravating factors. Limit sun exposure in cutaneous manifestations.
- **Diet:** rich in vegetables and fruits, low in Fe.
- **Supplements:**
  - — Vitamin E (mixed tocopherols): 400 to 1200 international units (IU) (mixed tocopherols) q.d.
  - — Mixed carotenes: 100,000 to 150,000 IU q.d.—vitamin C: 3000 to 5000 mg q.d.
  - — Vitamin D: 5000 to 10,000 IU q.d. (measure blood levels to determine optimal dose)
  - — Melatonin: 3 mg q.d.

Pregnancy Health and Primary Prevention of Adult Disease

OVERVIEW

A healthful environment will benefit the mother and positively affect future offspring health. Susceptibility to chronic disease in adulthood originates in part during fetal development. In utero epigenetic expression is sensitive to environmental changes, which can lead to altered function, metabolism, and hormone production. In utero environmental exposures alter phenotypic expression via DNA methylation, histone acetylation, messenger RNA expression, and chromatin structure modification. These epigenetic changes occurring in the womb are replicated throughout life and may even be passed to subsequent generations.

Preconception Work

Work with future mother before pregnancy—detoxify, restore deficient nutrients, and lower stress.

Pregnancy Death Rates and Premature Births

Pregnancy death rate has decreased owing to worldwide increase in training of midwives, improved medical technology, advances in obstetrics, and higher-quality pregnancy care.

Weight Gain

- Women should expect to gain 25 to 35 pounds during normal pregnancy, with 3- to 4-pound gain during first trimester.
- Low weight gain is associated with increased intrauterine growth restriction risk and perinatal mortality.
- Overall weight gain represents two components: (1) products of conception (fetus, amniotic fluid, and placenta); (2) maternal accretion of tissues (expansion of blood and extracellular fluid, enlarged uterus and mammaries, and adipose stores).

Current Recommendations for Weight Gain during Pregnancy

Prepregnancy Body Mass Index (BMI)	BMI (kg/m^2) (World Health Organization)	Total Weight Gain Range (lb)	Rates of Weight Gain in Second and Third Trimesters (lb/wk)
Underweight	<18.5	28-40	1 (1-1.3)
Normal weight	18.5-24.9	25-35	1 (0.8-1)
Overweight	25.0-29.9	15-25	0.6 (0.5-0.7)
Obese (includes all classes)	≥30.0	11-20	0.5 (0.4-0.6)

Data from the Institute of Medicine. Weight gain during pregnancy: reexamining the guidelines. Washington DC: National Academies Press; 2009.

Obesity in Pregnancy

- High maternal weight or weight gain during pregnancy changes the hypothalamus, pancreatic islet cells, fat tissue, endocrine physiology, and metabolic pathways affecting homeostatic weight control.
- Excessive gains are associated with gestational hypertension, labor augmentation, high birth weight, cesarean sections, and neonatal metabolic abnormalities, and fetopelvic disproportion complicates the risk.
- Babies born to obese women are three times more likely to die within first month of birth; stillbirth rates are doubled.
- Very obese women—body mass index (BMI) of 35 or higher—are three to four times as likely to deliver first baby by cesarean section.
- Weight gains of 6.7 to 11.2 kg (15 to 25 pounds) in overweight and obese women, and less than 6.7 kg (15 pounds) will reduce risk.
- Interestingly, in morbidly obese women, decreased weight gain was associated with 30% less use of epidural analgesia and overall reduction in negative outcomes.

Thyroid

- Preterm delivery, preeclampsia, hypertension, diabetic complications, placental abruption, miscarriage, and adverse fetal effects have all been reported with hypothyroidism or hyperthyroidism during pregnancy.
- Normal thyroid-stimulating hormone (TSH) levels alone do not ensure proper thyroid function. Normal TSH accompanying autoimmunity creates a twofold risk for pregnancy loss.

- Although TSH laboratory values range from 0.45 to 4.5 milli-international units (mIU) per liter, the upper range cutoff in pregnancy TSH should be around 2.5 mIU/L. Miscarriage and preterm delivery increase with higher levels.
- Women with positive antibodies and no replacement therapy have higher rates of miscarriage than women with positive antibodies and levothyroxine replacement.
- Women with otherwise unexplained previous pregnancy losses should be treated if TSH level is higher than 2.5 mIU/L and/or they have positive test for antibodies.
- Preeclamptic women are more likely to have hypothyroidism before conception or in late pregnancy. After the onset of preeclampsia, predelivery TSH increased 2.42 times above baseline versus 1.48 times in controls. Toward the end of pregnancy, women with preeclampsia had much higher levels of TSH than women with no history of preeclampsia.
- Iodine consumption in the United States has decreased 50% in the past 30 years; 14.9% of women of child-bearing age have a blood iodine level of less than 50 mcg/L, a level below which is associated with poorer infant outcomes.

Flu Shots and Vaccines

- In pregnancy care, it is recognized as reasonable to avoid any unnecessary treatment. Vaccination during pregnancy is a controversial topic.
- Vaccination is recommended in several countries; no studies demonstrate an increased risk of maternal or fetal adverse effects with inactivated, unadjuvanted shots.
- There is a 41% decreased incidence of flu in infants born to vaccinated women and a 39% decrease in influenza-like illness and hospitalization.
- Infant antibody titers were higher with vaccinated pregnant mothers.
- Newer vaccines (e.g., influenza H1N1 vaccine) now include adjuvant, which may induce stronger immune response in pregnant women, because they are more sensitive to proinflammatory stimuli than those who are not pregnant.
- An adjuvant is a substance that, when administered in combination with a specific antigen, enhances immune response against the antigen.
- Centers for Disease Control and Prevention CDC Advisory Committee on Immunization Practices in pregnancy supports

giving pregnant women a number of vaccinations during pregnancy and lists only two as contraindicated.

Adjuvant Ingredients

- Squalene
- Polysorbate 80
- Sorbitan trioleate
- Sorbitan oleate
- Polyethylene cetostearyl ether
- Mannitol
- Aluminum hydroxide
- Aluminum phosphate
- Aluminum hydroxyphosphate sulfate

Vaccination Recommendations from the Centers for Disease Control and Prevention Advisory Committee on Immunization Practices in Pregnancy

- Tetanus, diphtheria, pertussis
- Hepatitis A
- Hepatitis B
- Influenza
- Pneumococcus
- Polio
- Typhoid, nonlive
- Measles, mumps, rubella
- Varicella

Data from Zain A, Al-Safi Valerie I, Shavell VI, Gonik B. Vaccination in pregnancy. *Womens Health.* 2011;7(1):109-119.

LIFESTYLE FACTORS

Hydration

- Appropriate fluid intake provides a normal 40% volume expansion in the pregnant woman.
- About 32 ounces of fluid surround baby as amniotic fluid, replaced every third hour.
- Insufficient fluid intake can cause constipation, preterm labor, temperature dysregulation, cystitis, miscarriage, and fatigue. Proper hydration is important for subsequent breast milk production and flow.

- With 96 ounces of fluid loss via urination and perspiration per day, each pregnant women needs eight to 12 8-ounce glasses of water or other beverages per day.
- Weather that is warm and dry, cold weather increase moisture loss.
- Avoid heavily caffeinated drinks and sugary beverages.
- Drink at regular intervals; do not wait for feeling of thirst.

Energy Needs and Diet

- Pregnancy's anabolic state hormonally redirects nutrients to maternal reproductive tissues and developing infant.
- Pregnancy increases energy needs—90, 285, and 465 calories daily for first, second, and third trimesters, respectively, met by modest increases in consumption of a balanced diet.
- Minimum of 175 g carbohydrate per day for pregnancy; includes additional 33 g carbohydrate for fetal brain development.
- Dietary total fat intake, expressed as percentage of energy intake, need not differ from that of nonpregnant women.
- Micronutrient deficiencies are common during pregnancy (even in well-fed populations). Consider prenatal multivitamin with healthful diet.

Undernutrition and Overnutrition

- Undernutrition during pregnancy and low birth weight epigenetically increase risks of diabetes and cardiovascular disease.
- Fetal effects: higher weight and waist circumferences, higher adult BMI, increased risk of hypertension, impaired glucose tolerance, increased risk for cardiovascular disease and diabetes, and twofold increase in incidence of schizophrenia and both mood and schizoid personality disorders.
- Excess and unbalanced food choices lead to high birth weight, which increases risks for obesity, cancer and asthma later in life. A baby can be born with some adipose tissue, but excess fat is abnormal.
- Healthful dietary changes after baby is born may not reverse original fetal insult.
- Fatty diet may cause epigenetic DNA modifications that can be passed on to future generations.
- The brain and nervous system are also subject to epigenetic changes of a high-fat diet. Maternal diet will program brain changes that begin before birth; these cannot be reversed in offspring with a change in diet.

Healthy Foods

Fruits and Vegetables

- Pregnant women require more fruits and vegetables than usual because of extra demands on the body.
- Recommendation: seven servings of fruits and vegetables per day.

Folic Acid–Containing Foods

- Deficiency of folic acid during prenatal period is linked to spina bifida and other neural tube defects.
- Eat foods higher in folic acid, even before conception.
- Sources: fortified grains, spinach, lentils, chickpeas, asparagus, broccoli, peas, Brussels sprouts, corn, and oranges.
- Diet alone is unlikely to provide levels similar to those from folate-multivitamin supplements.

Apples

- Apples have a protective effect on children, with a 40% decreased rate of wheeze and 50% lowered risk of asthma at age 5.
- Apples contain flavonoids, isoflavonoids, and phenolic acids.

Vegetarian Diets

- Although vegetarian diets are associated with healthier pregnancy weight, strict vegan diets result in low vitamin B_{12} status, anemia, and delayed infant development.
- Properly planned vegetarian or vegan diets can be nutritionally adequate.

Soy

- The use of soy during pregnancy is controversial.
- Danish analysis: pregnancy diet lacking fish and meat is associated with fourfold increased risk of hypospadias, possibly because of increased soy intake.
- Suspected estrogenic effects may disrupt male masculinization through interference at the pituitary-gonadal axis.
- Animal perinatal genistein exposure resulted in alterations in male reproductive system (i.e., smaller anogenital distance and testis size, delayed preputial separation, lowered testosterone).
- Animal maternal exposure to daidzein during pregnancy masculinized female offspring with regard to memory and social behavior.

- Generations of Asian cultures have consumed **fermented soy.** As a prudent measure, balance soy protein with other sources of protein.

Fish

- Eating fish can support future brain development and reduce risk of asthma and atopy in offspring by 40%; it can also help to prevent postpartum mood disorders in the mother.
- Rich source of essential long-chain n-3 (omega-3) polyunsaturated fatty acids (PUFAs) for structural and physiologic support for neurologic, immune system, and cardiovascular development.
- Desired minimum intake: 200 mg docosahexaenoic acid (DHA) per day by consuming one to two portions of small wild oily ocean fish per week.
- Cautions: contaminants in large fish—methylmercury, dioxins and polychlorinated biphenyls (PCBs), brominated flame retardants, camphechlor, and organotin. Small, wild-caught, cold water fish are the best choice.

Mercury

- Greatest susceptibility to methylmercury and dioxin-like compounds occurs during fetal and early development.
- Methylmercury is toxic to developing brain and may adversely affect child growth.
- Reduce intake of contaminated foods in the months before and during pregnancy. Salmon is relatively low in mercury and 18 other trace metals; however, levels are three times higher in wild salmon than in farmed.

Mercury in Fish

Fish with High Mercury Levels

- Marlin
- Pike
- Swordfish
- Shark
- Tuna
- Halibut
- Mackerel
- Bass
- Lobster

Fish with Low Mercury Levels

- Salmon (farmed has less mercury than wild)
- Herring
- Anchovies
- Sardines
- Rainbow trout
- Calamari
- Flounder
- Tilapia
- Trout

Data from National Resources Defense Council. Consumer guide to mercury in fish. Available at www.nrdc.org/health/effects/mercury/guide.asp. Accessed February 15, 2012.

Dioxins

- Unwanted byproducts of industrial and combustion processes, dioxins are also in fish. Because they break down very slowly, avoiding them right before and during pregnancy will not decrease fetal exposure.
- Highest levels are present in herring and farmed salmon. Very high levels are present in Baltic Sea fish (and fish from other contaminated waters), and these fish should be avoided.

Polychlorinated Biphenyls

- Virtually all samples of human blood, fat, or breast milk show PCBs.
- Highest levels occur in farmed fish and inorganic butter; moreover, farmed salmon (Atlantic) contains higher levels than wild varieties.
- Adverse effects: low birth weight, small head circumference, earlier birth, a depressive response in the infant, and impaired vision and memory.
- At age 11, children who had been exposed to PCBs had thrice the risk of low verbal IQ and twice the lag in reading comprehension and attention issues as children who had not been so exposed.
- Benefits of eating fish may outweigh risks. Focus on fish with lower mercury and PCB content and avoid eating the skin and fat found along ventral, lateral, and abdominal areas, where PCBs are most heavily deposited.

Flaxseed

- Good source of fiber and omega-3 alpha-linolenic acid (ALA).
- Richest source of lignan secoisolariciresinol diglucoside (SDG), a phytoestrogen precursor.
- Beneficial for fetal brain development because of ALA content.
- Because of SDG, there has been concern about ingestion of flax during pregnancy.

Caffeine

- Sources: coffee or black and green tea.
- In pregnant women who consumed 200 mg of caffeine per day (amount in 10 ounces of coffee or 25 ounces of tea), there was doubling of risk of early miscarriage.
- Increased risk was associated with caffeine itself.
- No teratogenic consequences have been found.

Cocoa and Theobromines

- Maternal prenatal intake of cocoa could be associated with both hypospadias and testicular cancer in male offspring.
- Theobromine concentrations in cord serum from five or more servings of chocolate might be inversely associated with preeclampsia.

STEVIA

- Stevia is a small perennial shrub that yields a white crystalline compound (stevioside) used as a natural sweetener.
- With no calories, it is 100 to 300 times as sweet as table sugar.
- U.S. Food and Drug Administration (FDA) rates stevia as generally recognized as safe (GRAS).

Peanuts

- About 1% of population reports peanut or tree nut allergy.
- Babies of mothers who ate a greater number of peanut products during pregnancy were more likely to test positive for peanut allergies.
- All sensitized infants also tended to have either milk or egg allergy and/or eczema.

Sleep

- Pregnancy itself will affect quality of sleep, with difficulty in assuming usual sleep positions, discomfort from fetal movements, cramps, and poor sleep quality, with the last being influenced by the previous complaints.
- Pregnancy-specific sleep disorders: obstructive sleep apnea and restless legs syndrome.
- Decreases in rapid eye movement sleep during last trimester can be explained by progesterone and estrogen alterations.
- Sleep deprivation affects child renal development negatively.
- Human sleep deprivation (less than 8 hr/day) during pregnancy risks a 3.8-times increase in first-trimester miscarriage, impairs mother-infant relationship, and promotes postpartum depression.

Exercise

- Exercise during pregnancy improves well-being and psychological distress, reduces fatigue in second trimester, and lowers miscarriage and depression risk.

- Avoid contact sports. Engage in low-impact activities, wearing an athletic support bra, drinking ample water, and eating a snack 30 minutes before exercise to ensure adequate blood sugar.
- Avoid exercise if there is high blood pressure, asthma, or threat of miscarriage.
- Regular exercise during pregnancy can have positive effect on baby's birth weight without putting pregnancy or child at risk—lower birth weight (within normal range) and reduced cord concentrations of growth-related peptides—suggesting effects on endocrine regulation of fetal growth.

Recommendations for Exercise during Pregnancy

Agency	Recommendations
American College of Obstetricians and Gynecologists (ACOG)	• Not recommended if a woman has risk factors for preterm labor, vaginal bleeding, or premature rupture of membranes. • Safe exercises, even for women who did not exercise before pregnancy, include walking, swimming, cycling, and aerobics. • In women who are active before pregnancy, running, racquet sports, and strength training may be safe to continue in moderation. • Skiing, contact sports, and scuba diving should be avoided. • If just beginning to exercise, women should start with 5 minutes of exercise a day and add 5 minutes each week until 30 minutes of activity a day is tolerable. • Avoid exercises that require lying prone after the first trimester and exercises that may cause overheating or dehydration.
Department of Health, United Kingdom (DH-UK)	• If inactive before pregnancy, do not suddenly start strenuous exercise. • Keep active on a daily basis. Perform half an hour of activities a day, such as walking, keeping in mind that any amount is better than nothing. • Avoid strenuous exercise in hot weather. • If attending exercise classes, ensure the instructor is qualified and aware of the pregnancy and gestational age. • Swimming will support increased weight, and many pools offer aquanatal classes.

Recommendations for Exercise during Pregnancy—cont'd

Agency	Recommendations
• U.S. Department of Health and Human Services (HHS)	• Healthy women not already highly active or doing vigorous-intensity activity should get at least 150 minutes (divided) of moderate-intensity aerobic activity per week during pregnancy and the postpartum period. • Pregnant women who habitually engage in vigorous-intensity aerobic activity or are highly active can continue physical activity during pregnancy and the postpartum period provided that they remain healthy and discuss activity adjustment with a health practitioner.

Recommendations based on Yonkers KA, Wisner KL, Stewart DE, et al. The management of depression during pregnancy: a report from the American Psychiatric Association and the American College of Obstetricians and Gynecologists. *Gen Hosp Psychiatry.* 2009;31(5):403-413; American College of Obstetricians and Gynecologists (ACOG). Exercise during pregnancy. Washington, DC; American College of Obstetricians and Gynecologists; 2003; Department of Health, United Kingdom (DH-UK): The pregnancy book 2007. London: Department of Health; 2007; and U.S. Department of Health and Human Services (HHS). 2008 Physical activity guidelines for Americans. Washington, DC: U.S. Department of Health and Human Services; 2008.

Alcohol

- Fetal alcohol syndrome is a leading cause of mental retardation.
- Earlier gestational exposure to alcohol, often before awareness of pregnancy, may be most detrimental.
- Social factors—being single or divorced—and intimate partner violence increase alcohol consumption risk.
- Limiting alcoholic beverages during pregnancy to one or two per week causes offspring to be 30% less likely to have behavioral problems at age 5.
- There is still no precedent that any level of alcohol consumption is safe, because the long-term effects are unknown.

Smoking

- Smoking during pregnancy is a leading preventable cause of adverse maternal and fetal outcomes.
- Pregnancy smoking leads to fetal growth restriction, retroplacental hematoma, increased preterm birth, shorter fetal crown-to-rump lengths, placenta previa, and death in utero.

Cannabis

- Most frequently used illicit drug among pregnant women.
- Associated with fetal growth restriction, decreased birth weight, reduced length, smaller head circumference, and newborn cognitive, motor, and emotional issues.

- Increases in later tobacco use by offspring and adolescent psychosis have also been noted.

Betel Nut

- Fourth most commonly used drug in the world after tobacco, alcohol, and caffeine.
- Seed of areca palm of tropical Pacific, Asia, and parts of east Africa.
- Customarily wrapped in betel leaves and chewed.
- In mice, it causes skeletal immaturity; cases of human newborns showing withdrawal symptoms are documented.

Stress and Mind-Body Modalities

- High stress triples risk of pregnancy hypertension, causes adverse birth outcomes, and doubles preterm delivery risk.
- Low and moderate anxiety in first or early second trimester does not affect birth outcomes; anxiety in second and third trimesters is linked to smaller infant size, lower Apgar scores, increased obstetric complications, lower birth weight, and shorter birth length.
- Stress alters regulation of fetal hypothalamic-pituitary-adrenal (HPA) axis, with altered hippocampal glucocorticoid receptor density and sensitivity.
- Maternal anxiety or depression during pregnancy is linked with HPA axis overreactivity and higher cortisol in infants and children. Impaired HPA axis is associated with metabolic syndrome, fibromyalgia, depression, and posttraumatic stress disorder and likely increases susceptibility of offspring to stress-related disorders.
- Mind-body modalities may help balance HPA axis function. Pregnant women benefit from mind-body therapies used in conjunction with conventional prenatal care.
- Common approaches: progressive muscle relaxation, multimodal psychoeducation, yoga or meditation intervention.
- Treatment outcomes: healthier birth weight, shorter labor, fewer instrument-assisted births, and reduced perceived stress and anxiety.

Sunlight

- The birth month can affect birth weight and height of children.
- Mechanism: hours of sunlight may play a role.
- Higher temperature, more hours of sunlight, greater rainfall, and lower humidity are associated with greater birth length.
- Prenatal sunlight is a major determinant of height. Better nutrition and more-active lifestyles of pregnant women, with a longer warm period, may have beneficial outcomes.

- Diseases in offspring may be encouraged by minimal sun exposure. Low maternal exposure to sunlight during first trimester may increase risk of offspring later developing multiple sclerosis.
- Vitamin D: pregnancy increases physiologic need. Benefit of food sources is minimal in comparison with sun exposure.

Environmental Toxins

- Typical pregnant woman has dozens of toxic or cancer-causing chemicals in her body.
- Environmental factors trigger epigenetic changes in the fetus, which may not manifest until years later.
- Environmental pollutants may trigger genetic changes that can affect a person's health. This impairment can be passed on to future generations.
- Women in the top quintile of body load of persistent organic pollutants give birth to children with a 7-point lower IQ and doubled incidence of attention-deficit/hyperactivity disorder (ADHD).

Phthalates and Bisphenol A

- Bisphenol A (BPA), an estrogen-like industrial petrochemical found in 96% of pregnant women, affects brain, prostate, and behavioral development in children exposed both before and after birth.
- Phthalates are found in plastics, solvents, antifoam agents, alcohol denaturants, vinyl flooring, wall covering, pesticides, and personal care products (fragrances, shampoos, cosmetics, and nail polish). Human exposure occurs through inhalation, ingestion, and dermal contact.
- Phthalate are associated with poorer scores on aggression, conduct, attention, and emotional control, especially among boys.
- Prenatal phthalate exposure is linked to clinically diagnosed conduct disorders or ADHD.
- Organophosphate pesticide exposure has the strongest inverse correlation with child IQ.

Perchlorates

- Perchlorate in drinking water during pregnancy is linked to higher-than-normal neonatal TSH levels. Water filters can prevent exposure.

Arsenic

- Arsenic is poisonous to any organism, and arsenic exposure during pregnancy (metabolites of inorganic arsenic in maternal urine) was associated with increased morbidity from infectious diseases during infancy.

Lead

- Higher maternal lead levels can lead to preeclampsia or eclampsia, which can increase a woman's future risk of heart attack and cognitive deficits in her infant.
- Genomic methylation of developing fetus can be influenced by maternal cumulative lead burden, affecting long-term epigenetic programming and disease susceptibility.

Air Pollution

- Both outdoor and indoor air pollution affect fetal health via placental exposure and by effects on mother's health.
- Like maternal smoking, air pollution may encourage premature rupture of membranes, placental abruption, and lower birth weight.
- Indoor air pollutants are likely a stronger player in pregnancy health. Example: smoke secondary to cooking fuels in developing countries.
- Improve choices in cooking, cleaning products, paint, furniture, carpeting, and anything brought into the home.
- Recommend use of air filters.

Cell Phone Radiation

- Almost twice the incidence of behavioral problems occur in children who had possible prenatal or postnatal cell phone exposure.

GENERAL SUPPLEMENTATION

Multivitamins and Folic Acid

Supplements Used during Pregnancy

- Folate: 70%
- Iron: 38%
- Multivitamin: 27%
- Ginger: 7% to 20%
- Echinacea: 8%
- Raspberry leaf or pregnancy tea: 8% to 9%

Data from Maats FH, Crowther CA. Patterns of vitamin, mineral and herbal supplement use before and during pregnancy. *Aust N Z J Obstet Gynaecol.* 2002;42(5):494-496; and Tsui B, Dennehy CE, Tsourounis C. A survey of dietary supplement use during pregnancy at an academic medical center. *Am J Obstet Gynecol.* 2001;185(2):433-7.

- Folic acid and a multivitamin supplement among women of reproductive age reduced incidence of birth defects (anencephaly, myelomeningocele, meningocele, oral facial cleft, structural heart disease, limb defect, urinary tract anomaly, hydrocephalus).
- Folic acid at 5 mg daily will not mask a vitamin B_{12} deficiency (pernicious anemia).
- Folate sources: spinach, asparagus, romaine lettuce, turnip greens, mustard greens, calf's liver, collard greens, cauliflower, broccoli, parsley, lentils, and beets.
- Diet alone cannot provide levels similar to supplements.
- The more active the person, the greater the tendency toward deficiency.
- Folate is important in synthesis of purines and pyrimidines, in conversion of homocysteine to methionine, and in interconversion of serine and glycine.
- Prenatal folate deficiency may influence risk of schizophrenia in offspring by inhibiting neurogenesis and allowing homocysteine to accumulate in the fetal brain.
- Begin folate-multivitamins with 5 mg of folic acid at least 3 months before conception and continue until 10 to 12 weeks postconception. From 12 weeks postconception and continuing throughout pregnancy and postpartum period (4 to 6 weeks or as long as breastfeeding continues), supplement with multivitamin with folic acid (0.4 to 1.0 mg).
- The form of folic acid may affect efficacy. Metabolism of folic acid into active form 5-methyltetrahydrofolate may be impeded because of genetic mutations. L-Methylfolate may be more efficacious.

Three patient scenarios with specific folic acid recommendations are as follows:

1. Patients with no personal health risks, planned pregnancy, and good compliance:
   - Folate-rich diet
   - Multivitamin with folic acid (0.4 to 1.0 mg) daily for at least 2 to 3 months before conception and throughout pregnancy and postpartum period (4 to 6 weeks and throughout breastfeeding)
2. Patients with health risks, including epilepsy, insulin-dependent diabetes, obesity (BMI >35 kg/m^2), family history of neural tube defect:
   - Increased folate-rich foods
   - Multivitamins with 5 mg of folic acid daily, beginning at least 3 months before conception and continuing until 10 to 12 weeks postconception. From 12 weeks postconception and

continuing throughout pregnancy and the postpartum period (4 to 6 weeks and throughout breastfeeding), a multivitamin with folic acid (0.4 to 1.0 mg) daily

3. Medicated patients with a poor compliance history as well as poor diet, no consistent birth control, and teratogenic substance use (alcohol, tobacco, recreational nonprescription drugs):
   - Counseling regarding prevention of birth defects and health problems
   - Folic acid (5 mg) with a multivitamin daily

Essential Fatty Acids

- DHA is structural component of brain and retina, with uptake maximal during second half of gestation and infancy.
- Preterm infants have delayed mental development; third trimester is period of rapid brain growth that requires DHA for brain cell structure and communication.
- In totality, clinical studies support the use of fish oil in pregnancy.
- Fish oil supplements may be a healthier source of fatty acids than fish because of environmental toxins, which can be removed from fish oil. Except for belching and unpleasant taste, no adverse effects have been detected up to the highest intake of 2.8 g of total omega-3 fats.

Evening Primrose Oil

- Evening primrose oil (EPO) is rich in omega-6 fatty acids, linoleic acid (LA), and gamma-linolenic acid (GLA).
- Chronic ethanol intake causes depletion of essential fatty acids (EFAs). It is possible that in pregnant women who consume excess alcohol and will not cease, EPO may be protective by reducing alcohol's teratogenic potential.
- EPO may hasten cervical ripening, shorten labor, and decrease postdate pregnancy likelihood. One study supplementing from thirty-seventh gestational week until birth did not support this.
- Although EPO is rated as GRAS, oral EPO intake may be associated with increased incidence of prolonged rupture of membranes, oxytocin augmentation, arrest of descent, and vacuum extraction. Therefore EPO is not recommended except in case of alcohol intake with pregnancy.

Vitamin D

- Vitamin D is a preprohormone that supports calcium homeostasis, bone health, and general immune function.

- Vitamin D plays a role in pregnancy immune tolerance, insulin resistance, and preeclampsia risk.
- It appears to increase amount of blood flowing to placenta, bringing more oxygen and nutrients to fetus and promoting healthier growth. Effects of inadequate vitamin D in pregnancy are increased risk of the following:
  - — Adverse musculoskeletal effects
  - — Bacterial vaginosis
  - — Small-for-gestational-age babies
  - — Preeclampsia
  - — Flu
- Adequate vitamin D may prevent premature delivery, offspring wheezing, and multiple sclerosis.
- Prepregnancy obesity predicts poor vitamin D status in mothers and their neonates.
- Test serum 25(OH)D levels before pregnancy if possible and during early pregnancy to determine supplementation.
- Serum levels of 50 to 80 ng/mL are adequate.

Magnesium

- Low magnesium status may play a role vasospasm, coagulation defects, premature delivery, hypertension and eclampsia, intrauterine growth restriction, and muscle cramping.
- Low protein intake will negatively affect magnesium absorption.
- Magnesium intake of pregnant women must be increased by either dietary means or supplements, especially among low-income women in soft-water states. Excessive intake of calcium or phosphorus may be detrimental to magnesium absorption.

Vitamin A

- Vitamin A deficiency is common among pregnant women worldwide; supplementation can reduce infant mortality.
- Retinol (vitamin A) and other retinoids are essential for gene expression, cell differentiation, proliferation, and migration.
- Vitamin A is important in regulating early lung development and alveolar formation and in preventing night blindness.
- In central nervous system (CNS) morphogenesis, inadequate vitamin A can cause hydrocephalus, anencephaly, spina bifida, and underdeveloped posterior hindbrain.
- Retinoid antioxidants help to protect the developing brain from potential insults that generate free radicals.

- Excess vitamin A has potent teratogenic effects and is contraindicated during pregnancy. Isotretinoin and vitamin A–related acne medicines are responsible for malformations of the CNS, heart, and thymus and craniofacial defects. Dangerous dosage level: 25,000 international units (IU) or more daily as retinol or retinyl esters during pregnancy.
- National Research Council's recommended dietary allowance for vitamin A during pregnancy is 1000 retinol equivalents per day—equivalent to 3300 IU as retinol or 5000 IU of vitamin A obtained from diet as a combination of retinol and carotenoids (e.g., beta-carotene).
- Recommended daily allowance (RDA) established by FDA is 8000 IU/day. Supplementation of 8000 IU of vitamin A (as retinol or retinyl esters) per day should be considered the recommended maximum before or during pregnancy.
- Beta-carotene is not metabolized or stored in the same way as vitamin A and has not been associated with vitamin A toxicity in animals or humans, but may not have the ability to prevent deficiency issues because of differences in absorption and metabolism. However, genetic polymorphisms that impair conversion of carotenoid to vitamin A are common. Simply supplementing with carotenoids does not ensure adequate vitamin A levels.

Antioxidants

- Oxidative stress is implicated in pathologic processes during pregnancy, childbirth, and postnatal period; but possible preventive or therapeutic effects of antioxidants remain unclear.
- Overt deficiency of antioxidant status is a detriment to pregnancy.
- Maternal vitamin E intake helps prevent wheezing in second year of life.
- Maternal zinc intake during pregnancy can reduce risk for asthma and eczema in children at age of 5 years. Forty mg of zinc gluconate effectively increased mean birth weight among anemic and iron-deficient women but not among women with elevated iron stores in early pregnancy.
- Supplementing one or more antioxidants induces a 39% reduction in risk of preeclampsia and a 35% risk reduction of having a small-for-gestational-age infant.
- Supplementing vitamin C or vitamin E or both did not show any reduction of preeclampsia and was linked to higher rate of low-birth-weight infants.

- Overall, currently available data do not provide basis for recommending antioxidant intake for pregnant and lactating women in excess of reference nutrient intakes. Women with risk factors for preeclampsia may consider additional low-dose antioxidant support.

Iron

- During pregnancy, low iron and anemia can compromise oxygen delivery to fetus.
- Factors associated with deficiency: poor fetal brain and intrauterine development, prematurity, and low birth weight, leading to poor growth trajectory in infancy, childhood, and adolescence and low adult height.
- Indirect indicators of fetal hypoxia are linked to increased susceptibility to schizophrenia. Hippocampus is particularly vulnerable to hypoxia.
- Iron deficiency causes eightfold to tenfold increase in morbidity and mortality rates in pregnant women when hemoglobin falls below 5 g/dL.
- Iron is present in prenatal vitamins. Dose: 30 to 60 mg of elemental iron is common but may not be enough to prevent gestational anemia.

Probiotics

- The newborn gut is first colonized by microbes from mother as baby moves through birth canal; this is minimized with delivery by cesarean section. Newborns delivered in this way have higher rates of celiac disease.
- Strain of bacterium used is important to its effectiveness.
- *Lactobacillus* GG twice daily was associated with increased wheezing and bronchitis.
- Mixture of four probiotic species (*Lactobacillus rhamnosus* GG and LC705, *Bifidobacterium breve,* and *Propionibacterium freudenreichii* subsp. *shermanii*) for 4 weeks before delivery reduced frequency of respiratory infections.
- Oral and intravaginal yogurt and probiotics have been used to amelioriate bacterial vaginosis in pregnant patients. This is a first choice in pregnant patients to avoid antibiotic treatment.
- Safe during pregnancy; no increased neonatal morbidity, feeding-related difficulties (infantile colic), or serious adverse events.
- *Lactobacillus* and *Bifidobacterium* have demonstrated no ill effects.
- Safety of *Saccharomyces* during pregnancy is unknown.

Choline

- Rapid rate of cell division during pregnancy, expansion of maternal kidneys and uterus, growth of placental and fetal tissue, and increased lipoprotein required for nervous system development all deplete choline stores.
- Higher blood choline is linked to 2.5-fold reduction in risk for neural tube birth defects.
- Third-trimester fetal organ growth needs large amounts of choline for membrane biosynthesis, because neonates have choline levels three times higher than those in maternal blood.
- Certain genetic variants may increase requirements further.
- Recommended intake: 450 mg/day during pregnancy.
- Choline is not found in most varieties of prenatal vitamins; focus on choline-rich foods. Studies of choline supplementation in pregnancy are not available.

Dietary Sources of Choline

Food	Milligrams of Choline
Egg, large	115
Beef steak, 3 oz	110
Salmon, 3 oz	100
Baked beans, 1 c	70
Navy beans, 1 c	60
Brussel sprouts, 1 c	60
Kidney beans, 1 c	60
Broccoli cooked, 1 c	60

Data from Caudill MA. Pre- and postnatal health: evidence of increased choline needs. *J Am Diet Assoc* 2010;110(8):1198-1206.

Carnitine

- Essential constituent of intermediary metabolism.
- During gestation, plasma carnitine decreases precipitously. By delivery, levels are indicative of deficiency.
- Dose: 500 mg of L-carnitine L-tartrate from week 13 of gestation to term.
- Infant diets may have to supply supplemental carnitine to satisfy neonate's metabolic needs.

- L-Carnitine supplementation during pregnancy may help prevent gestational diabetes, especially in overweight women, by decreasing elevated free fatty acids. Lower L-carnitine downregulates expression of enzymes involved in fatty acid metabolism.
- Sources: meat, poultry, fish, and dairy products.

Botanicals

Raspberry Leaf *(Rubus idaeus)*

- Best known and oldest herb infusion in maternity.
- Relaxant effect on uterine musculature.
- Safe, with first stage of labor being shorter, as are second and third stages.
- No adverse effects for mother or baby. It allows for less intervention, with reduction in midwifery and medical time in labor and an increase in maternal satisfaction.
- Raspberry leaf does not cause preterm labor and birth.

Glycyrrhiza glabra **(Licorice)**

- Hepatoprotective and gives pulmonary support.
- There is no effect on maternal blood pressure or birth weight at the high exposure of 500 mg glycyrrhizin per week; but children show more behavioral problems, poor attention spans, and symptoms of ADHD in a dose-dependent manner.
- Salivary cortisol tests show higher offspring cortisol.
- Glycyrrhizin potently inhibits 11-beta-hydroxy-steroid dehydrogenase type 2. This enzyme blocks fetus from receiving maternal cortisol. Using licorice can induce higher cortisol levels in utero and may alter HPA axis function in children, contributing to altered mood and stress response.
- Ingestion of licorice is not recommended for pregnant women.

Gingko biloba

- Animal pregnancy studies have shown malformations in the eye and orbit; syndactyly; malformed pinnae, nostrils, lips, and jaws; and decreased weight and crown-rump length. Other studies indicate no problem.
- Given the lack of human data and suggestive teratogenicity in animal data, *Ginkgo* is not recommended during pregnancy.

Scutellaria (Scutellaria baicalensis)

- Anecdotal reports suggest fetal calming effects.
- Higher liver and kidneys weights in animal mothers who took *Scutellaria* in high doses.

Bitter Melon *(Momordica charantia)*

- Well used in Asian cultures for blood sugar regulation and cancer care.
- Bitter melon contains abortifacient proteins trichosanthin, alpha-momorcharin, and beta-momorcharin, which can inhibit cellular protein synthesis.
- Momorcharins and ribosome-inactivating proteins isolated from bitter melon seeds have abortifacient activity in pregnant mice.
- The use of bitter melon during pregnancy is not recommended.

Podophyllum

- Used topically to remove benign dermatologic lesions—warts.
- Anecdotal evidence suggests inducement of birth defects.

THERAPEUTIC APPROACH

Support

- Consider a midwife for optimal prenatal care, with conventional medical backup for urgent care if needed.
- Psychological therapy is beneficial for those with anxiety or mood disorders.

Foods

- Organic whole-foods diet with adequate hydration and protein and seven servings of fruits and vegetables daily.
- Fish with toxic contaminants and peanuts (minimal intake), flax, and caffeinated beverages are best avoided.

Sleep

- Eight hours each night.

Exercise

- Daily as appropriate for the individual.

Lifestyle

- Daily sunlight exposure.
- Cigarettes, cannabis, and betel nuts should be avoided.

- Meditation and relaxation work.
- Use filters to ensure toxin-free water and indoor air.

Nutritional Supplementation

- High-quality prenatal multivitamin with 1000 to 5000 mcg of folic acid, 1000 mg of calcium, and no more than 5000 IU of vitamin A.
- EFAs: 800 mg of DHA and corresponding eicosapentaenoic acid (EPA).
- Vitamin D: administered according to specific need based on laboratory findings.
- Probiotic.

Botanical Medicine

- According to specific health needs.

Premenstrual Syndrome

DIAGNOSTIC SUMMARY

- Recurrent signs and symptoms that develop during the late luteal phase of the menstrual cycle and disappear by end of full flow of menses
- Typical symptoms: decreased energy, tension, irritability, depression, headache, altered sex drive, breast pain, backache, abdominal bloating, edema of fingers and ankles

GENERAL CONSIDERATIONS

- Premenstrual syndrome (PMS) is cyclic constellation of symptoms appearing during the late luteal phase of the menstrual cycle and disappearing by the end of full flow of menses; they do not appear during the follicular phase.
- Most common symptoms: decreased energy, tension, irritability, anger, food cravings, depression, headache, altered sex drive, breast pain, muscle aches, abdominal bloating, edema of fingers and ankles.
- Affects 30% to 40% of menstruating women; 80% of women have emotional or physical changes without much difficulty. From 2.5% to 5% of women have severe symptoms that jeopardize home life and work. Peak occurrence is during the 30s and 40s.
- Premenstrual dysphoric disorder (PMDD) is a separate DSM-V *(Diagnostic and Statistical Manual of Mental Disorders, Fifth Edition)* diagnostic category of severe PMS with depression, irritability, and severe mood swings.
- Etiologic theory: interaction of cyclic changes in the ovarian steroids estrogen and progesterone causes changes in brain neurotransmitters, inducing emotional and physical symptoms. Why sensitivity to ovarian steroid–induced neurotransmitter changes differ among women is not known. Serotonin is most implicated. Whether PMS and PMDD are related to absolute serotonin levels, reduced blood levels, or serotonin transport remains unclear.

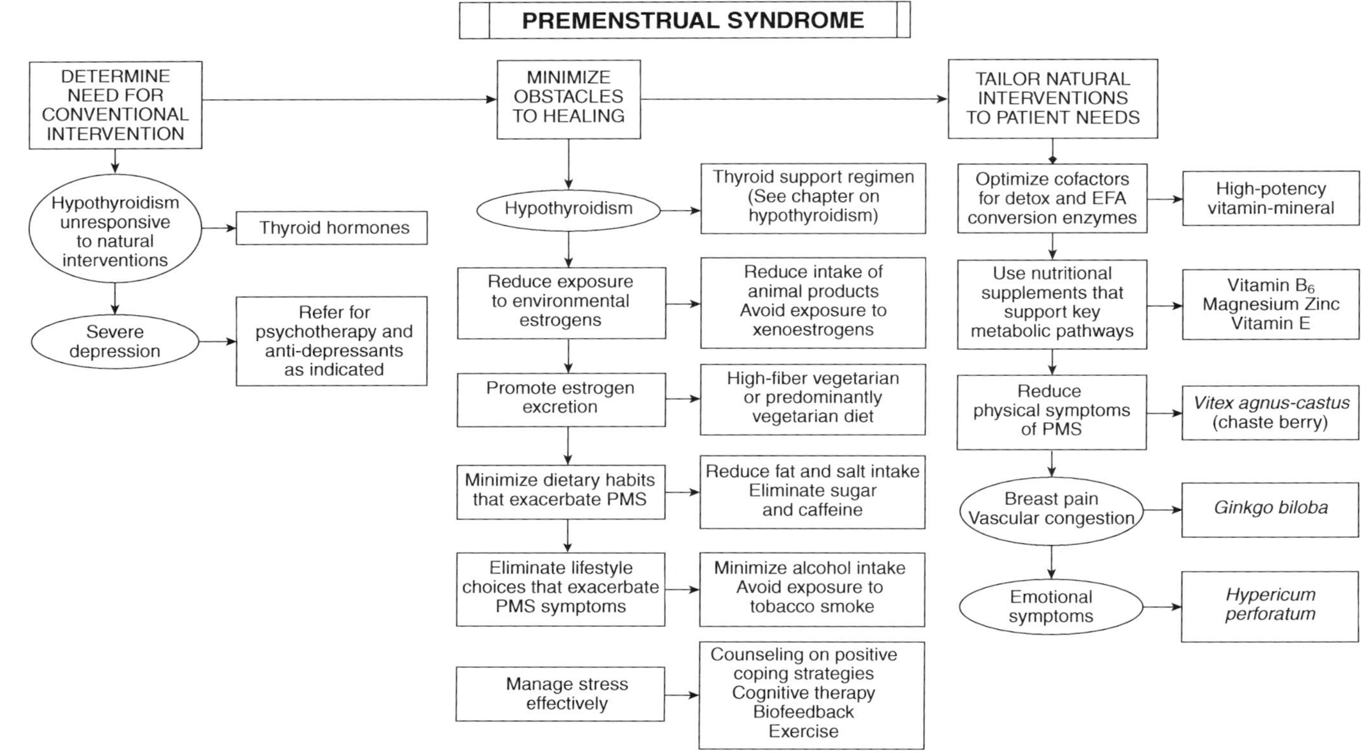
PREMENSTRUAL SYNDROME
DETERMINE NEED FOR CONVENTIONAL INTERVENTION
Hypothyroidism unresponsive to natural interventions
Thyroid hormones
Severe depression
Refer for psychotherapy and anti-depressants as indicated
MINIMIZE OBSTACLES TO HEALING
Hypothyroidism
Thyroid support regimen (See chapter on hypothyroidism)
Reduce exposure to environmental estrogens
Reduce intake of animal products Avoid exposure to xenoestrogens
Promote estrogen excretion
High-fiber vegetarian or predominantly vegetarian diet
Minimize dietary habits that exacerbate PMS
Reduce fat and salt intake Eliminate sugar and caffeine
Eliminate lifestyle choices that exacerbate PMS symptoms
Minimize alcohol intake Avoid exposure to tobacco smoke
Manage stress effectively
Counseling on positive coping strategies Cognitive therapy Biofeedback Exercise
TAILOR NATURAL INTERVENTIONS TO PATIENT NEEDS
Optimize cofactors for detox and EFA conversion enzymes
High-potency vitamin-mineral
Use nutritional supplements that support key metabolic pathways
Vitamin B_6 Magnesium Zinc Vitamin E
Reduce physical symptoms of PMS
Vitex agnus-castus (chaste berry)
Breast pain Vascular congestion
Ginkgo biloba
Emotional symptoms
Hypericum perforatum

- Other neurotransmitter systems include opioid and gamma-aminobutyric acid (GABA).
- Selective serotonin reuptake inhibitors (SSRIs) can alleviate psychological and physical symptoms in most patients with PMDD. Fluoxetine, sertraline, paroxetine, fluvoxamine, citalopram, and venlafaxine are more effective than placebo for PMDD.
- Other neurotransmitter systems that might be involved: adrenergic, opioid, GABA.

Diagnosis and Classifications

- **Diagnosis:** connecting symptoms attributed to PMS and occurrence during luteal phase of menstrual cycle.
- **Tools:** symptom questionnaire and menstrual symptom diary.
- **Key defining feature of both PMS and PMDD:** timing of symptoms; they appear only during the luteal phase and disappear before or during menstrual flow.
- **Rule out other disorders:** medical or psychiatric history (many mental and physical disorders mimic PMS, and many coexist).
- Only one of the following is required for diagnosis of PMS: mild psychological discomfort, bloating and weight gain, breast tenderness, swelling of hands and feet, various aches and pains, poor concentration, sleep disturbance, and change in appetite.
- Diagnosis of PMDD requires at least five of the following symptoms, with at least one being a core symptom, and symptoms must (1) occur only during the luteal phase, (2) peak close to menstruation, and (3) remit with menses or a few days after onset of menses for at least two cycles:
  - — Markedly depressed mood, hopelessness, self-defeating thoughts
  - — Marked anxiety or tension
  - — Marked affective lability
  - — Marked anger, irritability
  - — Decreased interest in usual activities
  - — Poor concentration—lack of energy, lethargy, fatigue
  - — Change in appetite, overeating, or food cravings
  - — Hypersomnia or insomnia
  - — Feeling overwhelmed
  - — Additional physical symptoms (breast tenderness, bloating, headache, joint or muscle pain)

THERAPEUTIC CONSIDERATIONS

Estrogen Metabolism

- Estrogen excess produces cholestasis—diminished bile flow or stasis of bile ("sluggish liver"). However, indicators of liver status (alkaline phosphatase, aspartate aminotransferase, alanine aminotransferase, gamma-glutamyl transpeptidase) are normal.
- Causes of cholestasis: estrogen excess or oral contraceptives, pregnancy, presence of gallstones, alcohol, endotoxins, hereditary disorders such as Gilbert's syndrome, anabolic steroids, various chemicals or drugs, nutritional deficiencies.
- Cholestasis reduces estrogen detoxification and clearance. A positive feedback scenario is produced.
- Estrogen excess during the luteal phase negatively affects endorphin levels. When the estrogen/progesterone ratio is increased, endorphins decline. Low endorphins during the luteal phase are common in women with PMS. Endorphins are lowered by stress and raised by exercise.

Estrogen Impairs Vitamin B_6 Function

Estrogens negatively affect vitamin B_6 function. B_6 is low in depressed patients, especially women taking estrogens (oral contraceptives or Premarin). B_6 supplementation positively affects all PMS symptoms (particularly depression) in many women. Improvement arises from reducing midluteal estrogen and increasing midluteal progesterone.

Dietary Considerations

- C-reactive protein: biomarker of inflammation that correlates with severity of physical and psychological symptoms. Foods that promote inflammation: sugar, poultry, eggs, cheese, milk, white flour, white rice, hydrogenated oils. Foods that reduce inflammation: fresh fruits (e.g., berries), green leafy vegetables, fish, nuts, seeds, turmeric, garlic, onions. Recommend a diet lower in saturated fat and cholesterol (by reducing animal foods) and higher in fiber-rich plant foods (fruits, vegetables, gluten-free grains, legumes).
- High intake of dairy, fat, starches, sugars, with low protein intake, may also contribute to some PMS symptoms.
- Food cravings are often also higher in women with PMS, perhaps because of decreased serotonin during the luteal phase in PMS. Thus serotonergic treatments may help control food cravings.

- Refined sugars: rapidly increase insulin, which then causes sodium and water retention, with swelling in hands and feet, abdominal bloating, and breast engorgement.

Seven most important dietary recommendations for PMS:

- Eat a vegetarian or predominantly vegetarian diet
- Reduce fat intake
- Eliminate sugar
- Reduce exposure to environmental estrogens
- Increase intake of soy foods
- Eliminate caffeine
- Keep salt intake low

Vegetarian Diet and Estrogen Metabolism

- Vegetarian women excrete two to three times more estrogen in their feces; have 50% lower blood levels of free estrogen; and have a lower incidence of breast cancer, heart disease, and menopausal symptoms compared with omnivores because of their lower fat and higher fiber intake.
- Reduce saturated fat and cholesterol (animal products) and increase fiber-rich plant foods (fruits, vegetables, grains, legumes).
- Limit animal protein to no more than 110 to 170 mg/day; recommend fish, skinless poultry, lean cuts of meat.
- Fiber promotes excretion of estrogens by favorable bacterial flora with less beta-glucuronidase activity.

Fat Intake and Estrogen Metabolism

- Fat intake is negatively associated with cravings and bloating.
- Decreasing fat intake, especially saturated fat, reduces circulating estrogen by 36%. Low-fat diet improves PMS symptoms and reduces the risk of cancer, heart disease, and stroke. Keep fat intake to less than 30% of calories.
- Easiest way is to eat less animal products and more plant foods.

Sugar

- Simple sugars increase insulin secretion and disturb glycemic control in hypoglycemics and diabetics. Sugar combined with caffeine has a detrimental effect on PMS and mood.
- Sugar impairs estrogen metabolism. PMS is more common in women eating a high-sugar diet. High sugar intake is associated with higher estrogen levels.
- Teach patients to read food labels carefully for clues about sugar content.

Caffeine

- Avoid caffeine, especially if anxiety or depression or breast tenderness and fibrocystic breast disease are major symptoms.
- Caffeine intake is linked to severity of PMS: anxiety, irritability, insomnia, depression.

Salt

- Excessive salt and diminished potassium stress the kidney's ability to maintain fluid volume.
- Salt sensitivity: high sodium intake increases blood pressure and/or water retention. Patients with water retention during midluteal phase may be sensitive to salt.
- Potassium intake must be concurrently increased with high-potassium foods (fruits and vegetables). Decrease high-sodium foods (processed foods). Keep total daily sodium intake below 1800 mg.

Lifestyle Choices

- Alcohol intake is negatively associated with anxiety, mood changes, and headaches during PMS.
- Cigarette smoke exposure, passive or active, is positively associated with menstrual cramps and back pain.

Hormone Therapy

Thyroid Function

- Hypothyroidism affects a large percentage of women with PMS.
- Many women with PMS and confirmed hypothyroidism who are given thyroid hormone have complete relief of symptoms (see the chapter on hypothyroidism).

Stress, Coping Style, and Depression

- Extreme, unusual, or long-lasting stress triggers brain changes by altered adrenal function and endorphin secretion or action. Domino effect alters normal physiology.
- Serotonin levels in women with PMS fall after ovulation. Those without PMS have much higher levels of serotonin during the last half of the menstrual cycle. Identify stressors and devise stress management approaches.
- Patients with PMS tend to use negative coping styles: feelings of helplessness, overeating, too much television, emotional outbursts, overspending, excessive behavior, dependence on chemicals, legal and illicit drugs, alcohol, and smoking.

- Depression is common feature of PMS. Symptoms are more severe in depressed women. Eighty percent of 12 million Americans on Prozac are women aged 25 to 50 years. Cause: decrease in brain neurotransmitters, especially serotonin and GABA.
- The most common pharmaceuticals recommended for moderate to severe PMS and PMDD are SSRIs—used daily for chronic depression or on days when PMS or PMDD symptoms are most problematic. The latter application suggests that SSRIs are not really increasing neurotransmitters, but rather altering brain neurophysiology and electrical conduction. SSRIs used: fluoxetine, sertraline, paroxetine. However, psychotherapy methods have been equally successful—biofeedback and short-term individual counseling (e.g., cognitive therapy). Cognitive therapy's advantage over drugs for PMS is learning coping skills that can produce excellent results sustainable over time.

Exercise

- Women who exercise regularly do not have PMS as often as do sedentary women. Regular exercisers get lower scores on impaired concentration, negative mood, behavior change, and pain.
- High exercisers have greater positive mood scores and the least depression and anxiety. Differences are most apparent during premenstrual and menstrual phases. Women who frequently exercise (but who are not competitive athletes) are protected from PMS. Exercise elevates endorphins, lowers cortisol, and modulates estrogen levels.

Nutritional Supplements

Supplements are widely used to treat PMS. Despite inconsistent evidence, positive results show that supplements can offer safe, affordable solutions.

Vitamin B_6

- Although PMS has multiple causes, B_6 supplementation alone benefits most patients, including those with premenstrual depression, fatigue, and irritability.
- Vitamin B_6 can increase synthesis of several brain neurotransmitters (e.g., serotonin, dopamine, norepinephrine, epinephrine, taurine, and histamine).

- Some women cannot convert B_6 to its active form, pyridoxal-5-phosphate (P5P), because of a deficiency in another nutrient (e.g., vitamin B_2 or magnesium [Mg]). Use a broader-spectrum nutritional supplement or injectable P5P.
- Therapeutic oral dose of B_6: 50 to 100 mg q.d. Divide doses greater than 50 mg into 50-mg doses throughout the day; 50 mg oral B_6 is all the liver can handle at once.
- Toxicity: one-time doses higher than 2000 mg/day can produce nerve toxicity (tingling sensations in feet, loss of muscle coordination, and degeneration of nerve tissue). Long-term administration of more than 500 mg q.d. can be toxic if taken daily for many months or years. Rare reports suggest toxicity with long-term administration as low as 150 mg/day. Supplemental B_6 overwhelms the liver's ability to add a phosphate group to produce the active form of P5P.
- Vitamin B_6 and Mg work together in many enzyme systems. B_6 may improve PMS by increasing accumulation of Mg within cells.

Magnesium

- Mg deficiency is a causative factor in PMS, accounting for a wide range of symptoms. Mg deficiency and PMS share many common features; Mg supplementation can effectively treat PMS.
- Study findings: plasma Mg does not differ between PMS patients and control subjects. Menstrual cycle does not affect plasma Mg. Patients with PMS have lower red blood cell Mg levels consistent across the menstrual cycle compared with control subjects. Mg measures do not correlate with severity of mood symptoms.
- Women with PMS have "vulnerability to luteal phase mood state destabilization." Chronic, enduring intracellular Mg depletion is a predisposing factor toward destabilization.
- Mg deficiency in PMS induces excessive nervous sensitivity with generalized aches and pains and lower premenstrual pain threshold.
- Better results are achieved by combining B_6 and other nutrients.
- Optimal intake for Mg: 6 mg/kg body weight. This is difficult to achieve by diet alone; supplementation is recommended. PMS dose: 12 mg/kg body weight.
- Mg bound to aspartate or Krebs cycle intermediates (malate, succinate, fumarate, or citrate) is preferred over oxide, gluconate, sulfate, and chloride for better absorption and fewer side effects (laxative effects).

Calcium

- Ca is a double-edged sword in PMS. High Ca intake from high milk consumption may be a causative factor; Ca, vitamin D, and phosphorus in milk may reduce the absorption of Mg.
- Ca supplementation (1000 to 1336 mg) can improve PMS symptoms. Ca and manganese supplementation (1336 and 5.6 mg, respectively) can improve mood, concentration, and behavior; 1000 mg/day can improve mood and water retention.
- Theory: Ca improves altered hormonal patterns, neurotransmitter levels, and smooth muscle responsiveness in PMS.
- Women with PMS have reduced bone mineral density (by dual-photon absorptiometry).

Zinc

- Zinc (Zn) levels are low in women with PMS.
- Zn serves as a control factor for prolactin secretion. When Zn levels are low, prolactin release increases; high Zn levels inhibit this release. In high-prolactin states, Zn is quite useful.
- Dose for elevated prolactin in women: 30 to 45 mg picolinate form.

Vitamin E

- Vitamin E has reduced breast tenderness, nervous tension, headache, fatigue, depression, and insomnia of PMS after 3 months of use. It also increased energy levels and reduced headaches and cravings for sweets.
- Dose: 400 international units (IU) (mixed tocopherols) q.d.

Essential Fatty Acids

- Women with PMS have decreased gamma-linolenic acid (GLA), which is derived biochemically from linoleic acid. This conversion requires B_6, Mg, and Zn as cofactors in the key conversion enzyme, delta-6-desaturase.
- Evening primrose, blackcurrant, and borage oils contain GLA, with typical levels being 9%, 12%, and 22%, respectively.
- Meta-analysis of clinical trials of evening primrose oil for PMS found little value in management of PMS. A better approach is to provide nutrients required for proper essential fatty acid metabolism plus adequate essential fatty acids and GLA.

Multiple Vitamin-Mineral Supplements

- Nutritional deficiency is common among women with PMS.
- High-potency multiple vitamin-mineral formulations produce significant benefits in PMS.
- Patients with PMS given a multivitamin-mineral supplement with high doses of Mg and B_6 have reductions (70% or more reduction) in both premenopausal and postmenstrual symptoms.

L-Tryptophan

Deficit in serotonin is a major factor in PMS. Tryptophan is a precursor to serotonin. L-Tryptophan in daily doses of 6 g/day for 17 days from ovulation to day 3 of menses can significantly reduce mood swings, insomnia, carbohydrate cravings, tension, irritability, and dysphoria. As 5-hydroxytryptophan (5-HTP) offers superior results to tryptophan in depression, it may also prove to be a more-effective option in PMS.

Botanical Medicines

Herbs traditionally used have a tonic effect on the female glandular system because of phytoestrogens or other compounds that improve hormonal balance of the female system and improve blood flow to female organs. Phytoestrogen activity is only 2% as strong as estrogen; thus phytoestrogens have a balancing action on estrogen effects. If estrogen levels are low, phytoestrogens will increase estrogen effect. If estrogen levels are high, phytoestrogens compete with estrogen, decreasing estrogen effects.

Often the same plant is recommended for PMS, menopause, and irregular menses. Many are termed uterine tonics because they nourish and tone female glandular and organ system. This nonspecific mode of action makes many herbs useful in a broad range of conditions affecting women.

Vitex agnus-castus (Chaste Tree)

- Used traditionally to suppress libido.
- Single most important herb for PMS. Graded as good or very good by physicians in the treatment of PMS. Thirty-three percent of women achieve complete resolution of symptoms; another 57% have significant improvement.
- Alters gonadotropin-releasing hormone (GnRH) and follicle-stimulating hormone–releasing hormone (FSH-RH), normalizing

secretion of other hormones, reducing prolactin, and reducing estrogen/progesterone ratio.

- Reduces irritability, mood changes, anger, headache, and breast tenderness. Bloating is only symptom that does not change significantly with *Vitex.*
- Studies comparing chaste tree extract to fluoxetine in decreasing PMS symptoms revealed comparable results, with the main difference being that fluoxetine is more effective in treating psychological symptoms and chasteberry is more effective with physical symptoms.
- PMS is also very common in perimenopausal women. A combination of St. John's wort and chasteberry can be helpful. St. John's wort daily dose: 5400 mg of St. John's wort standardized to contain 990 mcg hypericins, 9 mg hyperforin, and 18 mg flavonoid glycosides. The daily dose of chaste tree is 1000 mg of dried fruit. Clinical trials lasted for 16 weeks, demonstrating statistical superiority to placebo for total PMS-like symptoms and for PMS depression and food cravings.
- Dose: *Vitex* standardized extract (20-mg tablet standardized for casticin) daily.

Ginkgo biloba Extract

- Effective against congestive symptoms of PMS: breast pain or tenderness and vascular congestion.
- *Ginkgo biloba* extract (GBE) was evaluated using the Beck Depression Inventory, a daily symptom rating questionnaire containing 19 PMS symptoms according to DSM-V. Dose: 40 mg t.i.d. of a standardized GBE from day 16 of one cycle to day 5 of the next cycle. GBE was superior to placebo for overall severity of symptoms. Severity of psychological and physical symptoms also declined more significantly with GBE.
- Dose: GBE of 25% *Ginkgo* flavon glycosides at 80 mg b.i.d. from day 16 to day 5 of cycle.

Hypericum perforatum (St. John's Wort)

- Reduces emotional symptoms of PMS overall by 51%, with 67% of women tested having at least a 50% decrease in severity of symptoms.
- St. John's wort supports brain serotonin activity. St. John's wort (900 mg/day standardized to 0.18% hypericin and 3.38% hyperforin) is statistically more beneficial than placebo in relieving food cravings, swelling, poor coordination, insomnia,

confusion, headaches, crying, and fatigue. St. John's wort is not statistically more beneficial in anxiety, irritability, depression, nervous tension, mood swing, feeling out of control, and pain-related symptoms during two cycles of treatment. However, these pain-related symptoms appears to improve more than with placebo over time through several cycles. St. John's wort seems to have no effect on blood biochemical parameters: follicle-stimulating hormone (FSH), luteinizing hormone (LH), estradiol, progesterone, prolactin, testosterone, cytokine, interleukins (IL-1β, IL-6, and IL-8), interferon, and tumor necrosis factor-alpha.

Saffron (*Crocus sativus* L.)

Saffron has an antidepressant effect in women with mild to moderate depression through a serotonergic mechanism. Dose: 15 mg of saffron b.i.d. Saffron can induce a 50% reduction in severity of symptoms, far superior to placebo by the end of four cycles.

Bioidentical Progesterone Therapy

Bioidentical progesterone ("natural progesterone") is often made by extracting diosgenin from Mexican wild yam and chemically converting this into progesterone biochemically identical to human progesterone. It is neither wild yam nor an herbal product. Conventional synthetic progestin, found in birth control pills, as a hormonal treatment for PMS, has largely been replaced by select antidepressants for their effect on serotonin levels. Bioidentical progesterone has failed to prove superior to placebo for PMS (perhaps because of high placebo response in PMS). Study dose showing positive effects: 200 to 400 mg b.i.d. as a vaginal or rectal suppository from 14 days before expected onset of menstruation until onset of vaginal bleeding. Transdermal creams of natural progesterone are popular self-treatment products but vary greatly from herbal wild yam cream to wild yam cream with added bioidentical progesterone, up to 20 mg per ¼ tsp. Side effects are few and generally mild but may occur in 4% to 5% of women using transdermal creams that include 20 mg of United States Pharmacopeia (USP) progesterone per ¼ tsp. A positive study (progesterone at 400 mg b.i.d. via vaginal or rectal administration) reported adverse events in 51% of patients: irregularity of menstruation, vaginal itching, and headache.

THERAPEUTIC APPROACH

Seven key steps to consider are as follows:

1. Evaluate PMS symptoms by having patient complete a questionnaire.
2. Rule out psychiatric or other medical condition.
3. Implement dietary recommendations for PMS:
   a. Eat a high-fiber, vegetarian or predominantly vegetarian diet.
   b. Reduce fat.
   c. Eliminate sugar.
   d. Eliminate caffeine, especially if there is mastalgia.
   e. Keep salt intake low. Follow guidelines for nutritional supplementation given later.
4. Reduce exposure to environmental estrogens.
5. Select appropriate herbal support.
6. Establish a program for stress reduction; recommend regular exercise.
7. If after at least three complete periods the patient does not have significant improvement or complete resolution of symptoms, identify additional causative factors as detailed earlier, or change treatment program.

Nutritional Supplements

- Multivitamin-mineral supplement
- Vitamin B_6: 50 to 100 mg q.d. (total daily dose of vitamin B_6 in a single ingredient or in multiple vitamin should not exceed 150 mg)
- Mg (citrate, malate, aspartate, or glycinate): 250 mg b.i.d.
- Zn (picolinate): 15 to 20 mg q.d.
- Vitamin E (mixed tocopherols): 400 IU q.d.

Botanical Medicines

- *V. agnus-castus:* q.d.
  — Standardized extract (0.5% agnuside): 175 to 225 mg daily or 20 mg standardized to casticin
  — Liquid extract: 2 mL
- *G. biloba*
  — 80 to 160 mg standardized extract (24% *Ginkgo* flavon glycosides) b.i.d.
- *H. perforatum*
  — 900 to 1800 mg standardized extract (0.3% hypericin) q.d.

Proctologic Conditions

ANORECTAL ANATOMY

- Anorectal region:
  - Anus: extends from 3 to 4 cm above anal verge and merges with rectum
  - Rectum: 12 to 18 cm in length
  - Anal verge: demarcation point from perianal skin to anal skin
- Anal canal:
  - Dentate line: demarcation between ectoderm of external squamous epithelium and rectal entodermal mucosa. Anal canal does not contain sebaceous or sweat glands; it is innervated by somatic nerves up to and slightly beyond dentate line; it is sensitive to pain. Above the dentate line, rectal mucosa is relatively insensitive to pain but registers distention and inflammation as diffuse visceral pain.
  - Anorectal line: point above which rectum expands outward into pelvic bowl.
- Rectal columns, anal valves, anal glands, and anal crypts: occupy area between dentate and anorectal lines. Anal glands provide mucus to lubricate passage of stool and empty into anal crypts. This area is the locus of anal fistula or perirectal abscess if crypt becomes impacted, unable to discharge mucus. Anal fissures lie below the dentate line. Midway between dentate and anorectal lines lies the white line of Hilton, or pectinate line, the location of the intersphincteric groove, the region that lies between internal and external sphincters. The internal sphincter is controlled by the autonomic nervous system; the external sphincter is under somatic or voluntary control.
- Vascular supply: inferior mesenteric artery and internal iliac artery; superior, middle, and inferior rectal arteries; anastomosis between these branches. Venous return: superior and middle hemorrhoid veins that empty into inferior mesenteric veins and, subsequently, portal vein and internal iliac vein, vena cava, bypassing liver.
- Muscles: levator ani muscle forms the floor of the pelvis and helps form the puborectalis sling. The puborectalis sling causes

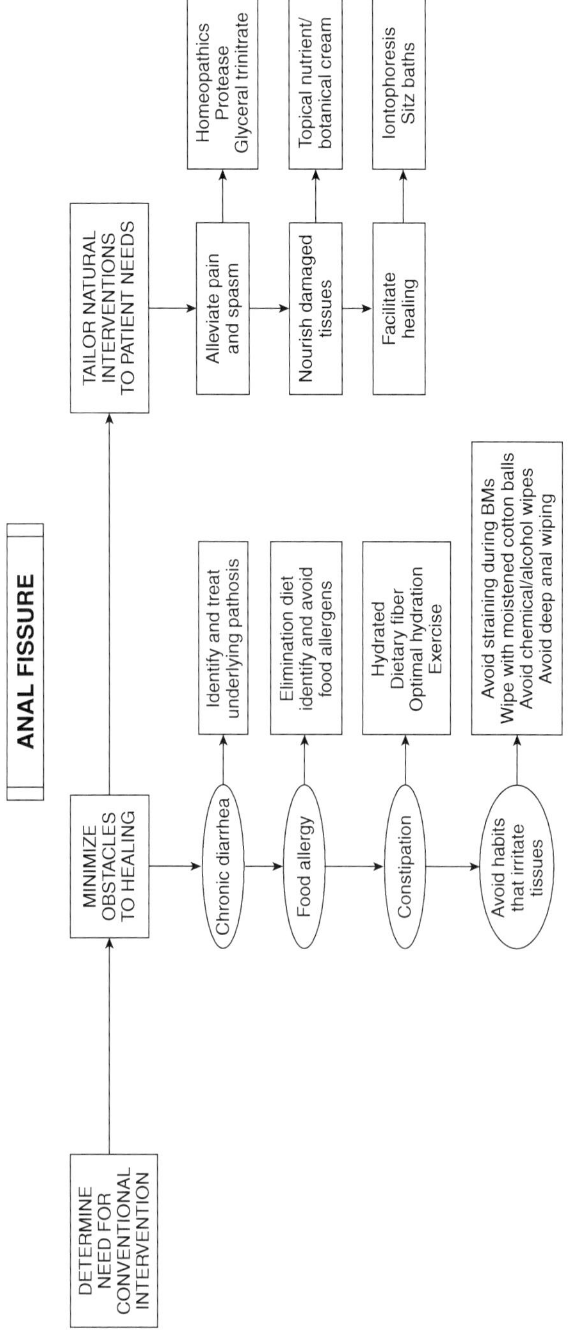
ANAL FISSURE
DETERMINE NEED FOR CONVENTIONAL INTERVENTION
MINIMIZE OBSTACLES TO HEALING
Chronic diarrhea
Identify and treat underlying pathosis
Food allergy
Elimination diet identify and avoid food allergens
Constipation
Hydrated
Dietary fiber
Optimal hydration
Exercise
Avoid habits that irritate tissues
Avoid straining during BMs
Wipe with moistened cotton balls
Avoid chemical/alcohol wipes
Avoid deep anal wiping
TAILOR NATURAL INTERVENTIONS TO PATIENT NEEDS
Alleviate pain and spasm
Homeopathics
Protease
Glyceral trinitrate
Nourish damaged tissues
Topical nutrient/ botanical cream
Facilitate healing
Iontophoresis
Sitz baths

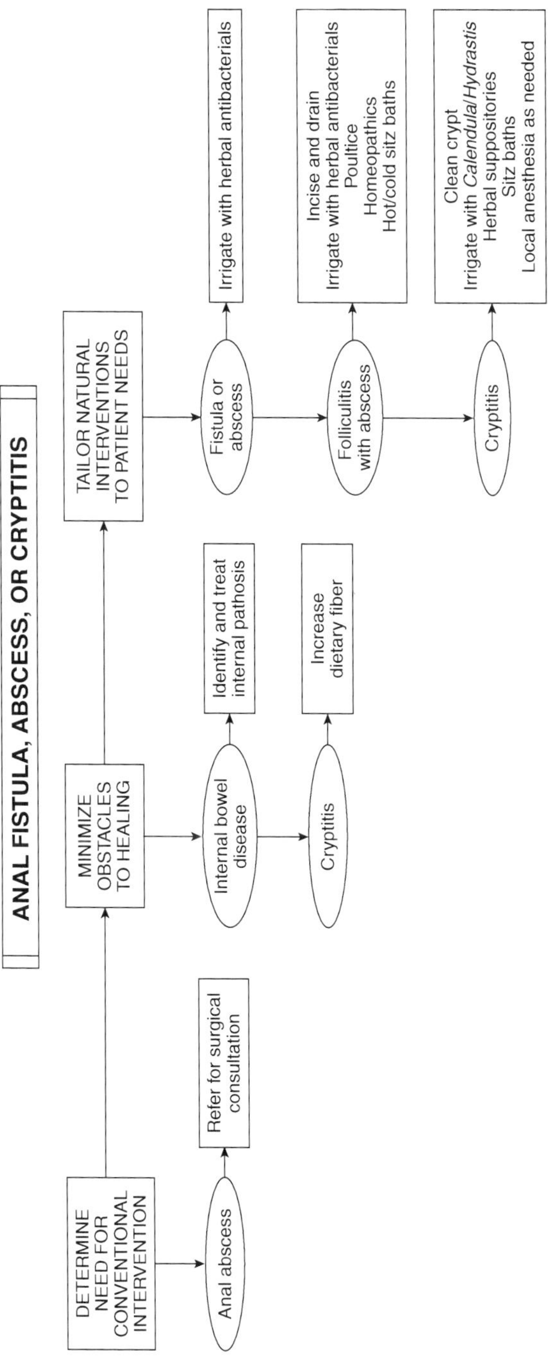
ANAL FISTULA, ABSCESS, OR CRYPTITIS
DETERMINE NEED FOR CONVENTIONAL INTERVENTION
Anal abscess
Refer for surgical consultation
MINIMIZE OBSTACLES TO HEALING
Internal bowel disease
Identify and treat internal pathosis
Cryptitis
Increase dietary fiber
TAILOR NATURAL INTERVENTIONS TO PATIENT NEEDS
Fistula or abscess
Irrigate with herbal antibacterials
Folliculitis with abscess
Incise and drain
Irrigate with herbal antibacterials
Poultice
Homeopathics
Hot/cold sitz baths
Cryptitis
Clean crypt
Irrigate with *Calendula*/*Hydrastis*
Herbal suppositories
Sitz baths
Local anesthesia as needed

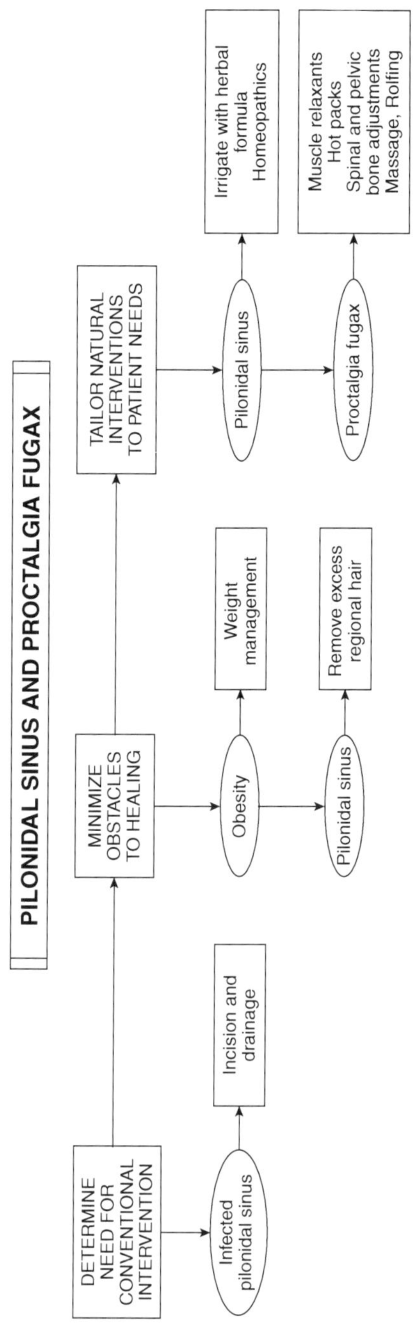
PILONIDAL SINUS AND PROCTALGIA FUGAX
DETERMINE NEED FOR CONVENTIONAL INTERVENTION
Infected pilonidal sinus
Incision and drainage
MINIMIZE OBSTACLES TO HEALING
Obesity
Weight management
Pilonidal sinus
Remove excess regional hair
TAILOR NATURAL INTERVENTIONS TO PATIENT NEEDS
Pilonidal sinus
Irrigate with herbal formula
Homeopathics
Proctalgia fugax
Muscle relaxants
Hot packs
Spinal and pelvic bone adjustments
Massage, Rolfing

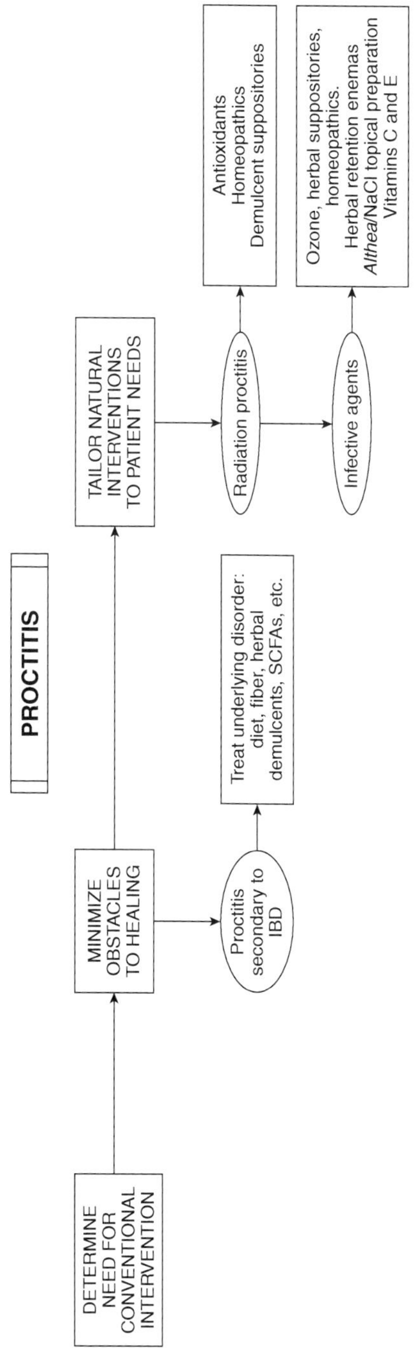
PROCTITIS
DETERMINE NEED FOR CONVENTIONAL INTERVENTION
MINIMIZE OBSTACLES TO HEALING
TAILOR NATURAL INTERVENTIONS TO PATIENT NEEDS
Proctitis secondary to IBD
Treat underlying disorder: diet, fiber, herbal demulcents, SCFAs, etc.
Radiation proctitis
Antioxidants
Homeopathics
Demulcent suppositories
Infective agents
Ozone, herbal suppositories, homeopathics.
Herbal retention enemas
Althea/NaCl topical preparation
Vitamins C and E

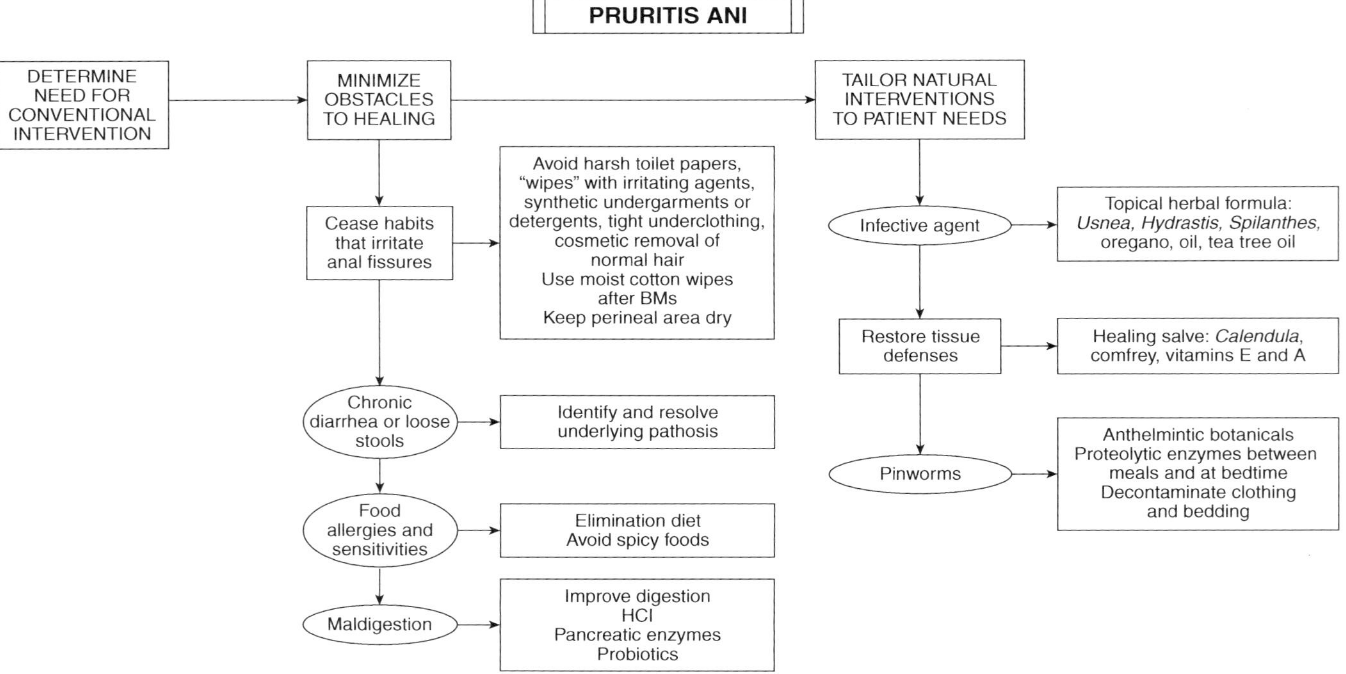
PRURITIS ANI
DETERMINE NEED FOR CONVENTIONAL INTERVENTION
MINIMIZE OBSTACLES TO HEALING
TAILOR NATURAL INTERVENTIONS TO PATIENT NEEDS
Cease habits that irritate anal fissures
Avoid harsh toilet papers, "wipes" with irritating agents, synthetic undergarments or detergents, tight underclothing, cosmetic removal of normal hair
Use moist cotton wipes after BMs
Keep perineal area dry
Chronic diarrhea or loose stools
Identify and resolve underlying pathosis
Food allergies and sensitivities
Elimination diet
Avoid spicy foods
Maldigestion
Improve digestion
HCl
Pancreatic enzymes
Probiotics
Infective agent
Topical herbal formula: *Usnea, Hydrastis, Spilanthes,* oregano, oil, tea tree oil
Restore tissue defenses
Healing salve: *Calendula*, comfrey, vitamins E and A
Pinworms
Anthelmintic botanicals
Proteolytic enzymes between meals and at bedtime
Decontaminate clothing and bedding

the bowel to change direction as it penetrates the pelvic floor, making passage of stool easier. The sphincter mechanism controls continence.

- Innervation of anal canal: pudendal nerves originating from S2, S3, and S4.
- Presenting symptoms: pain, tenderness, rectal spasm, bleeding, itching, protrusions, eruptions, discharges, constipation, diarrhea, changes in stool pattern, sacral backache, shooting pains down limbs, cramping and painful menses, urinary disturbances, anemia, prostatitis, restlessness (in children), foreign bodies. Seemingly unrelated symptoms may have their origin in the anorectal tract.

ANAL DISEASES

Anal Fistula and Anal Abscess

- Result of infection of an anal crypt whose distal end lies near the dentate line. Anal glands become infected because of impacted feces. Infection progresses into intersphincteric space but generally does not penetrate beyond the external sphincter. Most anal glands lie posteriorly; thus most abscesses drain from a line posterior to the ischial tuberosities; anterior ones drain radially from points of origin. Rectal fistula or abscess may indicate internal bowel disease: diverticulitis, trauma to area, or immune system incompetence such as with human immunodeficiency virus (HIV) infection.
- Weak points of highly vascularized rectal mucosa are anal glands impacted with feces. Surrounding tissue is swollen, red, and painful to touch. If infection remains in the intersphincteric space, rectal pain is seemingly without specific findings. Eliciting pain with pressure on examination provides a clue regarding the source. The patient may have a fever of unknown origin.
- Adjacent ischiorectal fossae have fatty tissue that allows distention of the rectum. An abscess can progress in many directions. In true perianal abscess, incision and drainage are contraindicated; bulk of lesion is untouched because of the invasion of underlying tissues and caverns of pus. Unlike other abscesses, do not allow perianal abscesses to come to a head and rupture to avoid excess necrosis of the anal sphincter.
- Obtain surgical consultation for rectal abscess. Surgery opens the tract, allowing healing by second intention. Localized treatment

helps abscess drain if it has ruptured or if patient is seen acutely and referral is not immediately possible. Irrigate with herbal antibacterial agents: *Hydrastis, Usnea,* and *Calendula succus* in 0.9% saline will help drainage.
- Folliculitis with abscess: incise and drain. This condition does not involve anal canal or ischiorectal fossa. Homeopathics: Calcarea sulphurica, silicea, Hepar sulphuris, *Myristica.* Poultices of onion, garlic, or potatoes have drawing action. Also use alternating hot and cold sitz baths. After abscess breaks open or is incised and drained, irrigate with these herbal solutions.

Anal Cryptitis

- Anal crypts are pockets between grooves formed by rectal columns at their distal point ending at the dentate line. Anal cryptitis, as separate from fistula, is debatable and rare. Symptom: pain worsened by bowel movement (BM). Signs: localized tenderness and redness at dentate line; rectal spasm. Rule out rectal fissure. Chronic cases suggest bacterial infection of gonorrhea.
- Treatment: herbal suppository, sitz baths, increased dietary fiber, local anesthesia as needed. Clean crypt with crypt hook if needed; irrigate with solution of *C. succus* and *Hydrastis* in normal saline.

Anal Fissure

- Anal fissure: slitlike separation of anal mucosa that lies below the dentate line. Majority (70% to 80%) are in the posterior midline region; anterior midline lesions (10% to 20%) are more common in women. Oval anal sphincter (rather than round), coming to a Y or narrow point at posterior midline, predisposes to fissure. Anal fissure also occurs in children with chronic diarrhea or hard stool. Fissure may also arise from congenital anal deformity. Lesions in anteroposterior vertical axis suggest internal bowel disease—Crohn's disease, squamous cell or adenocarcinoma of rectum, syphilitic fissure, and ulceration of tuberculosis (TB).
- Very painful because of the somatic innervation of spasm of the anal sphincter induced by stretching during BM. Anal fissure triggers vicious cycle—pain causing sphincter spasm with tightening of sphincter and increased pain with BM. Symptoms: severe pain during and after BM and bleeding. As lesion enlarges, it may ulcerate and become infected. Conventional treatment: rectal dilation, internal sphincterotomy, electrodessication, or surgical excision.

- Causes: passage of large, hard stools; childbirth trauma; chronic diarrhea; trauma; food allergy; prolonged straining to pass stool. High risk: infants and young children ingesting large amounts of cow's milk, with chronic constipation, especially if breastfed only a short time. Personality traits: intense, compulsive. Predisposing factors: previous anal or rectal operation, syphilis, Crohn's disease.
- Examination: difficult because of pain and spasm; anoscopic examination requires anesthesia. Local injection of 1% or 2% lidocaine into rectal sphincter at the 3 o'clock and 9 o'clock positions relaxes it enough for examination. Fissures are visible without anoscope; pull back anal skin and examine tissue. Sentinel pile or enlarged papillae suggest chronic anal fissure. Anal stenosis and fibrosis indicate chronic state.
- Differential diagnosis: Crohn's disease, especially if patient is younger or has history of periodic or chronic diarrhea or if fissure lies in anteroposterior vertical axis; squamous cell carcinoma; syphilitic ulcers; rarely TB. Spasm of levator ani muscle has no lesion.
- Treatment is challenging. Surgery removes the lesion and alleviates pain, but lesion will return if underlying cause is unresolved. Surgery predisposes to fecal incontinence later in life. Educate patient that healing will involve exacerbations and remissions.
- Initial treatment: alleviate pain and spasm. Homeopathics: promptly relieve if simillimum is found; aid healing process. Remedies: chamomile, graphite, nitric acid, ratanhia, Sepia, silicea, Thuja. Administer frequently. Proteases—315 mg, 2 capsules t.i.d. between meals and before bed—alleviate pain. Use preparation of 0.2% glycerol trinitrate topically to relieve rectal spasm and 5% lidocaine cream for local pain. Glycerol trinitrate relieves rectal spasm and increases blood flow to sphincter. (Decreased sphincter blood flow may be a precipitating mechanism of fissure.)
- Topical cream of vitamins A and E, panthenol, *Calendula,* and comfrey enhances healing by nourishing tissues. Some of the commercial preparations contain boric acid for a styptic effect. Apply cream topically after every BM and at bedtime. As healing occurs, twice-daily administration suffices until lesion resolves.
- Iontophoresis: use zinc electrode and apply positive current to facilitate healing by hardening underlying fissure, decreasing bleeding, and relieving pain. Patient lies on negative dispersing pad, and current is applied for 10 minutes at 10 mA.

- Patient should avoid straining during BM and use cotton balls moistened with water, rather than toilet paper or chemical or alcohol wipes; avoid wiping deep into anal canal.
- Sitz baths increase blood flow. Alternative: spray hot and cold water on perineal area.
- Increase dietary fiber if condition is caused by chronic constipation. If chronic diarrhea, identify cause. Dietary changes are mandatory in irritable bowel syndrome, Crohn's disease, and so forth. Higher rates of hemorrhoids and Crohn's disease occur with blood group O because of food intolerance.
- Frequent follow-up: assess healing; reassure patient. After healing, maintain proper bowel function and good dietary habits.

Hemorrhoids

- Hemorrhoids are rare in cultures with high-fiber, unrefined diets. Low-fiber diet leads to strain during BMs because of smaller, harder stools. Straining increases abdominal pressure, obstructing venous return, increasing pelvic congestion, and weakening veins.
- Begin to develop during age range 20 to 30 years; symptoms manifest during age range 30 to 40 years. Fifty percent of persons older than 50 years have symptomatic hemorrhoids; one third of total U.S. population have hemorrhoids to some degree.
- Causes: genetics, excessive venous pressure, pregnancy, long periods of standing or sitting, straining at stool, heavy lifting, portal vein lacking valves. Factors increasing venous congestion in perianal region can precipitate hemorrhoids: increasing intra-abdominal pressure (e.g., defecation, pregnancy, coughing, sneezing, vomiting, physical exertion, and portal hypertension from cirrhosis), straining during BM, and standing or sitting for prolonged periods.
- Presenting symptoms: itching, burning, irritation with BM, swelling of anus and perianal region, blood on toilet paper or in bowl, seepage of mucus. Rarely are internal hemorrhoids painful or itchy. Hallmark of hemorrhoids: bleeding or protrusion after passing stool. Pain of internal hemorrhoids occurs with strangulation from prolapse and thrombosis. Other pain is from a coexisting lesion, such as a fissure. Itching is rare with internal hemorrhoids except with excess mucus.
- Originate above anorectal line in the right anterior, right posterior, and left lateral quadrants. Other areas have secondary hemorrhoids. Occasionally, internal hemorrhoid enlarges enough to prolapse below anal sphincter.

- Classification of hemorrhoids:
  - According to location and degree of severity
  - External hemorrhoids: occur below the anorectal line; can be full of either blood clots (thrombotic hemorrhoids) or connective tissue (cutaneous hemorrhoids)
  - Thrombotic hemorrhoid: produced when a hemorrhoidal vessel ruptures and forms thrombus
  - Cutaneous hemorrhoid: contains fibrous connective tissue covered by anal skin; can be located anywhere on anal circumference; typically caused by resolution of thrombotic hemorrhoid, with thrombus transformed into connective tissue

Internal Hemorrhoids

- Occur above anorectal line
- Can enlarge enough to prolapse below anal sphincter
- Grading is according to degree of prolapse:
  - Grade I: no prolapse
  - Grade II: prolapse on defecation, but spontaneous reduction
  - Grade III: prolapse on defecation, and manual reduction
  - Grade IV: prolapse, and no reduction possible
- Internal-external, or mixed hemorrhoids: combination of contiguous external and internal hemorrhoids that appear as baggy swellings. Treating internal hemorrhoid may resolve external portion. If patient has external hemorrhoids, internal ones are probably present.
- Types of mixed hemorrhoids that can occur:
  - Without prolapse: bleeding possible, but no pain
  - Prolapsed: pain and possibly bleeding
  - Strangulated: prolapse to extent and for duration that blood supply is occluded by anal sphincter constriction; very painful; usually become thrombosed

Treatment

- High-fiber diet, rich in vegetables, fruits, legumes, and whole grains, promotes peristalsis and keeps feces soft, bulky, and easy to pass with less straining.
- Natural bulking compounds: well-hydrated milled flaxseed, chia seeds, psyllium seeds, and guar gum attract and hold water to form a gelatinous mass. They are less irritating than wheat bran and other cellulose fibers. They reduce symptoms (bleeding, pain, pruritus, prolapse) and improve bowel habits within 6 weeks.

- Breakfast: 7.5-fold increase in odds of hemorrhoids or anal fissures in persons who do not eat breakfast.
- Flavonoids: rutin and hydroxyethylrutosides (HERs) prevent and treat hemorrhoids by strengthening venous tissues. HERs (1000 mg q.d. for 4 weeks) relieve hemorrhoidal signs and symptoms in pregnant women. Micronized flavonoid combination (diosmin 90% and hesperidin 10%) for 8 weeks before delivery and 4 weeks after delivery also helps pregnant women. Treatment is well accepted and does not affect pregnancy, fetal development, birth weight, infant growth, or feeding.
- Topical treatments: suppositories, ointments, and anorectal pads provide only temporary relief. Natural ingredients: witch hazel *(Hamamelis),* cocoa butter, Peruvian balsam, zinc oxide, allantoin, homeopathics. Hydrocortisone cream relieves itching. Prolonged use can aggravate pruritus ani.
- Botanical medicines: used topically, as suppositories, or taken internally. Rectal suppositories after galvanic, infrared, or laser therapy facilitate healing and decrease bleeding.
- Hydrotherapy: warm sitz bath for uncomplicated acute flare-up; alternate hot and cold sitz baths for chronic conditions.
- Surgery: grade I and II are managed medically, especially if acute. Herbal suppositories and indicated homeopathics can calm flare-ups. Uncomplicated asymptomatic stage I and II hemorrhoids: treatment not recommended; increase dietary fiber and improve dietary choices. Injection of sclerosing agents: useful during stages I and II but contraindicated with anal fissure, inflammatory bowel disease, Crohn's disease, leukemia, portal hypertension. Sclerosing therapy is not usually effective in stages III and IV. Rubber band ligation: office procedure to remove redundant tissue and cause scarring replaced by new tissue. It induces sense of fullness and pressure; pain occurs if band is too close to pectinate line. Complications: bleeding; sometimes septicemia and death. Used for stage I, stage II, and occasionally stage III hemorrhoids; success is based on physician's skill in placing band.
- Cryosurgery: liquid nitrogen or nitrous oxide applied to hemorrhoid to destroy venous plexus, triggering scarring and tissue replacement. Used for stage II and III hemorrhoids and condylomata but contraindicated for stage IV hemorrhoids, chronic ulcers, and acutely thrombosed hemorrhoids. Sequelae: pain, swelling, and bleeding.

- Hemorrhoidectomy, the removal of redundant tissue, is the most invasive; requires outpatient surgical setting. Complications: pain and rectal sphincter instability.
- Monopolar direct current technique (inverse galvanism) of Keesey technique: treatment of choice in the United States; painless, effective, and safe outpatient treatment of all grades of hemorrhoids. It also relieves chronic anal fissures associated with internal hemorrhoids. Relief of chronic pain can occur after two treatments; anal fissures can heal in 4 weeks. This office procedure requires no anesthetic except locally for hypersensitive or nervous patients. Use 2% procaine solution injected directly into hemorrhoid. Chemicophysiologic action causes absorption and destruction of vein and permanent cure. Mechanism of action: introduced into interior of hemorrhoid, the negative pole of galvanic current generates H_2 gas and OH^- ions at contact with water of blood and tissues. Hydroxide destroys hemorrhoid and capillaries, producing hydrolysis and then hardening of hemorrhoid. Resolution: either absorption or rupture, with discharge of thrombosed elements into rectum, then contraction of residual tissues. Patient is freely ambulant after procedure. Hemorrhoid disappears 7 to 10 days after treatment. Treat each separate hemorrhoid; larger hemorrhoids may need more than one treatment. Treat only one or two hemorrhoids at one time to minimize bleeding and allow healing.
- Infrared coagulation (IRC): for stage I and II hemorrhoids and combined with Keesey treatment for stage III and IV hemorrhoids. Burst of intense heat is generated internally and shot through blue anodized sapphire tip to surface of hemorrhoid. IRC "coagulates" redundant tissue to a depth depending on the amount of time of light burst, 1 to 1.5 seconds. A 7- to 10-day period of healing is needed between treatments. Keesey treatment plus IRC usually reduces number of treatments needed per hemorrhoid. Compared with rubber band, laser, or cryotherapy, IRC gives better results and has less morbidity.
- Prevention: reduce straining during BM and sitting or standing for prolonged periods; address underlying liver disease. Eat a high-fiber diet for proper bowel activity, including nutrients and botanicals that enhance integrity of venous structures, proanthocyanidin- and anthocyanidin-rich foods (e.g., blackberries, cherries, blueberries) to strengthen vein structures. Supplements: vitamins A and B complex, antioxidant vitamins C and E, and zinc maintain vascular integrity and facilitate healing.

External Hemorrhoids

- External hemorrhoids arise from dilation of external rectal plexus or thrombosis after constipation, diarrhea, heavy lifting, or Valsalva from sneezing, coughing, or childbirth.
- Symptoms: often-painful perianal lump with bleeding; mild to little discomfort; resolve on their own if homeostasis is restored. External anal skin tags are remnants of previous external hemorrhoids. Thrombosis and increasing distention trigger cycle of acute edema and pain, worsened by BM or prolonged sitting, and bleeding after stool.
- Differential diagnosis: prolapsed internal hemorrhoid, perianal abscess, rectal fissure with sentinel pile, hypertrophied anal papillae, irritated skin tag, and condyloma latum or acuminata.
- Treatment: unless thrombosed or excessively painful, manage medically. Relieve pressure and dissolve thrombosis. Long-term management: patient education, dietary changes, enhanced vascular integrity. Initial treatment: enzyme protease 2400 milk clotting units (MCU), 2 capsules between meals t.i.d. and 2 capsules at bedtime, reduces thrombosis and decreases pain. Alternating sitz baths relieve pain and increase blood flow. Homeopathics: *Aesculus, Aloe, Hamamelis,* muriatic acid, ratanhia, and *Sepia* relieve pain and speed healing.
- Long-term management: dietary changes to eliminate offending foods; increase hydrated dietary fiber with fruits and vegetables or over-the-counter fiber supplement. Herbal medicines: *Aesculus, Collinsonia, Hamamelis, Althaea,* and *Ulmus* restore venous sufficiency and soothe inflamed tissues. Regulating bowel function with herbal laxatives may help normalize intestinal and colon function.
- Acute thrombosed external hemorrhoid: prompt surgical excision or incision is in order. Anesthesia before evacuation of clot is needed. Excision leaves wound that should not be sutured but allowed to heal, but this leads to increased postoperative pain. Incision and debridement of clot reduce pain but may close too early, reforming thrombus. Consult text on minor or rectal surgery.
- Herbal anodynes *Piscidia* and belladonna for pain of rectal spasm; *Hyoscyamus niger* facilitates postoperative management. Topicals: *Arnica, Hypericum,* and *C. succus.*
- Alternating sitz baths with ½ ounce of Betadine enhances healing and decreases chance of infection. Protease 2400 μU can give pain relief. Homeopathic *Arnica, Calendula,* and staphisagria also give pain relief.

PERIANAL DERMATOLOGIC DISORDERS

Condylomata Acuminata

- Symptoms: sticking or foreign body sensation perianally. Large lesion interferes with defecation; hygiene is problematic. Lesion is soft, moist, reddish pink, pedunculated. Differentiation: condylomata lata of secondary syphilis. Rapid plasma reagin (RPR) with reflexive fluorescent treponemal antibody (FTA) testing is warranted. If available, conduct darkfield microscopic examination. Diagnosis of condylomata acuminata is made by biopsy.
- Treatment: solution of 25% podophyllum applied topically 6 to 8 hours before patient washes it off. Several applications may be necessary. IRC after injection of subcutaneous 1% or 2% lidocaine. Proper homeopathics coupled with good nutritional program can prevent suppression of lesions contributing to deepening of the disease process. A number of homeopathics cover genital warts. Administering constitutional homeopathic medicine eradicates lesion and decreases susceptibility to reoccurrence.

Condylomata Lata

- Anogenital warts: caused by human papillomavirus (HPV) types 6, 11, 16, 18, 31, 33, and 35; transmitted by sexual contact. Appearance: soft, moist, pink to gray, flat to pedunculated excrescences, often in clusters. Location: warm, moist regions of anogenital region, often clustered around anus in homosexual men and women who practice receptive anal intercourse.
- Differential diagnosis: flat lesion of condyloma latum of secondary syphilis; squamous cell carcinoma if lesion does not respond to therapy or by biopsy.
- Treatment: 25% podophyllum, *Thuja* ointment, homeopathics, cryotherapy, infrared or electrosurgical desiccation.

Lymphogranuloma Venereum

- Infective agent: serotype of *Chlamydia trachomatis.*
- Appearance: papule lesion that ulcerates and heals rapidly. If in rectal mucosa, signs and symptoms of proctitis are present. Extremely painful inguinal adenitis or buboes subsequently arise. Later stages: fistulation, ulceration, fibrosis, rectal or anal stenosis, lymphedema of legs and genitalia. Non–lymphogranuloma venereum (LGV) *Chlamydia* serotypes can also be implicated in proctitis but without severity of symptoms.

- White blood cell (WBC) counts may reach 20,000/mL if lymphatic involvement; anemia is possible. Culture of chlamydial serotype from infected lesion is diagnostic, but complement fixation and immunofluorescent antibody tests are available.
- If treated promptly, prognosis is good. Cellular changes worsen prognosis. Allopathic treatment: antibiotics such as doxycycline, erythromycin, sulfisoxazole are effective. Homeopathic and herbals: see treatments under "Proctitis."

Herpes

- Most frequently encountered perianal lesion. Symptoms and signs: burning, searing pain; confused with rectal fissure. Examination: vesicles on erythematous base erode and form ulcers. With HIV or other immunocompromised condition, lesions can form deep ulcers of prolonged duration. Diagnosis: by Tzanck smear or viral culture.
- Treatment: address current eruption. Topicals: licorice root and *Melissa officinalis* extracts alleviate burning and pain and facilitate healing; zinc sulfate 2% is useful. Homeopathics address pain and eruptions and decrease susceptibility to outbreaks. Stress reduction: herpes eruptions often occur during excessive stress or other illness.
- Long-term strategies: decrease arginine-containing foods such as nuts, legumes (especially peanuts), chocolate. Increasing lysine to 500 to 1000 mg/day reduces outbreaks. Vitamins C, E, and B complex and zinc and copper are beneficial.

Pilonidal Sinus

- Definition: rare congenital tract that runs from coccyx or sacrum to perineum with constant drainage. Congenital and acquired factors contribute. Symptom: chronic discharge.
- Prevalence: most common in young white adults; rare in Africans; almost never seen in Asians. Predisposing factors: congenital postanal dimples, obesity, deep intergluteal cleft, excess body hair.
- Differentiated from anal fistula and furunculosis by its midline orientation and by passing probe through sinus, noting passage toward sacrum rather than anus.
- Treatment: if sinus is infected, incision and drainage may be needed but irrigation with herbal formula mentioned for abscess may help. Weight reduction and removal of excess regional hair reduce risk of infection and symptoms. Homeopathics silicea,

Calcarea sulphurica, Hepar sulphuris are useful. Homeopathic *Thuja* as intercurrent treatment has resolved obstinate cases.

Proctalgia Fugax

- Proctalgia fugax, or levator spasm syndrome: more common in men than women. Symptoms: searing pain near coccyx or rectum that is brief but intense; usually resolves on its own; awakes patient from sleep but may occur anytime.
- Cause: spasm of levator ani or pubococcygeal muscle, with deep-seated, often heavy, aching, or searing pain; feels localized in rectum and/or prostate in men.
- Signs: tense, tight levator ani muscle, tender with pressure, often drawn up above anal sphincter.
- Triggering mechanisms: poor posture, chronic anxiety, mental fixation on rectal area, misalignment of coccyx or other bones comprising pelvic bowl.
- Differential diagnosis: lumbar disk disease, coccygodynia, prostatitis, presacral tumor, developing ischiorectal abscess, spinal cord tumor, rectal lesion.
- Treatment: reassure patient of cause. Try muscle relaxants; hot packs; spinal and pelvic bone adjustments; massage to lower abdomen, lumbosacral spine, and perineum. Chronic cases respond to deep tissue work (Rolfing).

Proctitis

- Symptoms: rectal pain, tenesmus, rectal discharge, blood in stool.
- Signs: WBCs in large numbers seen on wet prep, Gram or Wright's stain. Conduct anoscopic examination for inflammation, mucopurulent discharge, mucosal friability, bleeding, and ulceration. Severe ulceration and bleeding suggest LGV chlamydial serotype.
- Causative agents: *Chlamydia* (genital and LGV immunotypes), yeast, bacteria (e.g., *Neisseria gonorrhoeae*), parasites, trauma, lectins, excessive fiber in diet, external radiation, syphilis, *Trichomonas,* Crohn's disease. Higher risk of ulcerative proctitis exists in smokers and persons who have had appendectomy.
- Treatment: based on cause. If caused by external-beam radiation for colon cancer or radium seed implants for prostate cancer, commence therapy before treatment and continue during and for several weeks after treatment has ceased. Radiation proctitis benefits from antioxidants. No ill effects on radiation occur

when combined with antioxidants. Concurrent homeopathic radium bromatum 200C potency before and after radiotherapy decreases skin burning. Other homeopathics: x-ray, sol, cadmium metallicum. Demulcent rectal suppositories soothe inflamed rectal mucosa and decrease pain.

- Proctitis secondary to inflammatory bowel disease: treat underlying disease with diet, fiber, herbal demulcents, enteric-coated peppermint oil. Short-chain fatty acids administered rectally alleviate symptoms of proctocolitis.
- Infective agents: bacteria, chlamydiae, yeasts, fungi, trichomonas, and parasites. Treatment: injection of ozone; herbal suppositories; homeopathics; retention enema consisting of *Hydrastis, Usnea, Echinacea,* yarrow if trichomonas is agent; *Althaea* in a base of 0.9% sodium chloride (NaCl) is effective. Apply this combination topically during initial examination to begin treatment. Vitamins C and E facilitate healing.
- Continue treatment for 10 to 14 days before reexamination and assessment. In ulcerative disease, treatment may be longer for complete healing.

Pruritus Ani

- Symptoms: chronic itching of perianal skin; excoriation from scratching; eventual thickening of chronically affected areas; scratching at night during sleep or being awakened from sleep by itching; intermittent to constant itching, burning, and soreness. Topical ointments give temporary relief. Signs: varying degrees of erythema, swelling, excoriation, thickening, and fissuring from scratching.
- Causes: excessive wiping with harsh toilet papers; "wipes" impregnated with drying alcohol, dyes, and antibacterial or antifungal agents; synthetic undergarments or detergents; tight underclothing that decreases air circulation; chronic diarrhea or loose stools. Cosmetic removal of normal hair disrupts normal bacterial flora.
- Infective agents: pinworms and *Candida.* Perianal itching, largely at night, suggests *Enterobius vermicularis* (pinworms), common in children and communicable to members of family. Wet prep reveals *Candida;* clear adhesive tape preparation reveals pinworms.
- Periodic and chronic diarrhea: itching caused by acidic stool and aggressive cleaning of area. Compulsive cleaners can use cotton wipes, bath or shower cleansers, or moist towels.

- Soaps, detergents, bleaches, dyes, perfumes: recent onset may be caused by a change in product. Aggravating foods: peanuts, coffee, colas, beer, spicy foods, acidic foods, food allergens.
- Diseases: psoriasis, contact dermatitis, precancerous or cancerous lesions, Bowen's disease (intraepithelial epithelioma), keratoacanthoma, melanoma, squamous cell carcinoma, basal cell carcinoma.
- Laboratory tests: culture and sensitivity if bacterial infection is suspected; potassium hydroxide (KOH) and/or wet prep for yeast or fungi; Wood's lamp examination for tinea cruris; punch biopsy of suspicious lesions.
- Treatments: eliminate spicy or offending foods, food allergens; improve patient's digestion. Infective agent identified: topical therapy for yeast, fungi, or bacteria. Initially wash with 3% hydrogen peroxide (H_2O_2), then apply topical herbal formula of *Usnea, Hydrastis, Spilanthes,* oregano, and tea tree oil; allow to dry. Reestablish skin defensive barrier: apply healing salve containing *Calendula,* comfrey, vitamins E and A. Resolution occurs within 7 to 10 days if underlying cause is removed.
- Pinworms: wash all clothing and bedding in warm to hot water to eliminate eggs laid outside rectum at night.
- Use moist cotton wipes after stool and eliminate excess moisture in the perineal area to break the cycle. Zinc oxide topically also has proven effective in the treatment of pruritus ani.

Botanicals for Anorectal Diseases

- *Aesculus hippocastanum* (horse chestnut): tonic, astringent, febrifuge, narcotic, and antiseptic, high in tannic acid and aesculin. Indications: pain relief of internal viscera, hemorrhoids, rectal irritation with marked congestion and sense of spasmodic closing of rectum as if foreign body were present; itching; sensation of heat, aching, or rectal pains; rectal neuralgia and proctitis.
- *Achillea millefolium* (yarrow): slightly astringent; alterative and diuretic; tonic on mucus membranes to stem mild hemorrhage. Indications: bleeding hemorrhoids with mucoid discharges.
- *Althaea officinalis* (marshmallow): high in mucilage; restores electrical charge to inflamed rectal mucosa. In rectal suppositories it decreases swelling, irritation, and inflammation.
- *Cinnamomum:* used in herbal rectal suppositories to stem hemorrhage.

- *Collinsonia canadensis* (stone root): alterative, tonic, stimulant, and diuretic. Indications: tones venous vascular tissue; hemorrhoids from chronic constipation and venous insufficiency; sense of constriction, weight, and heat in rectum with very dry stools; proctitis, anal fistulas, and rectal ulcer.
- *Hamamelis virginiana* (witch hazel): tonic and astringent; restores vascular integrity. Indications: varicose veins, hemorrhages, hemorrhoids; venous tissues that are pale and flaccid; deep redness because of vascular engorgement and stagnation of blood; hemorrhoids are very painful and may ulcerate.
- *Hydrastis canadensis* (goldenseal): antibacterial; contains hydrastine, berberine, canadine, and acrid resins. Actions: affects ulcerations on mucus membranes, controls mild hemorrhages; astringent effect on hemorrhoids. Indications: hemorrhoids from constipation with sinking feeling in stomach and dull headache; painful anal fissures with severe burning before, during, and after stool.
- *Ruscus aculeatus* (butcher's broom): reduces venous swelling; vasoconstrictive action reduces bleeding.

Treatment Summary for Hemorrhoids

- Primary treatment is prevention.
  - Reduce factors that increase pelvic congestion: straining during defecation, sitting or standing for prolonged periods, or underlying liver disease.
  - High-fiber diet for proper bowel regularity.
  - Supplements: fiber, flavonoids, botanical medicines (e.g., butcher's broom).
- Warm sitz baths and topical preparations ameliorate discomfort, but only temporarily.
- High–complex-carbohydrate diet, rich in fiber and liberal amounts of flavonoid-rich foods (e.g., blackberries, citrus fruits, cherries, blueberries) to strengthen vein structures.
- Nutritional supplements:
  - Milled flaxseed, chia seed, psyllium seed husks: 5 g (hydrated) at bedtime
  - Vitamin C: 500 to 1000 mg t.i.d.
  - Flavonoids (one of the following):
    - Citrus bioflavonoids, rutin, and/or hesperidin: 3000 to 6000 mg q.d.
    - Micronized diosmin: 500 to 1000 mg q.d.

  - o Grapeseed extract: (95% procyanidolic oligomers) 150 to 300 mg q.d.
  - o Pine bark extract: 150 to 300 mg q.d.
- Botanical medicine:
  - — Butcher's broom *(R. aculeatus)* extract (9% to 11% ruscogenin content): 100 mg t.i.d.
- Physical medicine:
  - — Hydrotherapy: warm sitz baths to relieve uncomplicated hemorrhoids

Psoriasis

DIAGNOSTIC SUMMARY

- Circumscribed red, thickened plaques overlying silvery white scale.
- Characteristically involves the scalp; the extensor surfaces of the wrists, elbows, knees, buttocks, and ankles; and sites of repeated trauma.
- Positive family history in 50% of cases.
- Nail involvement results in characteristic pitting. Other nail changes include onycholysis, discoloration, thickening, and dystrophy.
- Possible arthritis.

GENERAL CONSIDERATIONS

Psoriasis is an extremely common skin disorder. The rate of occurrence in the United States is 2% to 4%. It affects few blacks in the tropics but is more common among blacks in temperate zones. It is common among the Japanese and rare in Native Americans. It affects men and women equally. Mean age of onset is 27.8 years, but 2% have onset by age 2 years.

- Classic hyperproliferative skin disorder: rate of cell division is very high (1000 times greater than in normal skin), exceeding rate in squamous cell carcinoma. Even in uninvolved skin, number of proliferating cells is 2.5 times greater than in nonpsoriatics.
- Pathogenesis is incompletely understood—a complex, multifactorial disease with a genetic predisposition. It is a polygenic disorder involving oxidative stress, immune dysfunction, angiogenesis, and neuropeptides.
- Primary immune defect is increased cell signaling via chemokines and cytokines that act on upregulated gene expression and cause hyperproliferation of keratinocytes.
- Conventional targeted biologic treatments attempt to address these issues. HLA-Cw6, of the major histocompatibility region on chromosome 6, is considered the major genetic determinant

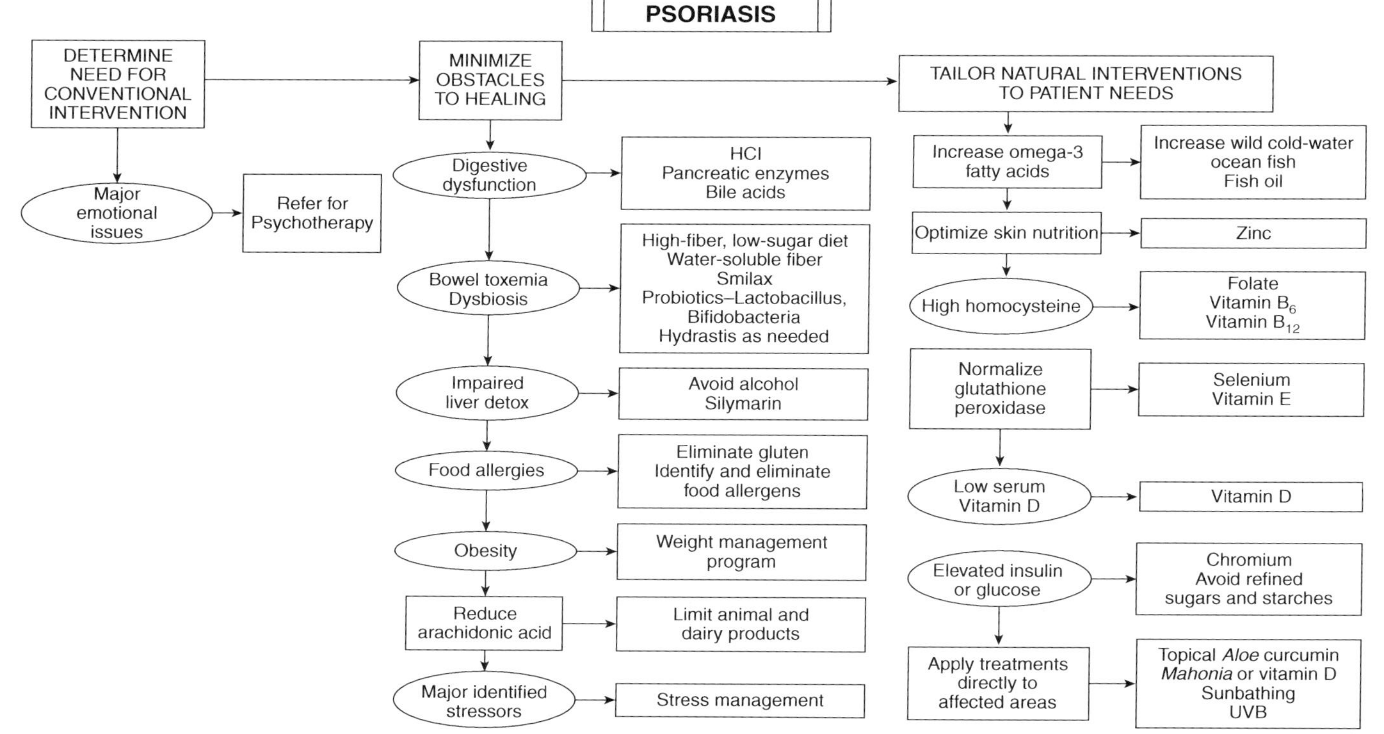
PSORIASIS
DETERMINE NEED FOR CONVENTIONAL INTERVENTION
MINIMIZE OBSTACLES TO HEALING
TAILOR NATURAL INTERVENTIONS TO PATIENT NEEDS
Major emotional issues
Refer for Psychotherapy
Digestive dysfunction
HCl
Pancreatic enzymes
Bile acids
Bowel toxemia
Dysbiosis
High-fiber, low-sugar diet
Water-soluble fiber
Smilax
Probiotics–Lactobacillus, Bifidobacteria
Hydrastis as needed
Impaired liver detox
Avoid alcohol
Silymarin
Food allergies
Eliminate gluten
Identify and eliminate food allergens
Obesity
Weight management program
Reduce arachidonic acid
Limit animal and dairy products
Major identified stressors
Stress management
Increase omega-3 fatty acids
Increase wild cold-water ocean fish
Fish oil
Optimize skin nutrition
Zinc
High homocysteine
Folate
Vitamin B_6
Vitamin B_{12}
Normalize glutathione peroxidase
Selenium
Vitamin E
Low serum Vitamin D
Vitamin D
Elevated insulin or glucose
Chromium
Avoid refined sugars and starches
Apply treatments directly to affected areas
Topical *Aloe* curcumin
Mahonia or vitamin D
Sunbathing
UVB

of psoriasis. Gene variants that encode interleukin cytokines or cytokine receptors are of interest. The gene product of the interleukin-12B gene *(IL12B)*, p40, is the target of monoclonal antibody therapy (ustekinumab). Other genes code for tumor necrosis factor-alpha (TNF-α). Many genetic variations also involve immune psoriatic disorders (e.g., Crohn's disease and diabetes).

- Psoriasis was once considered a disorder of keratinocytes; now it is seen as primarily an immune-mediated disorder. Skin cells include cytokine-synthesizing keratinocytes, antigen-presenting cells, epidermotropic and circulating T lymphocytes, dermal capillary endothelial cells, mast cells, tissue macrophages, granulocytes, fibroblasts, and non-Langerhans cells. They communicate via cytokines and respond accordingly via stimulation by bacteria, chemicals, ultraviolet light, and other irritants. The primary cytokine response to antigen presentation is TNF-α. Prolonged insult to skin induces imbalanced cytokine production in susceptible persons, leading to psoriasis. Activated keratinocytes in psoriatic lesions undergo accelerated turnover and are major sources of proangiogenic cytokines (e.g., vascular endothelial growth factor [VEGF], endothelial-cell stimulating angiogenesis factor, TNF-α, and platelet-derived growth factor [PDGF]). Other angiogenic mediators (e.g., hypoxia-inducible factors, angiopoietins, IL-8, and IL-17) are upregulated in psoriasis. Patients with psoriasis who are receiving anti-VEGF treatment for cancer showed complete remission of psoriasis.
- Initially, immature epidermal dendritic cells stimulate lymph node T cells in response to antigens. The lymphocytic infiltrate consists predominantly of CD4 and CD8 T cells. Adhesion molecules are highly expressed. After T cells are activated, mRNA for IL-2 increases IL-2 receptors. T-cell IL-2 and Langerhans cell IL-12 regulate genes for cytokines—for example, interferon-gamma (IFN-γ), TNF-α, and IL-2, which influence differentiation, maturation, and proliferation of T-cells into memory effector cells. T cells migrate to the skin, accumulate around dermal blood vessels, and produce proangiogenic factors.
- This immune response is a somewhat normal response to antigen stimulation. Unknown is why this response triggers accelerated cellular proliferation.
- Fibronectin (FN) is a cell adhesion molecule that anchors cells to collagen or proteoglycans and is involved in many cellular processes, including tissue repair, embryogenesis, blood clotting, and cell migration and adhesion. Transforming growth factor

beta (TGF-β) stimulates a form of FN, which in turn stimulates keratinocyte hyperproliferation, and through stimulation of Toll-like receptor 4 (TLR4) produces proinflammatory cytokines (e.g., TNF-α, IL-1, IL-6, and IL-12). These FN loops promote psoriatic lesions. A plausible link between heart disease and psoriasis may be the promotion of atherosclerosis and thrombotic heart disease by extra domain A (EDA-FN).

- Summary: psoriasis is caused by abnormal reactivity of specific T cells in the skin. Alterations in the epidermal barrier, innate defenses, and processing of inflammatory signals may all contribute to the triggering of a nonspecific innate immune mechanism, which, in combination with IL-23 signaling, may lead to the dysregulation of T cell–driven immune responses. Psoriasis develops in bone marrow transplant recipients from donors with psoriasis and clears in recipients from donors without psoriasis. Immunosuppressive drugs reduce psoriasis.
- Psoriasis is linked to celiac disease and Crohn's disease. Bowel mucosa of psoriatics without bowel symptoms has microscopic lesions and increased permeability. Factors leading to poor intestinal function encourage increased intestinal permeability and inflammation, allowing antigenic and endotoxic compounds to exit intestines, travel in bloodstream, and initiate activated immune cascades in susceptible tissues.

THERAPEUTIC CONSIDERATIONS

Decrease in sources of blood-borne antigenic immune activators is achievable by natural medicine. Controllable factors contributing to psoriasis are incomplete protein digestion, bowel toxemia, impaired liver function, bile deficiencies, alcohol consumption, excessive consumption of animal fats, nutritional deficiencies, and stress.

Gastrointestinal Function

Incomplete Protein Digestion

Incomplete digestion or poor absorption increases amino acids and polypeptides in bowel, where they are metabolized by bowel bacteria into toxins. Toxic metabolites of arginine and ornithine are polyamines (putrescine, spermidine, cadaverine) and are increased in psoriatics. Polyamines inhibit formation of cyclic adenosine monophosphate (cAMP), inducing excess cell proliferation. Lowered skin and urinary polyamines are linked to clinical improvement. Natural compounds inhibit formation of polyamines; vitamin A and berberine alkaloids of *Hydrastis canadensis* (goldenseal) inhibit bacterial decarboxylase enzyme, which converts amino acids into polyamines. Evaluate digestive function with Heidelberg gastric analysis and/or comprehensive digestive stool analysis. Reinforce digestion (hydrochloric acid, pancreatic enzymes).

Bowel Toxemia

Gut-derived toxins are implicated: endotoxins (compounds from cell walls of gram-negative bacteria), streptococci, *Candida albicans,* yeast, and immunoglobulin E (IgE) and IgA immune complexes. They increase cyclic guanosine monophosphate (cGMP) in skin cells, promoting proliferation. Chronic candidiasis may play a role in many cases.

- Low-fiber diet is linked to increased gut-derived toxins. Fiber of fruits, vegetables, milled flaxseed, chia seed, whole grains, and legumes bind toxins and promote their excretion.
- Aqueous extract of *Smilax* sarsaparilla is effective in psoriasis, particularly chronic, large plaque–forming variety. It improved psoriasis in 62% of patients and completely cleared another 18% (80% benefited). Benefit is from binding of endotoxins by sarsaparilla components, and their excretion. Severity and response correlate well with level of circulating endotoxins. Control of gut-derived toxins is critical. Support fecal excretion and proper handling of absorbed endotoxins by liver.

Liver Function

Correcting abnormal liver function is beneficial. The liver filters and detoxifies portal blood from the bowel. Structurally, hepatic architecture may be altered in psoriatics. If the liver is overwhelmed by excess bowel toxins or if the liver's detoxification ability is decreased, systemic toxin level increases and psoriasis worsens. Alcohol worsens psoriasis; it increases toxin absorption by damaging gut mucosa and impairs liver function. Eliminate alcohol. Silymarin, a flavonoid of *Silybum marianum,* is valuable in treating psoriasis by improving liver function, inhibiting inflammation, and reducing excess cellular proliferation.

Bile Deficiencies

- Bile acids normally present in intestines detoxify bacterial endotoxins. Bile acid deficiency allows endotoxins to translocate into bloodstream, inducing release of inflammatory cytokines that aggravate psoriasis.

- Hungarian study: oral bile acid (dehydrocholic acid) supplementation for 1 to 6 weeks plus diet high in vegetables and fruits and devoid of hot spices, alcohol, raw onion, garlic, and carbonated soft drinks alleviated symptoms in 78.8% of patients, whereas only 24.9% of those on conventional therapies recovered during treatment period. Bile acid effects were more pronounced in acute form of psoriasis; 95.1% of patients became asymptomatic. A total of 57.9% were asymptomatic 2 years later compared with 6.0% on conventional treatment. Product and dose: 2 or 3 Suprachol sugar-coated pills q.d. or dehydrocholic acid powder (acidum dehydrocholicum pulvis) at two or three doses of 0.25 g q.d.
- Theoretical risk of malignancy with sluggish intestinal function and long-term bile acid therapy causes researchers to recommend supplementation only after fatty meals after initial treatment period. Ursodeoxycholic acid may have protective effect on colon mucosa; it reduces risk of colon cancer, even in ulcerative colitis and primary sclerosing cholangitis. Consider bile acids for short-term treatment of psoriasis; monitor colon before and after treatment in patients at high risk for colon cancer.

Nutrition

Omega-3 fatty acids: serum free fatty acids are abnormal in psoriatics. Fish oil at 10 to 12 g (providing 1.8 g eicosapentaenoic acid [EPA] and 1.2 g docosahexaenoic acid [DHA]) improves symptoms. Equivalent amount of EPA is available in 150 g of salmon, mackerel, or herring. Wild cold-water fish plus 1 tbsp flaxseed oil daily may be advantageous because of the lipid peroxides in many fish oil products.

EPA improves psoriasis because of competition for arachidonic acid binding sites, thereby increasing anti-inflammatory leukotriene LTB5 from EPA, which is one tenth as potent as inflammatory LTB4 from arachidonic acid. LTB4 levels are elevated in psoriatic plaques, promote infiltration by leukocytes via chemotaxis, and enhance proliferation of keratinocytes.

Omega-3s suppress lymphocyte proliferation, CD4 cells, antigen presentation, adhesion molecule presentation, Th1 and Th2 responses, and proinflammatory cytokine production (e.g., IL-1, TNF-α, and PDGF), which prevents vascularization within psoriatic plaque.

- Cellular free arachidonic acid and 12-hydroxyeicosatetraenoic acid (HETE) (product of lipoxygenase metabolism of arachidonic acid) are 250 and 810 times greater, respectively, than in uninvolved epidermal tissue. A tissue-intrinsic unidentified inhibitor of cyclooxygenase is involved.

- Trauma releases free arachidonic acid. Plaques arise at sites of repeated trauma. Increased 12-HETE stimulates 5-lipoxygenase, promoting leukotriene formation. This pathway is inhibited by EPA and glutathione peroxidase (GP); selenium (Se) deficiency may contribute (see later in the section on individual nutrients).
- Cyclooxygenase inhibitors (aspirin, nonsteroidal anti-inflammatory drugs) may exacerbate psoriasis. Lipoxygenase inhibitors (benoxaprofen) may improve psoriasis. Natural substances (quercetin, ubiquitous plant flavonoid), vitamin E, onion, and garlic inhibit lipoxygenase. However, it is improbable that selective inhibition of one component or enzyme (e.g., a 5-lipoxygenase inhibitor) would do more than create an imbalance in this closely integrated network of mediators, which may not necessarily be beneficial.
- Arachidonic acid is found only in animal tissues; limit intake of animal fats and dairy. Diet, fasting, and food allergy control: psoriasis is positively linked to body mass index and inversely related to intake of carrots, tomatoes, fresh fruits, and index of beta-carotene intake. Fasting and vegetarian regimens help psoriatics, probably because of decreased gut-derived toxins and polyamines. Gluten-free and elimination diets are beneficial.

Individual Nutrients

- Decreased vitamin A and zinc, which are critical to skin health, are common in psoriasis.
- Chromium is indicated to increase insulin receptor sensitivity; psoriatics have increased serum insulin and glucose.
- Folate, B_6, and B_{12}: psoriasis is an independent risk factor for cardiovascular disease—whether risk factors are caused by psoriasis or share common pathogenesis. Inflammation, with proinflammatory cytokines and endothelial activation, is a common theme. Dyslipidemia, coronary calcification, increased highly sensitive C-reactive protein, decreased folate, and hyperhomocysteinemia are more common in psoriatics. Deficits of omega-3s, folate, and vitamin B_{12} are also found in cardiovascular disease. High homocysteine and low folate correlate with the Psoriasis Area and Severity Index (PASI) score. The rapid keratinocyte turnover in psoriasis may overconsume folate, inducing deficiency. To supplement folic acid or its active form 5-methyltetrahydrofolate, the recommended dose is 1 to 5 mg/day.

- GP is low in psoriatics, possibly because of alcohol abuse, malnutrition, and excess skin loss of hyperproliferation. GP is normalized with oral Se and vitamin E. Low concentrations in whole-blood Se are common in psoriasis. Lowest levels of whole-blood Se are found in male patients with widespread disease of long duration requiring methotrexate and retinoids.
- Active vitamin D (1,25-dihydroxycholecalciferol): patients with disseminated psoriasis have significantly lower serum levels of biologically active vitamin D compared with controls. Keratinocytes in the epidermis convert 7-dehydrocholesterol to vitamin D_3 in the presence of ultraviolet B (UVB). Sunlight, UVB phototherapy, oral calcitriol, and topical vitamin D and its analogues are effective therapy for psoriasis owing to vitamin D's antiproliferative and prodifferentiating actions on keratinocytes. Vitamin D analogues (e.g., calcipotriol) mediate expression of proinflammatory antimicrobial peptides (e.g., beta-defensin) and decrease IL-17A, IL-17F, and IL-8 in psoriatic lesions. Topical calcitriol reduces the number of dendritic cells in skin. Calcitriol binding to vitamin D receptors (VDRs) in skin modulates expression of many genes, including cell-cycle regulators, growth factors, and their receptors. Polymorphisms of *VDR* gene are linked to psoriasis and may predispose to its onset and resistance to calcipotriol therapy and may promote liver dysfunction in psoriatics. Recommendations for sun protection and skin cancer prevention may need to be reevaluated to allow for sufficient vitamin D status. However, studies conducted in Honolulu, Miami, and southern Arizona showed that abundant sun exposure does not ensure vitamin D adequacy. Vitamin D supplements may be needed nonetheless for adequate levels and to protect skin from sun damage and skin cancer. Administer vitamin D according to the dose that is necessary for patients to achieve adequate blood levels, which may require oral intake up to 5000 or 10,000 international units (IU) daily.
- Fumaric acid: oral dimethyl fumaric acid (240 mg q.d.) or monoethyl fumaric acid (720 mg q.d.) and topical 1% to 3% monoethyl fumaric acid are useful, but side effects (flushing of skin, nausea, diarrhea, malaise, gastric pain, mild liver and kidney disturbances) can occur. Use only if other natural therapies fail.

Psychological Aspects

Thirty-nine percent of psoriatics report specific stressful event within 1 month before initial episode. Such patients have better prognosis. Correlation occurs mostly in patients with repeated stressors four times or more in 1 year. Stress management can be beneficial. Listening to guided meditation tapes while undergoing phototherapy (UVB; and psoralen plus ultraviolet A [PUVA]) cleared lesions four times as quickly compared with phototherapy alone, based on three-part assessment: direct inspection by unblinded nurses, direct inspection by physicians blinded to patients' study group, and blinded physician evaluation of photographs of lesions. Psychotherapy is essential for patients with persistent unresolved psychological issues (e.g., anxiety, depression, and emotional stress of skin disease). A few cases have been successfully treated with hypnosis and biofeedback alone.

Physical Therapeutics

- Sunlight (ultraviolet light) is extremely beneficial. Outdoor 4-week heliotherapy promotes significant clearance of symptoms in 84% of subjects. Nonprescription commercial tanning beds have improved psoriasis severity and health-related quality of life. Combining retinoid acitretin (vitamin A derivative) with a 4- to 5-day per week tanning regimen induced complete or near complete recovery in 83% of 23 subjects. Specific UV exposure induces vitamin D synthesis in skin. The standard medical treatment is PUVA therapy at 320 to 340 nm. UVB (280 to 320 nm) alone inhibits cell proliferation and is as effective as PUVA with fewer side effects. UVB is the dominant light at the Dead Sea, where psoriasis in 80% to 85% of patients clears in 4 weeks. More study is needed to clarify risks, benefits, and specific UV therapy for varying presentations of psoriasis. UV deactivates vitamin D topicals; apply topicals only after UV treatment. Monitor light therapy carefully, especially in those at risk for skin cancer.
- Induction of elevation of temperature (42°C-45°C) to affected area by ultrasound and heating pads can be effective. Researchers have used hypotonic sulfate water (Leopoldine water) in a baleotherapeutic manner, yielding favorable immunohistologic profiles of affected tissues: decreased numbers of T lymphocytes, Langerhans cells, and markers of keratinocyte inflammation.

Topical Treatments

Botanical alternatives to hydrocortisone: glycyrrhetinic acid from licorice *(Glycyrrhiza glabra)*, chamomile *(Matricaria chamomilla)*, and capsaicin from cayenne pepper *(Capsicum frutescens)*.

- *Aloe vera:* topical extract in hydrophilic cream, applied three times daily, is highly effective in psoriasis vulgaris. It was well tolerated by all patients studied over 4 to 12 months of treatment, with no adverse drug-related symptoms and no dropouts.
- Curcumin gel: yielded 90% resolution of plaques in 50% of patients within 2 to 6 weeks; the remainder showed 50% to 85% improvement. Curcumin is twice as effective as calcipotriene cream (which takes 3 months for full effect). Curcumin is a selective phosphorylase kinase inhibitor, reducing inflammation by inhibiting nuclear factor kappa B (NF-κB). *Mahonia aquifolium:* topical cream, applied twice daily for 12 weeks, has proven effective in several open and placebo-controlled trials. Physician and patient assessments indicate that 71% to 81% of patients improved.
- Topical vitamin D: topical corticosteroids are commonly used to treat psoriasis; but with long-term side effects. Topical vitamin D modulators inhibit keratinocyte proliferation, normalize differentiation, and modulate immune cell activity with minimal effect on serum calcium. Calcipotriene is the most widely used. It is almost as effective as corticosteroids but not as quickly and may induce cutaneous irritation, especially on sensitive skin. Calcitriol ointment contains the naturally occurring active form of vitamin D3 and has fewer adverse effects. Topical nicotinamide: inhibits proinflammatory cytokines (IL-12, IL-23, and TNF-α), enhancing the efficacy of calcipotriene when used in combination.
- Emollients: help scaliness of psoriasis. Intercellular lipids (ceramides) help regulate homeostasis of skin water barrier and skin water-holding capacity. Ceramides are deficient in psoriatic epidermis. Newer ceramide-containing emollients (e.g., CeraVe, Mimyx, Aveeno Eczema Care) may improve skin barrier function and decrease water loss.

THERAPEUTIC APPROACH

Decrease bowel toxemia; rebalance fatty acid and inflammatory processes in skin; use therapeutic regimen to further balance abnormal cell proliferation.

- **Diet:** limit sugar, meat, animal fats, and alcohol. Increase dietary fiber and cold-water fish. Normalize weight. Eliminate gluten in gluten-sensitive patients. Identify and address food allergies.
- **Supplements:**
  — High-potency multiple vitamin-mineral formula
  — Fish oils: 3000 mg EPA plus DHA q.d.
  — Vitamin D: 5000 to 10,000 IU q.d. based on serum 25(OH)D level.
  — Vitamin E (mixed tocopherols): 400 IU q.d.
  — Chromium: 400 mcg q.d.
  — Se: 200 mcg q.d.
  — Zinc: 30 mg q.d.
- **Consider digestive enzymes and/or bile acids with meals.**
  — Water-soluble fiber (psyllium, pectin, guar gum): 5 g at bedtime.
- **Botanical medicines:**

Consider the following if indicated by impaired digestion or liver function:

  — *H. canadensis* (goldenseal): dose based on berberine content; standardized extracts three times daily are preferred—dried root or as infusion (tea), 2 to 4 g; fluid extract (1:1), 2 to 4 mL (0.5 to 1 tsp); solid (powdered dried) extract (4:1 or 8% to 12% alkaloid content), 250 to 500 mg
  — *Smilax* sarsaparilla (three times daily): dried root or by decoction, 1 to 4 g; liquid extract (1:1), 8 to 16 mL (2 to 4 tsp); solid extract (4:1), 250 to 500 mg
  — *S. marianum* (milk thistle): silymarin, 70 to 210 mg t.i.d.
- **Psychological: evaluate stress levels and use stress reduction techniques as appropriate.**
- **Physical medicine:**
  — Sunbathing: avoid becoming sunburned.
  — UVB: 295 to 305 nm, 2 mW/cm^2, 3 minutes, three times per week
- **Topical treatment:**
  — *Aloe vera*, curcumin, *M. aquifolium,* or vitamin D. Apply to affected areas b.i.d. or t.i.d.
  — Ceramide-containing emollient b.i.d. or t.i.d.

Rheumatoid Arthritis

DIAGNOSTIC SUMMARY

- Insidious onset of chronic, severe joint pain and inflammation.
- Polyarticular and symmetrical bilaterally.
- Begins in small joints and progresses to other joints.
- Systemic disease: fatigue, low-grade fever, weakness, weight loss, joint stiffness, and vague joint pain preceding painful, swollen joints by weeks or months.
- Extra-articular manifestations: vasculitis, subcutaneous and systemic granulomas, pleurisy, pericarditis, pulmonary fibrosis, lymphadenopathy, splenomegaly, anemia. Serum is usually positive for rheumatoid factor (RF) and/or anti–cyclic citrullinated peptide (anti-CCP) antibodies; but no single laboratory test is diagnostic.

GENERAL CONSIDERATIONS

Rheumatoid arthritis (RA) is the most common form of polyarthritis and is a chronic inflammatory condition affecting the entire body but especially synovial membranes of joints. Joints involved include the hands, feet, wrists, ankles, and knees. RA affects 0.3% to 1.0% of the population. Women outnumber men by 3:1. Age of onset is 40 to 50 years, but it may begin at any age. Onset is usually gradual but occasionally quite abrupt. Joints with greatest ratio of synovium to articular cartilage are most affected: knees, ankles, feet, wrists, and hands. Any joints may be affected eventually; however, distal interphalangeal joints are generally spared. Although confined to one or a few joints in one third of patients, initial presentation is often polyarticular and bilaterally symmetrical—both hands, both wrists, or both ankles. Affected joints are warm, tender, and swollen with prolonged morning stiffness. As RA progresses, bony erosion, subluxations, dislocations, and contractures develop, causing joint deformities, particularly in hands and feet. RA of the cervical spine dangerously destabilizes the atlantoaxial joint, risking spinal cord compression. Joint destruction

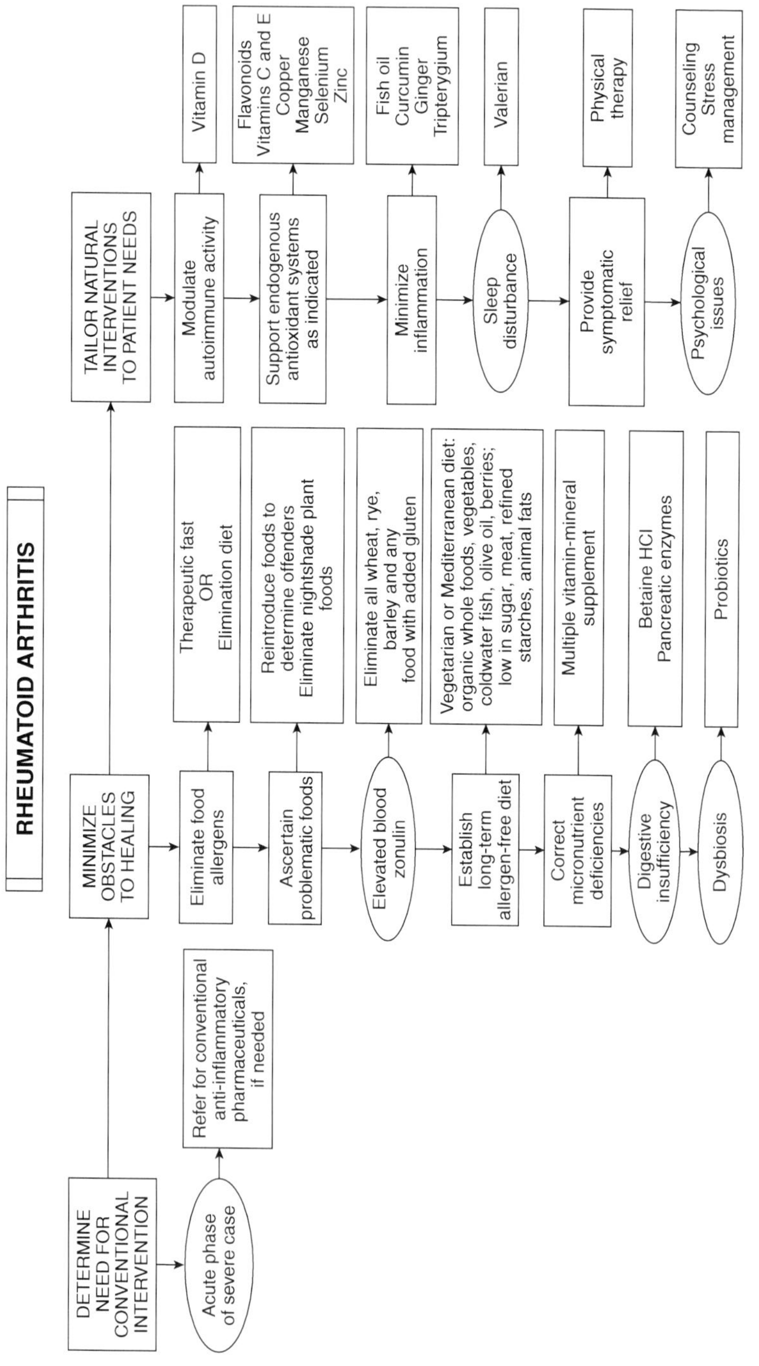

RHEUMATOID ARTHRITIS

DETERMINE NEED FOR CONVENTIONAL INTERVENTION

- Acute phase of severe case → Refer for conventional anti-inflammatory pharmaceuticals, if needed

MINIMIZE OBSTACLES TO HEALING

- Eliminate food allergens → Therapeutic fast OR Elimination diet
- Ascertain problematic foods → Reintroduce foods to determine offenders; Eliminate nightshade plant foods
- Elevated blood zonulin → Eliminate all wheat, rye, barley and any food with added gluten
- Establish long-term allergen-free diet → Vegetarian or Mediterranean diet: organic whole foods, vegetables, coldwater fish, olive oil, berries; low in sugar, meat, refined starches, animal fats
- Correct micronutrient deficiencies → Multiple vitamin-mineral supplement
- Digestive insufficiency → Betaine HCl; Pancreatic enzymes
- Dysbiosis → Probiotics

TAILOR NATURAL INTERVENTIONS TO PATIENT NEEDS

- Modulate autoimmune activity → Vitamin D
- Support endogenous antioxidant systems as indicated → Flavonoids; Vitamins C and E; Copper; Manganese; Selenium; Zinc
- Minimize inflammation → Fish oil; Curcumin; Ginger; Tripterygium
- Sleep disturbance → Valerian
- Provide symptomatic relief → Physical therapy
- Psychological issues → Counseling; Stress management

and immunosuppressive drugs predispose RA patients to septic arthritis, with a mortality rate as high as 11.5%. Such a case must not be confused with a flare of RA.

Pathogenesis

RA is far from idiopathic; it is multifactorial. An autoimmune reaction is a factor—antibodies against components of joint tissues. However, genetic, environmental, and immunologic factors contribute.

- **Genetic factors in susceptibility and disease expression:** female gender and positive family history are risk factors. There is a 15% concordance rate in monozygotic twins—four times that in dizygotic twins. There is a "shared epitope" in HLA-DR1 and HLA-DR4 subtypes in 80% of whites with RA. HLA-DRB1 and other factors might be linked to more-aggressive disease by affecting antioxidant, detoxification, and other processes that contribute to RA pathogenesis. Patients with RA also have undesirable fecal flora that may worsen pathogenesis (see later discussion). The flora of monozygotic twins is more similar than that of dizygotic twins, independent of other factors.
- **Environmental factors:** low penetrance in genetic studies indicates that environmental factors are contributory. Toxins in cigarette smoke interact with HLA-DRB1 shared epitope alleles, enhancing inflammation and increasing risk of seropositive RA. Smokers' RA risk is eightfold for carriers of shared epitope and sixteenfold for homozygous individuals. Smoking increases RA risk in general, threefold for men; and quitting decreases risk of seropositive disease. Low socioeconomic status increases morbidity and mortality in RA. Other factors (e.g., poor diet, drinking more than three cups of coffee daily, silicate exposure, and psychological factors) may affect levels of pain and physical disability. Contraceptives, tea intake, and increased vitamin D consumption might be protective. Other environmental factors (e.g., low temperature, high atmospheric pressure, and high humidity) correlate with increased RA pain.
- **Oxidative stress:** RA risk is highest in people with the lowest levels of nutrient antioxidants. Patients with both systemic lupus erythematosus (SLE) and RA have lower serum alpha-tocopherol, beta-carotene, and retinol than matched controls. Low antioxidant levels might be exacerbated by genetic factors; the shared epitope leads to increased nitrous oxide production and inhibition of antioxidative cellular pathways. Consequent

oxidative stress can produce free radical damage of DNA and mutations that may contribute to RA pathogenesis, which includes elevated synovial free radicals that accelerate inflammation and joint destruction.

- **Abnormal antibodies and immune complexes:** serum and joint fluid of nearly all RA patients contain RF and anti-CCP antibodies, contributing to pathogenesis. Serum titers often correlate with severity of symptoms and prognosis, but not in every case. The antibodies are not directly responsible for joint destruction. Autoantibodies may manifest 10 years before onset of clinical disease. Inflammatory markers (e.g., soluble tumor necrosis factor receptor 2) can be elevated 12 years before diagnosis and positively correlated with RA incidence. This suggests a "multiple hit" model: pathogenesis progresses in distinct stages, perhaps explaining why autoantibodies manifest years before clinical symptoms.
- **Microbial influences:** infection and cross-reactivity—the onset of RA is preceded by a specific inciting event (e.g., infection) in 8% to 15% of cases. Antimicrobials (e.g., metronidazole, clotrimazole, acyclovir, roxithromycin, tetracycline, sulfasalazine, and minocycline) have improved symptoms and in some cases induced complete remission. Many pathogens (e.g., Epstein-Barr virus, cytomegalovirus, parvovirus, rubella virus, *Mycoplasma,* amebic organisms, *Escherichia coli,* influenza AH2N2, *Porphyromonas,* and *Proteus*) are associated with RA. Although no single microbe has been consistently isolated in RA patients, a multitude of organisms might directly or indirectly induce pathogenesis by infection, antigen persistence, circulating immune complexes, or immune cross-reactivity. Reactive arthritis occurs secondary to an enteric, urogenital, or respiratory infection by a dozen different microbes in genetically susceptible persons and persists well beyond—or occurs even in the absence of—any clinically evident infection. The condition becomes chronic in 15% to 60% of cases. Some organisms (e.g., parvovirus B19) commonly produce RA-like arthritis and autoantibodies, including RF and antinuclear antibody (ANA), which may be positive in early infection. Although most patients clear the infection, chronic forms occur in up to 20% of cases, wherein viral DNA is recoverable from a variety of tissues for years postinfection. Thus RA development could be driven by chronic infection and/or persistence of parvovirus B19 antigens. Other pathogens (e.g., *Proteus mirabilis*) induce cross-reactive antibodies, elevated

in 90% of patients with active RA and positively correlated with markers of disease activity: erythrocyte sedimentation rate (ESR), C-reactive protein (CRP), and RF. These antibodies are homologous with type XI collagen found in hyaline cartilage; their immune complexes are present in synovia of RA patients. Other microbes inducing collagen cross-reactive antibodies are *Campylobacter, Salmonella,* and *Shigella.* Microbes inducing antibodies cross-reactive to other joint tissues are *Klebsiella pneumoniae, Proteus vulgaris,* and *Yersinia enterocolitica.*

- **Dysbiosis and small intestinal bacterial overgrowth (SIBO):** more important than specific pathogens is the subtler influence of commensal intestinal microflora. There are far more gut microflora than human cells in the body. The prevalence of hundreds of microbial species is affected by genetics, medical treatment, diet, and stress. Flora profoundly influence immune function, nutritional status, and stress response and affect many diseases. *Bacteroides thetaiotaomicron,* normal in humans, has an unexpected breadth of influence on intestinal function (e.g., improved nutrient absorption and processing, mucosal barrier fortification, influx of immunoglobulin A [IgA]–producing B cells, prevention of inflammatory response, and complement-mediated mucosal damage). Also affected are xenobiotic metabolism, neurotransmitter production, the enteric nervous system, gut motility, angiogenesis, and postnatal intestinal maturation. Many of these intestinal functions affect pathogenesis of RA. Fecal flora are significantly altered in RA (e.g., less bifidobacteria and *Bacteroides-Porphyromonas-Prevotella* group). Clinical improvement occurs with changes in microflora. Moreover, many RA patients (approximately 51%) have SIBO. The degree of SIBO correlates with the severity of symptoms and disease activity. Multifocal dysbiosis entails alteration in microflora not confined to the gut and cumulatively inducing immune dysregulation typical of autoimmunity. The concept of total pathogen burden correlates with increased CRP and cardiovascular risk and may contribute to pathogenesis of RA. Evidence to support this concept arises in patients with concurrent RA and periodontal disease—identical periodontal bacterial DNA in 100% of synovial fluid samples and 83.5% of serum samples of RA patients. In addition, severity of periodontitis correlates well with severity of RA symptoms. Antibodies to *Porphyromonas gingivalis* are linked to elevated anti-CCP antibodies and perhaps to breaking immune tolerance to citrullinated antigens and promoting the autoimmune response in RA.

- **Adverse food reactions:** about 10% of the population have food allergies. Consumption of allergenic foods is associated with elevated inflammatory markers (e.g., tumor necrosis factor-alpha [TNF-α], interleukin 1β [IL-1β], CRP, and ESR). Outcomes of food allergy studies in RA have been conflicting—allergen challenges were too small in quantity, frequency, or both, and serum antibody levels are not representative of mucosal immune response in the intestine. Furthermore, adverse food reactions (e.g., food intolerance, sensitivity, and dietary lectins) are not antibody mediated and thus are not apparent with antibody testing. Nevertheless, these reactions might be contributory. There is a positive correlation between RA and food allergies in 20% to 40% of patients. Although serum food antibodies do not correlate with RA, jejunal IgA, IgG, and IgM are elevated against nearly all food antigens in RA patients compared with controls, with cross-reactive antibodies. RA patients may have multiple modest hypersensitivity reactions, and the additive effect can lead to widespread antibody-mediated tissue destruction.
- **Xenobiotics and autoantibody production:** xenobiotics intersect with genetics, pathogenic organisms, and other dietary and environmental factors to stimulate autoantibody production and autoimmunity. Impaired metabolism of xenobiotics in acetylation pathways worsens the problem. A single genetic risk factor—the *N*-acetyltransferase 2 polymorphism—affects both acetylation of xenobiotics and susceptibility to RA. It also predicts disease severity: the slow-acetylator genotype involves 4.39 times greater risk of erosive RA than fast types. Other problematic toxins: bacterial toxins (e.g., streptokinase) and heat-shock proteins can bind to mucosal tissue enzymes and stimulate autoantibody production against peptides and tissue antigens. A similar response with gliadin peptides illustrates that food antigens can elicit responses comparable to bacterial superantigens. Streptokinase, gliadin, casein (a milk protein), and ethyl mercury (vaccine adjuvant in thimerosal) bind to lymphocyte receptors and tissue antigens, producing neoantigens that can induce production of cross-reactive autoantibodies.
- **Abnormal bowel permeability:** RA patients have increased intestinal permeability to dietary and bacterial antigens plus alterations in bowel flora. Chronic gut inflammation can increase intestinal permeability and is associated with joint inflammation. Adverse food reactions and bacterial endotoxins

may contribute greatly to chronic gut inflammation. Nonsteroidal anti-inflammatory drugs (NSAIDs), used to treat RA, can exacerbate hyperpermeability. This "leaky gut" facilitates the translocation of dietary and gut-derived antigens and bacterial gut flora to blood, mesenteric lymph nodes, the spleen, and the kidneys. In conjunction with dysbiosis and bacterial overgrowth, increased gut permeability to bacterial endotoxins and food antigens can produce immune activation and circulating immune complexes, many of which have been recovered in synovial fluid and could contribute to joint inflammation and degeneration. Newly emerging research is now showing that zonulin, released by the gliadin in gluten, is another cause of increased gut permeability in susceptible individuals. Those with haptoglobin type 1/2 produce modest amounts of zonulin after consumption of wheat, with increased gut permeability lasting about 1 hour. Those with haptoglobin type 2/2 release substantially more zonulin, with gut permeability typically lasting 3 hours after the consumption of wheat. RA is one of the autoimmune diseases shown to be associated with elevated blood zonulin levels.

- **Decreased androgen levels:** androgens and progesterone are natural immune suppressors involved in the apoptosis (cell suicide) of activated immune cells. Chronic deficits of testosterone and dehydroepiandrosterone (DHEA), an inhibitor of cytokines as a result of nuclear factor kappa B (NF-κB) inhibition, have been found in early and established RA. Testosterone replacement in male RA patients may decrease RF titers, the number of affected joints, and NSAID use. Although DHEA at 200 mg/day can be effective for SLE, DHEA has not proven effective for RA at the same dose. DHEA and testosterone may have to be modulated in concert with estrogens to be optimally effective in RA. Chronic inflammation and elevated TNF-α promote conversion of testosterone to estrogen by stimulating aromatase activity. Reduced androgen/estrogen ratio is common in both male and female RA patients.
- **Abnormal estrogen levels:** unlike androgens, estrogens may sustain inflammatory activity of activated T cells and humoral immunity. Estradiol levels are higher in RA patients than controls and are strongly and positively linked to indexes of inflammation. Gender is a major predictor of remission in early RA. Women have a lower androgen/estrogen ratio and, at 2 and 5 years, have more-severe disease and 16% to 22% fewer remissions than men.

DIAGNOSIS

The most commonly used criteria for diagnosing RA were issued by the American College of Rheumatology (ACR) in 1987; but they are low in sensitivity and specificity, especially in early disease. Earlier diagnosis allows earlier and aggressive treatment with better outcomes. Thus the ACR joined the European League Against Rheumatism to create new guidelines classifying definite RA based on the presence of synovitis in at least one joint, with no alternative explanation, and a score of 6 or greater in a four-tier rubric (see Section 6, Table 205-1 in Textbook).

Laboratory Findings

- **RF:** RF is a group of antibodies (IgM) that bind the Fc fragment of IgG. Although RF is present in 70% to 80% of RA patients, a variety of conditions can elevate RF, and 4% of apparently healthy persons test RF positive. Despite relatively low sensitivity and specificity of RF, its presence is confirmatory in diagnosing RA. Seropositivity is also associated with worse outcomes.
- **Anti-CCP antibodies:** much more-specific indicator of RA than RF and better predictor of clinical course. Sensitivity of anti-CCP antibodies is similar to that of RF (70% to 80%), but specificity exceeds 95%. These autoantibodies and RF have been identified 10 years before diagnosis. Their presence heralds more-aggressive disease and poorer prognosis. No single laboratory test is definitive for diagnosing RA. Patients can be seropositive for anti-CCP, RF, both, or neither.
- **ESR and CRP:** ESR and CRP are acute-phase reactants elevated during active inflammation. Although not specific to RA, they confirm diagnosis and monitor disease activity and response to treatment. Because RA patients are at increased risk for cardiovascular disease, CRP is a useful marker of cardiovascular risk as well.
- **Serum zonulin:** will be elevated in those with gliadin sensitivity, indicating that wheat, rye, and barley need to be scrupulously avoided.
- **Other laboratory abnormalities:** anemia is common—normocytic and normochromic or hypochromic. Decreased erythropoiesis is common in chronic inflammatory conditions. Serum iron (Fe) level and total Fe-binding capacity usually are low, but Fe supplements are of no value and may actually promote free radical damage. Because serum ferritin is an acute phase reactant,

Fe stores may appear falsely elevated in RA when ESR and/or CRP is elevated. ANAs may be present but at lower levels than in SLE. Joint aspiration is not necessary to diagnose RA but may be necessary to rule out crystalline arthropathies or septic arthritis.

- **Other diagnostic testing:** other conditions can mimic RA; these must be ruled out—vitamin D deficiency, hemochromatosis, hypothyroidism, and infections (e.g., Lyme disease and hepatitis B and C). Other tests to consider include the following:
  - — Hormone profiles: DHEA-S, testosterone, estradiol
  - — Food allergies (*Textbook,* "Food Allergies")
  - — Lactulose-mannitol test (*Textbook,* "Intestinal Permeability Assessment")
  - — Hydrogen-methane breath test (*Textbook,* "Bacterial Overgrowth of the Small Intestine Breath Test")
  - — Stool testing for digestive function and intestinal flora (*Textbook,* "Biomarkers for Stool Analysis")
  - — Urine testing (*Textbook,* "Urinary Organic Acids Profiling for Assessment of Functional Nutrient Deficiencies, Gut Dysbiosis, and Toxicity")
  - — Toxicity assessment (*Textbook,* "Functional Toxicology")

THERAPEUTIC CONSIDERATIONS

RA is a multifactorial condition that requires a comprehensive therapeutic approach addressing all the factors known to be involved in the inflammatory disease process. Foremost in this approach is the use of diet.

Diet

Population studies have demonstrated that RA is less common in societies that favor a more-primitive diet and is found at higher rates in societies consuming the Western diet. A diet rich in whole foods, vegetables, and fiber and low in sugar, meat, refined carbohydrates, saturated fat, and additives is protective against RA as well as holding promise for its treatment.

Adverse Food Reactions

Elimination of reactive foods can benefit some RA patients. The most common triggers: corn (56%), wheat (54%); bacon and pork (39%); oranges (39%); milk and oats (37%); rye (34%); egg, beef, and coffee (32%); malt (27%); cheese and grapefruit (24%); tomato

(22%); peanuts and cane sugar (20%); butter, lamb, soy, and lemon (17%). Nineteen percent of participants who avoided their reactive foods thereafter remained well without medication for up to 5 years. Dietary elimination and challenge can individualize identification of triggering foods.

Therapeutic Fasting

Patients with RA benefit from fasting. Short-term fasting for 3 to 5 days during acute flares reduces joint pain, swelling, and morning stiffness. It obviously eliminates reactive foods. Fasting increases serum DHEA-S and decreases serum IL-6, CRP, ESR, and disease activity. Fasting modulates intestinal permeability. Juice, broth, and water fasts of longer duration, up to 10 days, are also effective. Strict water fasting should be done only under direct medical supervision (*Textbook,* "Fasting").

Vegetarian Diet

Start with 7- to 10-day fast before transition to vegetarian diet. Fast components are herbal teas; garlic; vegetable broth; a decoction of potatoes and parsley; and carrot, beet, and celery juices. Follow with systematic reintroduction of a single food item every 2 days with elimination of foods that aggravated symptoms. Beyond allergen elimination, vegetarian diets increase fiber intake, improve gut flora, decrease antibodies to *P. mirabilis,* reduce SIBO, improve RA symptoms, increase potassium intake (which may improve biosynthesis and release of cortisol), improve fatty acid profile, and increase antioxidant intake.

The Mediterranean Diet

RA patients experience reduced inflammation, increased physical function and improved vitality after 12 weeks on a Mediterranean diet—a vegetarian diet plus fish, poultry, low to moderate use of red meat, dairy, red wine, and olive oil as the main lipid source. Although pasta and bread are commonly consumed in the Mediterranean diet, all wheat, rye and barley products should be avoided on a trial basis.

Dietary Antioxidants

Continuous production of free radicals within arthritic joints promotes joint degeneration, exhausts antioxidant systems, and worsens antioxidant deficits common in RA. Emphasize fresh fruit and vegetable sources of antioxidants. Antioxidants work synergistically. Single antioxidants can be helpful, but RA patients benefit from antioxidant-rich diets. Vegetarian and Mediterranean diets are rich in antioxidants.

Nutritional Supplements

- **Gamma-linolenic acid (GLA):** evening primrose oil (EPO), blackcurrant oil, and borage oil contain GLA, an omega-6 fatty acid and precursor to anti-inflammatory prostaglandins of 1-series, especially if omega-3 fatty acids are taken concurrently. An effective dose of GLA is 1.4 g/day. Two recent reviews found statistically significant improvements in pain and global function for GLA from data pooled from three randomized controlled trials. Conclusions in favor of GLA were even stronger than those for fish oil.
- **Omega-3 fatty acids:** rich sources of omega-3s are cold-water fish and flaxseed oil. Flaxseed oil alpha-linolenic acid (ALA) is converted to eicosapentaenoic acid (EPA) and docosahexaenoic acid (DHA), especially in the presence of zinc (Zn), a cofactor for conversion enzyme delta-6 desaturase. A low–omega-6 diet supplemented with 13 g (about 1 tbsp) of flaxseed oil a day plus Zn raises tissue EPA levels to an extent comparable with the effects of fish oil. Flaxseed oil supplementation can inhibit the autoimmune reaction as well as fish oil. Fish oil bypasses ALA conversion by directly supplying preformed EPA and DHA. Fish oil competitively inhibits cyclooxygenase-2 (COX-2; expressed in RA synovium) and decreases long-term use of NSAIDs. Fish oil improves morning stiffness and results in fewer tender or swollen joints and less joint pain and fatigue; and it reduces serum markers of inflammation (e.g., CRP, IL-1β, TNF-α, and leukotriene B_4 [LTB_4]). Fish oil must be consumed for at least 12 weeks at a minimum daily dose of 3 g of combined EPA and DHA before effects become apparent. Fish oil may also decrease cardiovascular risk. Insist on fish oil products that have been laboratory certified for purity and potency. (For more information about fish oils, *Textbook*, "Fish Oils")

Multivitamin and Multimineral Supplementation

Blood and/or tissue samples from RA patients reveal deficiencies of many nutrients (e.g., magnesium, folate, vitamin B_{12}, vitamin B_6, Zn, and selenium [Se]). Causes include decreased intake, decreased absorption because of impaired gut function, increased use of antioxidants because of elevated oxidative stress, and increased excretion as a result of stress and medicines. Supplementing individual nutrients may not be effective, but a multifactorial condition such as RA requires a multifaceted approach. It appears reasonable, safe, and—at least hypothetically—efficacious to address multiple deficiencies of multiple nutrients simultaneously.

- **Dietary antioxidants:** fresh fruits and vegetables are the best sources of dietary antioxidants. Vitamin C, beta-carotene, vitamin E, Se, and Zn are well recognized as antioxidants. Flavonoids neutralize inflammation and support collagen structures. Risk of RA is highest in people with lowest levels of nutrient antioxidants (serum alpha-tocopherol, beta-carotene, and vitamin C).
- **Se and vitamin E:** Se is a mineral cofactor for glutathione peroxidase and thioredoxin reductase, especially important for reducing production of inflammatory prostaglandins and leukotrienes and controlling free radical damage. SE or vitamin E alone may not be effective, but Se and vitamin E together have a positive effect. Food sources of Se: Brazil nuts, fish, and whole grains. The amount of Se in grains and other plant foods is related to amount of Se in soil.
- **Zn:** antioxidant and cofactor in antioxidant enzyme superoxide dismutase (copper [Cu]-Zn SOD) and cofactor for delta-6-desaturase, the rate-limiting enzyme in omega-3 fatty acid metabolism. Zn deficiency is linked to poor conversion of ALA to EPA and DHA. Zn deficiency is common in RA patients. Plasma Zn levels are inversely correlated with ESR, CRP, IL-1β, and TNF-α. Patients using corticosteroids may be Zn deficient because steroids decrease plasma Zn and increase urinary Zn. Zn has slight therapeutic effect alone. Zn picolinate, monomethionine, or citrate forms are preferred. Foods rich in Zn are oysters, whole grains, nuts, and seeds.
- **Manganese (Mn) and SOD:** Mn functions in a different form of SOD. Mn-SOD is deficient in RA patients. Injectable form of enzyme (available in Europe) is effective in treating RA. However, it has not been demonstrated that oral SOD affects SOD levels in tissue. Oral Mn supplements do increase SOD activity. No clinical studies have been conducted to determine efficacy of Mn in RA. RA patients are low in Mn. Dietary sources are nuts, whole grains, dried fruits, and green leafy vegetables. Meats, dairy, poultry, and seafood are poor sources of Mn.
- **Vitamin C:** antioxidant. WBC and plasma ascorbate are significantly decreased in RA patients. Vitamin C supplements increase SOD activity and decrease histamine levels and provide

some anti-inflammatory effects. There is a negative correlation between plasma vitamin C levels and RA disease activity, as well as CRP. Food sources are broccoli, Brussels sprouts, cabbage, citrus fruits, tomatoes, and berries.

- **Pantothenic acid:** whole-blood pantothenic acid is lower in RA patients than in normal controls. Disease activity is inversely correlated with pantothenic acid levels. Correcting low pantothenic acid levels to normal improves duration of morning stiffness, degree of disability, and severity of pain. The clinical research dose has been 2 g of calcium pantothenate per day. Dietary sources: whole grains and legumes.
- **Pyridoxine (vitamin B_6):** low levels of blood pyridoxal-5-phosphate (P5P) are linked to inflammatory indicators of RA. Plasma B_6 levels are lower in patients with high ESR, high CRP, more disabilities, more pain and fatigue, and more swollen joints. Low B_6 is caused by ongoing chronic inflammatory processes. Homocysteine is increased in these B_6-deficient patients, increasing risk of cardiovascular disease. RA patients have increased risk for comorbidity and death from cardiovascular disease—left ventricular diastolic dysfunction, pulmonary hypertension, and first-time myocardial infarction.
- **Cu:** Cu aspirinate (salicylate) yields better results in reducing pain and inflammation than standard aspirin. Wearing of Cu bracelets is a long-time folk remedy. Cu is absorbed through the skin and is chelated to another compound able to exert anti-inflammatory action. Cu is a component (with Zn) in one type of SOD (Cu-Zn SOD). Deficiency may increase susceptibility to free radical damage. Excess intake of Cu is detrimental because of its ability to combine with peroxides and damage joint tissues.
- **Vitamin D:** actually a steroid hormone with immunoregulatory and anti-inflammatory properties. Vitamin D deficiency is linked epidemiologically to autoimmunity, including RA. Low serum $25(OH)D_3$ correlates with worse RA symptoms. High intake of vitamin D is linked to decreased RA risk. Vitamin D supports calcium metabolism. There might be a disturbance in vitamin D metabolism in RA that might play a role in RA-associated osteoporosis.
- **Pancreatic enzymes and hydrochloric acid:** impaired digestion from pancreatic enzyme and/or hydrochloric acid insufficiency, common in RA patients, can contribute to the disease process. Incompletely digested food molecules can be absorbed, stimulating immune response. Eighty percent of untreated RA

patients have reduced maximal gastric acid output. Gastric acid affects passive immunity, and hypochlorhydric or achlorhydric patients may be predisposed to SIBO. Half of RA hypochlorhydric patients also had SIBO. Restoration of gastric pH helps resolve the overgrowth. Pancreatic enzymes may offer additional benefits when taken between meals: pancreatin reduces circulating immune complexes in RA. Clinical improvements usually correspond with decreases in immune complexes. (*Textbook,* "Pancreatic Enzymes")

- **Probiotics:** modulate immunity. Commensal organisms interact with Toll-like receptors in the intestinal mucosa to promote immune tolerance and regulatory T-cell formation and block NF-κB, inflammation, and allergies. These effects in RA patients may be strain specific. *Lactobacillus rhamnosus* GG has not proven effective, but *Bacillus coagulans* GBI-30, 6080 can improve pain scale, patient global assessment, self-assessed disability, CRP, ability to walk 2 miles, and participation in daily activities. Probiotics, prebiotics, and/or antimicrobial compounds may be indicated in cases of dysbiosis and SIBO in addition to dietary modification. (*Textbook,* "Prebiotics, Synbiotics, and Colonic Foods" and "Probiotics")

Botanical Medicines

- ***Curcuma longa*** **(turmeric):** curcumin is a yellow pigment of *C. longa,* which exerts excellent anti-inflammatory and antioxidant effects. Curcumin is as effective as cortisone or phenylbutazone in models of acute inflammation but without side effects. Molecular targets include transcription factors (e.g., NF-κB, peroxisome proliferator-activated receptor gamma (PPAR-γ), enzymes (e.g., COX-2, 5-lipoxygenase [5-LOX]), and cytokines (e.g., TNF-α, IL-1, IL-6). Curcumin may enhance endogenous corticosteroid activity, perhaps through increased synthesis and/or release, potentiation of receptor sites, or slowing of catabolic pathways. It inhibits formation of leukotrienes and other mediators of inflammation. In models of chronic inflammation, curcumin is much less active in adrenalectomized animals, suggesting that it enhances the body's own anti-inflammatory mechanisms. Its beneficial effects in human studies are comparable to those of standard drugs but without side effects at recommended doses. In a postoperative inflammation model for NSAIDs, curcumin has comparable anti-inflammatory action to phenylbutazone. It does not possess direct analgesic action.

Turmeric or curcumin is beneficial in acute exacerbations of RA. Dose of curcumin—400 to 600 mg t.i.d.; turmeric dose—8000 to 60,000 mg. New products and methods help resolve absorption issues. One entails using piperine, found in black pepper. Curcumin is also complexed with soy phospholipids to produce Meriva, which enhances absorption fivefold. Studies with the advanced form of curcumin, Theracurmin, have shown even greater absorption—27 times greater than regular curcumin.

- **Bromelain:** mixture of enzymes in pineapple. It reduces inflammation in RA. Mechanisms: it inhibits proinflammatory compounds and activates compounds that break down fibrin matrix that obstructs tissue drainage and causes edema. Fibrin forms a matrix that isolates the area of inflammation. This results in blockage of blood vessels and inadequate tissue drainage and edema. Bromelain blocks inflammatory production of kinin compounds that increase swelling and pain. A proteolytic enzyme product containing bromelain, papain (from papaya), trypsin, and chymotrypsin (pancreatic enzymes) decreases serum transforming growth factor beta, linked with progression of joint destruction in RA.
- ***Zingiber officinale* (ginger):** has antioxidant effects. It inhibits prostaglandin, thromboxane, and leukotriene synthesis. Fresh ginger may be more effective in RA than dried preparations; fresh contains protease with anti-inflammatory action similar to bromelain. It substantially improves RA symptoms—pain relief, joint mobility, and decreased swelling and morning stiffness. Recommended dose: 500 to 1000 mg q.d. Some patients have taken three to four times this amount with quicker and better relief. Forms: 1 g of dried powdered ginger root. Average daily dietary dose: 8 to 10 g in India; fresh (or freeze-dried) ginger root at equivalent dose may be better because of a higher gingerol level and active protease. Daily dose of 2 to 4 g of dried powdered ginger may be effective; it is equivalent to 20 g (⅔ oz) fresh ginger root (½-inch slice). Incorporate it into fresh fruit and vegetable juices. No side effects are apparent at these levels.
- ***Tripterygium wilfordii* Hook F:** in Chinese medicine, thunder god vine is used for RA and other autoimmune diseases. Both leaf and root have anti-inflammatory, analgesic, and immunosuppressive effects that may ameliorate RA. In patients with longstanding RA in whom conventional therapy had failed, 80% of patients on high dose (380 mg/day) of ethanol/ethyl acetate root extract had at least 20% improvement. Forty percent of the

low-dose (180 mg/day) group also responded positively. Furthermore, 180 mg of *Tripterygium* extract per day is more effective than sulfasalazine 1 g twice a day. Side effects include gastrointestinal upset, diarrhea, headache, hair loss, menstrual abnormalities, and hypertension. There are fewer adverse reactions from sustained-release products, topicals, and coadministration with *Glycyrrhiza glabra* (licorice) root. Coadministration of *Tripterygium* with methotrexate may improve efficacy and decrease side effects compared with methotrexate alone.

- ***Valeriana officinalis*** **(valerian):** 54% to 70% of RA patients report sleep disruptions. Valerian is a sleep aid that decreases the time between going to bed and the first cycle of deep sleep in RA patients. Valerian is a sedative and anxiolytic that sensitizes gamma-aminobutyric acid (GABA) receptors and may also affect the actions of serotonin and adenosine. All RA patients have marked sleep disturbances; overwhelming fatigue in RA might be undiagnosed sleep disturbance. This fatigue is often ignored by doctors. Morning symptoms of RA correlate with nonrestorative sleep disorder. Inadequate sleep can lead to inflammation (e.g., increased CRP). CRP and sleep problems are inversely related to RA pain thresholds.

Physical Medicine

- **Exercise:** improves strength and performance and maintains range of motion (ROM). It decreases cardiovascular risk, RA disease activity, and systemic inflammation (e.g., reduced ESR). Begin with progressive, passive ROM and isometrics, gradually introducing active ROM and isotonic exercises. High-intensity, long-term exercise in RA: over a 2-year period, intensive exercise did not increase radiographic damage of large joints, except possibly in patients with considerable baseline damage. High-intensity exercise improved functionality and created better mood and sense of well-being.
- **Hydrotherapy:** heat helps relieve stiffness and pain, relax muscles, and increase ROM. Moist heat (e.g., moist packs, hot baths) is more effective than dry heat (e.g., heating pad). Use paraffin baths if skin irritation from regular water immersion develops. Cold packs help during acute flares or after hot applications.
- **Constitutional hydrotherapy:** use of alternating hot and cold applications to the torso and back in combination with electrical stimulation. This creates an alternating vasodilation and

vasoconstriction—a "vascular pump"—intended to improve circulation of blood through viscera, promote detoxification, and tone the nervous system. This therapy focuses on causative factors underlying RA.

Psychological Aspects

Optimistic RA patients report better psychosocial and physical functioning than pessimistic ones with passive coping strategies (e.g., staying in bed). Patients who believe they can control and decrease pain by using spiritual or religious coping methods have less joint pain and negative moods and have higher social support. Positive support from a spouse or other family member is inversely related to depression and enhances quality of life. Patients who lack support or have other challenges (e.g., abuse, somatization disorders, obsession-compulsion) rely on health care providers for these needs. See RA patients as individuals, not mere diagnoses, to be believed concerning their pain and suffering, and to have their subjective experience acknowledged. Establish a supportive and validating doctor-patient relationship. Counseling is appropriate as needed to explore coping with pain, self-esteem, negative feelings, reflections on the past, focus on recovery, support, and so on.

THERAPEUTIC APPROACH

RA often requires aggressive treatment. In mild to moderate RA, the measures outlined here are extremely effective. Foremost interventions are diet to avoid causes and ameliorate symptoms. Relieve symptoms with physical medicine, botanicals, and nutrients. In severe cases, NSAIDs may be necessary in the acute phase. Never abandon natural measures because they enhance efficacy of drugs, allowing for lower doses.

- **Diet:**
  - — First step: therapeutic fast or elimination diet.
  - — Second step: carefully reintroduce individual foods to detect those that trigger symptoms. Most problematic foods: wheat, corn, dairy, beef, nightshade foods (tomato, potato, eggplant, peppers), pork, citrus, oats, rye, egg, coffee, peanuts, cane sugar, lamb, and soy.
  - — Third step: After eliminating allergens, start vegetarian or Mediterranean diet of organic whole foods, vegetables, coldwater fish (mackerel, herring, sardines, salmon), olive oil, and berries; low in sugar, meat, refined starches, animal fats.

- **Supplements:**
  - — High-potency multiple vitamin-mineral formula
  - — Fish oils: 3000 mg combined EPA plus DHA q.d.
  - — Vitamin C: 500 to 1000 mg q.d.
  - — Se: 200 to 400 mcg q.d.
  - — Vitamin E (mixed tocopherols): 200 to 400 international units (IU) (mixed tocopherols) q.d.
  - — Vitamin D_3: 2000 to 4000 IU q.d.

  Choose one of the following:
  - — Grapeseed extract (greater than 95% procyanidolic oligomers): 100 to 300 mg q.d.
  - — Pine bark extract (greater than 95% procyanidolic oligomers): 100 to 300 mg q.d.
  - — Another flavonoid-rich extract, "super greens formula," or other plant-based antioxidant providing oxygen radical absorption capacity (ORAC) of 3000 to 6000 units or higher q.d.
  - — Probiotic (*Lactobacillus* and *Bifidobacterium* species): at least 5 to 10 billion colony forming units q.d.
  - — Pancreatin (10× United States Pharmacopeia [USP]), 350 to 750 mg between meals t.i.d.; or bromelain, 250 to 750 mg (1800 to 2000 milk clotting units [MCU]) between meals t.i.d.
- **Botanical medicines:**

The following botanicals may be used alone or in combination with others. Severe inflammation and joint destruction require more-aggressive therapy.
  - — Curcumin: Choose one of the following:
  - — Curcumin: 400 mg t.i.d. between meals
  - — Meriva: 1000 to 2000 mg q.d.
  - — Theracurmin: 600 to 1200 mg q.d.
  - — Ginger: 8 to 10 g of dried ginger or ginger extracts standardized to contain 20% gingerol and shogaol at a dose of 100 to 200 mg t.i.d.
  - — *T. wilfordii* Hook F: 360 to 570 mg q.d of ethyl acetate extract
  - — *V. officinalis:* 1.5 to 3 g of dried herb q.d.
- **Physical medicine:**
  - — Heat (moist packs, hot baths): 20 to 30 min q.d. to t.i.d.
  - — Cold packs for acute flare-ups
  - — Paraffin baths (if hot water causes skin irritation)

  - Active (or in severe cases, passive) ROM exercises: three to 10 repetitions q.d. to b.i.d.
  - Progressive isometric (and isotonic as joints improve) exercise: three to 10 repetitions several times per day with generous periods of rest
- **Counseling and psychological therapy**
  - Establish supportive and validating doctor-patient relationship.
  - Prioritize stress management.
  - Evaluate for depression and social support.
  - Work with spouses and family members, if possible.
- Attend to other issues based on clinical and laboratory findings: DHEA, testosterone, vitamin D, intestinal permeability, SIBO, dysbiosis, and environmental toxicity.

Rosacea

DIAGNOSTIC SUMMARY

- Chronic acneiform eruption on the face of middle-aged and older adults associated with facial flushing and telangiectasia.
- The acneiform component is characterized by papules, pustules, and seborrhea; the vascular component by erythema and telangiectasia; and the glandular component by hyperplasia of the soft tissue of the nose (rhinophyma).
- The primary involvement occurs over the flush areas of the cheeks and nose.

GENERAL CONSIDERATIONS

- Rosacea is a chronic skin disorder; the nose and cheeks are abnormally red and may be covered with pimples similar to acne (see the chapter on acne). It was originally called acne rosacea because inflammatory papules and pustules closely mimic acne vulgaris. Rosacea inflammation is vascular, occurs between ages 25 and 70 years, and is more common in people with fair complexions. It is more common in women (3:1) but more severe in men. Thirteen million Americans are affected.
- Rosacea is divided into three stages, but because progression does not necessarily occur, it is also often divided into four subtypes (erythematotelangiectatic, papulopustular, phymatous, and ocular):
  - Stage I—erythematotelangiectatic rosacea: erythema triggered by hot beverages, spicy foods, and alcohol may persist for hours; telangiectasia is noticeable on central third of face; and burning, stinging, and itching occur after application of cosmetics, fragrances, and sunscreens.
  - Stage II—inflammatory papules and pustules, or papulopustular rosacea: flushing, telangiectasia, and seborrhea increase; facial pore enlargement is minimal.
  - Stage III—phymatous rosacea: deep inflammatory nodules, large telangiectatic vessels, markedly dilated facial pores,

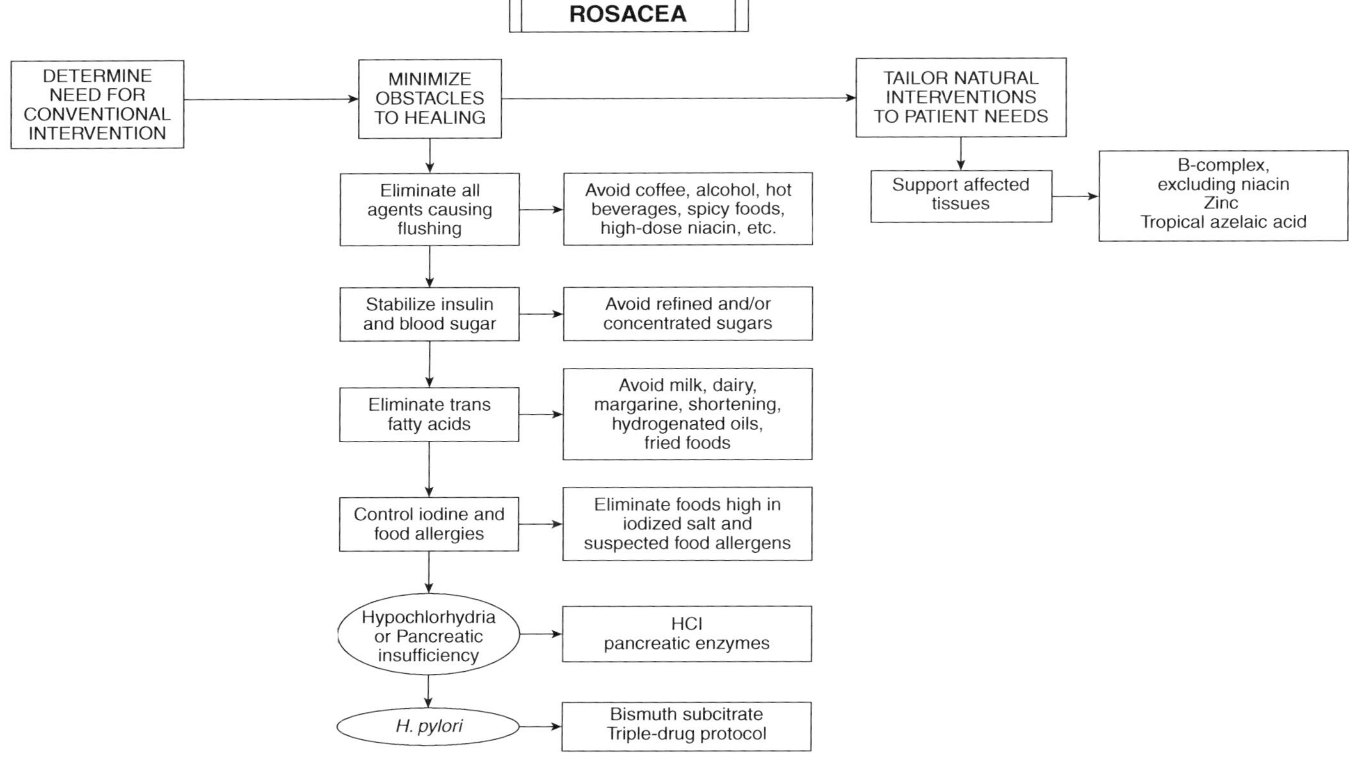
ROSACEA
DETERMINE NEED FOR CONVENTIONAL INTERVENTION
MINIMIZE OBSTACLES TO HEALING
TAILOR NATURAL INTERVENTIONS TO PATIENT NEEDS
Eliminate all agents causing flushing
Avoid coffee, alcohol, hot beverages, spicy foods, high-dose niacin, etc.
Support affected tissues
B-complex, excluding niacin
Zinc
Tropical azelaic acid
Stabilize insulin and blood sugar
Avoid refined and/or concentrated sugars
Eliminate trans fatty acids
Avoid milk, dairy, margarine, shortening, hydrogenated oils, fried foods
Control iodine and food allergies
Eliminate foods high in iodized salt and suspected food allergens
Hypochlorhydria or Pancreatic insufficiency
HCl
pancreatic enzymes
H. pylori
Bismuth subcitrate
Triple-drug protocol

and sebaceous gland hyperplasia and tissue hyperplasia, especially of nose (rhinophyma). Only a small number of cases progress to this stage.

- Ocular rosacea: spectrum of eye findings associated with skin problems. The eyes have a watery or bloodshot appearance, with sensation of foreign body, burning or stinging, dryness, itching, light sensitivity, or other signs and symptoms. Styes are a common sign of rosacea ocular disease. Some patients may have decreased visual acuity because of corneal complications.

Distinctions of rosacea flushing: prolonged nature and intensity. Nonrosacea flushing is evanescent flushing—occurs in response to embarrassment, exercise, or hot environments—and lasts from several seconds to a few minutes. Rosacea flushing typically lasts longer than 10 minutes, is more red than pink, with burning or stinging sensation. Triggering stimuli in rosacea flushing: acutely felt emotional stress, hot drinks, alcohol, spicy foods, exercise, cold or hot weather, hot baths or showers. However, some rosacea flushing episodes are without known stimuli.

Etiology

The cause of rosacea is poorly understood despite numerous theories. Causative factors suspected include the following:

- The mite *Demodex folliculorum*
- Alcoholism
- Menopausal flushing
- Vasomotor neurosis
- Seborrheic diathesis
- Local infection
- Food allergies
- B vitamin deficiencies
- Gastrointestinal disorders

Most patients display moderate to severe seborrhea, but sebum production is not increased in many. Vasomotor lability is prevalent; migraine headaches are three times more common than in matched control subjects.

- *Helicobacter pylori* infection in rosacea: increases vasoactive histamines, prostaglandins, leukotrienes, and cytokines. However, these mediators are found only with *H. pylori* strains that also produce specific cytotoxin—cytotoxin-associated gene A *(CagA)*. The presence of this *H. pylori* strain might be more etiologically important than other strains.

- Bottom line of rosacea etiology: because many implicated triggers are experienced by healthy persons who never develop symptoms or signs of rosacea, rosacea-prone individuals must have inherent sensitivity to these triggers.

THERAPEUTIC CONSIDERATIONS

- Avoid stimuli that exacerbate rosacea—exposure to extremes of heat and cold, excessive sunlight, ingestion of hot liquids, alcohol, spicy foods.
- Conventional treatment: oral tetracycline, especially for papular or pustular lesions; however, this treatment usually only controls rather than eradicates. Topical antibiotics or synthetic retinoids are less successful. Topical corticosteroids initially improve, but long-term therapy may actually lead to rosacea. Chronic skin changes and severe rhinophyma may require laser or surgical intervention, respectively.
- Natural approach: identify and eliminate contributing factors. Key factors: hypochlorhydria, eradication of *H. pylori,* elimination of food allergies, optimal intake of B vitamins.
  - Hypochlorhydria: gastric analysis of rosacea patients indicates hypochlorhydria. Psychological factors (worry, depression, stress) reduce gastric acidity. Hydrochloric acid supplements improve patients with achlorhydria or hypochlorhydria. Secretion of lipase also is decreased (bicarbonate and chymotrypsin are normal). Pancreatic supplements are beneficial.
  - *H. pylori:* high incidence of gastric *H. pylori* is found in rosacea patients. Flushing reaction in rosacea may be caused by gastrin or vasoactive intestinal peptides. Some histologically positive patients are serologically negative. Clinical success in treating rosacea with metronidazole and abatement of *H. pylori* isolates and serology after treatment provides evidence connecting rosacea with *H. pylori.* However, *H. pylori* might be associated with rosacea and not be causative; rosacea patients may have similar rates of *H. pylori* as do healthy subjects. Rosacea patients report "indigestion" more often and use more antacids than do individuals in the general population. Many studies confirm a strong link between *H. pylori* and rosacea and correlation between severity of rosacea and level of infection.
  - Food allergy: migraine headaches accompanying rosacea point to food intolerance, as does reflex flushing with vasodilator

substances. Rosacea might be a hypersensitivity disorder; dietary factors could exacerbate skin flushing.
— B vitamins: large doses of B vitamins are quite effective, with riboflavin (vitamin B_2) as key factor.

- Zinc: Supplementation is helpful in acne vulgaris and perhaps acne rosacea. At a dose of 23 mg zinc sulfate daily over a period of 6 months in placebo-controlled studies, zinc was found to be safe and effective and free of significant side effects.
- Topical azelaic acid (AzA): can be extremely effective in papulopustular rosacea. Initially, a 20% AzA cream proved effective for mild to moderate rosacea. A 15% AzA gel vastly improved delivery of AzA and proved superior to 20% AzA cream. It is equally as effective as metronidazole cream or gel. AzA decreases inflammatory lesion count and erythema severity better than placebo and is equal to metronidazole in papulopustular rosacea. However, AzA offers no significant decrease in severity of telangiectasia.
- Mite *D. folliculorum* is considered a factor, but it is a normal inhabitant of follicles. It may account for more-granulomatous response of some patients (researchers were able to infect skin of B_2-deficient rats with *Demodex,* but not skin of normal rats). Delayed hypersensitivity reaction in follicles is triggered by *D. folliculorum* antigens and stimulates progression of affection to papulopustular stage.
- Some patients' rosacea may be aggravated by large doses of these nutrients. Inflammation and exacerbations of acne related to vitamins B_2, B_6, and B_{12} are reported in European literature.

THERAPEUTIC APPROACH

Cause(s) are undetermined, but adequate treatment is possible for most patients. Eradicate *H. pylori* infection (when present). Control hypochlorhydria and food intolerance. Support with vitamin B complex and avoid vasodilating foods.

- General recommendations: see the chapter on acne.
- Treat *H. pylori* infection, if present. See the chapter on peptic ulcers.
- Diet: avoid coffee, alcohol, hot beverages, spicy foods, and any other food or drink causing flush. Eliminate refined and/or concentrated sugars, *trans* fatty acids (milk, milk products, margarine, vegetable shortening, synthetically hydrogenated vegetable oils, fried foods). Avoid foods high in iodized salt.

- Supplements:
  - Vitamin B complex: 100 mg q.d. (avoid niacin)
  - Pancreas extract (8× to 10× United States Pharmacopeia [USP]): 350 to 500 mg before meals
  - Hydrochloric acid (*Textbook,* "Hydrochloric Acid Supplementation: Patient Instructions")
- Zinc (prefer picolinate form): 60 to 75 mg/day for no more than 3 months, followed by 15 to 20 mg/day thereafter
- Topical AzA: application of 15% azelaic acid gel

Seborrheic Dermatitis

DIAGNOSTIC SUMMARY

- Branny or greasy scaling over erythematous skin patterned on sebum-rich areas of scalp, face, and trunk. Facial areas: forehead, eyebrows, eyelashes, nasolabial folds, beard. Truncal involvement: presternal region, umbilicus, axillae, inframammary and inguinal folds, and perineum.
- Scalp appearance varies from mild, patchy dandruff to widespread, thick, adherent crusts; may involve anterior and posterior hairline and periauricular skin. In infants: cradle cap.
- Usually nonpruritic, but active phases can manifest with burning and itching.
- Seasonal, worse in winter.

GENERAL CONSIDERATIONS

- Seborrheic dermatitis (SD) is a common papulosquamous condition with an appearance similar to psoriasis. It may be associated with excessive oiliness (seborrhea) and dandruff. Scale is yellowish and either dry or greasy. Erythematous, follicular, scaly papules may coalesce into large plaques or circinate patches. Flexural involvement often is complicated with *Candida* infection.
- Occurs in infancy (2 to 12 weeks of age) and in the middle-aged and elderly.
- Prognosis: lifelong recurrence.
- *Malassezia* yeast are probably not the cause but a cofactor linked to the following:
  - — Depressed helper T cells (SD is common in patients with acquired immunodeficiency syndrome [AIDS])
  - — Increased natural killer cells, which increase inflammatory cytokines
  - — Increased sebum levels
  - — Activation of alternate complement pathway
  - — Genetic susceptibility to skin barrier dysfunction

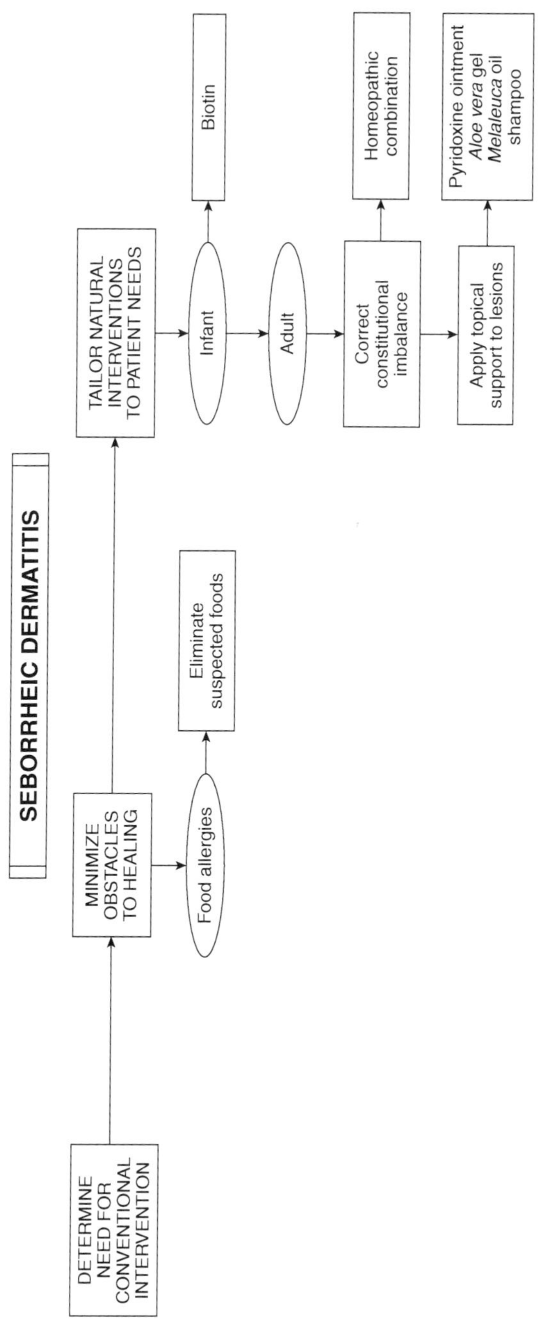
SEBORRHEIC DERMATITIS
DETERMINE NEED FOR CONVENTIONAL INTERVENTION
MINIMIZE OBSTACLES TO HEALING
Food allergies
Eliminate suspected foods
TAILOR NATURAL INTERVENTIONS TO PATIENT NEEDS
Infant
Biotin
Adult
Correct constitutional imbalance
Homeopathic combination
Apply topical support to lesions
Pyridoxine ointment
Aloe vera gel
Melaleuca oil shampoo

Malassezia species have lipases, which release inflammatory arachidonic acid.

- SD is aggravated by changes in humidity, scratching, emotional stress, diet, various medications, and androgen excess.

THERAPEUTIC CONSIDERATIONS

Nutrition

- **Food allergy:** SD begins as cradle cap. It is not primarily an allergic disease, but it is linked to food allergy (67% of SD patients have some form of allergy by age 10 years).
- **Biotin:** underlying factor in infants is biotin deficiency. Syndrome is clinically similar to SD induced in rats fed a diet high in raw egg white (high in avidin, a glycoprotein that binds biotin, making it biounavailable).
  - — Large portion of human biotin supply is provided by intestinal bacteria. Dysbiosis may cause biotin deficiency in infants. SD is successfully treated with biotin in nursing mothers and infants.
  - — In adults, biotin alone is ineffective.
- **Pyridoxine:** B_6 deficiency in human beings and rats causes lesions indistinguishable from SD.
  - — Treatment with oral and parenteral B_6 has been unsuccessful.
  - — In the sicca form of disorder (involving scalp [dandruff], brow, nasolabial folds, and bearded area with varying degrees of greasy, adherent scales on erythematous base), condition in all patients cleared completely within 10 days with a local water-soluble ointment containing 50 mg of pyridoxine per gram. Other types of SD (flexural and infected) are unresponsive.
  - — In patients with elevated urinary xanthurenic acid, oral, parenteral, and local B_6 all normalized excretion levels, implying transcutaneous absorption of B_6. However, improvement from topical B_6 may be caused by reducing sebaceous secretion rate from the ointment itself; adding B_6 had no effect.
  - — Check patient for exposure to B_6 antimetabolites: hydrazine dyes (U.S. Food, Drug, and Cosmetic Act [FD&C] yellow No. 5) and drugs (isoniazid and hydralazine), dopamine, penicillamine, oral contraceptives, and excessive protein intake.

Botanical Medicine

- *Aloe vera* **gel:** can be helpful topically. Thirty-percent crude aloe emulsion cream twice daily for 4 to 6 weeks improved scaling and itching in 62% of patients compared with only 25% using placebo.
- ***Melaleuca alternifolia*** **(tea tree) oil:** is active against *Malassezia* species and therefore beneficial for SD. Honey and cinnamic acid have similar activity. Study: 5% tea tree oil shampoo showed 41% improvement in severity versus 11% with placebo. Add tea tree oil to patient's shampoo to increase compliance.

Homeopathic Therapy

- Placebo, crossover study of homeopathic combination remedy for control of SD and chronic dandruff. The homeopathic therapy was Kali brom 1x, Natrum brom 2x, Niccolum sulf 3x, and Natrum mur 6x. After 10 weeks on active medicine, patients showed significant improvement compared with patients on placebo. Ten weeks after crossover, placebo patients experienced improvement as well.

THERAPEUTIC APPROACH

Optimal approach is unclear. Effective therapy, however, is available for most patients.

- Infants: alleviate biotin deficiency, control food allergies.
- Adults: use of *Aloe vera* and *M. alternifolia* oil constitutes primary therapy.

Maximize therapeutic results with a broad-spectrum approach.

The following doses are for adults; modify children's doses according to weight.

- **Diet**: detect and treat food allergies; in nursing infants, consider food allergies of mother.
- **Supplements**:
  — Biotin: 1 mg for infants
  — Homeopathic combination remedy once daily
- **Topical treatment:**
  — Pyridoxine ointment: 50 mg/g (in water-soluble base)
  — *Aloe vera* gel: apply twice daily to affected areas
  — *Melaleuca* oil: 5% solution (may be added to patient's shampoo)

Senile (Aging-Related) Cataracts

DIAGNOSTIC SUMMARY

- Clouding or opacity in the crystalline lens of the eye.
- Absence or altered red reflex (small cataracts stand out as dark defects).
- Gradual loss of vision.

GENERAL CONSIDERATIONS

- Leading cause of impaired vision and blindness in the United States; 4 million people have vision-impairing cataract, and 40,000 people in the country are blind because of cataracts. Cataract surgery is the most common major surgical procedure in the United States.
- Classified by location and appearance of lens opacities, cause or significant contributing factor, and age of onset.
- Causes and contributing factors: ocular disease, injury, surgery, systemic diseases (diabetes mellitus, galactosemia), toxin, ultraviolet and near-ultraviolet light, radiation exposure, and hereditary disease.
- Transparency of lens decreases with age. Most elderly people have some degree of cataract formation, including progressive increase in size, weight, and density of lens throughout life.
- Histopathology of cataract:
  - — Fibrous metaplasia of epithelium
  - — Liquefaction of fibers resulting in morgagnian globule formation (drops of fluid beneath capsule and between lens fibers)
  - — Sclerosis (melding of fibers)
  - — Posterior migration and swelling of epithelium
- Topoanatomic classification of cataracts:
  - — Anterior subcapsular cataract: fibrous metaplasia of lens epithelium (after iritis and adherence of iris to lens [posterior synechia])
  - — Anterior cortical cataract: liquefaction of lens fibers and morgagnian globules in cortex anteriorly

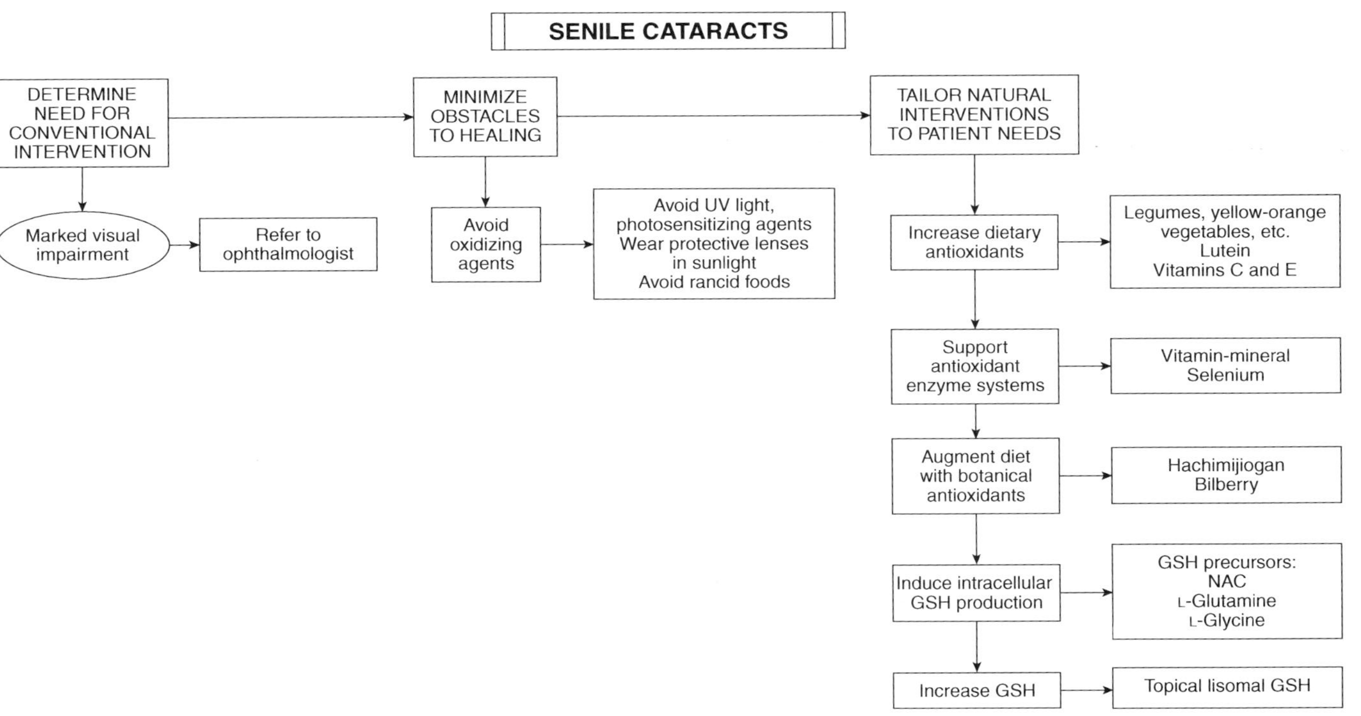
SENILE CATARACTS
DETERMINE NEED FOR CONVENTIONAL INTERVENTION
Marked visual impairment
Refer to ophthalmologist
MINIMIZE OBSTACLES TO HEALING
Avoid oxidizing agents
Avoid UV light, photosensitizing agents
Wear protective lenses in sunlight
Avoid rancid foods
TAILOR NATURAL INTERVENTIONS TO PATIENT NEEDS
Increase dietary antioxidants
Legumes, yellow-orange vegetables, etc.
Lutein
Vitamins C and E
Support antioxidant enzyme systems
Vitamin-mineral
Selenium
Augment diet with botanical antioxidants
Hachimijiogan
Bilberry
Induce intracellular GSH production
GSH precursors:
NAC
L-Glutamine
L-Glycine
Increase GSH
Topical lisomal GSH

  - Nuclear cataract: exaggeration of normal, aging-related, melding of fibers in nucleus
  - Posterior cortical cataract: liquefaction and globular degeneration of posterior lens cortex
  - Posterior subcapsular cataract: epithelial cells migrate posteriorly under capsule and form large, irregular nucleated cells
- Seventy-five percent of senile cataracts are cortical; 25% are nuclear. Cortical cataracts take three forms:
  - Spoke wheel, beginning in periphery and coursing anteriorly and posteriorly to nucleus
  - Perinuclear punctate opacities
  - Granular opacities under posterior capsule (subcapsular cataracts)

THERAPEUTIC CONSIDERATIONS

- Cause of cataract: inability to maintain normal homeostatic concentrations of sodium (Na^+), potassium (K^+), and calcium (Ca^{2+}) within lens, the result of decreased Na^+, K^+–adenosine triphosphatase (ATPase) activity—a defect from free radical damage to sulfhydryl proteins in the lens, including Na^+, K^+-ATPase, which contains a sulfhydryl component.
- Normal protective mechanisms are unable to prevent free radical damage; the lens depends on superoxide dismutase (SOD), catalase, glutathione (GSH), and accessory antioxidants vitamins E and C and selenium (Se) to prevent free radical damage.
- People with higher intake of vitamins C and E, Se, and carotenes have a much lower risk for cataracts.
- Nutritional supplements—such as multiple vitamin-mineral formulas, vitamins C and E, B vitamins (B_{12}, folic acid), vitamin A—also offer significant protection against nuclear and cortical cataracts. Age-Related Eye Disease Study Research Group conclusions: combination of all these nutrients produce better results than any single one alone or limited combinations in preventing both age-related macular degeneration and cataracts (see chapter on Macular Degeneration).

Antioxidants

- **Lutein:** yellow-orange carotene that protects against macular degeneration and cataract formation. Like the macula, the lens concentrates lutein. Spinach (high in lutein) consumption is inversely related to risk of cataract severe enough to require extraction. Intake of lutein is inversely associated with cataract extraction (20% to 50% risk reduction). Lutein (15 mg) given three times per week for up to 2 years to patients with age-related cataracts improved visual acuity and glare sensitivity.

- **Vitamin C:** high intake of vitamin C from dietary sources or supplements protects against cataract formation. Supplements can halt cataract progression and in some cases improve vision. Supplements reduced cataract development and number of surgeries required among cataract patients over a period of 11 years. Dose necessary to increase vitamin C content of lens: 1000 mg. Vitamin C in blood is 0.5 mg/dL, but in adrenal and pituitary glands the level is 100 times this, and in the liver, spleen, and lens of eye it is 20 times higher. Enormous amounts of energy are required to pull vitamin C out of blood against a tremendous gradient. Keeping blood vitamin C elevated with high doses reduces the gradient.
- **GSH:** GSH is a tripeptide composed of glycine, glutamic acid, and cysteine. It is present in very high concentrations in lens. GSH is a key protective factor against intralenticular and extralenticular toxins and is an antioxidant. It maintains reduced sulfhydryl bonds within lens proteins. It is a coenzyme of various enzyme systems. GSH participates in amino acid transport with gamma-glutamyl transpeptidase. It also is involved in cation transport. GSH is diminished in virtually all forms of cataracts.
- **Ascorbic acid (AA) and GSH interactions:** work in close conjunction as the most important host protective factors against induction of cataracts.
- **Se and vitamin E:** antioxidants that function synergistically. GSH peroxidase is Se dependent. Se content in lens with cataract is 15% of normal. Se in serum and aqueous humor is much lower in cataract patients than in controls, but Se in the lens itself did not differ much in cataract patients and normal individuals. Decreased Se in aqueous humor is a major finding. Excess H_2O_2 (25 times normal) is present in the aqueous humor of cataract patients and is associated with increased lipid peroxidation and altered lens permeability from damaged Na^+-K^+ pump. The lens is left unprotected against free radical and sun damage. Se-dependent GSH peroxidase breaks down H_2O_2. Vitamin E supplementation alone (500 international units [IU] q.d.) does not retard progression of cataracts. Vitamin E (400 IU) plus vitamin C (500 mg) and beta-carotene (15 mg) failed to affect the development or progression of cataracts in a 7-year trial.

- **SOD:** activity in human lens is lower than in other tissues because of increased ascorbate and GSH. Progressive SOD decrease parallels cataract progression. Oral SOD supplements do not affect tissue SOD activity. Trace mineral cofactors of SOD that are greatly reduced in cataractous lens are preferred (copper, 90%; manganese, 50%; zinc [Zn], 90%).
- **Catalase:** concentrated in epithelial portion of lens (anterior surface); very low levels are in the rest of lens. Primary function is to reduce (to water and oxygen) hydrogen peroxide formed from oxidation of ascorbate.
- **Tetrahydrobiopterin (BH_4):** pteridine compounds protect against cataract formation by preventing oxidation and damage by ultraviolet light. They prevent formation of high-molecular-weight proteins in lens. BH_4 is a coenzyme in hydroxylation of monoamines (phenylalanine hydroxylase, tyrosine hydroxylase, tryptophan hydroxylase). Decreased pteridine-synthesizing enzymes and BH_4 are found in senile cataracts. Supplemental folic acid may help compensate.

Other Nutritional Factors

- **Riboflavin:** lenticular GSH requires flavin adenine dinucleotide (FAD) as coenzyme for GSH reductase. Vitamin B_2 is a precursor of FAD. Vitamin B_2 deficiency may enhance cataract formation by depressed GSH reductase activity. Vitamin B_2 deficiency is common in the elderly (33%). Riboflavin status can be determined by red blood cell GSH reductase activity before and after FAD stimulation. Correction of the deficiency is warranted, but no more than 10 mg q.d. Vitamin B_2 should be prescribed for cataract patients because of a photosensitizing effect—superoxide radicals generated by interaction of light, ambient oxygen, and riboflavin and FAD. Vitamin B_2 and light (at physiologic levels) were used experimentally to induce cataracts. Excess vitamin B_2 does more harm than good in cataract patients.
- **Amino acids:** methionine is a component of lens antioxidant enzyme methionine sulfoxide reductase. It is a precursor of cysteine, a component of GSH. Cysteine and other amino acid precursors of GSH are helpful in cataract treatment.
- **Zinc, vitamin A, and beta-carotene:** antioxidants are vital for normal epithelial integrity. Beta-carotene may act as a filter, protecting against light-induced damage to fiber portion of lens. Beta-carotene is the most significant single oxygen free radical scavenger and is used to treat photosensitive disorders.

Long-term beta-carotene (50 mg on alternate days) on its own has no impact on cataract prevention in women and men.

- **Melatonin:** efficient free radical scavenger and antioxidant. It neutralizes hydroxyl and peroxyl radicals; enhances endogenous and exogenous antioxidant efficiency; and inhibits DNA damage, lipid peroxidation, and cataract formation in animals. It is present at significant levels in the cell nucleus, aqueous cytosol, and lipid-rich cell membranes.

Diet

Protective action is derived from some vegetables, fruit, Ca, folic acid, and vitamin E. Increased incidence arises with elevated salt and fat intake.

- **Dairy products:** cataracts often develop in infants with homozygous deficiency of either galactokinase or galactose-1-phosphate uridyltransferase. They also occur in laboratory animals fed a high-galactose diet. Abnormalities of galactose metabolism are identified by measuring activity of these enzymes in red blood cells. This is an important mechanism in 30% of cataract patients, but only diabetic cataracts. It is probably not relevant to senile cataracts (see the chapter on diabetes mellitus).

Toxic Metals

Increased concentrations are found in aging lens and cataractous lens; levels are higher in cataracts, but significance is unknown.

- Cadmium (Cd): concentration in cataractous lens is two to three times higher than in controls. Cd displaces Zn from binding in enzymes by binding to sulfhydryl groups. Cd contributes to deactivation of free radical quenching and other protective and repair mechanisms.
- Other elevated elements of unknown significance include bromine, cobalt, iridium, and nickel.

Botanical Medicines

- **Flavonoid-rich extracts:** *Vaccinium myrtillus* (bilberry), *Vitis vinifera* (grapeseed), *Pinus maritima* (pine bark), and curcumin from *Curcuma longa* (turmeric). Flavonoid components in well-defined diets may be protective. Bilberry anthocyanosides may offer the greatest protection; bilberry plus vitamin E stopped progression of cataract in 97% of patients with senile cortical cataracts.
- **Hachimijiogan:** ancient Chinese formula that increases antioxidant level of lens. It has been used in treating cataracts for

hundreds of years. Therapeutic effect is impressive in early stages; 60% of subjects noted significant improvement, 20% showed no progression, and only 20% displayed progression of cataract. It contains the following eight herbs (per 24-g dose):

— *Rehmannia glutinosa:* 6000 mg
— *Poria cocos sclerotium:* 3000 mg
— *Dioscorea opposita:* 3000 mg
— *Cornus officinalis:* 3000 mg
— *Epimedium grandiflorum:* 3000 mg
— *Alisma plantago:* 3000 mg
— *Alisma plantago-aquatica:* 2000 mg
— *Cinnamomum cassia:* 1000 mg

THERAPEUTIC APPROACH

Marked vision improvement is gained from cataract removal and lens implant. Prevention or treatment at an early stage is most effective. Free radical damage is the primary inducing factor; avoid oxidizing agents and promote free radical scavenging. Avoid direct ultraviolet light, bright light, and photosensitizing substances. Wear protective lenses outdoors. Greatly increase antioxidant nutrients. Progression can be stopped and early lesions can be reversed. Significant reversal of well-developed cataracts is unlikely. The elderly are especially susceptible to nutrient deficiencies; ensure they are ingesting and assimilating adequate macronutrients and micronutrients.

- **Diet:** avoid rancid foods and other sources of free radicals. Increase legumes (sulfur-containing amino acids methionine and cysteine), yellow vegetables (carotenes), and foods rich in vitamins C and E.
- **Supplements:**
  — High-potency multiple vitamin-mineral formula
  — Lutein: 5 to 15 mg q.d.
  — Vitamin C: 1 g t.i.d.
  — Vitamin E: 600 to 800 IU q.d. (mixed tocopherols)
  — Se: 400 mcg q.d.
  — *N*-acetylcysteine: 500 mg bid
  — L-Glutamine: 200 mg q.d.
  — L-Glycine: 200 mg q.d.
- **Botanical medicines:**
  — Bilberry extract (25% anthocyanidins): 80 mg t.i.d.
  — Hachimijiogan formula: 1000 mg t.i.d.
  — Topical liposomal GSH

Streptococcal Pharyngitis

DIAGNOSTIC SUMMARY

- Abrupt onset of sore throat, fever, malaise, nausea, and headache
- Throat red and edematous, with or without exudation
- Tender cervical lymph nodes
- Positive rapid detection of streptococcal antigen
- Group A streptococci on throat culture

GENERAL CONSIDERATIONS

Streptococcal pharyngitis ("strep throat") resembles viral pharyngitis. Of children with sore throat, 15% to 36% have group A beta-hemolytic *Streptococcus* (GABHS). The rate is less than 20% for adults. Ten percent to 25% of general, asymptomatic population are carriers for group A *Streptococcus.*

- Rapid streptococcal screens detect group A streptococcal antigens. Definitive positive culture takes 2 days. Antibiotics during this period lead to unnecessary development of antibiotic-resistant organisms and patient exposure to antibiotics. Second-generation rapid streptococcal screens (Strep A OIA test) have excellent sensitivity and specificity and will someday replace throat culture as the diagnostic gold standard. However, these tests remain underused because many doctors rely on antibiotics as a precaution against sequelae of GABHS even without positive diagnosis.
- Even if cultures are positive for *Streptococcus,* antibiotics may not be necessary; strep throat usually is self-limiting. Clinical recovery is similar in cases treated with antibiotics and those that were not.
- Concern with not using antibiotics: nonsuppurative poststreptococcal syndromes (rheumatic fever [RF], poststreptococcal glomerulonephritis [GN]). However, antibiotics do not significantly reduce incidence of sequelae. Most cases of sequelae are the result of the patient not consulting a physician. The dogma is

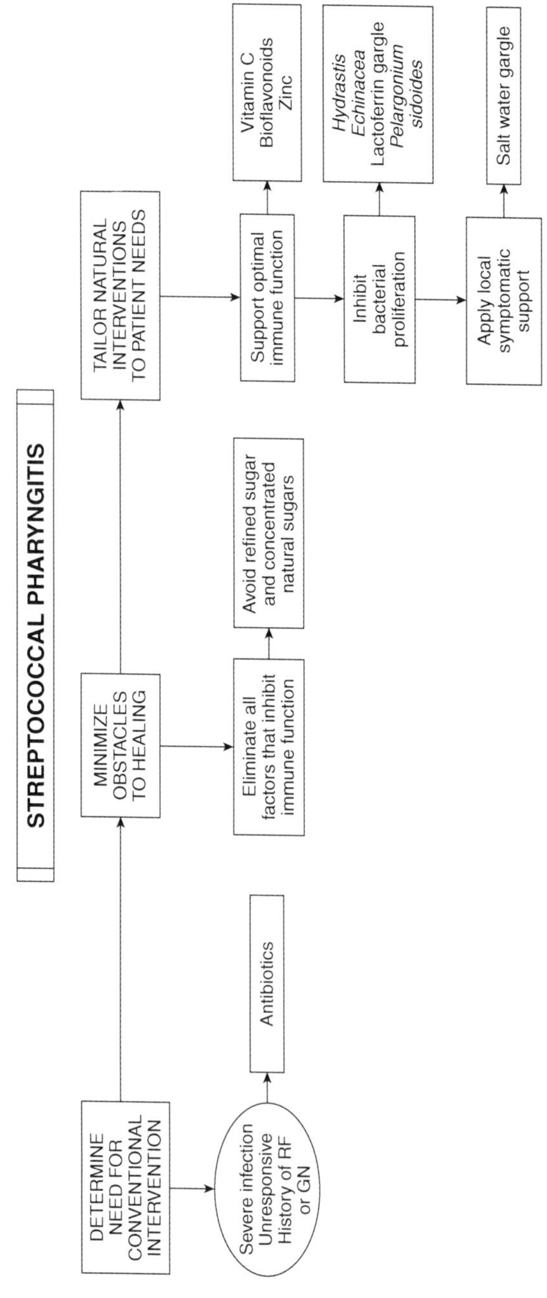
STREPTOCOCCAL PHARYNGITIS
DETERMINE NEED FOR CONVENTIONAL INTERVENTION
Severe infection
Unresponsive
History of RF or GN
Antibiotics
MINIMIZE OBSTACLES TO HEALING
Eliminate all factors that inhibit immune function
Avoid refined sugar and concentrated natural sugars
TAILOR NATURAL INTERVENTIONS TO PATIENT NEEDS
Support optimal immune function
Vitamin C
Bioflavonoids
Zinc
Inhibit bacterial proliferation
Hydrastis
Echinacea
Lactoferrin gargle
Pelargonium sidoides
Apply local symptomatic support
Salt water gargle

that acute RF can be caused only by GABHS infection of the upper respiratory tract, but streptococcal pyoderma is major cause in Aboriginal people of northern Australia and perhaps other high-incidence communities. In settings where RF is rare, group A streptococcal strains causing pharyngitis have lower virulence in causing RF.

- Penicillin, amoxicillin, erythromycin, and first-generation cephalosporins are recommended antibiotics for GABHS. Amoxicillin is most common for children for compliance reasons. Reserve antibiotics for patients with severe infection who are unresponsive to therapy (unresponsive after 1 week of immune support) and those with history of RF or glomerulonephritis (GN). Even then, antibiotics such as penicillin fail to eradicate streptococci in more than 20% of patients; beta-lactase–positive organisms (*Staphylococcus aureus* and *Bacteroides* species) deactivate penicillin. Stronger antibiotics (e.g., cephalosporin) may be required. Macrolides (erythromycin, cephalosporins) are the best first-line antibiotics.
- Dramatic decrease in incidence of RF began before advent of antibiotics. Improved socioeconomic, hygienic, and nutritional conditions are more important. Present attack rates after streptococcal infection are 0.4% to 2.8% for RF and 0.2% to 20% for GN.

THERAPEUTIC CONSIDERATIONS

Primary therapeutic consideration is status of patient's immune system. If immune function is good, illness is short-lived. Enhance immune function (*Textbook*, "Immune Support") to shorten course. If immune function is poor, make every effort to strengthen immune system.

- **Vitamin C:** vitamin C deficiency correlates with streptococcal sequelae. RF is virtually nonexistent in tropics, where vitamin C intake is higher. Eighteen percent of children in high-risk groups have subnormal serum vitamin C, which is preventive against RF in animals. Highly positive results arise when children are given orange juice supplementation. Promising research was dropped because of the advent of supposedly effective antibiotics.
- ***Hydrastis canadensis* (goldenseal) and *Echinacea angustifolia:*** these botanical medicines support immune function during GABHS infections. Berberine alkaloids of *Hydrastis* exert antibiotic activity against *Streptococcus* and inhibit attachment of

group A streptococci to pharyngeal epithelial cells. Streptococci secrete hyaluronidase to colonize tissue; this enzyme is inhibited by *Echinacea* and bioflavonoids. *Echinacea* inactivates and reduces proinflammatory response to GABHS; it also promotes increased phagocytosis, natural killer cell activity, and properdin levels (*Textbook*, "*Echinacea* Species [Narrow-Leafed Purple Coneflower]" and "*Hydrastis canadensis* [Goldenseal] and Other Berberine-Containing Botanicals").

- ***Pelargonium sidoides* (South African geranium):** extracts from rhizomes and tubers of *P. sidoides* are beneficial for upper respiratory tract infections (e.g., acute bronchitis). *P. sidoides* is immunity enhancing and antibacterial; it prevents adhesion of bacteria to epithelial cells. The product EPs 7630 was proven superior to placebo for non-GABHS tonsillopharyngitis in children, shortening duration of illness by 2 days. Although this study was in non-GABHS, the possibility remains that *P. sidoides* might benefit GABHS.
- **Bacteriotherapy:** colonizing throat with group A non–beta-hemolytic streptococci may prevent recurrent GABHS pharyngitis. Spray was used for at least 5 days; no side effects were reported. This therapy demonstrates superiority to placebo in preventing recurrences of GABHS throat infections.
- **Lactoferrin:** bovine lactoferrin (at even low concentrations) hinders in vitro invasion of cultured epithelial cells by GABHS from patients with pharyngitis. In tonsil specimens from children treated for 15 days before tonsillectomy with both oral erythromycin (500 mg t.i.d.) and lactoferrin gargles (100 mg t.i.d.), fewer intracellular GABHS organisms were found compared with children treated with erythromycin alone.

THERAPEUTIC APPROACH

If antibiotics are used, follow recommendations for *Lactobacillus acidophilus* (*Textbook*, "Probiotics").

- **Supplements:**
  — Vitamin C: 500 mg every 2 hours
  — Bioflavonoids: 1000 mg q.d.
  — Zinc: 30 mg q.d.
- **Botanical medicines:**
  — *Echinacea* species (t.i.d.): dried root (or as tea), 0.5 to 1 g; freeze-dried plant: 325 to 650 mg; juice of aerial portion of *E. purpurea* stabilized in 22% ethanol, 2 to 3 mL; tincture (1:5),

2 to 4 mL (½ to 1 tsp)/day; fluid extract (1:1), 2 to 4 mL (½ to 1 tsp)/day; solid (dried powdered) extract (6.5:1 or 3.5% echinacoside), 150 to 300 mg.

— *H. canadensis* (goldenseal) (dose based on berberine content; standardized extracts are preferred) (t.i.d.): dried root or as infusion (tea), 2 to 4 g; tincture (1:5), 6 to 12 mL (1½ to 3 tsp); fluid extract (1:1), 2 to 4 mL (½ to 1 tsp); solid (powdered dry) extract (4:1 or 8% to 12% alkaloid content), 250 to 500 mg.

— *P. sidoides* (dose for EPs 7630 or equivalent preparation): Adults—1.5 mL t.i.d. or 1 20-mg tablet t.i.d. for up to 14 days. Children—age 7 to 12 years, 20 drops (1 mL) t.i.d.; age 6 years or younger, 10 drops (0.5 mL) t.i.d.

- Local treatment: gargle with lactoferrin (100 mg) dissolved in water t.i.d. Alternatively, gargle with salt water as 1 tbsp salt/240 mL of warm water.

Trichomoniasis

DIAGNOSTIC SUMMARY

- Profuse, malodorous, white to green discharge from vagina.
- Discharge usually has a pH greater than 4.5, a weak amine odor, and large numbers of white blood cells and trichomonads on wet mount.
- Vulvovaginal pruritus, burning, and/or irritation.
- Vulva and introitus usually show erythema.
- Cervix may or may not have a mottled erythema "strawberry cervix" (less than 5%).
- Dysuria and/or dyspareunia may be present.
- Rule out trichomoniasis in men exhibiting signs of prostatitis, urethritis, or epididymitis.

GENERAL CONSIDERATIONS

Trichomoniasis ("trich") is common cause of vaginal irritation in women and the most common nonviral sexually transmitted disease. It affects one in five women in the United States during their lifetime. Five million cases appear each year. It is present in 3% to 15% of asymptomatic women treated at obstetric and gynecologic clinics and 20% to 50% of women treated at sexually transmitted disease clinics.

- Gonorrhea (GC) and trich commonly coexist; 40% of women with trich have GC, and vice versa.
- Trich frequently causes cervical erosion (90%), a factor in malignancy.
- Trich may complicate interpretation of Pap smears, increasing number of false-positive results.
- Trich increases sterility in women (salpingitis) and men (toxins decrease motility of spermatozoa).
- Increased postpartum fever and discharge in women with *Trichomonas vaginalis* at delivery.
- Neonates infected from passage through the birth canal may manifest serious illness (rare).
- Prostatitis and epididymitis are common in infected men.

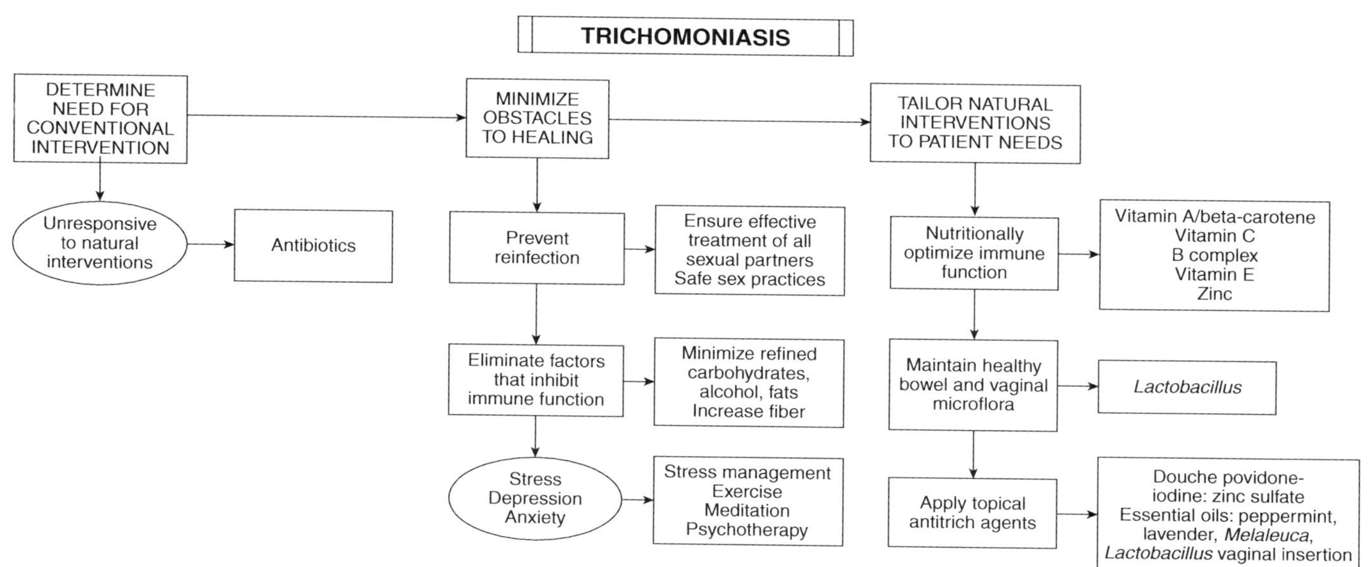
TRICHOMONIASIS
DETERMINE NEED FOR CONVENTIONAL INTERVENTION
Unresponsive to natural interventions
Antibiotics
MINIMIZE OBSTACLES TO HEALING
Prevent reinfection
Ensure effective treatment of all sexual partners
Safe sex practices
Eliminate factors that inhibit immune function
Minimize refined carbohydrates, alcohol, fats
Increase fiber
Stress
Depression
Anxiety
Stress management
Exercise
Meditation
Psychotherapy
TAILOR NATURAL INTERVENTIONS TO PATIENT NEEDS
Nutritionally optimize immune function
Vitamin A/beta-carotene
Vitamin C
B complex
Vitamin E
Zinc
Maintain healthy bowel and vaginal microflora
Lactobacillus
Apply topical antitrich agents
Douche povidone-iodine: zinc sulfate
Essential oils: peppermint, lavender, *Melaleuca*, *Lactobacillus* vaginal insertion

- Infection may confuse and/or complicate other genitourinary tract problems.
- Metronidazole (Flagyl) (most common antitrich agent) is carcinogenic and teratogenic in rodents.
- Trich increases human immunodeficiency virus (HIV) transmission and infectivity; HIV-seropositive men with concomitant trichomoniasis may have sixfold higher concentration of HIV RNA in seminal plasma.

DIAGNOSIS

T. vaginalis is a flagellate 15 to 18 mm long, shaped like a turnip, with three or four anterior flagella and one posterior flagellum mounted in undulating membrane. Transmission is through sexual intercourse; men and women are reservoirs. Diagnosis is by signs and symptoms (see earlier), saline wet mount, and culture. Trich cultures (Feinberg *Trichomonas* medium) increase diagnostic sensitivity. Fifty percent of women with *Trichomonas* (defined by positive culture) have the organism identified by microscopic wet mount. Although microscopic wet mount is commonly used and a quick method to identify trich compared with culture, sensitivity of wet mount ranges from only 45% to 60%. In men a reliable culture site has not been established, and cultures from urine and seminal samples give low yield. The organism can be cultured from vagina and paraurethral glands in 98%, the urethra in 82%, and endocervix in 13%. In only 56% to 65% is *T. vaginalis* seen on Pap smear; thus Pap smear is an unreliable form of diagnosis. DNA-based test called Affirm VP system uses synthetic oligonucleotide probes for detection of *T. vaginalis, Gardnerella vaginalis,* and *Candida* species from a single vaginal swab, with sensitivity of 92% and specificity of 98% compared with wet mount and sensitivity of 92% and specificity of 99% compared with culture. The positive predictive value of this test is acceptable for diagnosis of trichomoniasis when it is found incidentally on Pap smear, with a sensitivity of 57% and a specificity of 97%. Rapid point-of-care tests for trich vaginitis include the OSOM Trichomonas Rapid Test (Genzyme Diagnostics, Cambridge, MA), an immunochromatographic capillary-flow dipstick technology, and the Affirm VP III (Becton Dickinson, Franklin Lakes, NJ), a nucleic acid probe test that evaluates for trichomonal vaginitis, *G. vaginalis,* and *Candida albicans.* These tests are performed on vaginal secretions with a sensitivity exceeding 83% and a specificity exceeding 97%. Results of the OSOM are available in 10 minutes; Affirm VP III results are ready in 45 minutes.

Trichomonal Vaginitis

- Sexual transmission is the route of infection. Prevalence is highest among women with multiple partners and women with other sexually transmitted infections. Transmission rates are high from men to women; an 80% to 100% prevalence exists in female partners of infected men.
- In women, *T. vaginalis* infects the vagina and urethra and may involve the endocervix, Bartholin's glands, Skene's glands, and bladder.
  - Vagina is a good reservoir; estrogen causes walls to be glycogenated. Prepubescent and postmenopausal women seldom have trich symptoms.
  - Elevated pH increases susceptibility. Normal adult vaginal pH is 3.5 to 4.5 because of *Lactobacillus acidophilus* converting free glucose into lactic acid. Decreased lactobacilli increase pH. *Trichomonas* grow optimally at a pH of 5.5 to 5.8. Other conditions increasing vaginal pH are progesterone (latter half of menstrual cycle and during pregnancy), excess intravaginal secretions (cervical mucus), and bacterial overgrowth (*Streptococcus, Proteus*).

Trichomonas in the Male

Incidence is lower in men, but 5% to 15% of nongonococcal urethritis cases are caused by *Trichomonas.* Transmission rate of 70% exists among men having sexual contact with infected women in the previous 48 hours. Trich often is asymptomatic, but mild urethritis, prostatitis, and epididymitis are reported. Trich is a factor in male infertility, identified in semen, urethral discharge, and urine, in addition to prostatic fluid, prostatic secretions, and semen of 23% of men with chronic non-GC prostatitis. It persists in the male genitourinary tract; reinfection of sexually active treated women is well documented. Sexual partners must be treated. Among both women and men, *T. vaginalis* is linked to enhanced HIV acquisition and transmission.

THERAPEUTIC CONSIDERATIONS

- **Conventional therapy:** metronidazole and tinidazole, a second-generation nitroimidazole used for metronidazole-resistant infection. Both tinidazole (2-g single oral dose) and either metronidazole (2-g single oral dose) or short-course metronidazole have demonstrated parasitologic cure rates of 86% to 100% for all treatments, although tinidazole is slightly more effective but also more expensive. Comparing tinidazole and short-course therapy with metronidazole for trichomoniasis, metronidazole has higher rates of parasitologic failure, clinical failure, and adverse effects. To reduce recurrence, sexual partners must be treated concurrently. Side effects of metronidazole and tinidazole include nausea and vomiting, metallic taste, and gastrointestinal upset. Patients must avoid alcohol during therapy. As a long-term high-dose use for resistant trich, metronidazole rarely causes peripheral neuropathy—less than 1% in more than 35 years of use.

- **Probiotics:** if metronidazole or tinidazole is prescribed, supplement with probiotics. For bacterial vaginosis, vaginal insertion of *L. acidophilus* has cure rates superior to those of metronidazole. Vaginal probiotics may benefit vaginal trichomoniasis, given disruption of vaginal flora.
- **Diet:** affects body defenses. The "fertility of the soil," not the pathogenicity of the microbe, allows trich to flourish. Implement a well-balanced diet high in natural fiber (vegetables, fruits), and low in fat, sugar, and refined carbohydrates.
- **Lifestyle:** depression and anxiety are linked to exacerbations of trich infections. Reduce stress with exercise and meditation. Safe sex or abstinence (during infection) lowers incidence of infection and reinfection. Sixty-six percent of prostitutes not practicing safe sex have trich infection.

Nutritional Supplements

Consult (*Textbook*, "Immune Support").

- **Zinc:** has broad antimicrobial spectrum against genitourinary pathogens: gram-positive and gram-negative bacteria, *T. vaginalis, C. albicans, Chlamydia trachomatis,* viruses. Trichomonads are readily killed by Zn at concentration of 0.042% (6.4 mmol/L); Zn concentration in prostatic fluid ranges from 0.015% to 0.10% (2.3 to 15.3 mmol/L), suggesting persistent trichomonal infections in men may be caused by Zn deficiency. Zn sulfate (220 mg b.i.d. for 3 weeks) is a possible treatment for trich infections refractory to metronidazole. For women with drug-resistant trich, Zn douches plus metronidazole may relieve.

Topical Trichomonacides

- **Povidone-iodine:** iodine is a potent trichomonacide. Povidone-iodine (PVP) is a broad-spectrum antimicrobial for vaginal pathogens. PVP (iodine absorbed into polyvinylpyrrolidone) has advantages over iodine—little sensitizing potential, does not sting, water soluble, washes out of clothing. Success rate is 98.1% in intractable trichomonal, monilial, nonspecific, and mixed vaginitis with 2-week regimen with PVP preparations. A 28-day course of PVP pessaries is indicated if patient is using oral contraceptives.
- **Propolis:** ethanol extract of propolis (150 mg/mL) is 100% lethal in vitro on protozoa *T. vaginalis* and *Toxoplasma gondii* after 24 hours of contact. It diminishes inflammation associated with trichomonal vaginitis.
- **Essential oils:** diverse antimicrobial action of essential oils has been demonstrated. Strong antitrichomonal properties, found in *Mentha piperita* (peppermint) and *Lavandula angustifolia* (lavender) have the fastest killing effects (15 to 20 minutes).
- ***Melaleuca alternifolia* (tea tree) oil:** powerful topical antimicrobial agent (*Textbook, "Melaleuca alternifolia* [Tea Tree]"). A 40% solution is very effective with no irritation, burning, or other side effects. Daily douches (0.4% solution *Melaleuca* oil in 1 L water) also are effective.
- **Berberine botanicals:** contain the plant alkaloid berberine sulfate. They inhibit in vitro several protozoa: *Entamoeba histolytica, Giardia lamblia,* and *T. vaginalis.* No clinical trials have been reported in trichomoniasis (*Textbook, "Hydrastis canadensis* [Goldenseal] and Other Berberine-Containing Botanicals").

THERAPEUTIC APPROACH

- Given the risk of serious sequelae of trichomoniasis and the high success of pharmaceuticals, systemic metronidazole should be carefully considered as a possible first-line treatment, with simultaneous and subsequent naturopathic therapies to decrease risk of recurrence and treat underlying susceptibilities. Naturopathic therapies may be used as first-line therapy in cases of allergy to metronidazole or pregnancy. The safety of metronidazole during pregnancy remains controversial. Data have accumulated that, despite the role of *T. vaginalis* in perinatal morbidity, metronidazole treatment may actually increase the risk of preterm birth.

- *Trichomonas* is a sexually transmitted disease; treatment of the sexual partner(s) is mandatory to prevent reinfection. During treatment, avoid sexual intercourse. Use condom otherwise.
- **Diet:** decrease refined carbohydrates, alcohol, and fats; increase fiber.
- **Nutritional supplements**:
  — Zinc (picolinate): 10 to 15 mg q.d.
  — Vitamin E (mixed tocopherols): 200 international units (IU) q.d.
  — *L. acidophilus:* 5 to 10 billion live bacteria b.i.d. orally as well as intravaginal application in vaginal trichomoniasis
- **Topical treatment:**
  — Povidone-iodine douche, pessary, or saturated tampon b.i.d. for 14 days
  — *M. alternifolia* oil (40% solution): swab on affected area b.i.d.; or use as douche, 1 L of a 0.4% solution b.i.d.; or suppository, one at night
  — Zn sulfate douche: 1% solution b.i.d.
  — *Lactobacillus* insertions or douches daily, preferably in the morning

Urticaria

DIAGNOSTIC SUMMARY

- **Urticaria (hives):** the presence of well-circumscribed erythematous wheals with raised serpiginous borders and blanched centers that may coalesce to become giant wheals. Limited to the superficial portion of the dermis.
- **Angioedema:** similar eruptions to urticaria but with larger, well-demarcated edematous areas that involve subcutaneous structures as well as the dermis.
- **Chronic versus acute:** recurrent episodes of urticaria and/or angioedema of less than 6 weeks' duration are considered acute, whereas attacks persisting beyond this period are designated chronic. When no underlying cause is found, chronic urticaria is referred to as chronic idiopathic urticaria.
- **Special forms:** special forms have characteristic features—dermographism, cholinergic urticaria, solar urticaria, cold urticaria.
- Urticaria is experienced by 14% to 25% of the general population. Young adults (postadolescence through third decade) are most often affected. At least 40% of patients with idiopathic chronic urticaria have clinically relevant functional autoantibodies to high-affinity immunoglobulin E (IgE) receptor on basophils and mast cells. The term *autoimmune urticaria* is used for this subgroup of patients with continuous ordinary urticaria.

PATHOPHYSIOLOGY

Urticaria is named for the stinging nettle plant *(Urtica dioica),* which contains histaminic acid. Mechanism is the release of inflammatory mediators from mast cells or basophilic leukocytes, both of which have high-affinity receptors for IgE. Mechanisms involve agents other than IgE–anti-IgE complexes. The incidence of IgE-mediated urticaria is probably low compared with nonimmunologic factors in urticaria, including prostaglandins, leukotrienes, cytokines, and chemokines. Signs and symptoms are consistent despite diverse etiologic and initiating factors, yet pathogenesis is not ascribed to

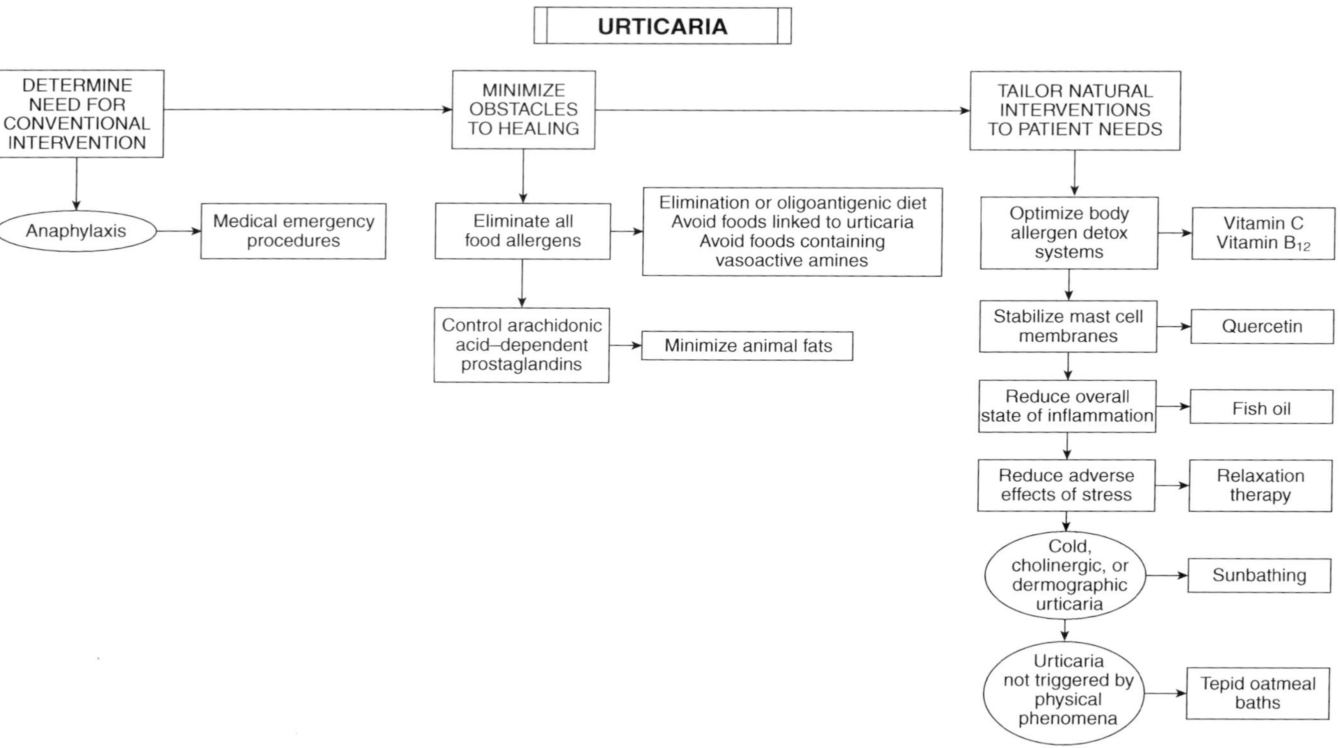
URTICARIA
DETERMINE NEED FOR CONVENTIONAL INTERVENTION
Anaphylaxis
Medical emergency procedures
MINIMIZE OBSTACLES TO HEALING
Eliminate all food allergens
Elimination or oligoantigenic diet
Avoid foods linked to urticaria
Avoid foods containing vasoactive amines
Control arachidonic acid–dependent prostaglandins
Minimize animal fats
TAILOR NATURAL INTERVENTIONS TO PATIENT NEEDS
Optimize body allergen detox systems
Vitamin C
Vitamin B_{12}
Stabilize mast cell membranes
Quercetin
Reduce overall state of inflammation
Fish oil
Reduce adverse effects of stress
Relaxation therapy
Cold, cholinergic, or dermographic urticaria
Sunbathing
Urticaria not triggered by physical phenomena
Tepid oatmeal baths

any one mechanism. Mast cells and mast cell–dependent mediators play the most prominent role.

- Three distinct sources of mediators:
  - **Preformed mediators:** contained in granules and released immediately
  - **Secondarily formed mediators:** generated immediately or within minutes by interaction of primary mediators and nearby cells and tissues
  - **Granule matrix–derived mediators:** preformed but slowly dissociate from granule after discharge and remain in tissues for hours
- Most common immunologic mechanism is mediated by IgE.
- Early vascular changes arise from mast cells—histamine and end products of arachidonic acid. Wheal and flare occur within minutes of initiation and last 30 to 60 minutes.
- Histamine and other mediators can be released by other nonallergic mechanisms as well. Neuropeptides can trigger mast cell degranulation and might be involved in dermographism and emotional exacerbation of urticaria.
- Prolonged and delayed reactions represent leukocytic infiltration in response to mast cell chemotactic factors. They develop over time—erythema, edema, and induration beginning within 2 hours and lasting 12 to 24 hours. Leukocyte infiltration may induce second wave of mast cell activation or release toxic lysosomal enzymes and mediators.
- Events triggered by mediators depend on type of mediator and tissues where they are released.
- *Helicobacter pylori* can be a causative agent in chronic urticaria. Testing for *H. pylori* seems reasonable; if positive, consider treatment options carefully in the context of relative harms or burdens and benefits as well as patient values and preferences.

CAUSES OF URTICARIA

Physical Urticaria

Urticaria can result from reactions to physical stimuli. Most common forms of physical urticaria are dermographic, cholinergic, and cold urticarias. Less-common types of physical urticaria or angioedema are contact, solar, pressure, heat contact, aquagenic, vibratory, and exercise induced.

Dermographism: defined as readily elicited wheals evolving rapidly after moderate pressure. Simple contact with furniture, garters, bracelets, watch bands, towels, or bedding can cause urticaria. Incidence of dermographism is 1.5% to 5%. This is the most frequent type of physical urticaria. Female/male ratio is 2:1. Average age of onset is in the third decade. Incidence is much greater among obese persons wearing tight clothing.

- **Lesions start within 1 to 2 minutes of contact:** erythema, replaced within 3 to 5 minutes by edema and surrounding reflex urticaria. Maximal edema occurs within 10 to 15 minutes. Erythema regresses within an hour; edema persists up to 3 hours.
- **Associated with other diseases and conditions:** parasitosis, insect bites, neuropsychiatric disorders, hormonal changes, thyroid disorders, pregnancy, menopause, diabetes, immunologic alterations, other urticarias, drug therapy (during or after), *Candida albicans,* angioedema, hypereosinophilia.

Cholinergic (Heat Reflex) Urticaria

- Heat reflex urticaria is the second most frequent physical urticaria. These lesions involve stimulation of sweat glands by cholinergic afferent fibers. Lesions are pinpoint wheals surrounded by reflex erythema. Wheals arise at or between follicles, preferentially on upper trunk and arms.
- **Three basic types of stimuli:** passive overheating, physical exercise, and emotional stress.
- **Eliciting activities:** physical exercise, warm bath or sauna, eating hot spices, drinking alcohol.
- **Lesions:** arise within 2 to 10 minutes and last 30 to 50 minutes.
- **Systemic symptoms:** suggest generalized mast cell release beyond skin—headache, periorbital edema, lacrimation and burning of eyes, nausea and vomiting, abdominal cramps, diarrhea, dizziness, hypotension, and asthmatic attacks.

Cold Urticaria

- Cold urticaria is an urticarial and/or angioedematous reaction of skin making contact with cold objects, water, or air. Lesions are restricted to area of exposure and develop within a few seconds to minutes after removal of cold object and rewarming of skin. The colder the object or element, the faster the reaction. Widespread local exposure and generalized urticaria are accompanied by flushing, headache, chills, dizziness, tachycardia, abdominal pain, nausea, vomiting, myalgia, shortness of breath, wheezing, unconsciousness.

— Cold urticaria accompanies a variety of clinical conditions, including viral infections, parasitic infestations, syphilis, multiple insect bites, penicillin injections, dietary changes, stress. Children with cold urticaria have higher risk of anaphylaxis, especially triggered by swimming.

— Associated with infectious mononucleosis, cryoglobulinemia, and myeloma, in which cold urticaria may precede diagnosis by several years.

Autoimmune Urticaria

- A minority of cases of chronic urticaria have an autoimmune basis, involving autoantibodies to IgE or the FcεRIα subunit of high-affinity IgE mast cell receptor. Autoimmune antibodies are found in 24% to 76% of patients with chronic urticaria. They have a more-severe, prolonged course of disease. Middle-aged women have higher rates of urticaria and autoimmunity, particularly for thyroid disease. Thyroid autoantibodies are found more frequently in patients with IgE-receptor autoantibodies (see the discussion of thyroid disease under "Therapeutic Considerations").
- Autoimmunity is linked to bowel permeabilities. Subclinical impairments of small bowel red blood cell function may induce higher sensitivity to histamine in the gastrointestinal tract. Naturopathic approach treats overt and subclinical gastrointestinal permeability to decrease systemic inflammatory responses to endotoxins.

Drug-Induced Urticaria

- Leading cause of urticaria in adults. In children, attributable to foods, food additives, or infections. Most drugs are small molecules incapable of inducing antigenic or allergenic activity by themselves. Typically they act as haptens binding to endogenous macromolecules, inducing hapten-specific antibodies. Alternatively, they interact directly with mast cells, inducing degranulation. Many drugs produce urticaria, most commonly penicillin and aspirin (ASA).
- **Penicillin:** antibiotics are most common cause of drug-induced urticaria. Population rate of allergenicity of penicillin is 10%, with 25% of these individuals displaying urticaria, angioedema, or anaphylaxis. Penicillin cannot be destroyed by boiling or steam distillation and is undetected in foods. Penicillin in milk

is more allergenic than in meat; penicillin can be degraded into compounds that are more allergenic in the presence of carbohydrate and metals.

- **ASA and nonsteroidal anti-inflammatory drugs (NSAIDs):** urticaria is a more-common indicator of ASA sensitivity than asthma (*Textbook,* "Asthma"). Incidence of ASA sensitivity in patients with chronic urticaria is 20 times greater than in normal controls. From 2% to 67% of patients with chronic urticaria are sensitive to ASA. ASA inhibits cyclooxygenase by shunting eicosanoids toward leukotriene synthesis and increasing smooth muscle contraction and vascular permeability. ASA and other NSAIDs increase gut permeability and may alter normal handling of antigens. Dosage of 650 mg ASA q.d. for 3 weeks may desensitize patients and reduce responsiveness to foods that typically cause a reaction. Effect also occurs in patients with asthma but disappears within 9 days after treatment is stopped, because of a loss of effect or possible placebo response. NSAIDs are associated with prolonged and more-pronounced autoreactivity in urticaria.

Food-Related Causes

IgE-mediated urticaria occurs on ingestion of a specific reaginic antigen. Most common are wheat, milk, fish, meat, eggs, beans, nuts, citrus, kiwis, peanuts, and apples. An atopic patient experiences urticaria triggered by IgE mechanisms, although pseudoallergic reactions can occur in which direct mast cell histamine release is involved. Basic requirement for food allergy is absorption of an allergen through the intestinal mucosa. Aromatic volatile ingredients in tomatoes, wine, and culinary herbs (basil, fenugreek, cumin, dill, ginger, coriander, caraway, turmeric, parsley, pepper, rosemary, and thyme) may be initiating factors in some non-IgE events.

- Factors increasing gut permeability: vasoactive amines in foods or produced by bacterial action on amino acids, alcohol, NSAIDs, and food additives (*Textbook,* "Intestinal Permeability Assessment").
- Food allergies may induce increased gut permeability in urticaria. Gut permeability is linked to autoimmunity. Chronic urticaria is partially related to autoimmune processes (see discussion of autoimmune urticaria on page 927); therefore, depending on genetic susceptibility, bowel permeability may play a key role in instigating and prolonging immune activity leading to chronic urticaria.

- Alterations occur in gastric acidity, intestinal motility, and function of the small intestine and biliary tract in 85% of patients with chronic urticaria, including selective IgA deficiency, gastroenteritis, hypochlorhydria, and achlorhydria. These changes may alter barrier and immune function of the gut wall.
- IgG reactions may cause the most adverse food reactions (*Textbook*, "Food Allergy Testing"). IgG antigen-antibody complexes can promote complement activation and anaphylatoxins triggering mast cell degranulation.

Food Colorants

- **Food colorants:** food additives are a major factor in chronic urticaria in children. Colorants (azo dyes), flavorings (salicylates, aspartame), preservatives (benzoates, nitrites, sorbic acid), antioxidants (hydroxytoluene, sulfite, gallate), and emulsifiers and stabilizers (polysorbates, vegetable gums) produce urticaria in sensitive people.
- **Tartrazine (azo dye, FD&C yellow No. 5):** first food dye reported to induce urticaria. Of the average daily per-capita consumption of certified dyes in the United States (15 mg), 85% is tartrazine. Children consume much more. Tartrazine sensitivity is present in 0.1% of the population and 20% to 50% of persons sensitive to ASA. Tartrazine is a cyclooxygenase inhibitor and inducer of asthma and urticaria in children. Tartrazine, benzoate, and ASA increase lymphokine leukocyte inhibitory factor, increasing perivascular mast cells and mononuclear cells; 95% of urticaria patients have increased perivascular mast cells and mononuclear cells. Eliminating food dyes from the diet is very beneficial.

Food Flavorings

- **Salicylates:** salicylic acid esters are used to flavor foods—cake mixes, puddings, ice cream, chewing gum, and soft drinks. Mechanism of action is similar to ASA. Daily salicylate intake from foods is 10 to 200 mg; level of salicylate used in clinical testing is 300 mg. Dietary sources are fruit (berries, dried fruits); raisins and prunes have the highest amounts. Also implicated are licorice and peppermint candies. Moderate levels are in nuts and seeds. Salicylate content is very high in some herbs and condiments such as curry powder, paprika, thyme, dill, oregano, and turmeric.

- **Other flavoring agents:** cinnamon, vanilla, menthol, and other volatile compounds may produce urticaria. Artificial sweetener aspartame can, as well.

Food Preservatives

- **Benzoates:** benzoic acid and benzoates are the most common food preservatives. Incidence of adverse reactions is less than 1% for the general population, but positive challenges in patients with chronic urticaria vary from 4% to 44%. Fish and shrimp may have very high levels of benzoates, triggering common adverse reactions to these foods in patients with urticaria.
- **Butylated hydroxytoluene (BHT) and butylated hydroxyanisole:** primary antioxidants in prepared and packaged foods. Fifteen percent of patients with chronic urticaria test positive to oral challenge with BHT.
- **Sulfites:** induce asthma, urticaria, and angioedema in sensitive persons. They are ubiquitous in foods and drugs. They prevent microbial spoilage, browning, and color change. They are sprayed on fresh foods (shrimp, fruits, vegetables) and used as antioxidants and preservatives in pharmaceuticals. Average per-capita intake is 2 to 3 mg/day. Wine and beer drinkers ingest up to 10 mg/day. Persons relying on restaurant meals ingest up to 150 mg/day. Enzyme sulfite oxidase metabolizes sulfites to safer sulfates excreted in urine. Those with poorly functioning sulfoxidation system have increased urine sulfite/sulfate ratio. Sulfite oxidase depends on the trace mineral molybdenum.

Food Emulsifiers and Stabilizers

Most foods containing emulsifiers and stabilizers also contain antioxidants, preservatives, and dyes. Polysorbate in ice cream can induce urticaria. Vegetable gums (e.g., acacia, gum arabic, tragacanth, quince, and carrageenan) induce urticaria in susceptible individuals.

Infections

Infections are a major cause of urticaria in children. In adults, immune tolerance occurs to many microbes from repeated exposure.

- **Bacteria:** *H. pylori* has been implicated in chronic urticaria. Bacterial infections contribute to urticaria in two other settings:
  - Acute *Streptococcus* tonsillitis in children: acute urticaria predominates.
  - Chronic dental infections in adults: chronic urticaria predominates.

- **Viruses:** hepatitis B is the most frequent cause of viral-induced urticaria. One study showed that 15.3% of patients with chronic urticaria had anti–hepatitis B surface antibodies. Urticaria is also linked to infectious mononucleosis (5%) and may develop several weeks before clinical manifestations.
- ***C. albicans:*** 19% to 81% of patients with chronic urticaria react positively to immediate skin test with *Candida* antigens. Sensitivity to *Candida* is an important factor in 25% of patients with chronic urticaria. Seventy percent of patients with a positive skin reaction also react to oral provocation with foods prepared with yeasts. Elimination of organism with nystatin can cure some individuals with positive skin tests, but more patients responded to a yeast-free diet than to elimination of organism. Thus it is prudent to eradicate yeast while implementing yeast-free diet. Yeast-free diet excludes bread, buns, sausage, wine, beer, cider, grapes, sultanas, Marmite, Bovril, vinegar, tomato, catsup, pickles, and prepared foods containing food yeasts. Use diet plus eliminate yeast with nystatin. Desensitizing patients to *Candida* by yeast cell wall extract was helpful in some, but treatment also included increasing gastrointestinal fermentation and acidity plus elimination of yeast.

THERAPEUTIC CONSIDERATIONS

- **Psychological factors (stress):** the most frequent primary cause in chronic urticaria. Stress decreases intestinal secretory IgA. Relaxation therapy and hypnosis may be beneficial for some patients.
- **Ultraviolet light therapy:** is of some benefit in chronic urticaria. Both ultraviolet A and B have been used. Cold, cholinergic, and dermographic urticaria respond most favorably.
- **Thyroid:** association of thyroid disease and autoimmunity with urticaria is well established. Prevalence of antithyroid antibodies in normal population is 3% to 6% and is commonly found with other autoimmune conditions (e.g., pernicious anemia and vitiligo). Subset of patients with chronic urticaria are best helped by thyroid hormone therapy (as described later), by surgery, or by antithyroid medication.
  — Subclinical hypothyroidism is an increasingly recognized entity and may underlie the thyroid-urticaria association in some cases.

— Some patients with presumed idiopathic chronic urticaria and angioedema also have thyroid autoimmunity. L-Thyroxine therapy has induced remission within 4 weeks in some. Thyroid hormone replacement therapy has dramatically improved chronic urticaria in patients with normal thyroid function but also thyroid autoimmunity. Antithyroid antibodies did not correlate with clinical response. Resolution of chronic urticaria associated with thyrotoxicosis has occurred in patients treated with antithyroid medication or radioactive iodine. With a fully diagnosed thyroid condition, do not treat presumptively with suppressive thyroid medication. Usefulness of thyroid hormone therapy in euthyroid patients with chronic urticaria has not been proven in controlled trials, but looking for thyroid autoimmunity is warranted in cases refractory to other therapies.

DIAGNOSIS

Physical Evaluation and History

- **Careful history:** identify all medicines, supplements, and botanicals; travel, recent infection, occupational exposure; timing and onset of lesions; morphology; associated symptoms; family medical history, preexisting allergies.
- **Contact sensitivities:** latex and exposure to physical stimuli.
- **History of tattoos.**
- **Diet and lifestyle diary:** date and time foods are eaten, major activities, bowel and urine habits, and stress, to characterize temporal relationships between urticaria and foods and activities.
- **Comprehensive physical examination:** to uncover clues and comorbidities.

Laboratory Testing

- No relationship exists between numbers of identified diagnoses and numbers of performed tests.
- Systemic diseases (excluding physical urticaria, allergens, infections, and psychological causes) were identified and believed to be related causally to urticaria in only 1.6% of patients. These diseases included vasculitis, thyroid disease, lupus, other rheumatic disease, hereditary angioedema, and hematologic or oncologic conditions.

- Screening skin testing for food allergies is controversial. Skin testing for foods in patient with chronic urticaria is fraught with false-positive and false-negative results. Without a specific history suggesting a particular food allergen (exposure and time course of subsequent symptoms consistent with food allergy), skin testing can be counterproductive, particularly in patients with dermatographism and "twitchy mast cells."
- If symptoms do not remit after proper history, physical examination, and the following therapies, run complete blood count with differential, urinalysis, erythrocyte sedimentation rate, liver function tests, antinuclear antibody titers, and thyroid panel with antithyroid autoantibodies to ferret out uncommon cases with detectable but unsuspected underlying cause (e.g., infectious and parasitic conditions, rheumatic conditions, thyroid conditions, hematologic conditions).
- Skin biopsy can rule out urticarial vasculitis when suspected. Research laboratories can focus on autoimmune urticaria and detect anti-FcϵRIα autoantibodies, but these tests are not standardized or routinely or widely available.
- Some specialists use autologous serum skin testing; patient's serum is centrifuged and used for skin prick testing in this form of a semiquantitative functional assay for autoimmunity to IgE or IgE receptors bound to cutaneous mast cells. This test is 75% sensitive and 74% specific for presence of autoantibodies.

Supplements

- **Vitamin B_{12}:** anecdotal reports indicate value in acute and chronic urticaria. Although serum B_{12} is normal in most patients, additional B_{12} is helpful. When injectable B_{12} is used, placebo effect cannot be ruled out (*Textbook,* "Placebo and the Power to Heal").
- **Quercetin:** in vitro, it is a mast cell stabilizer and inhibitor of many pathways of inflammation (*Textbook,* "Flavonoids—Quercetin, Citrus Flavonoids, and Hydroxyethylrutosides"). Sodium cromoglycate (200 to 400 mg q.d.) is a compound similar to quercetin that confers excellent protection against urticaria and angioedema in response to ingested food allergens.
- **Fish oil:** patients with salicylate-induced severe urticaria and asthma requiring systemic steroid therapy, and anaphylactic reactions were successfully treated with oral supplements of 10 g fish oil daily, providing 3000 mg eicosapentaenoic acid (EPA) and docosahexaenoic acid (DHA) for 6 to 8 weeks. They experienced

virtually complete resolution of symptoms, allowing discontinuation of steroids. Symptoms relapsed after dose reduction.

THERAPEUTIC APPROACH

Conventional management of chronic urticaria: patients often respond incompletely to antihistamines and often are uncomfortable and frustrated by chronic pruritus. Some patients respond to systemic steroids, but serious side effects preclude safe long-term use. A wide variety of drugs used singly or in combination testifies to the inability of pharmaceuticals to address and treat symptoms and underlying causes of urticaria fully.

Identify and control all factors that can potentially promote a patient's urticarial response. Thorough history is paramount. Acute urticaria is usually self-limiting, especially after eliciting agent is removed or reduced. Chronic urticaria responds to removal of eliciting agent(s). In severe anaphylaxis, emergency measures are imperative.

- **Diet:** elimination or oligoantigenic diet is paramount in chronic urticaria (*Textbook,* "Food Allergy Testing" and "Food Reactions"). Eliminate suspected allergens and all food additives.
  - Strictest elimination diets allow only water, lamb, rice, pears, and vegetables. Avoid foods most commonly linked to urticaria (milk, eggs, chicken, fruits, nuts, additives). Avoid foods containing vasoactive amines, even if no direct allergy to them is noted. Primary foods to eliminate are cured meat, alcohol, cheese, chocolate, citrus fruits, and shellfish.
  - Control arachidonic acid–dependent prostaglandins with a diet low in animal fat.
- **Supplements:**
  - Vitamin C: 1 g t.i.d.
  - Vitamin B_{12}: 1000 mg intramuscularly per week
  - Quercetin: 250 to 400 mg 20 minutes before meals
  - Fish oil: 3000 mg EPA plus DHA daily
- **Psychological:** relaxation techniques daily, including audiotaped relaxation programs. Appropriate mind-body management approaches, leading to good clinical outcomes for chronic urticaria, are dependent on the clinician's ability to discern unique patient stories.

Physical Medicine

- Daily sunbathing for 15 to 20 minutes or ultraviolet A solarium, especially in chronic physical urticaria
- Tepid oatmeal baths
- *Caution:* with physical modalities when symptoms have physical triggers such as heat, cold, or water

Traditional Chinese Medicine: Acupuncture

Acupuncture can work quite well together with naturopathic therapies to treat underlying causes and symptoms of urticaria.

Uterine Fibroids

DIAGNOSTIC SUMMARY

- Most are asymptomatic.
- Symptoms include vague feeling of discomfort, pressure, congestion, bloating, heaviness; pain with vaginal sexual activity; urinary frequency; backache; abdominal enlargement; and abnormal bleeding.
- Abnormal bleeding occurs in 30% of women with fibroids.
- Fibroids can degenerate with necrosis, resulting in cystic degeneration.
- Calcification can occur.
- Examination by pelvic palpation and/or pelvic ultrasonography.
- Main diagnostic consideration: differentiating fibroid from ovarian malignant tumor, abscess in fallopian tube or ovarian region, diverticulum of colon, pelvic kidney, endometriosis, adenomyosis, congenital anomalies, and uterine sarcoma.

GENERAL CONSIDERATIONS

- Uterine fibroids consist of smooth muscle cells and connective tissue. Growth is stimulated by estrogen. Fibroids arise during reproductive years, grow during pregnancy, and regress after menopause. Growth spurt can happen in perimenopausal years—anovulatory cycles with irregular relative estrogen excess.
- Incidence is 20% to 25% of women by age 40 years; more than 50% of women overall; African American women have higher incidence. Fibroids are the most common indication for major surgery in women and the most common solid tumor in women.
- Cause is poorly understood. Factors include increased local estradiol concentration within fibroid itself, higher estrogen receptor density in fibroid tissue than in surrounding myometrium but lower than in endometrium.
- From 50% to 80% of fibroids are asymptomatic. Abnormal bleeding, including menorrhagia and metrorrhagia, occurs in 30% of women

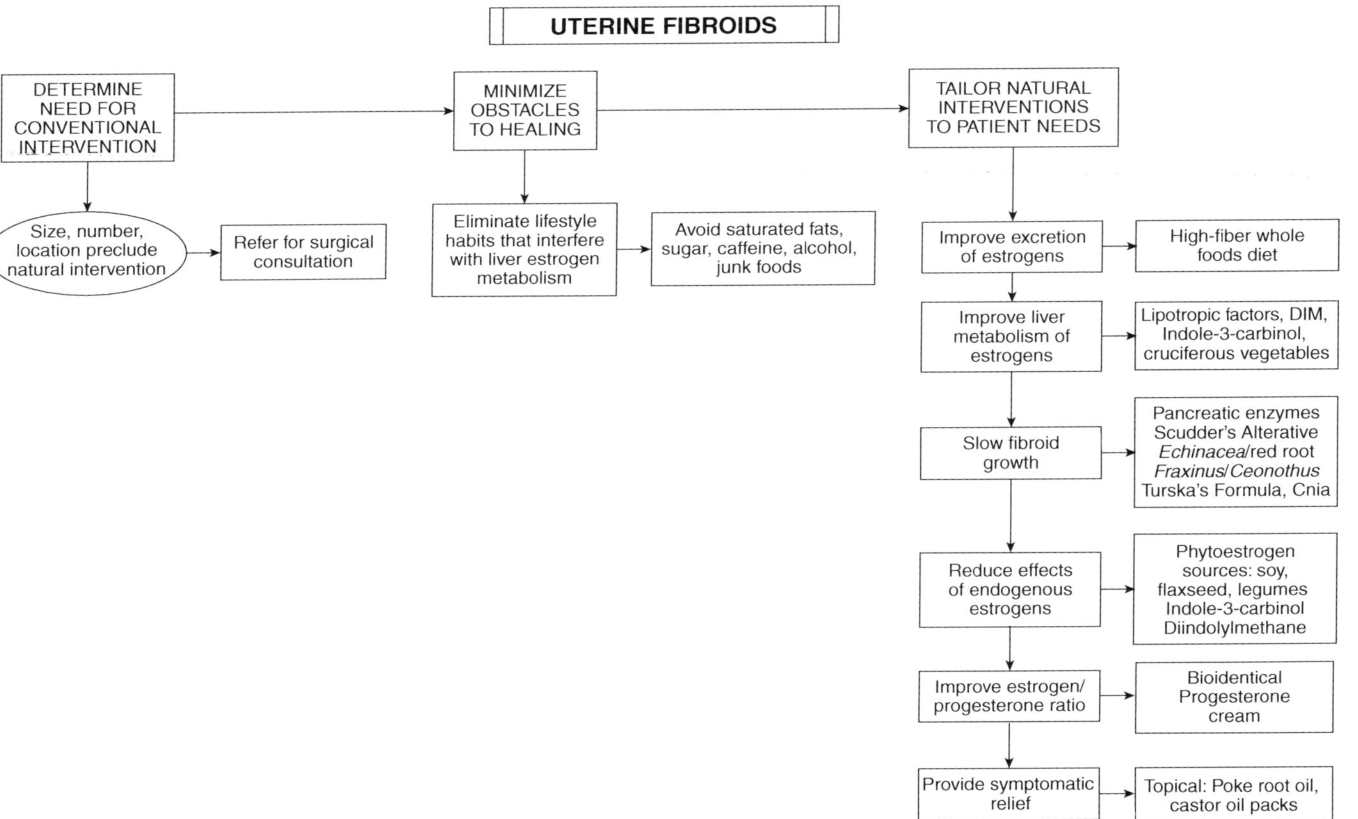
UTERINE FIBROIDS
DETERMINE NEED FOR CONVENTIONAL INTERVENTION
Size, number, location preclude natural intervention
Refer for surgical consultation
MINIMIZE OBSTACLES TO HEALING
Eliminate lifestyle habits that interfere with liver estrogen metabolism
Avoid saturated fats, sugar, caffeine, alcohol, junk foods
TAILOR NATURAL INTERVENTIONS TO PATIENT NEEDS
Improve excretion of estrogens
High-fiber whole foods diet
Improve liver metabolism of estrogens
Lipotropic factors, DIM, Indole-3-carbinol, cruciferous vegetables
Slow fibroid growth
Pancreatic enzymes
Scudder's Alterative
Echinacea/red root
Fraxinus/*Ceonothus*
Turska's Formula, Cnia
Reduce effects of endogenous estrogens
Phytoestrogen sources: soy, flaxseed, legumes
Indole-3-carbinol
Diindolylmethane
Improve estrogen/progesterone ratio
Bioidentical Progesterone cream
Provide symptomatic relief
Topical: Poke root oil, castor oil packs

with fibroids. Hydronephrosis can occur from compression of ureter. Fibroids cause of 2% to 10% of infertility cases. Large fibroids can interfere with pregnancy by interfering with fetal growth and being associated with premature rupture of membranes, retained placenta, postpartum hemorrhage, abnormal labor, or abnormal lie of fetus. Incidence of miscarriage from fibroids is two to three times greater than that in women without fibroids.
- Degenerative changes: fibroid outpaces blood supply; cellular detail is lost from decreased vascularity of tumor. Necrosis results in cystic degeneration. Calcification can occur over time, especially in postmenopausal women.

DIAGNOSIS

- Based on mitotic count, nuclear atypia, and other morphologic features, uterine smooth muscle tumors can be classified as leiomyomas, smooth muscle tumors of uncertain malignant potential, and leiomyosarcomas.
- Presumptive diagnosis of fibroids: thorough history and pelvic examination. Palpation findings: enlarged, firm uterus or uterus with irregular edges.
- Differentiate possible fibroid from ovarian malignant tumor, fallopian tube or ovarian region abscess, diverticulum, pelvic kidney, endometriosis, congenital anomaly, pelvic adhesions, or rare retroperitoneal tumors. Not all of these can be distinguished by medical history, physical examination, and pelvic ultrasound. Submucosal pedunculated fibroids can be visualized with laparoscopy. Laparoscopy can visualize intramural and subserous fibroids.
- Uterine fibroids are classified by location:
  - — Submucosal: just under the endometrium
  - — Intramural: within the uterine muscle wall
  - — Subserosal: from the outer wall of the uterus
  - — Interligamentous: in the cervix between the two layers of the broad ligament
  - — Pedunculated: on a stalk, either submucosal or subserous

THERAPEUTIC CONSIDERATIONS

Natural therapies manage troublesome symptoms. No reliable alternative to surgery shrinks fibroids. Natural therapies help keep fibroid from growing larger and usually resolve or improve most symptoms. Do not expect size reduction despite individual case reports. Reduction in fibroid size as a result of treatment is difficult to assess, especially in perimenopausal women in their 40s, who at some point will have lower endogenous estrogen production with resultant diminution of the fibroid.

Diet

- Although no dietary approach is known to prevent or shrink uterine fibroids, there are strong rationales for several dietary interventions. High intake of saturated fats is associated with higher blood levels of estrogen. Low-fiber diets are linked to estrogen elevation and poor estrogen excretion. Dietary improvement may reduce gastrointestinal symptoms associated with large or pedunculated fibroids and an enlarged uterus.
- Natural therapies work best in context of healthy lifestyle and diet. These changes can decrease heavy bleeding or pain and discomfort.
- Liver metabolizes estradiol for elimination by converting it to estrone, then to estriol, a weaker estrogen with little influence on the uterus.
- Saturated fats, sugar, caffeine, alcohol, and junk foods are problematic because they interfere with metabolism of estradiol to estrone to estriol and are deficient in B vitamins or interfere with B-vitamin metabolism. B vitamins facilitate metabolic processes and help regulate estrogen levels.
- Whole grains are excellent sources of B vitamins and help excretion of estrogens through the bowel. Vegetarian women who eat a high-fiber, low-fat diet have lower blood estrogen than omnivores with low-fiber diets. Fiber may prevent and perhaps reduce fibroids by reducing estrogen influence on uterine tissue.
- High-fiber diet may relieve bloating and congestion. Bulking stool and regulating bowel movements may improve bloating.
- Uterine fibroids are linked to a fourfold increased risk of endometrial cancer. Three dietary imperatives are to increase fiber, lower dietary fat, and increase soy products and other legumes. Higher fat intake is linked to increased risk for endometrial cancer, higher fiber intake reduces risk for endometrial cancer, and higher soy and legume intake decreases risk of endometrial cancer.
- Increase intake of other sources of phytoestrogens (whole grains, vegetables, fruits, seaweeds).

- Soy phytoestrogens do not have estrogenic effect on uterus. They are selective of tissues estrogenically affected. In the uterus, soy isoflavones have antiestrogen effect.

Nutritional Supplements

Supplement recommendations are based on tradition, theory, logic, and clinical experiences rather than scientific evidence of clinical trials.

- **Lipotropic factors:** inositol and choline exert lipotropic effect, promoting removal of fat from the liver. Lipotropics combine vitamins, herbals, and animal liver extract to support liver function in metabolizing and excreting estrogens.
- **Indole-3-carbinol (I3C), diindolylmethane (DIM), and *Brassica* (cruciferous) vegetables:** anticancer phytonutrients in cabbage-family vegetables (e.g., I3C, DIM, and sulforaphane) help to metabolize cancer-causing forms of estrogens to nontoxic forms.
- **Pancreatic enzymes:** treat pancreatic insufficiency with symptoms of abdominal bloating, gas, indigestion, undigested food in stool, and malabsorption. Pancreatic enzymes help digest fibrous and smooth muscle tissue and dissolve fibroids. Supplement must be taken between meals rather than with meals when used for this purpose.

Botanical Medicines

Traditional Herbs

Attempt to reduce uterine fibroids or slow their growth as prescribed based on anecdotal reports of modest success reducing size and number of fibroids.

- **Scudder's Alterative:** 30 to 40 drops in a small amount of warm water t.i.d.
  — *Dicentra canadensis* (*Corydalis* tubers)
  — *Alnus serrulata* (black alder bark)
  — *Podophyllum peltatum* (mayapple root)
  — *Scrophularia nodosa* (figwort flowering herb)
  — *Rumex crispus* (yellow dock root)
- **Compounded *Echinacea*/red root**
  — *Echinacea* species
  — *Ceanothus americanus* (red root)
  — *Baptisia tinctoria* (*Baptisia* root)
  — *Thuja occidentalis* (*Thuja* leaf)
  — *Stillingia sylvatica* (*Stillingia* root)

— *Iris versicolor* (blue flag root)
— *Zanthoxylum clava-herculis* (prickly ash bark)

- **Compounded *Fraxinus/Ceanothus***
  — *Fraxinus americana* (mountain ash bark)
  — *C. americanus* (red root)
  — *Packera aurea* (life root)
  — *P. peltatum* (mayapple root)
  — *Chamaelirium luteum* (helonias root)
  — *Hydrastis canadensis* (goldenseal root)
  — *Lobelia inflata* (lobelia)
  — *Zingiber officinale* (ginger root)
- **Compounded *Gelsemium/Phytolacca* (Turska's Formula)**
  — *Gelsemium sempervirens* (*Gelsemium* root)
  — *Phytolacca americana* (poke root)
  — *Aconitum napellus* (aconite)
  — *Bryonia dioica* (*Bryonia* root)
- **Other herbal extracts to consider:**
  — *Vitex agnus-castus* (chaste tree)
  — *Urtica dioica* (nettles)
  — *Arctium lappa* (burdock root)
  — *Taraxacum officinale* (dandelion root)
  — *Berberis aquifolium* (Oregon grape)
- **Crila (*Crinum*):** traditional botanical medicine of Vietnam. Of the 12 varieties of Crila, *Crinum latifolium* (or Tram, named after the leading researcher) has decreased the size or stopped the growth of fibroid tumors in 79.5% of women. In 20.5%, tumor growth continued at a very slow rate. Crila may even reduce heavy menstrual flow in such cases. Side effects are slight—nausea, headache, vaginal dryness, and hot flashes—but decrease over time.

Topical Applications

- **Poke root oil:** rub on belly over uterus nightly before bed
- **Castor oil packs:** apply over pelvis three to five times per week

Herbal Phytoestrogens

- Three types of phytoestrogens are found in medicinal plants: resorcylic acid lactones, steroids and sterols, and phenolics.
  — **Resorcylic acid lactones:** not true phytoestrogens because they are from plant mold contamination.
  — **Steroids:** classic steroidal estrogens estradiol and estrone are found in very minute amounts in apple seed, date palm, and

pomegranate—1 to 10 parts per billion. Diosgenin is a steroid derivative found in 20 plants (e.g., wild yam species). Beta-sitosterol is the most common phytosterol; found in plant oils such as wheat germ oil, cottonseed oil, and soybean oil. Beta-sitosterol is the dominant phytosterol in garlic and onions. Herbal sources include licorice root, saw palmetto, and red clover. Stigmasterol is related to beta-sitosterol. Soybean oil is a source of stigmasterol and a better source for laboratory synthesis of progesterone than is beta-sitosterol. Herbal sources include burdock, fennel, licorice, alfalfa, anise, and sage.
  - **Phenolic phytoestrogens:** are flavonoids. Phenolics include isoflavones, which are highest in legumes, especially soybeans. Coumestans have one estrogenic member, coumestrol, which is six times more estrogenic than isoflavones. Lignans are high in grains and highest in flaxseed.
- Phytoestrogens reduce incidence of uterine cancer.
- Red clover contains the highest concentrations of phytoestrogens. Both coumestans and isoflavones change typical stimulation with steroidal hormones (e.g., estradiol) in all target organs. Coumestrol temporarily enhances uptake of estradiol by the uterus and vagina but inhibits uptake of estradiol by the uterus long term by competing with estradiol for receptor sites.
- Estrogenic effect of phytoestrogens is dose dependent. Given in high enough doses, they have estrogenic effects on all the same target tissues as estradiol.
- Soy phytoestrogens are not estrogen stimuli for endometrium; they are estrogen antagonists associated with low rates of endometrial cancer in countries where soy phytoestrogen intake is high.
- *Tripterygium wilfordii* Hook F: traditional Chinese herbal therapy for uterine fibroids. A clinical study showed that treatment was effective and time dependent; 28% responded in 3 to 4 months and 52% in 5 to 6 months. Therapy induced an increase in luteinizing hormone and follicle-stimulating hormone and a decrease in estradiol and progesterone. Treatment effect may be caused by a reversible inhibitory effect on the ovary.

Natural Progesterone

- Progesterone may inhibit growth of uterine fibroids. Progesterone administered to guinea pigs prevents formation of tumors induced by estrogen. Clinically diagnosed uterine fibroids have regressed after progesterone therapy.

- Dr. John Lee: many women in their mid-30s have nonovulating cycles, producing less progesterone but normal (or more) estrogen. Indications of estrogen dominance and progesterone deficiency: retention of water and salt, fibrocystic swollen breast tissue, weight gain (hips and torso), depression, decreased libido, bone mineral loss, and fibroids. Natural progesterone replacement causes fibroid growth to cease (generally decrease in size) until menopause, after which fibroids atrophy.
- Preferred form of natural progesterone for treating fibroids (unless heavy bleeding is present): topical cream with 400 mg progesterone per ounce. Apply ¼ tsp q.d. or b.i.d. for 1 week after menses, and ¼ to ½ tsp b.i.d. for next 2 weeks (second half of cycle). Progesterone cream is not used for 1 week during menstrual flow. Apply cream to inner arms, chest, inner thighs, and/or palms.
- Dr. Mitchell Rein: no evidence shows that estrogen directly stimulates myoma growth, but progesterone and progestins promote fibroids. Development and growth of myomas involve multistep chain of events.

THERAPEUTIC APPROACH

Diet: high fiber, low fat, whole grains, high flaxseeds and soy foods; avoid saturated fats, sugar, caffeine, alcohol.

Nutritional Supplements

- **Lipotropic factors:** 1000 mg choline and 1000 mg methionine and/or cysteine daily. Alternatively, if high homocysteine (methionine supplementation will elevate homocysteine): 200 to 400 mg *S*-adenosylmethionine (SAM) daily.
- Choose one or a combination of the following:
  — I3C: 300 to 600 mg daily
  — DIM: 100 to 200 mg daily with food
- **Proteolytic enzymes:** for example, mixed enzyme preparations or pancreatin (8× to 10× United States Pharmacopeia [USP]), 350 to 750 mg between meals t.i.d.; or bromelain 250 to 750 mg (1800 to 2000 milk clotting units [MCU]) between meals t.i.d.

Herbal Medicines

- **Scudder's Alterative:** 30 to 40 drops in small amount of warm water t.i.d.

- ***Echinacea*/red root compound:** 30 drops in small amount of warm water t.i.d.
- ***Fraxinus*/*Ceanothus* compound:** 30 drops in small amount of warm water t.i.d.
- **Turska's Formula:** 5 drops in small amount of warm water t.i.d.

Topical

- Bioidentical progesterone cream: ¼ tsp b.i.d. from day 15 to day 26
- Topical poke root oil over uterus every night for 1 month, then one to three times a week

Conventional Medicine Therapies

- Fibroids causing heavy bleeding: progestogens or oral contraceptives may help manage bleeding.
- Fibroids and uteri large enough for presurgical treatment with leuprolide acetate (Lupron) may facilitate less radical surgical option.
- High-intensity focused ultrasound: new nonmedical technique for fibroids.
- Selective progesterone receptor modulators: new experimental treatment for fibroid pain and bleeding and for reducing the size of fibroids.

Consider surgical options based on size, number, and location of fibroids.

- Myomectomy
- Laparoscopic surgery for subserous and pedunculated fibroids
- Uterine embolization
- Hysteroscopic resection
- Supracervical hysterectomy
- Laparoscopic-assisted vaginal hysterectomy

Vaginitis

DIAGNOSTIC SUMMARY

- Increased volume of vaginal secretions.
- Abnormal color, consistency, or odor of vaginal secretions.
- Vulvovaginal itching, burning, or irritation.
- Introitus may show patchy erythema, and vaginal mucosa may exhibit congestion or petechiae.
- Dysuria or dyspareunia may be present.

GENERAL CONSIDERATIONS

Vaginitis is a common complaint in women, accounting for 7% of all visits to gynecologists and being the most common gynecologic problem encountered by primary care providers for women. Seventy-two percent of young, sexually active women have one or more forms of vulvovaginitis. Vaginal infections are six times more common than urinary tract infections (UTIs); dysuria is more likely caused by vaginitis than a UTI. Most women can distinguish "internal" dysuria of UTI from "external" dysuria felt when urine passes over inflamed labial tissues; question patients with dysuria more specifically about symptoms of vaginal discharge or irritation. Medical importance of vaginitis is as follows:

- Symptoms could overlie serious problem (e.g., chronic cervicitis or sexually transmitted disease). If infectious, agent may ascend the genital tract, leading to endometritis, salpingitis, and pelvic inflammatory disease (PID), leading to tubal scarring, infertility, or ectopic pregnancies.
- Implicated in recurrent UTIs by acting as reservoir of infectious agents.
- Some vaginal infections during pregnancy increase the risk of miscarriage and, if present at delivery, cause neonatal infections.
- Some forms of vaginitis are linked to cervical cellular abnormalities and increased risk of cervical dysplasia.

Vaginal ecosystem is governed by the relationships among normal endogenous microflora, metabolic products of microflora

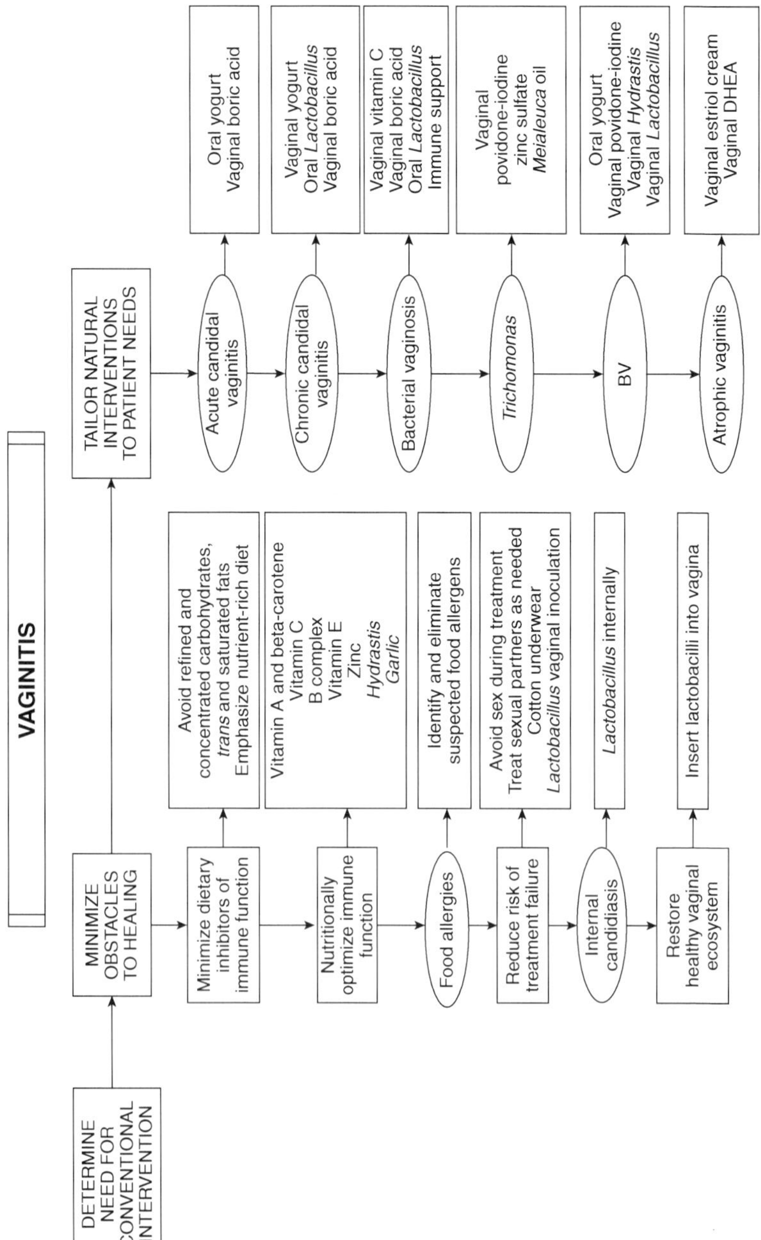
VAGINITIS
DETERMINE NEED FOR CONVENTIONAL INTERVENTION
MINIMIZE OBSTACLES TO HEALING
TAILOR NATURAL INTERVENTIONS TO PATIENT NEEDS
Minimize dietary inhibitors of immune function
Avoid refined and concentrated carbohydrates, trans and saturated fats
Emphasize nutrient-rich diet
Nutritionally optimize immune function
Vitamin A and beta-carotene
Vitamin C
B complex
Vitamin E
Zinc
Hydrastis
Garlic
Food allergies
Identify and eliminate suspected food allergens
Reduce risk of treatment failure
Avoid sex during treatment
Treat sexual partners as needed
Cotton underwear
Lactobacillus vaginal inoculation
Internal candidiasis
Lactobacillus internally
Restore healthy vaginal ecosystem
Insert lactobacilli into vagina
Acute candidal vaginitis
Oral yogurt
Vaginal boric acid
Chronic candidal vaginitis
Vaginal yogurt
Oral Lactobacillus
Vaginal boric acid
Bacterial vaginosis
Vaginal vitamin C
Vaginal boric acid
Oral Lactobacillus
Immune support
Trichomonas
Vaginal povidone-iodine
zinc sulfate
Melaleuca oil
BV
Oral yogurt
Vaginal povidone-iodine
Vaginal Hydrastis
Vaginal Lactobacillus
Atrophic vaginitis
Vaginal estriol cream
Vaginal DHEA

and host, estrogen, and pH. Normal microflora include *Candida, Lactobacillus* species, gram-negative aerobic bacteria, facultative bacteria (*Mycoplasma* species and *Gardnerella vaginalis*), and obligate anaerobic bacteria (*Prevotella, Peptostreptococcus* species, *Eubacterium* species, *Mobiluncus* species). Lactobacilli dominate the healthy vagina of a reproductive-age woman: *Lactobacillus plantarum, Lactobacillus reuteri, Lactobacillus acidophilus.* Normal microflora inhibits adhesion and growth of pathogens, depletes nutrients available to pathogens, and modulates host immune response and vaginal environment. Lactobacilli act via three mechanisms: (1) producing lactic acid from glycogen in vaginal vault cells and providing normal acidic environment of 3.5 to 4.5, hostile to pathogens; (2) producing hydrogen peroxide; and (3) competing with pathogens for adherence to vaginal epithelium.

TYPES OF VAGINITIS

Traditional classifications—yeast, bacterial vaginosis (BV), *Trichomonas vaginalis,* or atrophic vaginitis—leave gaps in diagnosis and treatment of atypical scenarios. New categories: desquamative inflammatory vaginitis (DIV), *Mobiluncus* vaginitis, lactobacillosis, noninflammatory vaginitis (NV), and inflammatory vaginitis (IV).

- **Atrophic vaginitis:** usually affects perimenopausal and postmenopausal women but can also occur in prepubertal girls, owing to poorly estrogenized vaginal and vulvar tissue, and in postpartum women because of sudden declines in hormone levels. The structure and function of vaginal tissues undergo change with declining estrogenic stimulation, including estrogen loss after oophorectomy. Vaginal epithelium atrophies from a lack of estrogenic stimulation; this may cause a decrease in *Lactobacillus* in the vagina, more-alkaline pH, vaginal thinning, less lubrication, more-easily irritated and inflamed tissue, adhesions, dyspareunia, and increased susceptibility to infection. Most common symptoms are itching or burning and thin, watery discharge, occasionally blood tinged (any vaginal bleeding in postmenopausal women requires complete workup to rule out endometrial hyperplasia and endometrial carcinoma; see baseline evaluation in the chapter on menopause). The pH is typically equal to or greater than 5.5, but there is no infection. Other common complaints: dyspareunia and/or vaginal dryness with vaginal sexual activity.

- **Increased vaginal discharge:** increased normal secretions in the absence of other symptoms. Diagnosis of physiologic vaginitis often is applied but is inappropriate because no inflammation exists. Increased discharge often reflects increased hormonal stimulation (pregnancy or some stages of menstrual cycle). This is primarily a diagnosis of exclusion after ruling out other causes. Usually no further treatment is required other than reassurance. Overly zealous douching or washing briefly alleviates symptoms but may aggravate the condition by causing irritant vaginitis.
- **Irritant vaginitis:**
  - — Caused by physical or chemical agents damaging delicate vaginal membranes. Identified by careful history and examination.
  - — **Chemical vaginitis:** medications or hygiene products can irritate vaginal mucosa. Allergic vaginitis is damage elicited by immunologic reaction to a product rather than direct toxic reaction. Perfumed toilet paper, douches, spermicides, condoms, and lubricants can be irritating agents.
  - — **Traumatic vaginitis:** injury caused by physical agents or sexual activity.
  - — **Foreign body vaginitis:** foul discharge may indicate foreign body in vagina. Most common are forgotten tampons, contraceptive devices, and pessaries. Very young girls and adolescents may leave foreign bodies in their vaginas from exploring their bodies; they either forget or are too embarrassed to tell someone that they cannot retrieve the item. Also, semen may be an irritant in some women.
- **Infectious vaginitis:**
  - — Ninety percent of vaginitis in reproductive-aged women is caused by BV, candidiasis, or trichomoniasis. BV is most common. Less-common causes include herpes simplex virus, gonorrhea (GC), and chlamydia. Infections of the vulva can cause local itching and/or discharge: folliculitis, hidradenitis, scabies, condyloma, herpes, syphilis, human papillomavirus (HPV), *Candida*. Rare conditions of vulva causing itching and/or discharge include chancroid, lymphogranuloma venereum inguinale, and molluscum contagiosum.
  - — May be sexually transmitted or a result of a disturbance of the delicate ecosystem of the healthy vagina. It often involves common organisms found in the cervix and vagina of healthy, asymptomatic women.

- — Unifying factor in pathogenesis of pelvic infections is not which microbes are present, but rather the cause of patient susceptibility.
  — Factors influencing vaginal environment are pH, glycogen content, glucose level, presence of other microbes (lactobacilli), estrogen, semen exposure, nonoxynol-9 spermicide exposure, douching, menstrual blood, and antibodies and other compounds in vaginal secretions; all are affected by a woman's internal milieu and general health.
  — Immune dysfunction predisposes to increased vaginal infections: nutritional deficiencies, medicines (e.g., steroids), pregnancy, or serious illness (e.g., human immunodeficiency virus [HIV] infection).
  — Other predisposing factors are diabetes mellitus, hypothyroidism, leukemia, Addison's disease, Cushing's syndrome, pregnancy, and *Candida* infections.
  — Predisposing factors for sexually transmitted disease: high number of partners, unsafe sex, birth control (barriers reduce risk), birth control pills, steroids, antibiotics, tight-fitting garments, occlusive materials, douches, chlorinated pools, perfumed toilet paper, and decrease in lactobacilli in vagina.
- ***T. vaginalis:*** flagellated protozoan found in the lower genitourinary tract of men and women. Human beings are the only host. Sexual intercourse is the primary mode of dissemination. *Trichomonas* does not invade tissues and rarely causes serious complications.
  — Most common symptoms are leukorrhea, itching, and burning. Discharge is malodorous, greenish yellow, and frothy.
  — "Strawberry cervix" with punctate hemorrhages is found in only a small percentage of *Trichomonas* cases.
  — Grows optimally at pH of 5.5 to 5.8. Conditions elevating pH (e.g., increased progesterone) favor *Trichomonas* growth. Vaginal pH of 4.5 in women with vaginitis suggests agent other than *Trichomonas.*
- Saline wet mount of fresh vaginal fluid shows small motile organisms, confirming diagnosis in 80% to 90% of symptomatic carriers.
- ***Candida albicans:*** 2.5-fold increase in candidal vaginitis has occurred in the past 20 years, paralleling the declining incidence of GC and *Trichomonas.* Contributing factors are increased use of antibiotics, which changes the vaginal ecosystem to favor *Candida.*
  — 100% correlation between genital and gastrointestinal *Candida* cultures: significant intestinal colonization with

Candida may be the single most significant predisposing factor in vulvovaginal candidiasis. However, this has not been confirmed by adequate research. Steroids, oral contraceptives, and diabetes mellitus contribute. Candidiasis is 10 to 20 times more frequent during pregnancy because of elevated vaginal pH, increased vaginal epithelial glycogen, elevated blood glucose, and intermittent glycosuria.

— Candidiasis is three times more prevalent in women who wear pantyhose than in those who wear cotton underwear; pantyhose prevent drying of area.

— Four or more episodes of vulvovaginal candidiasis in 1 year classify the patient as having recurrent disease. Cause may be non-*albicans* strains of *Candida*—resistant strains generated by antifungals. Three main theories of why women get recurring yeast vaginitis: (1) intestinal reservoir migrating into vagina, (2) sexual partner is source of recurrence, and (3) vaginal relapse forms small residual numbers of yeast after treatment. Research supports the third theory. Women with recurrent infections have an abnormal immune response, increasing susceptibility.

— Allergies can cause recurrent candidiasis, which resolves after allergies have been treated.

— Primary symptom of candidiasis is vulvar itching (sometimes severe). Burning of vulva, exacerbated by urination or vaginal sexual activity, also occurs. Thick, curdy or "cottage cheese" discharge that adheres to vaginal walls may be present. Such discharge is strong evidence of yeast infection, but its absence does not rule out *Candida*. Less than 20% of symptomatic candidiasis displays classic thrush patches. In addition, an increase or change in the consistency of the vaginal discharge is common.

— Other clues include erythema of vulva and excoriations from scratching. Vaginal pH is not usually altered.

— Neither the character of discharge nor the symptoms are sufficient alone for diagnosis of *Candida*. Wet mount in saline or 10% potassium hydroxide (KOH); mycelia are confirmatory. Budding forms of yeast are found in normal and symptomatic vaginas, but mycelial stage is found only in symptomatic women.

- **BV:** shift in flora predominance from lactobacilli to anaerobes and facultative bacteria that degrade mucins of natural gel barrier on vaginal epithelium, causing characteristic vaginal discharge. Destruction of mucins exposes cervical epithelium and allows other organisms to affect cervix, resulting in appearance of clue cells. Epithelial surface disruption causes immunologic shifts: upregulation of interleukin 1β (IL-1β) and decrease in protectant molecules (e.g., secretory leukocyte protease inhibitor).

- Three factors shift dominance from lactobacilli to anaerobes and facultative bacteria: sexual activity, douching, and absence of peroxide-producing lactobacilli. A new sexual partner or frequent sexual activity increases incidence of BV. Routine douching is linked to loss of vaginal lactobacilli and occurrence of BV. Women who regularly douche for hygiene purposes have BV twice as often as women who do not routinely douche. Women lacking vaginal peroxide–producing lactobacilli may not have had normal lactobacilli at menarche, or lactobacilli were eliminated by broad-spectrum antibiotics.
- Other factors increasing risk for BV: cigarette smoking suppresses immune response. Racial background: Hispanic women have a 50% greater risk and African American women have twice the risk. African American women practice douching twice as often as white women; African American women also are less likely to have vaginal lactobacilli.
- Examination for BV: medical history; observe discharge to determine vaginal pH. Symptomatic BV releases fishy odor. Discharge is thin, dark, or dull gray. Itching is uncommon in BV unless discharge is profuse. Perform whiff test and wet mount to detect clue cells and observe vaginal flora. Abundance of various bacteria and absence of or decrease in lactobacilli suggests BV. Numbers of bacteria increase from 100-fold to 1000-fold. Diagnosis of BV requires three of four criteria:
  1. Thin, dark, or dull gray, homogeneous, malodorous discharge that adheres to vaginal walls
  2. Vaginal pH above 4.5
  3. Positive KOH (whiff or amine) test result
  4. Clue cells on wet mount microscopic examination
- pH is elevated to 5.0 to 5.5; correlation exists between elevated pH and presence of odor
- Patient having four or more BV episodes per year (recurrent BV) has an underlying problem—the inability to reestablish normal *Lactobacillus* vaginal ecosystem. Thirty percent of women have recurrence of symptomatic BV within 1 to 3 months; 70% have recurrence within 9 months. Whether this is a relapse or reinfection is unclear. One possibility includes chronic underlying abnormal vaginal ecosystem, sometimes asymptomatic, sometimes symptomatic. Asymptomatic women lacking

lactobacilli have a four-times-greater risk for BV. No proven treatment benefit exists for asymptomatic women.

- Other potential consequences of altered vaginal flora:
  - Increased susceptibility to HIV and GC. PID is linked to BV. Organisms in pregnant women with BV can ascend the genital tract, causing preterm delivery and postpartum endometritis. BV increases risk for infection after gynecologic surgery.

THERAPEUTIC CONSIDERATIONS

Dietary Considerations

Vaginal secretions are continuously released and contain water, nutrients, electrolytes, and proteins (secretory immunoglobulin A) and are altered by hormonal and dietary factors. Prescribe a well-balanced diet low in fats, sugars, and refined foods. Nutrients for proper immune function are zinc (Zn), vitamin A, vitamin C, vitamin E, manganese, and vitamin B complex. Diet high in lysine and low in arginine reduces number and severity of herpetic outbreaks, but many foods high in lysine are animal products high in fats. A low-arginine diet plus lysine supplements is a viable alternative.

- ***Lactobacillus* yogurt:** the most specific medicinal food for BV. Daily ingestion of 8 oz of *L. acidophilus* yogurt by women with recurrent candidal vaginitis induced a threefold decrease in infections and candidal colonization compared with women who did not eat yogurt.

Nutritional Supplements

A high-quality multivitamin-mineral supplement is a low-cost compensation for dietary inadequacies.

- **Vitamin A and beta-carotene:** are necessary for epithelial tissues of the vaginal mucosa. Vitamin A is needed for adequate immune response and resistance to infection. Secretory immunoglobulin A is a major factor in resistance to infection. Beta-carotene is a nontoxic vitamin A precursor that enhances T-cell number and ratio. Excessive vitamin A is toxic and teratogenic; use caution in women of reproductive age. Limit total vitamin A intake to 5000 international units (IU) q.d. Use mixed carotenoids rather than synthetic beta-carotene.
- **B vitamins:** needed for carbohydrate metabolism, protein catabolism and synthesis, cell replication, and immune function. B_2 and B_6 have estrogen-like effects and act synergistically with

estradiol. B_1 and pantothenic acid enhance estradiol activity without having estrogenic activity themselves. B vitamins are useful in estrogen deficiency (atrophic vaginitis), especially if combined with phytoestrogens.

- **Vitamin C and bioflavonoids:** vaginal vitamin C has been used to treat BV. Vitamin C deficiency reduces phagocytic activity of leukocytes. Vitamin C and bioflavonoids improve connective tissue integrity, reducing spread of infection and frequency and severity of herpetic outbreaks. A 250-mg vitamin C tablet inserted vaginally once daily for 6 days can help eliminate BV, including bacteria and clue cells, and restore lactobacilli.
- **Vitamin E:** supplemental vitamin E increases resistance to *Chlamydia*. It regulates retinol in human beings; an inadequacy of vitamin E hinders use of vitamin A. Vitamin E is used to treat atrophic vaginitis. Excess vitamin E intake may be immunosuppressive (more than 1200 IU q.d.) and may transiently elevate blood pressure. It improves glycogen storage and tone of heart muscle. Use extra caution in patients with diabetes, hypoglycemia, hypertension, or heart disease. In high-risk patients, begin with a daily dose of 100 IU. Monitor blood sugar and/or blood pressure and increase dose slowly over time (e.g., 50 IU q.d.).
- **Zn:** all DNA and RNA polymerases and repair and replication enzymes require Zn. It enhances prostaglandin E_1 synthesis, normalizes lymphocyte activity, and enhances epithelial growth. Zn deficiency is linked to depressed immunity and thymic atrophy, which are corrected when Zn is replenished. Zn is essential for use of vitamin A. Topical and oral Zn reduces duration and severity of herpes outbreaks because of its antiviral activity. High levels are toxic to *Chlamydia* and *Trichomonas* and are effective in some cases unresponsive to antibiotics.

Botanical Medicines

- ***Glycyrrhiza glabra:*** licorice is antiviral against RNA and DNA viruses. It is effective in treating herpes. The number and severity of recurrences are reduced by the repeated application of gel to active lesions. 18-Beta glycyrrhetinic acid in licorice is effective against *Candida* (*Textbook, "Glycyrrhiza glabra* [Licorice]").
- **Chlorophyll:** has a bacteriostatic and soothing action. Water-soluble chlorophyll added to douching solutions offers symptomatic relief.

- ***Allium sativum:*** garlic is antibacterial, antiviral, and antifungal and is effective against some antibiotic-resistant organisms. Major growth inhibitory component is allicin; therefore, garlic products with the highest amount of allicin are preferred. A garlic clove may be carefully peeled so as not to nick the clove, pierced with thread, and inserted into the vagina. Garlic capsules may also be inserted into the vagina.
- ***Hydrastis canadensis* (goldenseal) and *Berberis vulgaris* (barberry):** contain berberine, a broad-range antibacterial. Berberine enhances immune function when taken internally and offers symptomatic relief when used in douching solutions; it soothes inflamed mucous membranes (*Textbook, "Hydrastis canadensis* [Goldenseal] and Other Berberine-Containing Botanicals").
- ***Melaleuca alternifolia:*** alcoholic extract of tea tree oil diluted to 1% in water is a strong antibacterial and antifungal. It is effective in treating trichomoniasis, candidiasis, and cervicitis. Use daily as a douche and weekly in saturated tampons. No adverse reactions have been reported. It has soothing effect. Tea tree oil preparations have antimicrobial activity against *Staphylococcus aureus* and *C. albicans* (*Textbook, "Melaleuca alternifolia* [Tea Tree]").
- **Botanical mixture:** cream containing *Azadirachta indica* (neem) seed oil, *Sapindus mukorossi* (reetha) saponin extract, and quinine—effective and proven better than placebo. It is applied intravaginally at bedtime for 14 days for *Chlamydia trachomatis* vaginitis and BV. It offers no benefit for candidal or trichomonal infections.

Other Agents

- ***Lactobacillus* species:** dominant organisms in vagina of healthy reproductive-aged premenopausal women. Beneficial properties: adhesiveness; synthesis of acids, hydrogen peroxide, bacteriocidins, biosurfactants. Antipathogenic strains: *Lactobacillus rhamnosus* GG, *L. acidophilus* NCFM, *Lactobacillus casei* Shirota, *L. reuteri* MM53, *L. casei* CRL 431, *L. rhamnosus* GR-1, *Lactobacillus fermentum* RC-14 (now called *L. reuteri*), *L. plantarum* 299v, *Lactobacillus salivarius*. Others: *Lactobacillus* strains *Lactobacillus johnsonii* LC1, *L. plantarum* 299v, and *Lactobacillus crispatus* CTV-05. Administer vaginally and orally. Weekly intravaginal *L. acidophilus* in HIV-positive women, susceptible to recurrent yeast vaginitis, is as effective as antifungal drug after just two treatments. After conventional antibiotics, restore vaginal lactobacilli by coadministering *Lactobacillus* and low-dose vaginal estriol. When *L. rhamnosus* GR-1 and *L. fermentum* RC-14 are given orally, they colonize the vagina and/or reduce vaginal candidiasis. Vaginally or orally administered *Lactobacillus* can colonize the vaginal ecosystem. Supplementation must continue for 2 to 6 months to sustain colonization. Use alone or in combination with other vaginal or oral therapies.

- **Iodine:** used as douche, it is effective against many organisms *(Trichomonas, Candida, Chlamydia)* and nonspecific vaginitis. Povidone-iodine (Betadine) does not sting or stain. It is effective in treating 100% of cases of candidal vaginitis, 80% of *Trichomonas,* and 93% of combination infections. Although douching in recent years is not as recommended, one study used a douching solution diluted to 1 part iodine to 100 parts water (1½ to 3 tsp povidone-iodine to 1 quart water) b.i.d. for 14 days.
- **Boric acid:** suppositories are both antibacterial and antifungal. Exact mechanism of action is unclear. Capsules of boric acid treat candidiasis almost as well as nystatin. Women with chronic resistant yeast vaginitis who did not respond to extensive, prolonged conventional therapy were treated with 600 mg boric acid vaginal suppositories b.i.d. for 2 or 4 weeks. This regimen cured 98% of these women. Boric acid cure rates vary from 40% to 100%. Recurrence rates vary from 0% to 45.5%. Vaginal burning sensation occurs in less than 10% of patients. Watery discharge during treatment and vaginal erythema may also occur.
- **Kudzu *(Pueraria mirifica):*** *P. mirifica,* given as 20, 30, or 50 mg capsules daily for 24 weeks, reduced average vaginal dryness symptoms after 12 weeks; and the maturation index increased after 24 weeks. This indicates an estrogenic effect on vaginal tissue and applicability for vaginal dryness and dyspareunia resulting from vaginal atrophy.
- **Hops:** a combination gel containing phytoestrogens from hops extract, hyaluronic acid, liposomes, and vitamin E. In postmenopausal women with vaginal dryness and related symptoms, one vaginal suppository inserted daily for the first 14 days and then one suppository every other day for 14 days: the average vaginal dryness scale score decreased from 7.92 to 0 by the end of treatment. Itching and burning disappeared progressively. Dyspareunia also improved progressively. Inflammation and irritation of vulvar and vaginal mucosa also improved significantly.

- **Estrogens:** estrogen therapy is the most effective treatment for moderate to severe atrophic vulvovaginitis. Systemic estrogen therapies and estrogen-progestogen therapies are effective for treating these symptoms. However, when urogenital atrophy is the main or only indication for estrogen, local vaginal estrogen therapy is recommended and not systemic hormone therapy.
- **Vaginal dehydroepiandrosterone (DHEA):** daily local intravaginal DHEA ovules (13 mg DHEA) were studied for 12 weeks in postmenopausal women relative to sexual dysfunction parameters of libido, arousal, orgasm, and dyspareunia. The ovules contained Prasterone, in a lipophilic agent manufactured by Recipharm of Sweden. Compared with placebo, DHEA improved symptoms by 68% in the abbreviated sex function/arousal/sensation domain, in the arousal/lubrication domain by 39%, orgasm by 75%, and dryness during intercourse by 57%. DHEA proved better than placebo in the desire domain of menopause-specific quality-of-life inventory. Serum levels of vaginal DHEA showed no or minimal changes during treatment, indicating therapeutic safety.

DIAGNOSTIC APPROACH

- Question women directly regarding pruritus, vaginal discharge, dysuria, and so on.
- Complete gynecologic and sexual history: sexual activity and practices of patient and partner(s), method of contraception, personal hygiene, self-medication. Rule out associated symptoms suggesting PID or systemic infection. Ascertain previous occurrences: diagnosis, treatment, and resolution.
- Identify causative agent; avoid douching, intercourse, and vaginal medications for 1 to 2 days before office visit.
- Determine by speculum examination whether discharge emanates from vagina or cervix, condition of vaginal mucosa, and character of discharge. Collect specimens and place on slides for saline and KOH examination. Use pH paper, amine testing strips, and microscopy of wet mounts.
- Assess pH.
- Use microscopy when needed for diagnosis (e.g., KOH wet prep).
- Perform abdominal bimanual examination.
- Genital culture can diagnose group B Streptococcus, yeast, BV (not well), *S. aureus,* and *Escherichia coli.* Yeast culture with request to identify strains of *Candida* can be done. Group B

streptococcal DNA probe or group B streptococcal culture is indicated for pregnant patients.

- Affirm VP III test is used to diagnose *Candida* species, BV, and trichomoniasis.
- Thin prep can test for many different pathogens—HPV and its genotype HPV 16/18, *Chlamydia*, gonococcus, *Trichomonas*, yeast, *Actinomyces*, herpesviruses 1 and 2, group B *Streptococcus*, BV, syphilis, *Ureaplasma*, and *Mycoplasma*.
- Culture if diagnosis remains in question or if screening for GC or *Chlamydia*.
- Best time to test for low-level persistent infection *(Candida)* is just before menstrual period.

THERAPEUTIC APPROACH

Keep in mind the following natural medicine concepts:

- Remove or limit obstacles to cure.
- Improve vaginal immunity.
- Support systemic immunity.
- Restore vaginal pH.
- Restore vaginal microenvironment.
- Restore gut ecology.
- Decrease inflammation and irritation.
- Provide symptom relief.
- Correct coexisting medical conditions.

Focus of this protocol is on *Candida*, *Trichomonas*, and BV. (For atrophic vaginitis, see the chapter on menopause; for herpes simplex, see the chapter on herpes simplex.) Immune support (diet, nutritional supplements, and botanical medicines) is an important aspect of the therapy.

- **Diet:** nutrient-dense diet; avoid refined foods and simple carbohydrates. Minimize trans and saturated fats. Determine and eliminate suspected food allergens.
- **Supplements:**
  - **Vitamin A:** 5000 IU q.d. or beta-carotene 50,000 IU q.d.
  - **Vitamin C:** 500 to 1000 mg q4h.
  - **Vitamin B complex:** balanced B complex averaging 20 to 50 mg of each major component.
  - **Zn:** 10 to 15 mg q.d.
  - **Vitamin E (mixed tocopherols):** 200 IU q.d.
  - ***Lactobacillus* species:** orally and vaginally; dose depends on duration and kind of infection.

- **Botanical medicines:**
  - — *H. canadensis* (goldenseal)
  - — Doses t.i.d. as follows:
    - Dried root or infusion (tea): 2 to 4 g
    - Tincture (1:5): 6 to 12 mL (1.5 to 3 tsp)
    - Fluid extract (1:1): 2 to 4 mL (½ to 1 tsp)
    - Solid (powdered dry) extract (4:1 or 8% to 12% alkaloid content): 250 to 500 mg
  - — *A. sativum* (garlic): dose equivalent to 4000 mcg allicin.

Other Botanicals

Traditional texts and modern practitioners find efficacy in treating vaginitis with the following herbs, used alone or with other agents in capsules or suppositories placed into vagina: *H. canadensis* (goldenseal); *Eucalyptus; Calendula officinalis* (marigold; use succus); and chlorophyll.

General Recommendations

- In all cases of chronic vaginitis, *Lactobacillus* capsules or *Lactobacillus* yogurt should be used daily, at least orally if not vaginally, to reinoculate the vagina. Continue oral intake for 2 to 6 months to ensure colonization.
- Treatment failures may be a result of incorrect diagnosis, reinfection, failure to treat predisposing factors, or patient resistance to treatment.
- *Trichomonas* infections in women require concurrent treatment of male partners.
- In cases of recurrent or chronic BV or yeast vaginitis, consider treating both male and female partners.

Specific Recommendations and Treatments

- **Acute candidal vaginitis**
  - — Boric acid capsules (600 mg) inserted b.i.d. into vagina for 3 to 7 days
  - — Daily ingestion of 8 oz of *L. acidophilus* yogurt
- **Chronic candidal vaginitis**
  - — 8 oz of *Acidophilus* yogurt daily
  - — *Lactobacillus* species (e.g., *L. rhamnosus, L. reuteri*): 1 to 5 billion; b.i.d. for 1 to 6 months
  - — Boric acid: 600-mg vaginal suppositories b.i.d. for 2 weeks (4 weeks if patient is not symptom free). To prevent vulvar

irritation from the boric acid, vitamin E oil or petroleum jelly can be applied to external genitalia.

- **BV**
  - — Vitamin C vaginal tablet for 6 days and then boric acid suppositories once daily for 1 week
  - — Multiple *Lactobacillus* species or strains: at least 2 billion daily for 2 weeks
  - — Systemic immune support
- ***Trichomonas***
  - — Povidone-iodine: applied b.i.d.
  - — Zn sulfate: applied daily
  - — *M. alternifolia:* oil applied daily
- **Atrophic vaginitis**
  - — Intravaginal estriol cream (1 mg/g): insert 1 g q.d. for 2 weeks, then 1 g twice weekly as maintenance. Other vaginal estrogen options: vaginal estradiol 0.1% cream, Premarin cream, Estring, Vagifem.
  - — Consider vaginal DHEA ovules 13 mg/day for 12 weeks, then twice a week.

Varicose Veins

DIAGNOSTIC SUMMARY

- Dilated, tortuous, superficial veins in the lower extremities.
- May be asymptomatic or associated with fatigue, aching discomfort, feeling of heaviness, or pain.
- Edema, pigmentation, and ulceration of the skin of the distal leg may develop.
- Women are affected four times as often as men.

GENERAL DISCUSSION

Veins are frail structures. Defects in the venous wall allow dilation of vein and damage to valves. Valve damage increases static pressure, causing bulging known as varicose veins.

- Fifty percent of middle-aged adults are affected.
- Subcutaneous veins of legs are most commonly affected because of gravitational pressure that standing exerts on veins. Standing for long periods increases pressure up to 10 times. Occupations requiring long periods of standing are greatest risk for varicose veins.
- Women are affected four times as often as men. Obesity greatly increases risk. Risk increases with age because of the loss of tissue tone and muscle mass, weakening vein walls. Pregnancy increases risk by increasing venous pressure in legs.
- Pose little harm if involved vein is near surface, but they are cosmetically unappealing. Significant symptoms are uncommon, but legs may feel heavy, tight, and tired.
- If varicose veins are associated with chronic venous insufficiency, leg ulcers may form that are often difficult to resolve.
- Serious varicosities involve obstruction and valve defects of deeper veins of the leg. This can lead to thrombophlebitis, pulmonary embolism, myocardial infarction, and stroke. Phlebography and Doppler ultrasonography are the most accurate methods of diagnosing deep vein involvement.

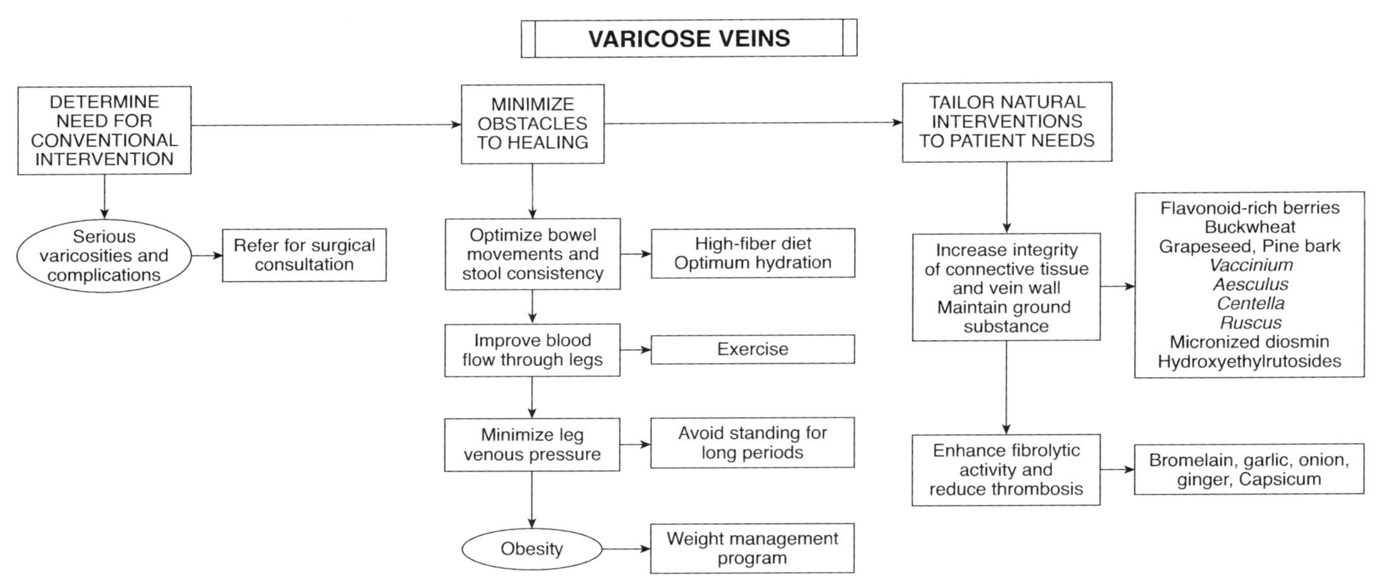
VARICOSE VEINS
DETERMINE NEED FOR CONVENTIONAL INTERVENTION
Serious varicosities and complications
Refer for surgical consultation
MINIMIZE OBSTACLES TO HEALING
Optimize bowel movements and stool consistency
High-fiber diet Optimum hydration
Improve blood flow through legs
Exercise
Minimize leg venous pressure
Avoid standing for long periods
Obesity
Weight management program
TAILOR NATURAL INTERVENTIONS TO PATIENT NEEDS
Increase integrity of connective tissue and vein wall Maintain ground substance
Flavonoid-rich berries Buckwheat Grapeseed, Pine bark *Vaccinium* *Aesculus* *Centella* *Ruscus* Micronized diosmin Hydroxyethylrutosides
Enhance fibrolytic activity and reduce thrombosis
Bromelain, garlic, onion, ginger, Capsicum

Etiology

- Genetic weakness of veins or venous valves.
- Excess venous pressure from increase in straining during defecation because of a low-fiber diet.
- Long periods of standing and/or heavy lifting.
- Damage to veins or venous valves as a result of thrombophlebitis.
- Weakness of vascular walls from abnormalities in proteoglycans of interendothelial cement substance or excessive release of matrix metalloproteinases (MMPs)—beta-*N*-acetylglucosaminidase, beta-glucuronidase, and arylsulfatase, which degrade extracellular matrix proteins and structural integrity of the vein wall.
- MMPs affect endothelium and smooth muscle components of the vein wall, inducing changes in venous constriction and relaxation.
- Endothelial cell injury triggers leukocyte infiltration, activation, and inflammation, worsening damage to the vein wall.

THERAPEUTIC CONSIDERATIONS

Severely affected veins may require more-aggressive treatment. Conventional surgery involves removal—vein stripping. Newer treatments seal the main leaking vein at the highest point of valvular dysfunction on the thigh (e.g., ultrasound-guided foam sclerotherapy, radiofrequency ablation, and endovenous laser treatment). Most blood in the legs returns via deep veins; therefore these interventions might not cause harm. In sclerotherapy with segmental phlebectomy (vein stripping), a sclerosing agent is injected at the highest portion of the affected vein and only the worst segments are removed.

Dietary Factors

- **Fiber:** varicose veins are rarely seen in parts of world with high-fiber, unrefined diets. A low-fiber diet contributes to the development of varicose veins because of the need to strain more during bowel movements (smaller, harder stools are more difficult to pass). Straining increases abdominal pressure, obstructing return of blood through the legs. Long-term increased pressure may weaken the vein wall, causing varicosities or hemorrhoids, or may weaken wall of large intestine, producing diverticuli. A high-fiber diet is the most important treatment and preventive measure for varicose veins (and hemorrhoids).

- **Bulking agents:** psyllium seed, pectin, and guar gum have a mild laxative action. They attract water and form a gelatinous mass, keeping feces soft, promoting peristalsis, and reducing straining during defecation.
- **Flavonoid-rich berries:** hawthorn berries, cherries, blueberries, blackberries contain proanthocyanidins and anthocyanidins—flavonoids that improve the integrity of ground substance.
- **Buckwheat** ***(Fagopyrum esculentum):*** contains rutin. Dose: tea standardized to contain 5% total flavonoids, yielding 270 mg of rutin daily.

These extracts are effective because they do the following:

- Reduce capillary fragility
- Increase integrity of venous wall
- Inhibit breakdown of ground substance compounds
- Improve venous muscular tone

Use of berries and their extracts or grapeseed or pine bark is indicated to treat varicose veins and to prevent them.

Botanical Medicines

- ***Centella asiatica:*** extract containing 70% triterpenic acids (asiatic acid, madecassic acid, asiatoside) is impressive in treating cellulite, venous insufficiency of lower limbs, and varicose veins. It exerts normalizing action on metabolism of connective tissue. It enhances tissue integrity by stimulating glycosaminoglycan (GAG) synthesis without promoting excessive collagen synthesis or cell growth. GAGs are major components of amorphous intercellular matrix (ground substance) in which collagen fibers are embedded. Net effect is normal tissue. Effect in venous insufficiency and varicose veins is to enhance connective tissue structure, reducing sclerosis and improving blood flow through affected limbs.
- ***Aesculus hippocastanum*** **(horse chestnut):** seeds of the horse chestnut tree were traditionally used to improve hemorrhoids and varicose veins. Horse chestnut seed extract (HCSE) contains escin (a triterpenic saponin), proanthocyanidin A2, and esculin. All three active components are vasoprotective and venotonic—provide antioxidant effects combined with the ability to inhibit enzymes that destroy venous structures (collagenase, hyaluronidase, beta-glucuronidase, elastase), thus shifting equilibrium between degradation and synthesis of proteoglycans and other venous structures toward net synthesis. HCSE prevents

accumulation of leukocytes in varicose vein–affected limbs and their subsequent activation. Ultimate effect of HCSE treatment is prevention of vascular leakage and increasing venous tone.

— **Venotonic:** substance improving venous tone by increasing contractile potential of elastic fibers in the vein wall. HCSE's venotonic activity is confirmed in the treatment of varicose veins and thrombophlebitis.

— HCSEs standardized for escin are as effective as compression stockings without the nuisance.

— Can be given orally, or escin/cholesterol complex can be applied topically. Topical formula is beneficial in treatment of bruises by decreasing capillary fragility and swelling.

- ***Ruscus aculeatus* (butcher's broom):** a subshrub of the lily family native to the Mediterranean region. Active ingredients are ruscogenins, with anti-inflammatory and vasoconstrictive effects. Extracts are used internally and externally in Europe for treating varicose veins and hemorrhoids. Clinical trials have confirmed benefits in both symptomatic relief and improved venous blood flow.
- **Micronized diosmin:** the most useful single flavonoid for varicose veins. Micronization reduces size of particles for superior absorption, increased bioavailability, and greater clinical efficacy. Micronized diosmin improves signs and symptoms of chronic venous insufficiency. It decreases levels of some plasma markers of endothelial activation—soluble endothelial adhesion molecules. It promotes healing of venous ulcers and hemorrhoids.
- **Bromelain and other fibrinolytic compounds:** persons with varicose veins have a decreased ability to break down fibrin. Fibrin is deposited in tissue near the varicosity. Skin then becomes hard and "lumpy" from fibrin and fat. Decreased fibrinolysis increases risk of thrombi and thrombophlebitis, myocardial infarction, pulmonary embolism, and stroke. Herbs increasing fibrinolytic activity of blood are capsicum (cayenne), garlic, onion, ginger; all increase fibrin breakdown. Use them liberally in food. Bromelain (proteolytic enzyme from pineapple) is also indicated. Vein walls are an important source of plasminogen activator, which promotes breakdown of fibrin. Varicose veins have decreased plasminogen activator. Bromelain acts in a similar manner to plasminogen activator, causing fibrin breakdown. It may help prevent hard and lumpy skin (lipodermatosclerosis) found around varicose veins.

THERAPEUTIC APPROACH

- **Diet:** rich in dietary fiber; liberal amounts of proanthocyanidin- and anthocyanidin-rich berries; garlic, onions, ginger, and cayenne liberally
- **Botanical medicines**:
  — *A. hippocastanum:* bark of root, 500 mg t.i.d.
  — Escin: 50 mg t.i.d.; alternatively an escin preparation may be applied topically in a 1% concentration.
  — *C. asiatica* extract (70% triterpenic acid content): 30 mg t.i.d.
  — *R. aculeatus* extract (9% to 11% ruscogenin content): 100 mg t.i.d.
  — Grapeseed *(Vitis vinifera)* extract (95% procyanidolic oligomers): 150 to 300 mg /day.
  — Pine bark extract *(Pinus pinaster):* 150 to 300 mg/day.
  — Micronized diosmin: 500 to 1000 mg/day.
  — Hydroxyethylrutosides: 1000 to 3000 mg/day.
- **Useful adjunct:**
  — Bromelain (minimum 1500 milk clotting units [MCU]): 500 to 750 mg t.i.d. between meals

Index

Page numbers followed by "*f*" indicate figures, "*t*" indicate tables, and "*b*" indicate boxes.

B

E

F

G

H

I

J

K

M

P

T